AF866517

CLINICAL ANESTHESIOLOGY: STRATEGIES AND TECHNIQUES

Dr. (Prof.) Samarendra Pratap Singh

ALLIED HEALTH PRESS

Clinical Anesthesiology: Strategies and Techniques

Author: **Dr. (Prof.) Samarendra Pratap Singh**

Allied Health Press
4164 Lakeshore Road
Burlington ON L7L 1A4
Canada
www.alliedhealthpress.com
Email: orders@arclereducation.com

ISBN: 978-1-77956-787-1

ABOUT THE AUTHOR

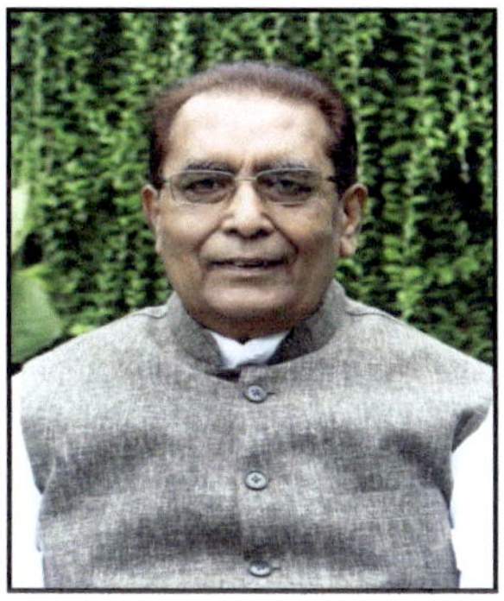

Dr. (Prof.) Samarendra Pratap Singh, born on April 20, 1947, is a distinguished academician, administrator, and medical professional whose career spans decades of excellence in medicine, higher education, and institutional leadership. He began his medical journey at Darbhanga Medical College, Darbhanga, where he earned his MBBS in 1969, followed by a Diploma in Anesthesia in 1974, an MD in Anesthesia in 1978, and later a Diploma in Acupuncture from Saurashtra in 1980, reflecting his commitment to advancing both mainstream and alternative medical practices.

He served as an Anaesthetist, Associate Professor, and ultimately Professor & Head of the Department of Anaesthesia at Darbhanga Medical College & Hospital, contributing significantly to medical education and clinical services. Beyond teaching, he mentored five Ph.D. scholars and 27 M.D. students, leaving a lasting academic legacy. His leadership roles were equally prominent—he held the position of Vice-Chancellor at Lalit Narayan Mithila University, Darbhanga (2010–2013) and Aryabhatta Knowledge University, Patna, where he guided institutional reforms and higher education development. He also served as Superintendent and Principal of Darbhanga Medical College Hospital and as Principal, Dean, and Chief Superintendent of Saraswati Institute of Medical Sciences, Ghaziabad. Nationally, he rose to become President of the Indian Society of Anaesthesiologists in 1995, having earlier served as its Vice-President, and chaired the Specialty Board of Anesthesiology, National Board of Examination, New Delhi.

His contributions extended to policy and governance as a member of the Standing Committees of AIIMS Patna, the Medical Council of India, State Higher Education Council of Bihar, and several expert and selection committees across India. A prolific academic, he authored the book Higher Education in India: Issues & Concerns (2013) and published more than 16 research articles. His efforts were recognized through numerous honors, including the Amity Academic Excellence Award (2012), Bharat Academic Excellence Award, Lifetime Academic Achievement Award by World Management Congress (2011), Bharat Mata Award (2012), and the Best University Administrator of the Year Award (2012). Beyond academics, Dr. Singh actively engaged in community service through free medical camps, health awareness programs, and welfare initiatives, embodying a spirit of service to society. His academic tours to Singapore, Dubai, and Nepal further enriched his international perspective. Dr. S. P. Singh's journey is a testament to a lifetime dedicated to medicine, education, leadership, and social service, marking him as a towering figure in both healthcare and academia.

Brief Table of Contents

1. Introduction to Clinical Anesthesiology 1
2. Pharmacology of Anesthetic Agents 27
3. Anatomy and Physiology Relevant to Anesthesia 59
4. Preoperative Assessment and Preparation 85
5. Airway Management and Techniques 111
6. General Anesthesia: Induction and Maintenance 137
7. Regional Anesthesia: Spinal, Epidural, and Peripheral Nerve Blocks 163
8. Monitored Anesthesia Care (MAC) and Sedation 189
9. Pediatric Anesthesia 215
10. Obstetric Anesthesia 241
11. Geriatric Anesthesia 265
12. Anesthesia for Patients with Comorbid Conditions 293
13. Intraoperative Monitoring and Crisis Management 317
14. Post-Anesthesia Care and Pain Management 347
15. Anesthetic Complications 371
Index 393

Getting Started with This Book

Chapter Openers

A list of Chapter Outline is presented providing a brief Introduction to what will be covered in the chapter.

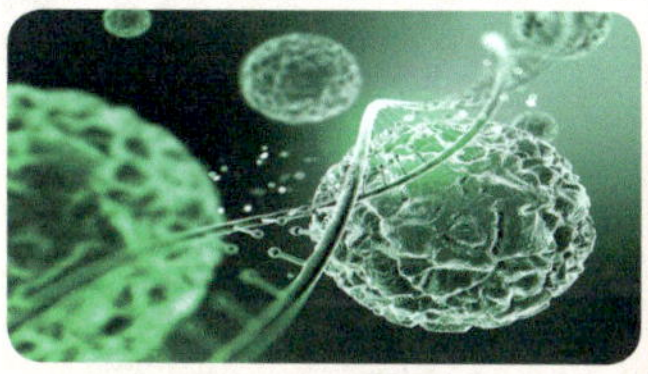

Introduction

Often referred to as the science of life, biology is a broad field of study aimed at comprehending the several kinds of life on Earth, from tiny creatures to sophisticated multicellular entities. Comprising several subfields, including molecular biology, ecology, and evolutionary biology, each of which advances our knowledge of living systems, this field clarifies the mechanisms controlling life events, including development, reproduction, and interaction with the surroundings, which is the central goal of biology. Moreover, biology fills in the void between the natural sciences and medicine by offering a necessary understanding of health, illness, and the interactions between organisms and their environments. Dealing with urgent global issues such as climate change, biodiversity loss, and new diseases depends on an awareness of these complex biological interactions, therefore highlighting the critical part biology plays in modern civilization. Fundamentally, biology explores and tests ideas about the living world using the scientific method. Through methodical observation and experimentation,

LEARNING OBJECTIVES

After studying this chapter, you will be able to:

1. Discuss the scientific method in biology;
2. Explain the cell theory;
3. Discuss the genetics and heredity;
4. Evolution and natural selection;
5. Focus on ecology and ecosystems;
6. Learn about human biology;
7. Evaluate the plant biology;
8. Explain the microbiology;
9. Focus on current trends in biology.

1.1. The Scientific Method in Biology

Learning Outcome

1. Describe the steps of the scientific method;
2. Focus on hypothesis formation;
3. Learn about experimental design.

Learning Outcomes

The beginning of each section of every chapter contains a set of Learning Outcomes that inform students of concepts they should understand. These outcomes help students understand what they should be able to do if they have mastered the material in that section.

Test Your Knowledge

Throughout each chapter, Test Your Knowledge cues you to note which topics have been covered and to self-test your understanding of the material presented.

Test Your Knowledge

1. Explain why correlation does not imply causation in scientific experiments.
2. How does the scientific method help reduce the influence of personal opinions in research?

Chapter Summary

The Summary Section appear at the end of each chapter and summarize main concepts covered throughout the chapter. These points provide key concepts in an engaging and meaningful way.

Summary

The investigation of biological principles highlights the importance of a comprehensive view of life by reflecting the intricate interactions that occur within living systems. The complexity of biology goes beyond individual species or systems, as this essay highlights; it also includes the interactions that mold ecosystems and affect biodiversity. Researchers can conduct in-depth analyses of metabolomic data using sophisticated technologies like MetaboAnalyst, which offer insights into the molecular mechanisms underlying these interactions. As demonstrated by the developments in MetaboAnalyst, for example, the integration of diverse omics data promotes a thorough understanding of metabolic pathways and helps identify important biological markers necessary for research on development and disease (Chong et al., 2018). Additionally, the phenomenon of ecological invasions is a key component of biological research and a vital field of study. The introduction of non-native species into unfamiliar habitats has significant ramifications and calls for multidisciplinary management strategies. Examining the origins and effects of these biological incursions, invasion science has become a crucial field that highlights the need to comprehend ecological dynamics and community interactions. As interest in biological invasions increases, new findings are emerging that put conventional ecological theories and practices to the test. The importance of incorporating various scientific viewpoints is shown by this developing discipline, which also highlights how invasive species shape ecosystems and advances our knowledge of ecological resilience (David et al., 2013). When taken as a whole, these discoveries from invasion science and metabolomics highlight the value of multidisciplinary biology research. Fostering cross-disciplinary collaboration and utilizing technological breakthroughs to improve our comprehension of intricate biological interactions are crucial as we look to the future of biological research. In addition to deepening our understanding of the complexities of life, this method lays the groundwork for tackling urgent environmental issues. Future studies can ensure the continued relevance of biology in a world that is constantly changing by acknowledging the interconnection of biological systems and opening the door to creative solutions that support sustainability and biodiversity conservation. We might imagine a thorough comprehension of life that serves both academia and society at large through ongoing investigation and integration of scientific knowledge.

Knowledge Assessment

The chapter includes material designed to review and reinforce each content. It includes Critical Thinking Questions to help test of your understanding of information presented in the chapter and Short answer Questions to review your understanding of the key concepts presented in the chapter.

Critical Thinking Questions

1. **Who is known as the "Father of Modern Biology"?**
   a. Aristotle
   b. Charles Darwin
   c. Gregor Mendel
   d. Louis Pasteur
2. **What is the basic unit of life?**
   a. Atom
   b. Molecule
   c. Cell
   d. Organism
3. **Which branch of biology studies the interaction of organisms with their environment?**
   a. Genetics
   b. Ecology
   c. Physiology
   d. Botany
4. **Which macromolecule is the main source of energy for living organisms?**
   a. Proteins
   b. Lipids
   c. Carbohydrates
   d. Nucleic acids
5. **DNA is primarily responsible for which function in living organisms?**
   a. Energy production
   b. Protein synthesis
   c. Storing genetic information
   d. Regulating body temperature

Short Answer Questions

1. What is biology, and why is it important to study biology?
2. What are the three main domains of life, and how are they different from one another?
3. Define homeostasis and give an example of how it works in living organisms.
4. What is the cell theory, and why is it fundamental to biology?
5. How do autotrophs and heterotrophs differ in the way they obtain energy?
6. What is the scientific method, and how is it applied in biological research?
7. Discuss how biology helps address global challenges such as climate change, disease, and food security.
8. Explain the levels of biological organization from the smallest unit to the largest. Provide examples at each level.
9. Describe the relationship between structure and function in biology, giving specific examples from cells or organs.
10. How has the discovery of genetics shaped our understanding of inheritance and variation among organisms?

Supplementary Materials

Key Terms: A list of key terms is given for quick reference

KEY TERMS FROM THIS CHAPTER

Annotation enrichment analysis	Biological structure	Cell
Cell theory	Cellular structure	Ecology
Ecosystems	Genetics	Human biology
Microbiology	Natural selection	Organism
Plant biology		

Further Resources: Recommendations for additional readings, websites, and multimedia resources.

References

1. Argelaguet, R., Velten, B., Arnol, D., Dietrich, S., Zenz, T., Marioni, J. C., Buettner, F., et al. (2018). Multi-omics factor analysis—A framework for unsupervised integration of multi-omics data sets. *Molecular Systems Biology, 14*. https://doi.org/10.15252/msb.20178124.
2. Bacher, S., Blackburn, T. M., Essl, F., & Genovesi, P. (2017). *Socio-Economic Impact Classification of Alien Taxa (SEICAT)*. https://core.ac.uk/download/286567949.pdf (accessed on 8th March 2025).
3. Barnett, R., Brace, S., Cucchi, T., & Dobney, K. (2013). *Divergent Evolutionary Processes Associated with Colonization of Offshore Islands*. https://core.ac.uk/download/20664364.pdf (accessed on 8th March 2025).

Detailed Table of Contents

List of Figures *xv*
Preface *xxiii*

CHAPTER 1

Introduction to Clinical Anesthesiology 1

Introduction **1**
1.1. Types of Anesthesia **4**
1.1.1. General Anesthesia (GA) 5
1.1.2. Regional Anesthesia (RA) 6
1.1.3. Local Anesthesia 6
1.2. Preoperative Assessment **8**
1.2.1. Patient History and Physical Examination 8
1.2.2. Risk assessment and Stratification 9
1.2.3. Preoperative Optimization Strategies 10
1.3. Intraoperative Management **11**
1.3.1. Monitoring Techniques and Equipment 13
1.3.2. Anesthetic Administration Protocols 13
1.3.3. Management of Intraoperative Complications 14
1.4. Postoperative Care **15**
1.4.1. Recovery Room Protocols 16
1.4.2. Pain Management Strategies 16
1.4.3. Monitoring for Postoperative Complications 17
Summary **19**
References **22**

CHAPTER 2

Pharmacology of Anesthetic Agents 27

Introduction **27**
2.1. Classification of Anesthetic Agents **30**
2.1.1. General Anesthetics 30
2.1.2. Local Anesthetics 32
2.1.3. Adjunctive Anesthetic Agents 32
2.2. Mechanisms of Action **33**
2.2.1. Interaction with Neurotransmitter Systems 34
2.2.2. Effects on Ion Channels 35
2.2.3. Influence on Central Nervous System Activity 36
2.3. Pharmacokinetics of Anesthetic Agents **37**
2.3.1. Absorption and Distribution 38
2.3.2. Metabolism and Elimination 39
2.3.3. Factors Affecting Pharmacokinetics 40
2.4. Clinical Applications **41**
2.4.1. Surgical Procedures 41
2.4.2. Pain Management 42
2.4.3. Emergency Medicine 43
2.5. Side Effects and Complications **44**
2.5.1. Common Side Effects 45
2.5.2. Serious Adverse Reactions 45
2.5.3. Risk Factors for Complications 46
2.6. Advances in Anesthetic Pharmacology **47**

2.6.1. Development of New Anesthetic Agents 48
2.6.2. Innovations in Delivery Methods 49
Summary 51
References 54

CHAPTER 3

Anatomy and Physiology Relevant to Anesthesia 59

Introduction 59
3.1. Basic Anatomy of the Human Body 61
3.1.1. Major organ Systems Involved in Anesthesia 62
3.1.2. Anatomical Landmarks Relevant to Anesthesia Administration 63
3.1.3. Variations in Anatomy Among Patients 63
3.2. Physiology of the Nervous System 64
3.2.1. Role of the Central Nervous System in Anesthesia 65
3.2.2. Peripheral Nervous System and Its Significance 66
3.2.3. Mechanisms of Pain Perception and Modulation 67
3.3. Cardiovascular System and Anesthesia 68
3.3.1. Heart Anatomy and Its Function During Anesthesia 68
3.3.2. Blood Pressure Regulation and Its Implications 69
3.3.3. Effects of Anesthetic Agents on Cardiovascular Dynamics 70
3.4. Respiratory System Considerations 71
3.4.1. Anatomy of the Respiratory Tract Relevant to Intubation 72
3.4.2. Gas Exchange Processes and Anesthetic Implications 73
3.4.3. Impact of Anesthesia on Respiratory Function 74
3.5. Patient Assessment and Monitoring 75
3.5.1. Preoperative Assessment of Anatomy and Physiology 75
3.5.2. Monitoring Techniques During Anesthesia 76
3.5.3. Postoperative Considerations Related to Anatomy and Physiology 77
Summary 78
References 81

CHAPTER 4

Preoperative Assessment and Preparation 85

Introduction 85
4.1. Objectives of Preoperative Assessment 88
4.1.1. Identifying Patient Risks 88
4.1.2. Establishing Baseline Health Status 89
4.1.3. Enhancing Surgical Outcomes 90
4.2. Components of Preoperative Assessment 91
4.2.1. Medical History Evaluation 91
4.2.2. Physical Examination 92
4.2.3. Laboratory and Diagnostic Tests 93
4.3. Role of Anesthesia in Preoperative Assessment 94
4.3.1. Anesthesia Consultation 94
4.3.2. Assessment of Anesthesia Risks 95
4.3.3. Patient Education Regarding Anesthesia 96
4.4. Multidisciplinary Approach to Preoperative Preparation 97
4.4.1. Involvement of Healthcare Professionals 97
4.4.2. Coordination Among Surgical Team Members 98
4.4.3. Role of Nursing in Preoperative Care 99
4.5. Challenges in Preoperative Assessment 100
4.5.1. Patient-Related Challenges 100
4.5.2. Systemic and Logistical Challenges 101
4.5.3. Strategies to Overcome Challenges 101
Summary 103
References 106

CHAPTER 5

Airway Management and Techniques 111

Introduction 111
5.1. Anatomy of the Airway 113

5.1.1. Upper Airway Structures 114
5.1.2. Lower Airway Structures 115
5.1.3. Physiological Functions of the Airway 116
5.2. Assessment of Airway Patency 117
5.2.1. Signs of Airway Obstruction 117
5.2.2. Techniques for Airway Assessment 118
5.2.3. Importance of Early Recognition 119
5.3. Basic Airway Management Techniques 120
5.3.1. Head Tilt-Chin Lift Maneuver 120
5.3.2. Jaw Thrust Maneuver 121
5.3.3. Use of Oropharyngeal Airways (OPA) 122
5.4. Advanced Airway Management Techniques 123
5.4.1. Endotracheal Intubation 124
5.4.2. Supraglottic Airway Devices 124
5.4.3. Surgical Airway Management 125
5.5. Special Considerations in Airway Management 126
5.5.1. Pediatric Airway Management 127
5.5.2. Airway Management in Trauma Patients 127
5.5.3. Considerations for Patients with Obesity 128
Summary 130
References 133

CHAPTER 6

General Anesthesia: Induction and Maintenance 137

Introduction 137
6.1. Mechanisms of Action 140
6.1.1. Pharmacodynamics of Anesthetic Agents 140
6.1.2. Effects on the Central Nervous System 141
6.1.3. Role of Neurotransmitters in Anesthesia 142
6.2. Induction of General Anesthesia (GA) 143
6.2.1. Preoperative Assessment and Preparation 144
6.2.2. Common Induction Agents 145
6.2.3. Techniques for Induction 145
6.3. Maintenance of General Anesthesia 146
6.3.1. Monitoring During Surgery 147
6.3.2. Maintenance Agents and Their Administration 148
6.3.3. Adjustments Based on Patient Response 148
6.4. Risks and Complications 150
6.4.1. Common Side Effects of General Anesthesia (GA) 150
6.4.2. Serious Complications and Their Management 151
6.4.3. Risk Factors Influencing Anesthesia Safety 152
6.5. Advances in Anesthesia Technology 153
6.5.1. Development of New Anesthetic Agents 153
6.5.2. Innovations in Monitoring Equipment 154
6.5.3. Future Trends in Anesthesia Practice 155
Summary 156
References 159

CHAPTER 7

Regional Anesthesia: Spinal, Epidural, and Peripheral Nerve Blocks 163

Introduction 163
7.1. Mechanism of Action 166
7.1.1. How Regional Anesthesia (RA) Works 166
7.1.2. Differences in Mechanisms Among Spinal, Epidural, and Peripheral Nerve Blocks 167
7.1.3. Pharmacology of Anesthetic Agents Used 168
7.2. Spinal Anesthesia (SA) 169
7.2.1. Indications for Spinal Anesthesia (SA) 169
7.2.2. Procedure and Technique 170
7.2.3. Advantages and Disadvantages 171
7.3. Epidural Anesthesia 172
7.3.1. Indications for Epidural Anesthesia 172
7.3.2. Procedure and Technique 173
7.3.3. Advantages and Disadvantages 174
7.4. Peripheral Nerve Blocks (PNBs) 175
7.4.1. Indications for Peripheral Nerve Blocks (PNBs) 175
7.4.2. Procedure and Technique 176
7.4.3. Advantages and Disadvantages 177
7.5. Complications and Risks 178
7.5.1. Common Complications Associated with Regional Anesthesia (RA) 179
7.5.2. Risk Factors Influencing Complications 180
7.5.3. Management and Prevention Strategies 180

Summary 182
References 185

CHAPTER 8

Monitored Anesthesia Care (MAC) and Sedation 189

Introduction 189
8.1. Types of Sedation 192
8.1.1. Minimal Sedation 192
8.1.2. Moderate Sedation 193
8.1.3. Deep Sedation 194
8.2. Indications for Monitored Anesthesia Care (MAC) 195
8.2.1. Surgical Procedures Requiring Sedation 196
8.2.2. Diagnostic Procedures and Interventions 197
8.2.3. Patient-Specific Factors Influencing MAC Use 197
8.3. Benefits of Monitored Anesthesia Care (MAC) 198
8.3.1. Enhanced Patient Comfort and Satisfaction 199
8.3.2. Reduced Recovery Time Compared to General Anesthesia (GA) 200
8.3.3. Flexibility in Managing Patient Sedation Levels 200
8.4. Risks and Complications 202
8.4.1. Potential Adverse Effects of Sedation 202
8.4.2. Monitoring Requirements During MAC 203
8.4.3. Strategies for Minimizing Risks 203
8.5. Role of Anesthesia Providers 205
8.5.1. Responsibilities of Anesthesiologists and Nurse Anesthetists 205
8.5.2. Importance of Preoperative Assessments 206
8.5.3. Postoperative Care and Monitoring 207
Summary 208
References 211

CHAPTER 9

Pediatric Anesthesia 215

Introduction 215
9.1. Physiological Differences in Children 218
9.1.1. Differences in Anatomy and Physiology 218
9.1.2. Impact on Drug Metabolism 219
9.1.3. Considerations for Anesthetic Dosage 219
9.2. Types of Anesthesia Used in Pediatrics 220
9.2.1. General Anesthesia (GA) 221
9.2.2. Regional Anesthesia (RA) 222
9.2.3. Sedation Techniques 222
9.3. Preoperative Assessment 224
9.3.1. Importance of Medical History 224
9.3.2. Physical Examination Protocols 225
9.3.3. Psychological Considerations for Pediatric Patients 226
9.4. Intraoperative Management 227
9.4.1. Monitoring Techniques 227
9.4.2. Anesthetic Agents and Their Effects 228
9.4.3. Role of the Anesthesiologist 228
9.5. Postoperative Care 230
9.5.1. Recovery Room Protocols 230
9.5.2. Pain Management Strategies 231
9.5.3. Potential Complications and Their Management 232
Summary 233
References 236

CHAPTER 10

Obstetric Anesthesia 241

Introduction 241
10.1. Types of Obstetric Anesthesia 244
10.1.1. Epidural Anesthesia 244
10.1.2. Spinal Anesthesia (SA) 245
10.1.3. General Anesthesia (GA) 246
10.2. Indications for Use 247
10.2.1. Pain Management During Labor 248
10.2.2. Surgical Interventions (e.g., Cesarean Sections) 249
10.2.3. Special Considerations for High-Risk Pregnancies 250
10.3. Benefits of Obstetric Anesthesia 251
10.3.1. Enhanced Maternal Comfort 251
10.3.2. Improved Fetal Outcomes 252
10.3.3. Reduction of Stress and Anxiety During Labor 253

10.4. Risks and Complications 254
10.4.1. Potential Side Effects for the Mother 255
10.4.2. Risks to the Fetus 255
10.4.3. Long-Term Implications of Anesthesia Use 256
Summary 258
References 261

CHAPTER 11

Geriatric Anesthesia 265

Introduction 265
11.1. Physiological Changes in the Elderly 267
11.1.1. Cardiovascular System Adaptations 268
11.1.2. Respiratory System Considerations 269
11.1.3. Neurological Changes Affecting Anesthesia 270
11.2. Common Anesthetic Agents Used in Geriatric Patients 271
11.2.1. Inhalational Anesthetics 272
11.2.2. Intravenous Anesthetics 273
11.2.3. Regional Anesthesia Techniques 273
11.3. Preoperative Assessment in Geriatric Patients 274
11.3.1. Comprehensive Medical History Review 275
11.3.2. Evaluation of Functional Status 276
11.3.3. Risk Assessment Tools 277
11.4. Intraoperative Management Considerations 279
11.4.1. Monitoring Techniques for Elderly Patients 280
11.4.2. Dosage Adjustments for Anesthetic Agents 280
11.4.3. Management of Comorbidities 281
11.5. Postoperative Care and Complications 282
11.5.1. Common Postoperative Complications in the Elderly 283
11.5.2. Pain Management Strategies 284
11.5.3. Importance of Early Mobilization 284
Summary 286
References 289

CHAPTER 12

Anesthesia for Patients with Comorbid Conditions 293

Introduction 293
12.1. Common Comorbid Conditions 295
12.1.1. Cardiovascular Diseases 295
12.1.2. Respiratory Disorders 296
12.1.3. Diabetes Mellitus 298
12.2. Preoperative Assessment 299
12.2.1. Medical History Evaluation 300
12.2.2. Physical Examination 300
12.2.3. Diagnostic Testing 301
12.3. Anesthetic Considerations for Specific Conditions 303
12.3.1. Adjustments for Cardiovascular Patients 303
12.3.2. Strategies for Managing Respiratory Issues 304
12.3.3. Protocols for Diabetic Patients 306
12.4. Risks and Complications 307
12.4.1. Potential Complications of Anesthesia 307
12.4.2. Increased Risks in Patients with Comorbidities 308
12.4.3. Strategies to Mitigate Risks 308
Summary 310
References 313

CHAPTER 13

Intraoperative Monitoring and Crisis Management 317

Introduction 317
13.1. Types of Intraoperative Monitoring 320
13.1.1. Physiological Monitoring (e.g., Heart Rate, Blood Pressure) 321
13.1.2. Neuromuscular Monitoring 321
13.1.3. Depth of Anesthesia Monitoring 322
13.2. Technologies Used in Intraoperative Monitoring 323

13.2.1. Electrocardiography (ECG) 324
13.2.2. Pulse Oximetry 325
13.2.3. Capnography 325
13.3. Role of Anesthesiologists in Monitoring 327
13.3.1. Responsibilities During Surgery 328
13.3.2. Communication with the Surgical Team 328
13.3.3. Decision-Making in Response to Monitoring Data 329
13.4. Common Intraoperative Crises 330
13.4.1. Anaphylactic Reactions 331
13.4.2. Cardiac Arrest 332
13.4.3. Hemorrhage 334
13.5. Crisis Management Protocols 335
13.5.1. Immediate Response Strategies 335
13.5.2. Use of Emergency Medications 336
13.5.3. Team Coordination During Crises 337
Summary 339
Critical Thinking Questions 341
References 342

CHAPTER 14

Post-Anesthesia Care and Pain Management 347

Introduction 347
14.1. The Role of Post-Anesthesia Care Units (PACUs) 350
14.1.1. Purpose and Function of PACUs 351
14.1.2. Staffing and Resources in PACUs 351
14.1.3. Monitoring Protocols in the PACU 352
14.2. Pain Assessment Techniques 354
14.2.1. Subjective Versus Objective Pain Assessment 354
14.2.2. Common Pain Scales Used in Clinical Practice 355
14.2.3. Importance of Timely Pain Assessment 356
14.3. Pain Management Strategies 357
14.3.1. Pharmacological Interventions for Pain Relief 357
14.3.2. Non-Pharmacological Approaches to Pain Management 358
14.3.3. Multimodal Pain Management Techniques 359
14.4. Challenges in Post-Anesthesia Care 360
14.4.1. Variability in Patient Responses to Anesthesia and Pain 360
14.4.2. Managing Complications and Side Effects 361
14.4.3. Addressing the Opioid Crisis in Pain Management 362
Summary 363
References 366

CHAPTER 15

Anesthetic Complications 371

Introduction 371
15.1. Common Anesthetic Complications 374
15.1.1. Allergic Reactions 374
15.1.2. Respiratory Complications 375
15.1.3. Cardiovascular Complications 376
15.2. Risk Factors for Anesthetic Complications 377
15.2.1. Patient Health History 378
15.2.2. Type of Surgery 379
15.2.3. Anesthetic Technique Used 379
15.3. Prevention Strategies 380
15.3.1. Preoperative Assessment 381
15.3.2. Monitoring During Anesthesia 382
15.3.3. Postoperative Care 382
15.4. Management of Anesthetic Complications 383
15.4.1. Immediate Response Protocols 384
15.4.2. Long-Term Management Strategies 385
15.4.3. Role of the Anesthesiologist 385
Summary 387
References 390

Index 393

LIST OF FIGURES

Figure 1.1. Clinical anesthesiology
Figure 1.2. Anesthesiology
Figure 1.3. Importance of anesthesia in modern medicine
Figure 1.4. Types of anesthesia
Figure 1.5. Regional anesthesia
Figure 1.6. Local anesthesia
Figure 1.7. Preoperative assessment clinic
Figure 1.8. Patient history form
Figure 1.9. Preoperative optimization strategies
Figure 1.10. Intraoperative management
Figure 1.11. Monitoring techniques and equipment
Figure 1.12. Anesthetic administration protocols
Figure 1.13. Postoperative care
Figure 1.14. Pain management strategies
Figure 2.1. Anesthesia: how anesthesia works.
Figure 2.2. Anesthetic agents
Figure 2.3. Importance of anesthetics in medical practice
Figure 2.4. General anesthetics
Figure 2.5. Laceration wound injecting local anesthetics
Figure 2.6. Adjunctive Anesthetic Agents.
Figure 2.7. Interaction with neurotransmitter systems
Figure 2.8. Importance of ion channels in the body
Figure 2.9. Pharmacokinetics
Figure 2.10. Pharmacokinetics (absorption, distribution, metabolism, and elimination)
Figure 2.11. Anesthetic medications.
Figure 2.12. Surgical procedures
Figure 2.13. Pain management.
Figure 2.14. Emergency medicine
Figure 2.15. Anesthesia side effects and complications
Figure 2.16. Allergic bursts
Figure 2.17 . Anesthetic Pharmacology.

Figure 2.18. Innovations in anesthetic delivery
Figure 2.19. Personalized Anesthesia.
Figure 3.1. Anesthesia.
Figure 3.2. Anatomy of the human body
Figure 3.3. Organ systems in humans
Figure 3.4. Nervous system
Figure 3.5. Central nervous system
Figure 3.6. Peripheral nervous system
Figure 3.7. Cardiovascular system
Figure 3.8. Heart anterior exterior view
Figure 3.9. Regulation of blood pressure
Figure 3.10. Respiratory system
Figure 3.11. Understanding airway anatomy for intubation
Figure 3.12. Gas exchange processes
Figure 3.13. Anesthesia patient monitoring.
Figure 3.14. Monitoring techniques during anesthesia
Figure 4.1. Preoperative Assessment and Preparation.
Figure 4.2. Preoperative assessment
Figure 4.3. Importance of patient preoperative preparation
Figure 4.4. Patient safety risks
Figure 4.5. Surgical outcomes
Figure 4.6. Medical history
Figure 4.7. Physical examination
Figure 4.8. Laboratory and diagnostic tests
Figure 4.9. Anesthesia consultation
Figure 4.10. Anesthesia risk assessment
Figure 4.11. The importance of patient education in anesthesia
Figure 4.12. Healthcare professionals
Figure 4.13. Role of nursing in preoperative care
Figure 4.14. Surgery underway at the Red Cross Hospital in Tampere, Finland during the 1918 Finnish Civil War.
Figure 4.15. Iapyx removing an arrowhead from the thigh of Aeneas using a forcepts (Virgil Aeneid XII.383-440) Roman fresco from the Casa di Sirico in Pompeii.
Figure 5.1. CPR patient airway management.
Figure 5.2. Airway management
Figure 5.3. Anatomy of the airway

Figure 5.4. Functional upper airway
Figure 5.5. A diagram of the lower airway
Figure 5.6. Airway patency
Figure 5.7. Techniques for airway assessment
Figure 5.8. The importance of early detection recognizing signs of respiratory issues.
Figure 5.9. Basic airway management techniques
Figure 5.10. Head tilt-chin lift
Figure 5.11. Jaw thrust
Figure 5.12. Use of oropharyngeal airways
Figure 5.13. Advanced airway management techniques
Figure 5.14. Endotracheal tube intubation procedure
Figure 5.15. Supraglottic airway devices
Figure 5.16. Surgical airway management
Figure 5.17. Pediatric airway management
Figure 5.18. Strategies for airway management in trauma cases
Figure 6.1. General Anaesthesia: A Professional Overview.
Figure 6.2. General anesthesia
Figure 6.3. Importance of general anesthesia in surgical procedures
Figure 6.4. Anesthetic drugs.
Figure 6.5. Synaptic transmission is the biological process by which neurotransmitters are released by a neuron and activate the receptors of another neuron.
Figure 6.6. Propofol induction dose for general anesthesia
Figure 6.7. Induction agents
Figure 6.8. To maintain upper airway patency, the pediatric anesthesiologist holds the anesthesia mask snugly to the patient's face and performs the triple airway maneuver—neck extension, jaw thrust, and mouth opening—without applying pressure to the soft tissue or causing pain.
Figure 6.9. Monitoring during surgery
Figure 6.10. Laryngeal mask airway.
Figure 6.11. Side effects of general anesthesia
Figure 6.12. Complications of general anesthesia (GA)
Figure 6.13. Technological advancements and emerging trends in anesthesia
Figure 6.14. Anesthesia monitoring equipment
Figure 6.15. Future of Anesthesiology.
Figure 7.1. Understanding Regional Anesthesia.
Figure 7.2. Regional anesthesia
Figure 7.3. Importance of regional anesthesia (RA) in modern medical practice
Figure 7.4. How Is Regional Anesthesia Used During Surgery?

Figure 7.5. Anesthetic Drugs.
Figure 7.6. Spinal anesthesia
Figure 7.7. Procedure and technique of spinal anesthesia
Figure 7.8. Epidural anesthesia
Figure 7.9. Anesthesiologist performing an epidural anesthesia injection
Figure 7.10. Peripheral nerve block (upper limb)
Figure 7.11. Peripheral nerve blocks.
Figure 7.12. Procedure and technique of peripheral nerve blocks
Figure 7.13. Pain.
Figure 7.14. Complications of regional anesthesia
Figure 7.15. Peripheral nerve blocks allow providers to forgo, or at least lessen, the use of general anesthesia in surgical cases.
Figure 8.1. Understanding Monitored Anesthesia Care.
Figure 8.2. Monitored anesthesia care (MAC)
Figure 8.3. An Overview of Procedural Sedation.
Figure 8.4. Minimal sedation
Figure 8.5. Moderate conscious sedation for dental anxiety
Figure 8.6. Deep sedation
Figure 8.7. Indications for Monitored Anesthesia Care.
Figure 8.8. Surgical procedures requiring sedation
Figure 8.9. Diagnostic Procedures and Interventions.
Figure 8.10. Benefits of monitored anesthesia care (MAC)
Figure 8.11. Patient comfort and satisfaction
Figure 8.12. Managing patient sedation levels
Figure 8.13. Monitoring requirements during MAC
Figure 8.14. Role of anesthesia providers
Figure 8.15. Responsibilities of nurse anesthetists
Figure 8.16. Post-anesthesia monitoring
Figure 9.1. Pediatric anesthesia
Figure 9.2. Importance of anesthesia in pediatric surgery
Figure 9.3. Anatomy of adults versus pediatric airway
Figure 9.4. Anesthesia for kids.
Figure 9.5. General anesthesia for children during dental procedures
Figure 9.6. Pediatric regional anesthesia (RA)
Figure 9.7. Sedation techniques for children
Figure 9.8. Pediatric preoperative assessment

Figure 9.9. Physical examination
Figure 9.10. Intraoperative Management.
Figure 9.11. Anesthesiologist
Figure 9.12. Postoperative care for kids
Figure 9.13. Recovery room protocols
Figure 9.14. Avoiding anesthesia complications for kids.
Figure 10.1. Obstetric anesthesia
Figure 10.2. Definition of Obstetric Anesthesia.
Figure 10.3. Types of Obstetric Anesthesia.
Figure 10.4. Epidural anaesthesia
Figure 10.5. Spinal anesthesia in labor and childbirth
Figure 10.6. General anesthesia (GA) used during labor
Figure 10.7. Managing pain during labor
Figure 10.8. Caesarian section
Figure 10.9. High-risk pregnancy
Figure 10.10. Comfort and pain relief during labor
Figure 10.11. Reduction of stress and anxiety during labor
Figure 10.12. C-section injuries: Risks and complications
Figure 10.13. C-Section delivery side effects
Figure 10.14. Obstetric Anesthesia Patient Safety: Practices to Ensure Adequate Venous Access and Safe Drug Administration During Transfer to the Operating Room for Emergency Cesarean Delivery.
Figure 11.1. Geriatric anesthesia
Figure 11.2. Definition of Geriatric Anesthesia.
Figure 11.3. Factors that increase and decrease age-related changes in the kidney
Figure 11.4. Respiratory system
Figure 11.5. Clinical pharmacology of anesthetic agents in elderly
Figure 11.6. Inhaled anesthetics
Figure 11.7. Intravenous anesthetics
Figure 11.8. Techniques of regional anesthesia
Figure 11.9. Medical history review
Figure 11.10. Treating older patients under anesthesia
Figure 11.11. Intraoperative management
Figure 11.12. Anesthesia monitoring in geriatric surgeries
Figure 11.13. Managing multiple comorbidities
Figure 11.14. Post operative care for elderly patients
Figure 11.15. Common postoperative complications in the elderly

Figure 11.16. Importance of early mobilization
Figure 12.1. Anesthesia for Patients with Comorbid Conditions.
Figure 12.2. Anesthesia.
Figure 12.3. Cardiovascular diseases
Figure 12.4. Respiratory disorders
Figure 12.5. Diabetes mellitus
Figure 12.6. Preoperative Assessment.
Figure 12.7. Physical exam before surgery
Figure 12.8. Diagnostic testing
Figure 12.9. Caring for patients with cardiovascular disease
Figure 12.10. The respiratory system
Figure 12.11. Dietary guidelines for diabetic patients
Figure 12.12. Spine surgery
Figure 12.13. Strategies to Mitigate Risks.
Figure 13.1. Equipment used for anaesthesia in the operating room.
Figure 13.2. Intraoperative monitoring
Figure 13.3. Crisis management in critical care and surgery
Figure 13.4. Arterial blood pressure monitoring during surgery
Figure 13.5. Neuromuscular monitoring
Figure 13.6. Anesthesia depth monitoring
Figure 13.7. Electrocardiogram
Figure 13.8. Capnography: Assessing ventilation during anesthesia
Figure 13.9. Anesthesia and the vital role of an anesthesiologist
Figure 13.10. Responsibilities of anesthesiologist during surgery.
Figure 13.11. The importance of communicating in surgery
Figure 13.12. Schematic overview of a capnograph.
Figure 13.13. Allergic reactions: The secret danger of anesthesia
Figure 13.14. Cardiac arrest
Figure 13.15. Hemorrhage
Figure 13.16. U.S. Navy sailors assigned to the aircraft carrier USS Carl Vinson treat a baby injured by 2010 Haiti earthquake.
Figure 13.17. Emergency medicine
Figure 13.18. Team coordination during crises
Figure 14.1. Post Anesthesia Care Unit (PACU).
Figure 14.2. Post-anesthesia care
Figure 14.3. The importance of proper pain management after surgery

Figure 14.4. Role of post-anesthesia care units (PACUs)
Figure 14.5. PACU nurse
Figure 14.6. The importance of patient monitoring in the PACU
Figure 14.7. Subjective versus objective pain assessment
Figure 14.8. Importance of Timely Pain Assessment.
Figure 14.9. Post-surgical pain management strategies for a smooth recovery
Figure 14.10. Pain control after surgery: pain medicines
Figure 14.11. Multimodal analgesia pain management
Figure 14.12. Post-surgery psychological challenges for seniors
Figure 14.13. Reduce your risk of side effects from anesthesia
Figure 15.1. Anesthetic Complications.
Figure 15.2. Anesthetics.
Figure 15.3. Postoperative pain
Figure 15.4. Allergic reactions
Figure 15.5. Post-surgery respiratory complications
Figure 15.6. Cardiovascular complications
Figure 15.7. Patient health history
Figure 15.8. Type of surgery
Figure 15.9. Anesthetic Technique.
Figure 15.10. Preoperative Assessment.
Figure 15.11. Importance of post-operative care
Figure 15.12. Immediate response protocols
Figure 15.13. Role of the Anesthesiologist.

PREFACE

Clinical anesthesiology is a medical specialty focused on making surgical and diagnostic patients comfortable, safe, and stable. Practitioners apply general knowledge of pharmacology, physiology, and leading-edge monitoring to design patient-tailored plans of care that control pain, support critical processes, and facilitate quick recovery. During surgery, anesthesiologists carefully monitor hemodynamic variables and respiratory mechanics and subtly adjust them to maintain homeostasis. Over the decades, technological advances such as high-tech ventilators, ultrasound-guided nerve blocks, and multimodal analgesia have transformed everyday practice. These developments have expanded the scope of techniques available, reduced complication rates, and improved outcomes in diverse patient populations.

For each patient encounter, a comprehensive evaluation begins with risk factor identification, history, and procedure needs. The anesthetic regimen may include regional techniques, intravenous sedation, or general anesthesia, selected according to safety profiles and surgical stress anticipated. Vigilance in care entails serial observation of cardiovascular and respiratory parameters, temperature control, and neuromuscular blockade monitoring. Successful postoperative pain control and careful monitoring of recovery by an expert after surgery are required to prevent either respiratory depression or hemodynamic instability. With every new generation of anesthetic agents and equipment, clinicians refine protocols to maximize comfort with minimal side effects. This ongoing process of analysis and improvement demonstrates the field's commitment to patient-centered practice and to clinical excellence.

In order to provide an overview and a practical guide, the book *Clinical Anesthesiology: Strategies and Techniques* utilizes opinion and evidence-based practice techniques that can be applied to present-day anesthetic practice. It addresses principles that are essential—drugging action to patient assessment—along with reporting detailed descriptions of airway management and regional block methods. The theory is applied to real-world situations, with clinical pearls to lead the reader through anticipating and successfully responding to problems. Important learning points are presented through illustrative case vignettes, and references to landmark trials form the basis for evidence-based decision-making. Details on contemporary perioperative monitoring technology and procedures reflect current standards for safety and efficiency. Contemporary trends in multimodal analgesia, opioid-sparing, and pathways of optimized recovery are also covered.

The book has 15 chapters, each addressing a particular aspect of anesthesiology practice. Chapter 1 has a general overview of clinical anesthesiology, including its history, professional role definitions, and anesthesia care continuum. Chapter 2 gives a summary of major anesthetic agents, including pharmacokinetics, pharmacodynamics, routes of administration, interactions, and safety concerns. Chapter 3 discusses cardiovascular, respiratory, neuroanatomy, and physiology and emphasizes functional changes under anesthesia. Chapter 4 describes preoperative evaluation methods like airway evaluation, comorbidity evaluation, fasting guidelines, and optimization guidelines.

Chapter 5 teaches airway management techniques, ranging from basic mask ventilation to roto probe fiberoptic intubation and emergency surgical airways. Chapter 6 details the induction and conservation of general anesthesia, comparing volatile-based balanced with total intravenous techniques, and addresses hemodynamic control. Chapter 7 teaches spinal, epidural, and peripheral nerve block techniques involving ultrasound guidance, calculation of dose, and prevention of complications. Chapter 8 covers monitored anesthesia care and procedural sedation, including sedation scales, patient selection, and monitoring standards. Chapter 9 covers pediatric anesthesia, where age-related pharmacological considerations, airway anatomy, and intraoperative fluid management are addressed.

Chapter 10 discusses anesthesia for labor and cesarean delivery, with emphasis on maternal physiology, neonatal evaluation, and analgesic options. Chapter 11 discusses anesthetic issues in geriatric patients, with emphasis on impaired drug metabolism, cognitive protection, and fall prevention strategies. Chapter 12 provides solutions for patients with cardiac, pulmonary, renal, hepatic, and endocrine disease, including perioperative risk reduction and multidisciplinary planning.

Chapter 13 outlines intraoperative monitoring modalities—such as capnography, invasive blood pressure, neuromuscular monitoring, and processed EEG—and illustrates crisis management algorithms. Chapter 14 outlines postoperative care, pain control modalities—such as regional techniques, multimodal regimens, and enhanced recovery protocols—and recovery area management. Chapter 15 addresses the recognition, prevention, and management of complications such as malignant hyperthermia, anaphylaxis, residual neuromuscular blockade, and post-dural puncture headache.

This book is written for anesthesiology residents preparing for board examinations and clinical practice, practicing anesthesiologists seeking a quick review, and nurse anesthetists looking to strengthen their knowledge foundation. It will also be valuable for anesthesia fellows and critical care doctors who require an integrated approach to perioperative management. The operating room nurse and surgical residents can use specific chapters to learn fundamental principles and prepare for intraoperative management changes. Medical students with an interest in anesthesia will find the initial chapters and case examples helpful for building foundational knowledge. Beyond the perioperative environment, emergency physicians, pain medicine physicians, and intensivists can apply principles of sedation, monitoring, and pain management within various clinical practice environments. Educators and program directors can use chapter outlines and representative cases to design curricula and simulation exercises. Practitioners from across the globe will appreciate the consideration of internationally accepted guidelines with adaptable protocols for low-resource settings. The combination of evidence-based guidelines, simple algorithms, and concise clinical pearls is appropriate for teaching and rapid decision-making at the bedside. With discussion of both routine and difficult scenarios given in an easily accessible manner, it aims to be a useful companion throughout an anesthesia provider's career.

INTRODUCTION TO CLINICAL ANESTHESIOLOGY

1

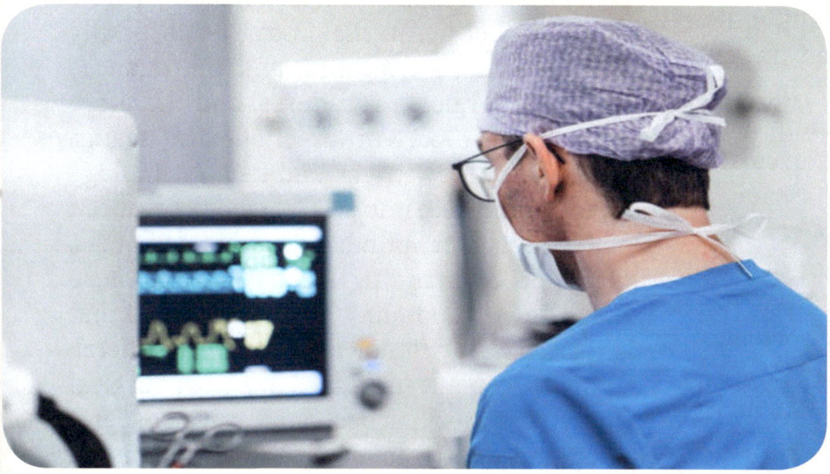

LEARNING OBJECTIVES

After studying this chapter, you will be able to:

1. Describe the types of anesthesia.
2. Understand the preoperative assessment.
3. Describe the intraoperative management.
4. Explain the postoperative care.

Introduction

Anesthesiology is at the forefront of modern medicine, and its role extends far beyond keeping patients stable during procedures. In operating theaters around the globe, comfort and safety involve more than technical know-how—it involves overseeing pre-surgery evaluations, the administration of care while patients are anesthetized, and post-surgery recovery. Sometimes, however, things get complex; postoperative residual curarization (PORC), for instance, can occur after the use of non-depolarizing muscle relaxants. Research in general links PORC with higher risks—longer recovery times and more costs for hospitals (Hassim et al., 2016). Monitoring anesthesia patients is, therefore, a must; anesthesiologists need to remain alert and be cognizant of how muscles and nerves work in tandem. Beyond learning such technical processes, there's been a palpable shift in priority to the well-being of students learning the trade. The majority of anesthesiology residency programs now lean in the direction of supporting the mental and emotional health of residents, as well as their clinical performance. The evidence suggests that residents are prone to burnout and even substance abuse issues, so program directors must take proactive steps to safeguard their staff (Dilorenzo et al., 2020). In most cases, this is not a nice-to-have. Rather, creating resilience and a support system is seen as a priority—so that, as residents learn the art, they're also better resilient in the face of actual practice pressures in the real world. The balance between technical knowledge and emotional strength is influencing the future of anesthesiology gradually but definitely. With emerging technology advances and constantly changing protocols, staying up to date is definitely necessary. For example, a new call for interventions like neuromuscular monitoring with acceleromyography has been welcomed as a smart move to enhance operating room safety on a larger scale (Hassim et al., 2016). At the same time, the integration of wellness programs in training is an important, more integrated measure of equipping future doctors. When both practitioners and residents are emotionally nurtured and provided with the latest clinical competencies, patient care, as well as general health services, are bound to flourish—showing that it is the combination of science and compassion that creates the difference (Figure 1.1).

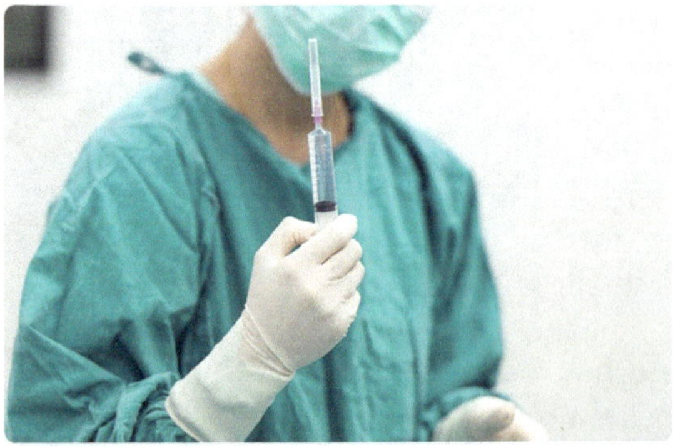

Figure 1.1. Clinical anesthesiology.

Source: https://d2jx2rerrg6sh3.cloudfront.net/image-handler/picture/2017/8/shutterstock_209570263.jpg.

Definition and Scope of Anesthesiology

Anesthesiology is more than administering drugs to knock you out for surgery—it's deeply involved in every step of the surgical process. It starts with pre-op evaluations, glides into a period of careful watching as the procedure goes along, and ends with recovery measures meant to keep patients safe and, in most cases, comfortable. Professionals in practice reconcile challenging comprehension of how drugs interact with the body, what bodily responses can be triggered, and the nuances of complex surgical procedures, and therefore are an intrinsic part of larger medical teams. More recently, new tricks and new technology have taken the field into steadily more advanced practices aimed at optimizing patient outcomes. One of the outstanding facets of what these experts do is responding to complications that might arise with or following surgery. In general, keeping an eye out for issues like post-surgical cognitive changes has become a grave concern. Having the ability to quantitatively measure and track changes in the mental sharpness of a patient is considered a critical point because it can dictate the ease of recuperation. In fact, most patients only have small, short-term bumps in their memory or concentration, but there are fewer who have longer-lasting problems that can complicate the recovery process and even increase the risk of other problems. This awareness makes it even more important to depend on prudent, evidence-based screening both before surgery and afterwards, confirming the manner in which anesthesiologists help guide procedures safely (Newman et al., 2019). Yet another area where anesthesiology leaves its mark is in controlling complications such as pulmonary edema—a situation that can sabotage the patient's recovery process. Detection of risk factors, either cardiac or inflammatory, is a major component of optimizing preoperative screening. Rapid, accurate diagnosis and early treatment are critical here, and technologies such as lung ultrasonography and transpulmonary thermodilution have provided them with a serious advantage in preventing such problems from taking hold. These advances lend a hand not only through the course of the procedure but also in regards to adjusting post-op therapy, showing how expansive and expansive the field can be through all phases of patient care (Assaad et al., 2018) (Figure 1.2).

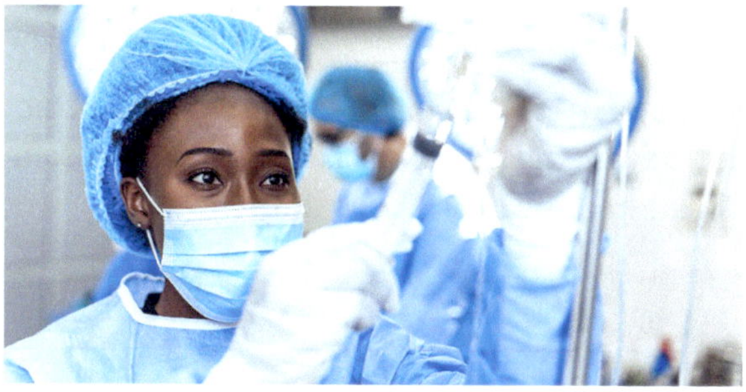

Figure 1.2. Anesthesiology.

Source: https://woodburysurg.com/wp-content/uploads/sites/241/surgeons-scahealth-1306095509-550-3.jpg.

Historical Development of the Field

Clinical anesthesiology actually took off in the 19th century—remember when ether and chloroform hit the scene? Before those breakthroughs, surgery was a ghastly experience with nothing better than primitive pain control, leaving patients dazed and often leading to very high mortality rates. Volatile anesthetics changed the image, permitting surgeons to perform longer and more complex procedures and maintaining patient distress to a minimum. They even began closely monitoring vital signs and creating simple techniques that, in the majority of instances, eventually developed into the standard practices of today. It's an irony of fate that those early techniques set the stage for contemporary anesthesiology and contributed to how surgery care improved. New drugs and gadgets started disrupting the field even further by the 20th century. Muscle relaxants and the development of gases to be inhaled gave doctors a finer degree of control over patients' physical responses while under the knife. Regional anesthesia (RA), for example, developed and offered a distinction from general anesthesia (GA) and expanded the anesthesiologist's toolkit. As increasing attention was given to safety, guides and manuals emerged to help prevent postoperative complications, and the continuous stream of complication data gradually infused practice with evidence-based origins. Overall, this movement away from less research-informed practices armed practitioners with better know-how for managing what happens around surgery time. Today, technology advances have a profound impact on anesthesiology practice. Modern technology like the Anesthesiology Control Tower (ACT) integrates telemedicine and decision support to increase intraoperative care—sometimes in almost sci-fi fashion. Clinical settings now depend on smart monitoring systems to dial up patient management during procedures, a transition no wonder considering conditions like obstructive sleep apnea (OSA) affecting many patients (Doghramji et al., 2012). All of this eloquently argues in favor of personalized medicine, where calculating each patient's risk equals more closely customizing anesthesia than ever before. It's a testament to persistent innovation and a commitment to not just making surgery safer, but more effective in contemporary medical practice.

Importance in Modern Medicine

Anesthesia changed the face of the hospital and how patients are treated today. Those days when, before any effective method to block pain was discovered, going under the knife was a ferocious process—surgery meant intractable NOT bearable pain, and too common mortality is now a thing of the past. With all the many different numbing drugs combined with inventive techniques, modern anesthesiology makes surgery safer and less painful. Not only does this advance make d on pain obsolete, it also brings the prospect of complex, once-too-perilous procedures. Anesthesia permits patients to be kept completely unconscious and effortlessly pain-free, and in most cases, this has broadened the range of treatments that can be offered and improved survival rates. Outside the operating room, too, the impact of anesthesiology is being felt in other areas of medicine. In the management of pain, practitioners employ local and general numbing methods; in some instances, nerve blocks or spinal anesthesia (SA) are employed in combination—methods that have increasingly unraveled the grip of chronic pain from most patients. In intensive care and emergency medicine, anesthesiologists generally work with other clinicians to keep patients at a stable level during crucial moments of life. Their work in managing sedation and observing vital signs illustrates just how highly their specialty coincides with the broader universe of modern medicine.

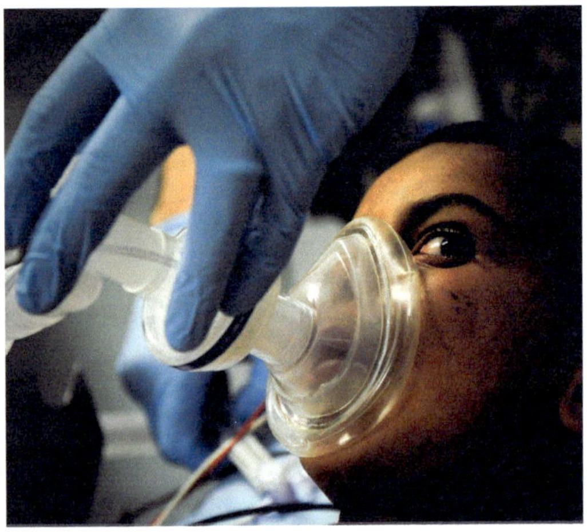

Figure 1.3. Importance of anesthesia in modern medicine.

Source: By ISAF Headquarters Public Affairs Office - originally posted to Flickr as 100410-F-7713A-002, CC BY 2.0, https://commons.wikimedia.org/w/index.php?curid=10958712.

Although ongoing innovation in the practice of anesthetics and technology ongoingly continues to illustrate the discipline's ongoing vitality in scholarship and pedagogy, for the most part, when new information on drug effects, monitoring methods, and safety protocols becomes available, the need for continuous learning arises. Several medical schools and training institutions are today more dedicated than ever to developing future anesthesia experts (Edgar et al., 1956; Outlook Magazine, 2011). Through prioritizing education and research, the medical fraternity is working diligently to improve patient care—an endeavor which, in the majority of instances, reinforces the notion that advancing anatomy is key to progressing overall healthcare (Figure 1.3).

1.1. Types of Anesthesia

Learning Outcome

1. Understand the general anesthesia.
2. Describe the regional anesthesia.
3. Explain the local anesthesia.

Clinical anesthesiology relies on establishing different forms of anesthesia (Figure 1.4), and this is crucial to having uneventful surgery as well as good patient care., there is a mix of general, regional, and local methods that each have specific applications depending on the operation and the overall health of the patient. GA, by contrast, induces patients into a deep state of unconsciousness by a combination of IV drugs and inhaled anesthetics—a method most often chosen for major invasive surgery where muscle relaxation is total, and pain relief is total. RA, by contrast, inspects an area of a block of sensation while often having the patient awake or lightly sedated; this can be satisfactory with situations such as cesarean section or orthopedic reconstruction. Local anesthesia targets more specifically by anesthetizing a small area, which suits procedures of small sizes like dental work or skin biopsies. It's administered fairly easily—sometimes injected or put on topically as a cream—and tends to have fast recovery times. Of course, choosing which type to use is dependent upon a variety of factors, such as the nature of the surgery, the duration it's likely to last, and the patient's clinical history. Taking a personalized strategy for every patient will generally enhance safety and normally leads to an improved surgical outcome. Innovations like ultrasound-guided surgery for RA illustrate how the specialty is always evolving, giving clinicians even better tools to deliver pain relief. There's also been a very real attempt to wed artificial intelligence (AI) and machine learning into anesthesia techniques. Overall, these technologies can build on current practices and even develop entirely new practices. As an example, anesthesiologists might utilize previous data to predict how an individual would respond to anesthesia, which in most cases would lead to better results. Naturally, the challenge is to integrate these new technology solutions with actual clinical, patient-focused care, so clinicians and data scientists have to work closely together to ensure that these innovations actually meet clinical requirements. Ongoing research, such as observations captured by relational interviewing (Marinkovic et al., 2018), keeps shedding light on the nuances of patient experience and pain management in the operating room.

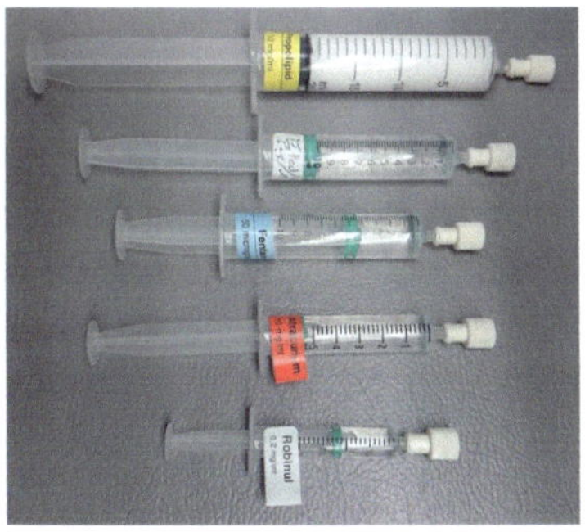

Figure 1.4. Types of anesthesia.

Source: By Mikael Häggström - work, CC0, https://commons.wikimedia.org/w/index.php?curid=44903688.

1.1.1. General Anesthesia (GA)

GA has changed a great deal—it now matches new technological innovation with a more grounded approach to how drugs work within the body. Clinicians don't blindly apply standard methods anymore; now they choose a cocktail of inhaled agents, IV drugs, and other support medications, each chosen to fit an individual patient's profile. One might argue that the foundations of contemporary anesthesia are spread out over a vast array of texts—consider, for example, Smith and Aitkenhead's Textbook of Anaesthesia, which provides readers with an insider's glimpse into the way drugs act and interact with bodily systems. Adhering to established protocols, particularly when dealing with high-risk cases, is frequently the difference maker; in most instances, this combination of hands-on evidence and hard-earned know-how constitutes the very foundation of safe practice. Although GA is generally quite safe, it is attended by intrinsic risks that demand constant monitoring and meticulous preparation. You cannot ignore potential complications like slows in breathing, heart irregularities, or a recovery that is slower than expected—and, in the process, thorough preoperative evaluations become a necessity. Sometimes, some challenges also present themselves; for example, patients with challenging airways sometimes need very specialized procedures for intubation (one of these procedures is awake tracheal intubation, outlined in modern policy documents). These procedures, seemingly too painstaking at first, not only augment patient safety and improve an anesthesiologist's capacity for averting unintended catastrophes in the operating room. But GA's story doesn't conclude at the operating room; its impact carries forward into postoperative care and recovery too. Pain management, for instance, is both directly critical to patient comfort and fewer complications after the procedure, and today's team works hand-in-hand with RA techniques on a routine basis to achieve effective pain management. Changing guidelines and ongoing education have reshaped the way care is provided at each step—from pre-op screening through the recovery room—so that rigorous monitoring standards inform every decision where patient safety and quality are concerned. As attested to in works like Smith and Aitkenhead's definitive compilation, a broad, sound foundation of knowledge helps anesthesiologists navigate the intricacies of the delivery of anesthesia while juggling the varied needs of patients along the course of their surgical treatment.

1.1.2. Regional Anesthesia (RA)

Regional anesthesia (RA) has changed everything about how anesthetics are performed and brought the art of anesthetic care to an entirely new level. Not only is it a safer pain management method; it's a whole new system that needs you to know a lot about how our bodies work, from physiology and anatomy to how drugs interact, and, of course, you must consider each patient's idiosyncrasy. The COVID situation, overall, did not enhance learning for the majority of residents, so advanced education became all the more important. Ultrasound, for instance, has turned around by enabling clinicians to see inside the body in real-time, which enhances local anesthetic injection precision and seems to reduce complications (Whizar-Lugo et al., 2022). For pediatric conditions, RA plays just as important a role. Kids derive a great deal of value from these techniques during recovery from surgery, and the ESPA Pain Committee has even created guidelines that break roughly into easy and then more complicated stages. This tiered model is helpful because European hospitals vary in resources and drugs on hand – so it's helpful to have an idea that's common but also which will be adaptable, as things work out (Adamek et al., 2018). The advantages don't stop there with pain management early on, though. Regional block patients often need fewer other pain medications, can leave the hospital earlier, and recover more quickly. When used with GA, they can also alleviate some of the side effects typically caused by strong opioids, like bouts of nausea or sleepiness. That said, as with anything, there is a very small chance for complications like nerve injury or infection. Overall, following ongoing education and best practices is most critical to keeping benefits high and risks low, and this remains a very big area of emphasis in the advancement of anesthesiology (Whizar-Lugo et al., 2022) (Figure 1.5).

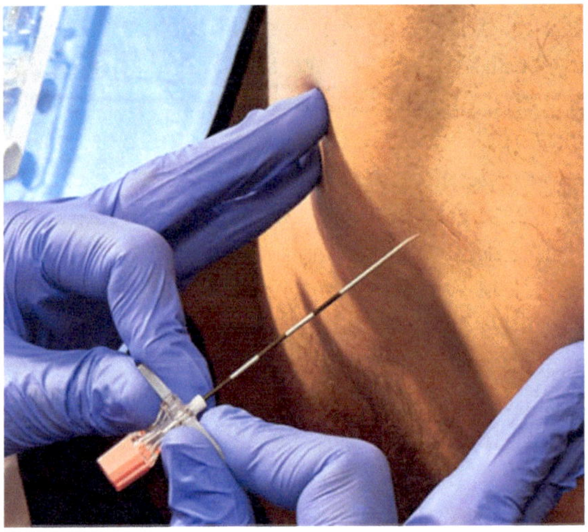

Figure 1.5. Regional anesthesia.

Source: https://www.citizenshospitals.com/static/uploads/bba76359-fd58-4e3e-bd43-433b7e9cb9c9-1709044256544.jpg.

1.1.3. Local Anesthesia

Local anesthesia has come a long way too. It now revolutionizes pain management for surgeons. Many procedures today make use of ultrasound so experts have improved visualization of nerves and other structures that are vital, making it much easier to find the right target. This seems to improve how well and how safely RA works—research, in most cases, still indicates that these technologies benefit high-risk patients substantially. Research shows that even the choice of the right anesthetic can even flip outcomes completely. For instance, although both Ropivacaine and Levobupivacaine are common options, recent research indicates that Ropivacaine might actually take hold more quickly, blocking sensation and movement more than the other, finally allowing for better pain management during and after the procedure (Chakrabarti, 2022). Physicians are no longer wed to a single type of local anesthetic; instead, a series of agents have appeared to meet different requirements. Older stalwarts like lidocaine persist, but newer agents, like Ropivacaine, offer alternatives with, on average, a kinder safety profile. Interesting is that the combination of these anesthetics with other agents—like dexmedetomidine (DEX)—can extend pain relief while keeping systemic risk low. This match-and-mix approach implies that there are greater avenues for research, and as their personalities emerge more distinctly in each agent, understanding them becomes essential in developing the optimal anesthesia regimen available (Zink, 2018).

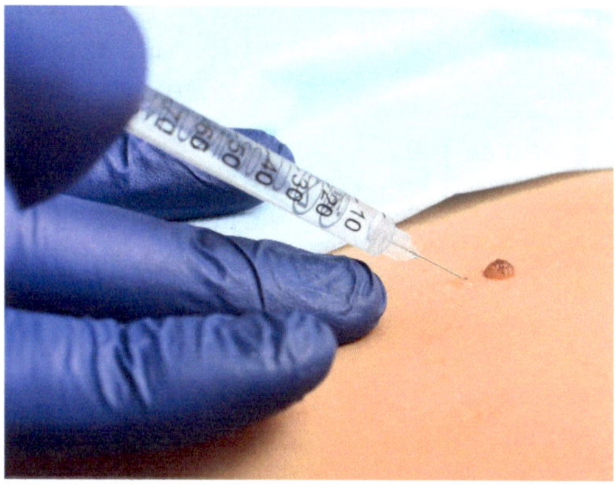

Figure 1.6. Local anesthesia.

Source: https://www.verywellhealth.com/thmb/OBM5z6-W9C0GVNtf_plkBIGdwTo=/3190x2125/filters:no_upscale():max_bytes(150000):strip_icc()/local_anesthesia_mole-b56769a7261945d2ba813c91f24767e2.jpg.

Although these apparent advantages exist, there is always room for caution. Infrequent but grave complications—nerve trauma, hematomas, infections—dictate the need to have a thorough understanding of anatomy and careful technique. New books and guides on RA complications still highlight the necessity of proper information to prevent and manage such failures. Clinicians can enhance their approach by knowing the causes of such failures. With local methods being the norm in most specialties, medical staff need to remain aware of safety norms even as they take advantage of the several benefits of local anesthesia, for the sake of better patient outcomes (Zink, 2018) (Figure 1.6).

Test Your Knowledge

1. What happens during general anesthesia?
2. Explain the regional anesthesia.
3. Describe the local anesthesia.

1.2. Preoperative Assessment

Learning Outcome

1. Understand the patient's history and physical examination.
2. Know the risk assessment and stratification.
3. Describe the preoperative optimization strategies.

Performing a careful examination is important in the hectic arena of surgeries so that outcomes end up being as best as possible. This assessment isn't merely revealing a tiny medical past—it also explores personal circumstances, past anesthesia experience, and current medication regimen. Mostly, anesthesiologists are weighing risks by spotting potential hiccups in the OR while monitoring other issues like heart and lung problems that may completely change the plan of anesthesia. Directing these variables initially helps to establish a firm foundation for directing care pre-operatively, intra-operatively, and even post-operatively. In all seriousness, these are measures towards individualized anesthesia techniques that are derived from each patient's unique requirements, with an overall boost in security and efficiency of the operation. Postoperative pain relief matters—in addition to making patients comfortable, it prevents recovery complications too. Unrelieved pain can open up an entire kit of challenges, including extended hospital stays, increased levels of anxiety, and in some instances even a downward slide into chronic pain. Generally speaking, the preoperative evaluation is a critical step in building an intelligent pain management program that considers both a patient's opioid tolerance and pain history. Anesthesiologists are not only focused in the operating room but also try to foresee pain pathways and map out intervention strategies ahead of time in response. Putting a broad, well-thought-out plan of analgesics well ahead of time usually straightens out the surgical procedure somewhat—keeping patients less agitated while dialing back dangers of uncontrolled pain (Wenzel et al., 2016). Switching a bit to the mental side of things, the cognitive effects after surgery are worth sincere consideration even before the operation is underway. Cognitive glitches can occur in any number of ways—sometimes simply small, others more pronounced—where some patients do have an especially hard time recovering. Numerous anesthesiologists test patient's cognitive baselines pre-surgery, which is extremely useful background for follow-up testing. They depend on established neuropsychological assessments to track how mental acuity recovers over time. In fact, it's not a simple thing to quantify and comprehend cognitive ability; it takes a process that takes into account both the individual quirks of patients and the overall surgery variables. When those subtleties are factored in, they are used to blunt cognitive risks and allow for a more supportive recovery pathway (Newman et al., 2019) (Figure 1.7).

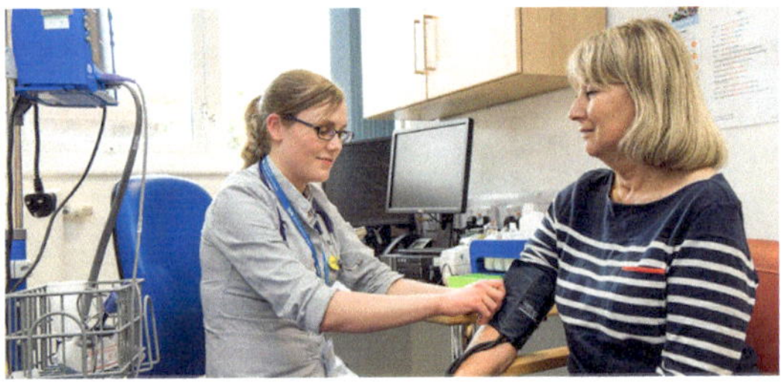

Figure 1.7. Preoperative assessment clinic.

Source: https://www.torbayandsouthdevon.nhs.uk/uploads/peripoperative_medicine_patient_having_blood_pressure_taken.jpg.

1.2.1. Patient History and Physical Examination

Understanding a patient's history is a big aspect of anesthesia—it opens the door for what is carried out during surgery. Ancient charts, details regarding medications, and even a list of other ailments all get integrated to decide the best course of action; as an example, someone with heart issues might be given an entirely different plan than someone with no major issues. A quick, hands-on exam can also flag things that the history might have missed—those immediate clues sometimes pop up unexpectedly. Lately, extra tests before surgery (Firde et al., 2024) have been shown to sometimes complicate matters even more, meaning that both doctors and patients have to talk things through to agree on the plan. In all, the back-and-forth between digging up a patient's history and conducting a physical exam makes care feel personalized and intimate. In critical care, though, the tug-of-war between old medical records and an exam in the present moment takes on even more meaning. For patients with complex medical problems that might need extra attention in the ICU, getting all of the background information is essential to planning the appropriate anesthesia strategy. Respiratory complications and cardiovascular issues—these change the risk profile (Handrawan et al., 2021). It is worth it for doctors to note everything carefully so they can more precisely individualize anesthesia for safety. The physical exam itself is not just routine; it has a tendency to catch little things that point toward possible bumps (or complications) in surgery. Understanding these subtleties, doctors can then make better decisions that ultimately result in patients faring better. Furthermore, monitoring patients closely during the anesthesia stage directly follows back from what was discovered in pre-op assessments. With a solid foundation of a complete history and a fresh physical, anesthesiologists can even catch subtle variations in vital signs or overall condition as they occur within the operating room. This ongoing monitoring is especially crucial when the patient is already known to have risks—essentially, being able to pick up on any slight change sooner can lead to earlier remediation. These thorough preoperative assessments guarantee that, in the event of complications arising, the surgical team has a plan to intervene, even if things get a little chaotic. Finally, merging deep historical insight with real-time monitoring not only makes it possible to individualize anesthetic technique but also provides the feeling of constant vigilance and active management that's required for best surgical outcomes (Firde et al., 2024; Handrawan et al., 2021) (Figure 1.8).

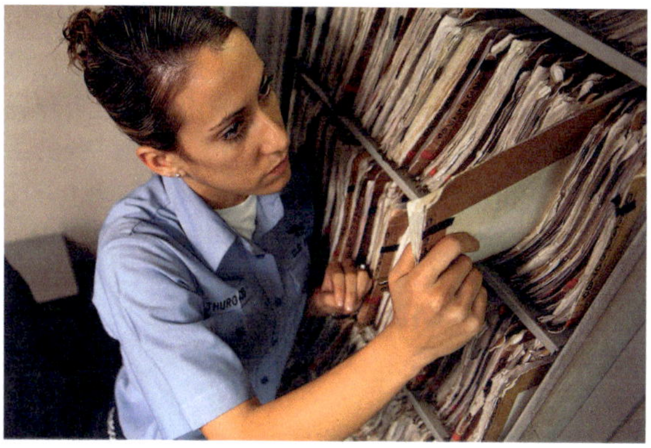

Figure 1.8. Patient history form.

Source: By U.S. Navy photo by Photographer's Mate 3rd Class Jason T. Poplin - This image was released by the United States Navy with the ID 041019-N-5821P-019 (next). This tag does not indicate the copyright status of the attached work. A normal copyright tag is still required. See Commons:Licensing.العربية · বাংলা ·Bahaso Jambi ·Deutsch · Deutsch (Sie-Form) · English · español · euskara · فارسی · français · italiano · 日本語 · 한국어 · македонски · മലയാളം · Plattdüütsch · Nederlands · polski · پښتو · português · русский · slovenščina · svenska · Türkçe · українська · 简体中文 · 繁體中文 · +/−, Public Domain, https://commons.wikimedia.org/w/index.php?curid=8231755.

1.2.2. Risk assessment and Stratification

During surgery, knowing how much risk a patient poses is the way to avoid future trouble. Anesthesiologists are using equipment that extracts bits of information from computerized health records—like vital signs and medical history—to make educated guesses that simply feel intuitive for each patient. Take the AGES score (Yap et al., 2025) for example; it pulls EHR data to forecast whether elderly patients would develop complications in 30 days after surgery, something that helps make improved choices in the operating room. As personalized medicine continues to grow, these models of risk are slowly turning the whole approach to perioperative care on its head, especially among the most vulnerable. On another related note, recent research using cardiovascular markers is generating new perspectives on patient levels of danger. High-sensitivity cardiac troponin (hs-Tn) has emerged as a favorite marker for identifying early heart dangers—even in individuals who seem symptom-free but could have hidden artery disease.

This marker, generally better than previous models of risk by detecting problems prior to their occurrence, gives doctors a chance to step in and avert heart complications under anesthesia (Akbar et al., 2025). Studies show that as levels of hs-Tn rise, so too does the likelihood of cardiac complications, and therefore anesthesiologists can adjust their treatment regimens based on each patient's needs, combining clinical judgment with these new markers. Closing the divide between risk assessment and using that data to utilize in the clinic is still in the works. This hinges on how versatile these tools are in relating to various bumps and patient scenarios. Merging past clinical data and markers like hs-Tn seems to hone the risk image—improving overall management guidelines (Akbar et al., 2025). Prospective investigations, in turn, must keep refining such methods so they hold true in a large number of patients, and not merely in special groups. And when anesthesiologists, surgeons, and primary care physicians work together—even if the details get a bit complicated—the end result usually ends up being a more integrated appraisal of risk that creates wiser surgery decisions and better patient results.

1.2.3. Preoperative Optimization Strategies

Optimal surgical outcomes depend on a knowledge of how to optimize a patient's status prior to surgery even beginning. Preoperative optimization is not a box to check; it is a process of getting a patient's body into the optimal condition for both surgery and anesthesia. A check-up can review a patient's history, conduct a physical, and include diagnostic testing to reveal potential issues; for most, these steps help to recognize complications in advance. Clinical guidelines generally recommend that risk must be analyzed by considering patients' overall health and any other conditions, and this helps to direct how anesthesia is managed and care is coordinated around the surgery. And then there is fluid management perioperatively—a puzzle piece that is critical. Following fluid protocols can reasonably reliably improve how quickly a patient bounces back while reducing other complications. Look, for instance, to the Clinical Practice Guidelines for Perioperative Fluid Therapy in Chinese Adult Patients; the guideline offers a usable template that speaks both to preoperative hydration and to monitoring volume during the operation. With over 50 evidence-based recommendations aimed mostly at individualizing fluid management to prevent excessive or insufficient fluid—especially for high-risk patients—it quietly advises clinicians that adherence to these guidelines is a top priority for safe, smooth recoveries in Enhanced Recovery After Surgery (ERAS) precepts. Pediatric anesthesiology adds another complexity to preoperative planning. Kids need extra-special care, and that requires staff to need to adjust their technique and even their training. In Colombia, some experts have already stressed the necessity to enhance competencies in pediatric anesthesiology by strengthening educational trajectories and training. Qualitative studies, for instance, illustrate real challenges in everyday practice and reveal the need for more expertise so that children's unique responses to anesthesia can be dealt with accordingly. In short, when teams move to methods suited particularly to children—often with long, continuous training—it serves to make surgery as secure and suitable as possible for children (Sebasti et al., 2025) (Figure 1.9).

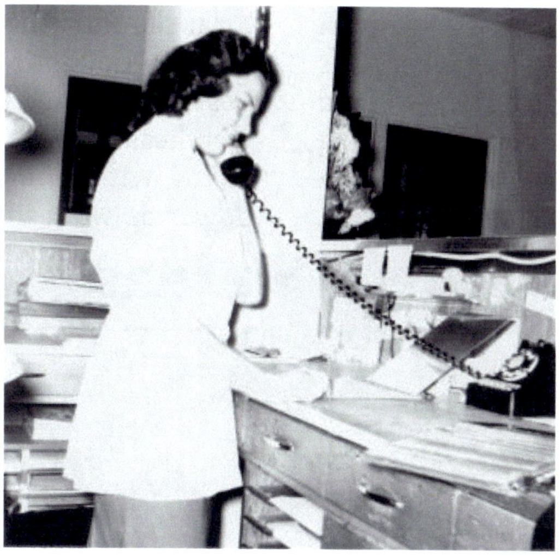

Figure 1.9. Preoperative optimization strategies.

Source: By Mennonite Church USA Archives - https://www.flickr.com/photos/mennonitechurchusa-archives/24648175876/, No restrictions, https://commons.wikimedia.org/w/index.php?curid=53024024.

Test Your Knowledge

1. Describe the patient's history and physical examination.
2. Explain the risk assessment and stratification.

1.3. Intraoperative Management

Learning Outcome

1. Monitor intraoperative techniques and equipment.
2. Describe the anesthetic administration protocols.
3. Understand the management of intraoperative complications.

Keeping all of it in balance in the operating room is crucial – patient safety and success are at stake. There are many things packed into this, including vital sign monitoring, properly dosing anesthetic medications, and following procedures everyone knows to work best. A simple example is measuring endotracheal tube cuff pressure. This is usually achieved by touch and not by measurement, and such subjectivity can sometimes result in problems like ventilator-associated pneumonia or even airway obstruction. In recent years, there's been an effort to bridge the existing literature and establish one single method of achieving this (Dixon et al., 2018). Most often, this method defends the individual patient as well and smoothes out practice variation across many operating rooms. A couple of pre-surgery preparatory steps can be beneficial as well, though. For instance, prewarming the patients eliminates d on the possibility of them getting too cold during the procedure – a drop in temperature that could lead to complications such as higher infection or issues with blood clotting. In one large teaching hospital, pressing time sometimes left the perioperative team unable to always use active warming techniques. To overcome this glitch, a training module with effective visual reminders was instituted and piloted to promote these evidence-based practices of warming (Dixon et al., 2018). On balance, this little program demonstrates how formal education can promote better use of best practices by staff. It is not necessarily the technical process that matters but the human factor within the OR which wields gigantic power as well.

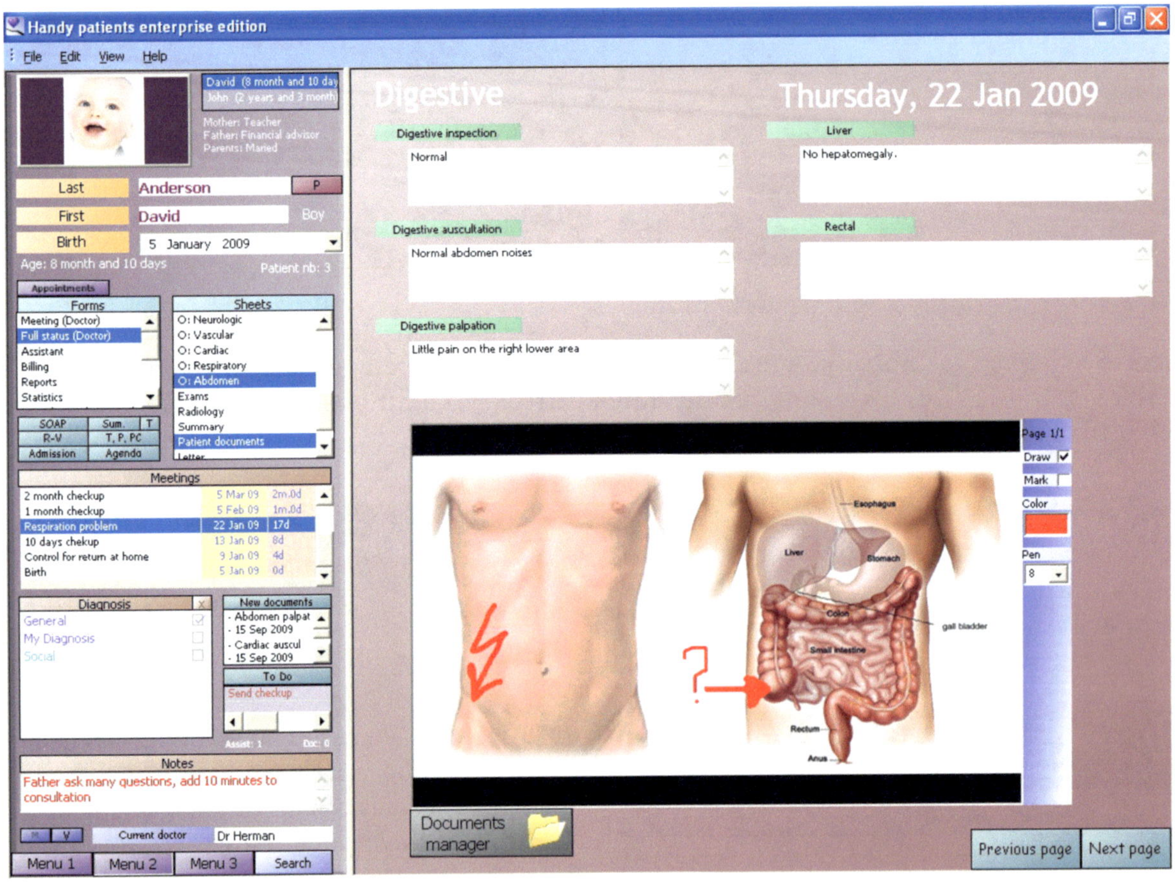

Figure 1.10. Intraoperative management.

Source: By Oguntoye patients electronic medical record (free open source version), GPL, https://commons.wikimedia.org/w/index.php?curid=8894074.

Open communication and actual collaboration between the surgical and anesthesia teams keep everyone's feet on the ground and abreast of the patient's status at all times. Frequent contact, regular but sometimes loose-worded recording, and integration of interdisciplinary input all serve to create a composite view of what the patient needs. Evidence shows that good open communication is linked with fewer complication rates (Comans et al., 2021). By facilitating a culture where colleagues freely exchange ideas, intraoperative management is that much more responsive and attuned to each specific case – and that, in turn, will yield improved results for surgery (Figure 1.10).

1.3.1. Monitoring Techniques and Equipment

Precise monitoring is the foundation of safe surgery. Anesthesiologists depend upon a combination of devices – monitoring vital signs, oxygen status, and cardiac function – that deliver real-time data and even alert them if something is wrong. For example, pulse oximetry is used early to quantify oxygenation while capnography tracks carbon dioxide levels, offering clues to respiratory status during anesthesia. These devices, which have been refined considerably over the decades, allow clinicians to act rapidly and thus improve the level of care in a wide range of surgical sites. Modern anesthetic practice is seeing more sophisticated technology being introduced into everyday routines in unexpected ways. Electroencephalography (EEG) signals, for instance, are used to approximate a patient's depth of anesthesia—a technique that goes beyond simply looking at a number. Monitoring systems such as the Bispectral Index, or BIS, interpret these brain wave patterns and give feedback on a patient's state of consciousness in general terms. Recent studies even derived new indicators from EEG recordings that not only correlate with BIS values but also reflect the findings of veteran anesthesiologists. This merging of innovation and technology inspires practitioners to keep pace with new equipment that may further improve their techniques (Liu et al., 2015). Even with these improved methods, upholding the same degree of quality in different healthcare settings is still a challenge. Professional organizations like the European Society for Pediatric Anesthesiology (ESPA) have advocated for guidelines that can smooth out differences, particularly for pediatric care. The ESPA Pain Management Ladder, for instance, offers a practical guideline specific to the various surgeries and available resources in a given institution. Such guidelines are essential in bridging the gaps in equipment and proficiency from one facility to the next. By adhering to these established guidelines, clinicians help develop a culture of safety and reliability—ensuring that all patients have solid, quality monitoring and care regardless of where they are treated (Adamek et al., 2018) (Figure 1.11).

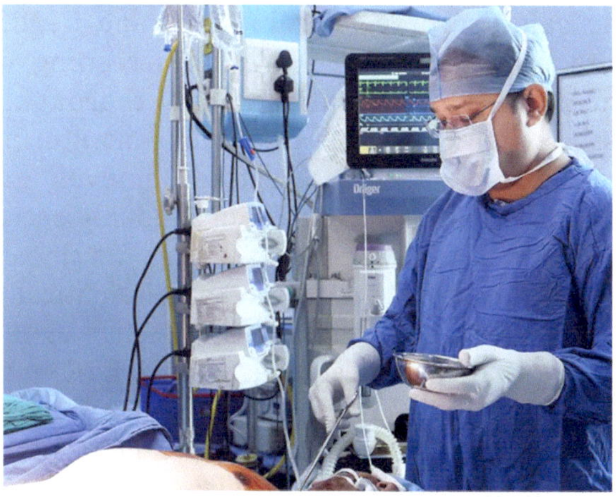

Figure 1.11. Monitoring techniques and equipment.

Source: https://www.mgmch.org/images/cardic_img2.webp.

1.3.2. Anesthetic Administration Protocols

Clinical anesthesiology calls for protocols well in hand to safely and effectively administer anesthetics. Every member of the surgical team should be aware of his or her function and be ready to roll with the punches of unexpectedness. Proper communication and artful tech form the basis for these protocols—this synergy has nothing to do with check-boxing but really reducing risks. For instance, an individualized intraoperative escalation procedure helps to apprehend "near-misses" promptly through close monitoring and strict adherence to guidelines. Computerized decision support systems also give anesthesiologists that extra push to maintain quality care, thereby promoting a culture of patient safety and quality improvement in general (Thakrar et al., 2024). In the administration of anesthetic drugs, particularly newer ones such as IV Ketamine, it is essential to adhere to safety guidelines to achieve best results. Ketamine, popular for its sedative properties, is now also targeted for treatment-resistant depression—so the guidelines must be stringent. In general, the safety protocol for IV Ketamine begins with an attentive pre-infusion screening to exclude high-risk patients and thoroughly assess vital signs. Even continuous monitoring is necessary, because dizziness or even the slightest deviation in taste can suddenly occur. With a stringent monitoring setting, the chance of severe complications decreases dramatically. The conservative approach is reflective of the reality that anesthesiologists no longer just sedate patients but are being asked more and more to play a central role in treating sophisticated psychopathologies (Argitis et al., 2024). Creating and enforcing such anesthetic standards is mandatory to improve the quality of care industry-wide. Procedures are refined over time by combining information gained through day-to-day clinical experience with results from research so they're continuously evolving to what works. Each surgical procedure has its own set of challenges, so being flexible but methodical pays when it's not predictable. Interdisciplinary collaboration also ensures the guidelines are up-to-date despite changing technology and treatment approaches. In the future, there is a pattern towards harmonizing machine learning and data analysis to produce more personalized care plans—bringing together the need for safety and best treatment. Ultimately, all these innovations result in a more responsive model of healthcare that is directed towards better outcomes for every patient undergoing surgery (Thakrar et al., 2024) (Figure 1.12).

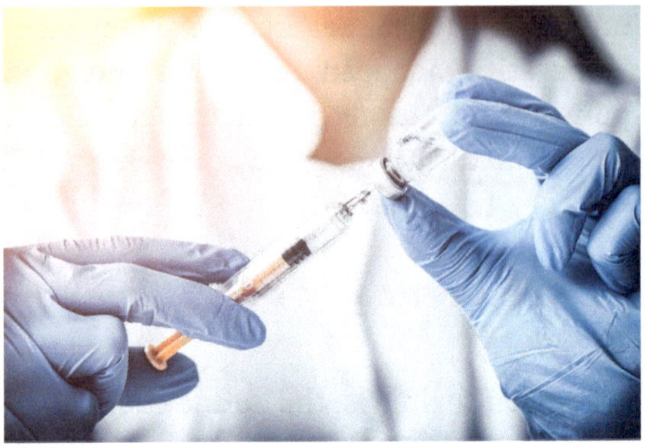

Figure 1.12. Anesthetic administration protocols.

Source: https://madeforthismoment.asahq.org/wp-content/uploads/2017/10/iStock-627196908.jpg.

1.3.3. Management of Intraoperative Complications

Surgical procedures invariably accompany an unruly set of complications that need to be resolved promptly – e.g., the sudden falls in blood pressure, respiration problems, or sudden shifts in a patient's baseline status. These speed bumps sometimes call for a nearly custom response from the anesthesia team. As a whole, one useful method of avoiding such complications has been to utilize advanced decision support systems – i.e., the Anesthesiology Control Tower (ACT). This real-time tracking and discerning algorithm-based system prompts clinicians toward interventions based on robust evidence. The system targets difficulties such as managing blood sugar and body temperature and tries to reduce major setbacks such as acute kidney injury (AKI) and postoperative respiratory complication (Gregory et al., 2018). In most instances, this type of pre-emptive management shows just how important a flexible, pro-active attitude can be when conducting surgery. A re-evaluation of ventilatory strategies is also an important factor in staying ahead of complications, particularly for those patients who may have issues with their lungs. More recent research on the matter indicated that establishing tailored positive end-expiratory pressure (PEEP) settings is able to minimize postoperative lung complications. For instance, the Driving pressure throughout GA for Open abdomen surgery trial (Designation) is determining whether a personalized high PEEP is superior to the standard low PEEP strategy, with the aim of best maintaining lung function. The trial is seeking to discover merely the right level of PEEP that restores driving pressure and, ultimately, the overall risk of surgery complications (Aarts et al., 2020). These intense explorations remind us that anesthesiologists do and are able to make subtle adjustments in their approach to better accommodate the needs of each individual patient, thereby improving surgical safety. Having an ever-present, if not necessarily infallible, observation of patient status—and being ready to adjust the plan as events unfold—is categorically integral for reducing on patient issues and optimizing recovery. At the moment, when the vital signs of the patient are all over the place and unexpected physiological changes are the norm, establishing a climate of vigilance and adaptability in the OR is crucial. In most cases, more training in dealing with complications, coupled with the technologies of telemedicine support devices, makes the anesthesia practitioner more self-assured and prepared to manage unexpected trouble. It's a reminder that by staying in touch with the latest research and guidelines, the practice can go on improving, therefore reducing intraoperative errors and improving overall care outcomes (Gregory et al., 2018). Short of that, the balance of know-how clinical expertise and state-of-the-art technology continues to act as a foundation in how we handle and treat the unpredictable nature of surgery.

Test Your Knowledge

1. Discuss the anesthetic administration protocols.
2. Explain the management of intraoperative complications.

1.4. Postoperative Care

Learning Outcome

1. Understand the recovery room protocols.
2. Describe the pain management strategies.
3. Monitor postoperative complications.

Postoperative care is at the heart of a speedy recovery and acceptable surgical results. Pain control is not simply an issue of treating physical pain – it also touches upon people's general well-being. Quite often, techniques like TENS (transcutaneous electrical nerve stimulation) fall into view; the literature, in the majority of cases, reveals its benefits despite underuse. A lot of that seems to derive from a deficiency of guidelines and training gaps, which may lead to excessive dependence on opioids (Diwan et al., 2025). Enhanced education and more clear-cut routines could simply maximize the extent to which patients have a sense of control over their recuperation. Other than pain, following the patient directly after surgery can be somewhat of a roller coaster. Patients can develop unforeseen respiratory issues or heart problems, and those risks demand vigilant, constant monitoring. Anesthesiologists tend to take over at those moments of crisis, moving swiftly—especially in complicated, high-acuity cases like gunshot wounds (Walters et al., 2024). In real practice, it is timely interventions that count for safety; indeed, a well-balanced and versatile monitoring approach can catch complications while they are not yet too severe. As patients are exiting the operating room, getting them to recovery is not as simple as it sounds. The whole team – nurses, anesthesiologists, and everyone involved – needs to know what occurred during surgery, what anesthetics were given, and what issues may be encountered down the road. This open, if sometimes imperfect, line of communication is especially critical in difficult cases such as gunshot wounds (Walters et al., 2024). Finally, the synthesis of evidence-based practice and collaboration on a daily basis works to tie all the loose ends together, and care is seamless and supportive throughout the path of recuperation (Figure 1.13).

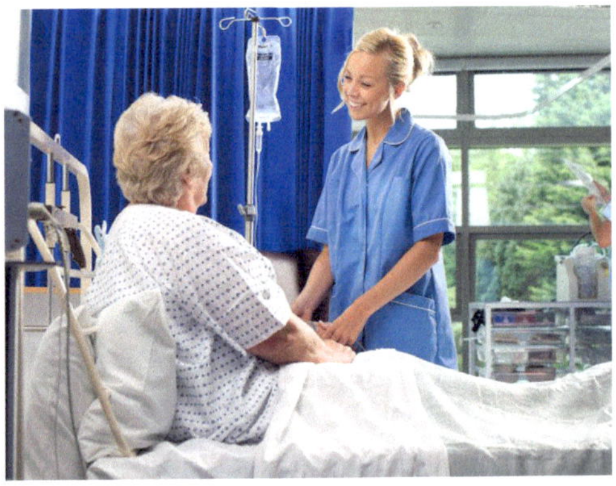

Figure 1.13. Postoperative care.

Source: https://media.post.rvohealth.io/wp-content/uploads/2020/08/postoperative-care_thumb.jpg.

1.4.1. Recovery Room Protocols

As the patients are rolled out of surgery, the scene is transformed. Recovery isn't a stroll down the corridor—it's a high-stakes moment when each beat and breath is watched with rigorous scrutiny as patients slowly come around from anesthesia. Blood pressure, levels of alertness, and even pain are checked repeatedly, making certain that no hitch like shallow breathing or a sudden decrease in blood pressure goes unnoticed. The majority of recovery rooms use scores—i.e., the Aldrete score—to help determine if someone's ready to go, and while these systems are in place to maximize outcomes, they always need a human touch to fit the patient's story. It's all about tailoring the process to reduce complications and improve the entire experience post-op. Managing pain in those seconds is downright critical. Patients can suffer the entire range of discomfort after surgery, and overall, the mixing and matching of different pain management strategies can reduce opioid dependency. Instead of depending on one type of drug, doctors often mix modalities—some by combining systemic drugs with local drugs like anesthetics, non-steroidal anti-inflammatory drugs, and other non-opioid drugs—to tackle pain from multiple directions. Increasingly, reports of opioid side effects like ongoing pain or even addiction highlight the necessity of protocols that stick strictly not only to clinical standards but to what each patient individually needs (Schwenk et al., 2018). Such a thoughtful protocol makes recovery smoother and more individualized. Education also plays a significant role in getting these recovery room protocols in line. Generally, keeping healthcare professionals informed about the latest multimodal pain management techniques is important because it's not just knowledge in theory but applying it when it matters most. Anesthesiologists and nurses, for instance, can benefit from repeat workshops and refresher courses covering current trends and practical tips so that postoperative treatment becomes effective and humane. Without this kind of training, even the best tactics occasionally miss the mark—possibly affecting patient satisfaction and recovery time. Thus, with investment in continuing education, healthcare providers not only treat immediate conditions but lay the foundation for overall wellness (Brennan et al., 2024).

1.4.2. Pain Management Strategies

Postoperative pain is still a tremendous problem for anesthesiologists today. New ideas keep arising to make patients recover more comfortably. One idea is the use of RA—solutions like the erector spinae plane block (ESPB) and the transversus abdominis plane block (TAPB) are being tried to reduce opioids. Some studies show that ESPB can reduce overall morphine consumption by a considerable amount and achieve better visual analog scale (VAS) scores compared to TAPB. Generally, RA seems to simplify recovery and even shorten the healing process, which is very much in line with modern anesthetic care goals (Liu et al., 2025). In chronic pain management, especially in syndromes like Bladder Pain Syndrome (BPS), there does not exist any fit-for-all plan. Each patient's symptoms are unique, and therefore doctors prefer to start with fundamental remedies such as modification of daily habits, stress management, and addition of therapeutic exercises. Medications like pentosan polysulfate are typically added as supplementary aid in most cases, even though they have different effects from person to person. Such complexity necessitates that treatment strategies be rethought and readjusted on a daily basis, and it underlines the reasons why teams of clinicians must keep learning together when attempting to treat difficult pain syndromes like BPS (Qiu et al., 2025). Today, blending drug therapies with other modalities of pain management highlights a movement towards greater individuality in style for anesthesiology. Where the conventional methods lag behind, newer techniques like neuromodulation or even minimally invasive procedures step in to offer alternatives. Doctors also now attempt to personalize their treatment based on how patients respond, which is vital to getting the best results. As new studies illuminate us more on the workings of pain and recovery, the majority of anesthesiologists are using the novel information to refine their technique and update their regimens. On the other hand, these advances not only boost patient satisfaction but also reduce the overall strain on healthcare systems, making intelligent pain management a pillar of anesthesia practice today (Liu et al., 2025) (Figure 1.14).

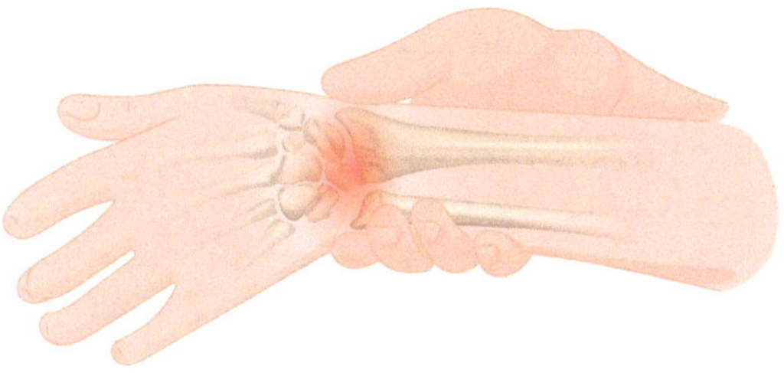

Figure 1.14. Pain management strategies.

Source: By Injurymap - InjuryMap - Free Human Anatomy Images and Pictures., CC BY 4.0, https://commons.wikimedia.org/w/index.php?curid=78335761.

1.4.3. Monitoring for Postoperative Complications

Post-op monitoring for complications is only key in anesthesiology—it determines the extent of recovery of patients. Anesthesia takes center stage during surgery, but the minutes following might bring surprises that need close monitoring. The individual may see early warning signs such as respiratory distress, unstable rhythm of the heart, or unexplained blood glucose changes if a person is kept awake. Think about intraoperative fluid management; older, static approaches to monitoring have a knack for missing what is really happening with a patient's fluid balance—something that a case of severe abdominal surgery has shown. In many cases it's possible to transfer to a less invasive, dynamic approach to monitoring, enhancing the overall quality of care, reducing on later complications, and helping recovery (Gutierrez et al., 2013). That initial amount of time postoperatively still demands continuous monitoring, especially to prevent complications like labile blood pressure and dysglycemia. It's surprising how elevated blood sugar levels generated intraoperatively can cause injury, resulting in added complications and longer stays. Overall studies show that the stress of surgery can provoke acute insulin resistance—a condition that would usually hit diabetic patients a bit harder. For example, in a study of elderly patients undergoing elective surgery, over half of the patients were revealed to have evident dysglycemia, which was therefore associated with poorer post-op outcomes (Knaak et al., 2019). This points to the need to keep a vigilant eye on blood sugar levels and other similar risk factors so that their resolution can be undertaken at the earliest if required. Multidisciplinary approaches seem to improve postoperative care. When anesthesiologists, surgeons, and nurses all pitch in—coordinating such essentials as airway management, heart rate control, and rough metabolic balance—it provides a safety net that can catch issues early. Technology-intensive evidence-based practices, such as continuous blood glucose monitors, can then finish fine-tuning the reaction as complications evolve. Of course, it's important that everyone stays well-trained and follows these monitoring routines (even if there's the occasional lapse) because a safety-first attitude cuts down on risks. In the end, postoperative monitoring is not another routine task; it's the quintessential element of good-quality anesthetic care that has a profound impact on surgical outcomes and patient overall well-being.

Test Your Knowledge

1. What are recovery room protocols?
2. Explain the pain management strategies.

SUMMARY

Anesthesiology isn't just about high-tech equipment—it's a question of balancing new technology with old-fashioned clinical acumen. Take Trial Sequential Analysis (TSA), for example; it arises as a useful tool that works to strengthen the overall validity of scientific findings. Instead of getting bogged down by the usual meta-analysis pitfalls—like publication bias or too-low statistical power—TSA kind of leads the way toward better clinical practices. Not only does it sharpen the decision-making process, but it also drives us into a mindset that values good, evidence-based practice. Interestingly enough, its use raises its head even in certain Russian anesthesiology-resuscitation journals, where the tool seems perfectly positioned to back up outcomes and drive standards for the future (Yadgarov et al., 2024). Switching what we're looking at, the rise of AI tools also is shifting the scene in anesthesiology. Departments are now building inventive web apps that help with everything from searching through literature to deciding research protocols. These AI-driven solutions don't merely smoothen out the paperwork; they make critical info way more accessible for both clinicians and researchers. As individuals work assiduously to test and apply these tools in everyday practice, there is a growing sense that they might revolutionize the way professionals learn and, ultimately, patients are cared for (Melvin et al., 2024). Overall, the prospects of clinical anesthesiology look very promising. The compounding of pressure to validate research findings with the latest wave of innovations driven by AI proves the field resilient, even in the face of emerging threats. By adopting evidence-based practices and embracing modern technology, anesthesiology will advance patient outcomes and reimagine its role in medicine. In a way, such efforts blend innovation and tradition—a synthesis of sorts that keeps the field both innovative and responsive to contemporary worldly needs (Melvin et al., 2024; Yadgarov et al., 2024).

Clinical anesthesiology is not so straightforward as it looks. There is this mix of problems, from safety with the patient to perioperative success in general, which all feed on one another in unknown ways. For example, an aging population of patients tends to move the prevalence of neurocognitive complications closer to surgery – something which cannot be stopped. Neuroinflammation due to trauma among older patients is a serious issue in general, and therefore the rationale for a full preoperative assessment with an accommodating, multi-modality strategy. In most cases, the literature suggests the merits of individualized interventions to mitigate such risks (Arcadipane et al., 2018). That is, when anesthesiologists comprehend the changes brought about by age and surgical stress, they are more likely to work around these challenges and eventually enhance patient outcomes. The emotional well-being of the anesthesiologists themselves also significantly contributes. It so happens that the emotional well-being of a physician can have an impact on the way care is provided. Latest literature has also pointed out some quite alarming burnout rates, especially in high-risk areas like cardiology anesthesiology, where the emotional toll strikes both doctors and patients alike (Arcadipane et al., 2018). Crushing workload – with emotional exhaustion and detachment finding their way in – shows how high the stakes are when working with critically ill patients. It is worth noting that while many experts remain firmly committed, a serious burnout danger remains in the wings, calling for some overdue systemic changes in the medical establishment. In most cases, giving precedence to mental health has the impact of keeping staff sustainable as well as effective. Merging solid clinical experience with some real emotional resilience seems to be the magic formula. Since the field of anesthesiology continues to evolve (and at increasingly speedy rates), constant education and reliable support structures propel not just career satisfaction but also maintain patient care consistently. Anesthesiologists must juggle sophisticated methods and cutting-edge technologies with self-care and coping strategies to buffer against stress (Lai et al., 2019). As these pieces fall together in harmony, it works to help guarantee that anesthesiology remains current with quality care, regardless of the ever-growing challenges of our modern-day medical environment.

KEY TERMS FROM THIS CHAPTER

- Airway management
- Anesthesiology
- Emotional health
- Heart irregularities
- Lung ultrasonography
- Patient safety
- Anesthesia techniques
- Anesthesiology control tower
- General anesthesia
- Local anesthesia
- Modern medicine
- Recovery process

CRITICAL THINKING QUESTIONS

1. **What is the primary purpose of the ASA Physical Status Classification System?**
   a. To estimate surgical difficulty
   b. To predict patient mortality
   c. To assess a patient's physical fitness before surgery
   d. To classify the type of anesthesia to be used
2. **Which agent is commonly used for rapid sequence induction of anesthesia?**
   a. Propofol
   b. Ketamine
   c. Thiopental sodium
   d. Etomidate
3. **Which of the following is a contraindication for spinal anesthesia?**
   a. History of severe headaches
   b. Hypovolemia
   c. Pregnancy
   d. Lower limb surgery
4. **Capnography monitors the concentration of which of the following gas in exhaled air?**
   a. Oxygen
   b. Nitrous oxide
   c. Carbon dioxide
   d. Volatile anesthetics
5. **What is the most common cause of postoperative hypoxemia in the recovery room?**
   a. Atelectasis
   b. Pulmonary embolism
   c. Aspiration
   d. Bronchospasm

Short Answer Questions

1. What is anesthesiology?
2. Name the three types of anesthesia.
3. Why is anesthesia important in modern medicine?
4. Explain the preoperative optimization strategies.
5. What kind of tools do anesthesiologists use?

Answers to Critical Thinking Questions

1. (c); 2. (d); 3. (b); 4. (c); 5. (a)

REFERENCES

1. Abbod, M. F., Chang, H. C., Chiu, Y. F., Chuang, et al. (2015). Sample entropy analysis of EEG signals via artificial neural networks to model patients' consciousness level based on anesthesiologists' experience. https://core.ac.uk/download/29140453.pdf (accessed on 20 May 2025).
2. Adamek, A., Akin, A., Al-Zaben, K., Alm, S., Amminnikutty, J., Amoli, M., Anderson, B., et al. (2018). Postoperative pain management in children: Guidance from the pain committee of the European Society for Pediatric Anesthesiology (ESPA Pain Management Ladder Initiative). https://core.ac.uk/download/157582937.pdf (accessed on 20 May 2025).
3. Agledahl, K. M., & Pedersen, R. (2024). Ethics in the operating room: A systematic review. *BMC Medical Ethics, 25*, 128. https://doi.org/10.1186/s12910-024-01128-7.
4. Ahmad, I., El-Boghdadly, K., Bhagrath, R., Hodzovic, I., McNarry, A. F., Mir, F., O'Sullivan, E., et al. (2019). Difficult Airway Society guidelines for awake tracheal intubation (ATI) in adults. *Anesthesia, 75*, 509–528. https://doi.org/10.1111/anae.14904.
5. Akbar, H. A., Khan, J., Khan, W., Subhan, M., Iftikhar, R., Naz, S., Musthafa, H., et al. (2025). High-sensitivity troponin for cardiovascular risk stratification in asymptomatic individuals with subclinical atherosclerosis: Insights into sex-specific differences and emerging clinical applications: A meta-analysis with crucial implications for cardiovascular risk assessment. *Insights–Journal of Health and Rehabilitation*. https://www.semanticscholar.org/paper/750a7f86648895fbbb1208d6ff1908a70e8a01ba (accessed on 20 May 2025).
6. Arcadipane, A., Bignami, E., Blangetti, I., Cattaneo, et al. (2018). Burnout in cardiac anesthesiologists: Results from a national survey in Italy. https://core.ac.uk/download/188829816.pdf (accessed on 20 May 2025).
7. Argitis, P., Karampas, A., Peyioti, M., Koukouras, T., Karavia, S., & Chaviaras, Z. (2024). Half a decade of intravenous ketamine administration: Our observation results and insights regarding its safety. *European Psychiatry, 67*(S347–S348). https://www.semanticscholar.org/paper/3092826f12d8b02c23ef6c0c9cc8987ed97b4141 (accessed on 20 May 2025).
8. Assaad, S., Friedman, M. B., Kratzert, W. B., Perrino, et al. (2018). Assessment of pulmonary edema: Principles and practice. https://core.ac.uk/download/145643671.pdf (accessed on 20 May 2025).
9. Bogoń, A., Górska, M., Ostojska, M., Kałuża, I., Dziuba, G., & Dobosz, M. (2024). Artificial intelligence in anesthesiology–A review. *Journal of Pre-Clinical and Clinical Research*. https://www.semanticscholar.org/paper/f0675c7d4ce9e68003a85b778c5e4c0872e48443 (accessed on 20 May 2025).
10. Brennan, L., & Kaye, A. (2024). Evidence-based educational module on management of multi-modal analgesia for perioperative providers. https://core.ac.uk/download/614443183.pdf (accessed on 20 May 2025).
11. Cabrera Hernández, J. S., & Reinoso Chávez, N. (2025). Perception of pediatric anesthesiology training in Colombia: A qualitative study. *Colombian Journal of Anesthesiology*. https://www.semanticscholar.org/paper/90cbf155613e3d094f2026f85da20774eaf95340 (accessed on 20 May 2025).

12. Central Administration, Medical Public Affairs. (2011). *Outlook Magazine*. Bernard Becker Medical Library Archives, Washington University School of Medicine, Saint Louis, Missouri. https://core.ac.uk/download/70380426.pdf (accessed on 20 May 2025).
13. Chakrabarti, A. (2022). Comparison between ropivacaine 0.5% and levobupivacaine 0.5% in axillary brachial plexus block for upper limb surgeries in a tertiary healthcare center of Tripura—An observational study. *RA Journal of Applied Research*. https://www.semanticscholar.org/paper/ff8f0b0afa261089eb64052b261d08fb73d1073b (accessed on 20 May 2025).
14. Comans, T., Hays, Z., & Leach, C. (2021). Barriers to preoperative warming: Best practice guideline. https://core.ac.uk/download/483691872.pdf (accessed on 20 May 2025).
15. Dilorenzo, A. N. (2020). Leading well: Anesthesiology program directors as servant leaders and their development of resident wellness programs. https://core.ac.uk/download/346141152.pdf (accessed on 20 May 2025).
16. Diwan, S., Olausson, A., Andréll, P., Wolf, A., & Jildenstål, P. (2025). Knowledge, attitudes, and practices of transcutaneous electrical nerve stimulation in perioperative care: A Swedish web-based survey. *Scandinavian Journal of Pain, 25*(1). https://doi.org/10.1515/sjpain-2024-0078.
17. Dixon, M. J. (2018). Analysis of current practices for measuring endotracheal cuff pressures. https://core.ac.uk/download/301292694.pdf (accessed on 20 May 2025).
18. Doghramji, K., Grewal, R. G., Vasu, et al. (2012). Obstructive sleep apnea syndrome and perioperative complications: A systematic review of the literature. https://core.ac.uk/download/83049558.pdf (accessed on 20 May 2025).
19. Edgar, D. J., Heverly, I. K., Prevost, M. C., Rake, et al. (1956). *Nurses' Alumnae Association Bulletin, May 1956*. https://core.ac.uk/download/46974789.pdf (accessed on 20 May 2025).
20. Ermakov, A. V., Dubina, E. A., Khramova, M. A., Ustinova, E. A., & Trusov, Y. A. (2025). On the issue of choosing anesthesia methods: A comparison of general medicine and clinical dentistry. *Stomatology, 104*(1), 76–80. https://www.semanticscholar.org/paper/8f583a4ce2fbe39701710dd0498353d6e8a5db08 (accessed on 20 May 2025).
21. Feitosa, G. de A., Soares, R. A., Feitosa, J. V. A., Santos, F. N. M. dos, Nascimento, I. S. B. do, Campos, K. L., Carvalho, K. R. P., Melo, F. D. de A., & Formiga, J. J. D. (2024). Innovations in anesthesia: Advances and ethical considerations. *Research, Society and Development, 13*(3), e14513345320. https://doi.org/10.33448/rsd-v13i3.45320.
22. Firde, M., & Yetneberk, T. (2024). Preoperative investigation practices for elective surgical patients: Clinical audit. *BMC Anesthesiology, 24*, 184. https://doi.org/10.1186/s12871-024-02557-y.
23. Gregory, S., Murray-Torres, T. M., Fritz, B. A., et al. (2018). Study protocol for the Anesthesiology Control Tower—Feedback Alerts to Supplement Treatments (ACTFAST-3) trial: A pilot randomized controlled trial in intraoperative telemedicine [version 2; peer review: 2 approved]. *F1000Research, 7*, 623. https://doi.org/10.12688/f1000research.14897.2.
24. Gutierrez, M. C., Liu, H., & Moore, P. G. (2013). Goal-directed therapy in intraoperative fluid and hemodynamic management. https://core.ac.uk/download/323069925.pdf.
25. Handrawan, S. E., Lestari, M., & Zulkifli. (2021). Herbicide intoxication: Still a threat in developing countries. *Journal of Anesthesiology & Clinical Research*. https://jurnalkedokteranunsri.id/index.php/JACR/index (accessed on 20 May 2025).

26. Hassim, S. (2016). The occurrence of residual curarisation in postoperative patients at an academic hospital. https://core.ac.uk/download/188773225.pdf (accessed on 20 May 2025).

27. Kampi, R., Okello, C., Ochieng, J., & Mwaka, E. (2024). Informed consent in cancer clinical care: Perspectives of healthcare professionals on information disclosure at a tertiary institution in Uganda. *PLOS ONE, 19*. https://www.semanticscholar.org/paper/82bb1b016e9ad1c7ead9930c3f41b951721f568d (accessed on 20 May 2025).

28. Knaak, C., Kuenz, S., Kurpanik, M., Lachmann, et al. (2019). Risk factors of intraoperative dysglycemia in elderly surgical patients. https://core.ac.uk/download/225124691.pdf (accessed on 20 May 2025).

29. Lai, I. K., Li, R., Maze, M., Saxena, A., et al. (2019). Neuroinflammation is a putative target for the prevention and treatment of perioperative neurocognitive disorders. https://core.ac.uk/download/287623880.pdf.

30. Liu, M., Mo, X., Zhan, R., et al. (2025). Erector spinae plane block versus transversus abdominis plane block with rectus sheath block for postoperative analgesia in laparoscopic hepatectomy: A randomized clinical trial. *BMC Anesthesiology, 25*, 162. https://doi.org/10.1186/s12871-025-03031-z.

31. Lonsdale, H., Jalali, A., Gálvez, J. A., Ahumada, L., & Simpao, A. F. (2020). Artificial intelligence in anesthesiology: Hype, hope, and hurdles. *Anesthesia & Analgesia, 130*, 1111–1113. https://doi.org/10.1213/ane.0000000000004751.

32. Marinkovic, A., & Lee, S. M. (2018). Interviewing in social science research: A relational approach. *Anesthesia & Analgesia, 127*(Suppl 1), e13–e14. https://doi.org/10.1213/ane.0000000000003462.

33. Medvedeva, A. A., Malyshev, A. A., Vlasenko, A. V., Rodionov, E. P., Evdokimov, E. A., Makarov, O. V., Lykhin, V. N., et al. (2025). Clinical cases of the use of ESPB as a component of combined anesthesia in patients with liver resection operations. *Medical Alphabet,* (35), 50–55. https://www.semanticscholar.org/paper/839150ea991d504679aa6ea6877dad1fad9590a4 (accessed on 20 May 2025).

34. Melvin, R., & Godwin, R. (2024). AI-powered web applications for enhanced clinical, research, and professional development. *Physiology, 39*(S1). https://www.semanticscholar.org/paper/bdfed36372bbeb1d0c041f0c1dfa045bb16b0b36 (accessed on 20 May 2025).

35. Newman, S. P., & Piggin, L. H. (2019). Measuring and monitoring cognition in the postoperative period. https://core.ac.uk/download/169434531.pdf (accessed on 20 May 2025).

36. Nono, D., Mwebesa, E., Bagenda, G., Okullo, I., Rwenyonyi, C., & Williams, S. (2024). Assessment of the knowledge, attitude and practices of the informed consent process in oral healthcare among dental students in Makerere University Dental Hospital, Uganda. *BMC Medical Education, 24*. https://www.semanticscholar.org/paper/e508d0df77f473cef156c11b90b202521371dc7d (accessed on 20 May 2025).

37. Qiu, M., Nico, A., Rahman, A., Ponen, K., & Kiosoglous, A. (2025). Bladder pain syndrome: Clinical diagnosis and management strategies. *Journal of Surgery, 10*, 11285. https://doi.org/10.29011/2575-9760.011285.

38. Saeed, M., Swaroop, M., Yanagawa, F. S., et al. (2018). Avoiding fire in the operating suite: An intersection of prevention and common sense. In *Vignettes in Patient Safety–Volume 3*. InTech. https://doi.org/10.5772/intechopen.76210.

39. Schwenk, E. S., & Mariano, E. R. (2018). Designing the ideal perioperative pain management plan starts with multimodal analgesia. *Korean Journal of Anesthesiology, 71*(5), 345–352. https://doi.org/10.4097/kja.d.18.00217.

40. Thakrar, S. P., Kim, C., Suarez-Winowiski, O., Navarrete, S. B., Potter, K. F., Prasanna, P., Graham, J. P., Diallo, M. S., Lahaye, L., & Coombs, A. A. T. (2024). A process-based standardization of an intraoperative escalation protocol in anesthesiology. *Anesthesia and Analgesia, 139*(4), 851–856. https://doi.org/10.1213/ANE.0000000000006782.

41. The DESIGNATION Investigators. (2020). Driving pressure during general anesthesia for open abdominal surgery (DESIGNATION): Study protocol of a randomized clinical trial. *Trials, 21*, 198. https://doi.org/10.1186/s13063-020-4075-z.

42. Walters, A. M., Aichholz, P., Muldey, M., van Cleve, W., Hess, J. R., Stansbury, L. G., & Vavilala, M. S. (2024). Emergency anesthesiology encounters, care practices, and outcomes for patients with firearm injuries: A 9-year single-center US Level 1 trauma experience. *Anesthesia and Analgesia*. https://www.semanticscholar.org/paper/9e8b682b5760f79fb3f93724f7bde84fbde0844b (accessed on 20 May 2025).

43. Wang, M., & Argalious, M. (2020). *Smith and Aitkenhead's Textbook of Anesthesia* (7th ed., Vol. 130, pp. e103–e104). *Anesthesia & Analgesia*. https://doi.org/10.1213/ane.0000000000004649.

44. Wenzel, J. T., Schwenk, E. S., Baratta, J. L., & Viscusi, E. R. (2016). Managing opioid-tolerant patients in the perioperative surgical home. *Anesthesiology Clinics, 34*(2), 287–301. https://doi.org/10.1016/j.anclin.2016.01.005.

45. Whizar-Lugo, V. M., Saucillo-Osuna, J. R., & Castorena-Arellano, G. (n.d.). *Topics in Regional Anesthesia*. https://core.ac.uk/download/534901319.pdf (accessed on 20 May 2025).

46. Yadgarov, M., Berikashvili, L., Polyakov, P., Kadantseva, K., Smirnova, A., Kuznetsov, I., Yakovlev, A., et al. (2024). Trial sequential analysis in anesthesiology and intensive care: A systematic review. *Pathology Krovoobrashcheniya I Kardiokhirurgiya*. https://www.semanticscholar.org/paper/f287a1f45659e7a6992c95133d793964f71a485a (accessed on 20 May 2025).

47. Yap, E. N., Huang, J., Chiu, J., Chang, R. W., Cohn, B. R., Hwang, J. C. F., & Reed, M. E. (2025). Development and validation of an EHR-based risk prediction model for geriatric patients undergoing urgent and emergency surgery. *BMC Anesthesiology, 25*. https://www.semanticscholar.org/paper/25f20e96555b75f0ba7b8fd736d1d1b7fd396777 (accessed on 20 May 2025).

48. Zink, W. (2018). *Complications of Regional Anesthesia* (3rd ed.). *Anesthesia & Analgesia*. https://www.semanticscholar.org/paper/e089ac5a414b0561b221020cb9e956faaa69e963 (accessed on 20 May 2025).

PHARMACOLOGY OF ANESTHETIC AGENTS

2

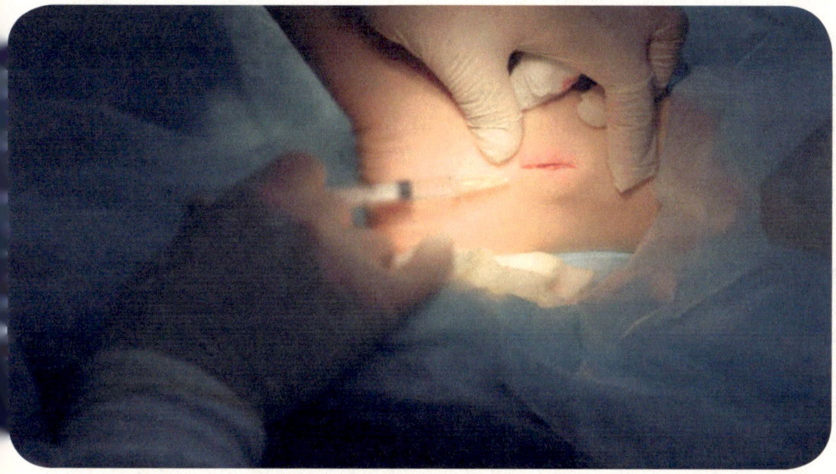

LEARNING OBJECTIVES

After studying this chapter, you will be able to:

1. Explain the classification of anesthetic agents.
2. Understand the mechanism of action.
3. Understand the pharmacokinetics of anesthetic agents.
4. Explain the clinical applications.
5. Describe the side effects and complications.
6. Describe the advances in anesthetic pharmacology.

Introduction

Anesthetic medicine is evolving quickly—new drugs and changing care routines are turning everything upside down. Anesthetics no longer just belong in a surgical setting; they are applied to pain relief and calming nerves in many locations. Caregivers, never ones to look for something safer and smarter, now blend the old inhaled or IV with new chemicals that sometimes work in fully unexpected ways. For example, greater use of topical drugs mirrors growing need to minimize whole-body side effects while obtaining good local relief, especially for refractory neuropathic pain (Coderre, 2018). Use of topical anesthetics is evidence of how target-based action can improve patient benefit. They directly act on nerves in the involved area and, in most cases, offer a better choice for patients with neuropathic pain—where traditional systemic medications get remiss by triggering unwanted side effects (Coderre, 2018). Localized methods not only target pain directly but also reduce the risks associated with medicines that affect the whole body. Interestingly, the clinics are now mixing various types of anesthetics based on each drug's mechanism of action and how they may even complement each other, which speaks of a change in strategy. This trend—particularly crucial when dealing with children who have special needs—is typically asking for more studies to better refine these strategies. Taking a closer examination of anesthetic selection, it is obvious that individual patient care is paramount. Understanding the way a drug acts in the body and how the body processes it is the foundation for enhanced decision-making under procedure scenarios. Continual monitoring and real-time adjustments (things won't always work out exactly as planned, after all) show a genuine commitment to reducing complications and improving overall safety. As every patient reacts in his or her own individual way, customized anesthetic planning to accommodate distinctive features and surgical requirements continues to take center stage. By combining state-of-the-art drug developments with age-old methods, the profession of anesthesiology will keep operations safer and more effective well into the future (Figure 2.1).

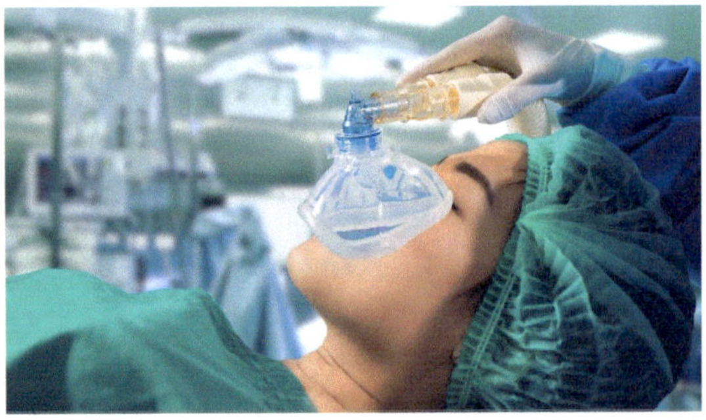

Figure 2.1. Anesthesia: how anesthesia works.

Source: https://cdn.britannica.com/78/240878-138-E9CB8517/How-Does-Anesthesia-Work.jpg.

Definition of Anesthetic Agents

In modern medicine, especially where performing surgeries and other operations are concerned, understanding how certain substances actually work is crucial. Anesthetic drugs—commonly called anesthetics in most cases—have completely revolutionized the discipline by making it possible to perform painless operations. They generally work by causing a strictly controlled form of unconsciousness or deep sedation in patients, which has the effect of silencing both sensation and physical response. This kind of drug effect not only aids in carrying out intricate procedures but also functions to make patients more comfortable and safer as a whole, their effectiveness comes from altering the central nervous system—specifically targeting neural circuits and pathways—to get desired results. In most cases, it's this very manipulation that necessitates the constant changing and refining of anesthetic use in the hospital environment. These agents come in all shapes and sizes, and they're typically separated into groups based on their mechanism of action and how they're administered. So, for example, there are the inhalational anesthetics—like isoflurane and nitrous oxide—that have a quick onset and are usually renowned for their ease; and then there are the intravenous ones—like propofol—that allow a physician to very carefully regulate just how deep the anesthesia will be. Each class is defined by its journey through the body, affecting how potent, how long-lasting, or even which side effects will occur. More recently, there's been a growing trend towards the use of multimodal anesthesia—an approach that incorporates many different kinds of anesthetics. Generally speaking, the idea is to reduce the amount needed of each agent, with the hope of reducing on unwanted effects while still blocking pain effectively. It's a balancing act of sorts that also opens the window to how various drugs can combine in unforeseen ways. If you look at the bigger picture of clinical practice, the action of anesthetic agents goes well beyond their immediate effect during a procedure. They need to balance unconsciousness, immobility, and control of automatic body reactions to the stress of surgery—while keeping patient comfort levels high. This balancing act, and it can be a real balancing act, means doctors have to remain current on how each anesthetic functions, how much to administer, and how it will interact with other drugs, particularly in groups like special needs children. More attention is being given as well to what occurs once the procedure has been completed, with more focus on recovery and post-anesthesia outcomes. For most circumstances, as new research continues to emerge, clinicians are forced to re-examine the safety and effectiveness of these agents in an effort to guide patient care in the face of an ever-evolving surgical landscape (Coté et al., 2019; Egan et al., 2018) (Figure 2.2).

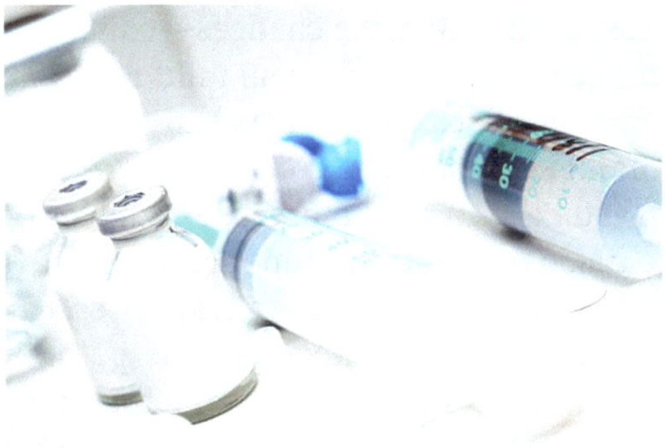

Figure 2.2. Anesthetic agents.

Source: https://media.istockphoto.com/id/531440475/photo/professional-medicines-anesthetic-drugs-and-syringes.jpg?s=612x612&w=0&k=20&c=4iIhpz6cFQ82A5PuC_s_hM8E58mCp8lviPu13BQlrYY=.

Importance of Anesthetics in Medical Practice

Not only do anesthetics numb pain. They calm patients and keep them comfortable during surgeries and diagnostic procedures both. Doctors select them based on a patient's overall health, sensitivities, and what the procedure entails—even if that means reconciling a few difficult variables. You can liken it to custom fitting; knowing how these drugs behave inside the body (pharmacodynamics and pharmacokinetics, for simplicity's sake) is key. For example, the American Academy of Pediatrics typically recommends checking a child's medical history and analyzing the effect of the drug in depth. This preparation minimizes unwanted interactions and maintains adequate depth of sedation, yielding quick return to baseline. Continuing education for medical professionals is most commonly required as anesthesia techniques are ongoing (Coté et al., 2019). The elderly put their own twist on things. With diminishing physiological reserves and comorbidities, risk of complications—such as delirium, for instance—increases considerably. Planned anesthetic with prudence becomes necessary; it's merely a question of achieving a proper balance between successful pain relief and avoiding side effects that might fog an older person's recovery. The American Geriatrics Society has quoted that delirium is still a very present danger, its development depends on the method of anesthesia used and the patient's pre-existing degree of mental function. Paying attention to these nuances enables clinicians to adjust their practice, ensuring appropriate pain management while maximizing chances of easier recovery (Ags et al., 2015). Advanced monitoring now goes hand-in-hand with administering anesthesia—a synergy that optimizes patient safety. Real-time systems enable anesthesiologists to monitor vital signs, thus enabling them to step in when things don't seem quite right. Transitioning to a blend of modalities, like the addition of RA with other meds, not only improves pain control but also reduces on opioid use and its effects. All of this aligns with the current patient care environment of today, especially for those who need extra care. Whether trauma interventions or procured procedures, understanding the do's and don'ts of these meds is the key to better outcomes, shaping a greater experience overall. Ultimately, careful selection and maintenance of anesthetic drugs pave the way to safer and more efficient healthcare delivery (Coté et al., 2019) (Figure 2.3).

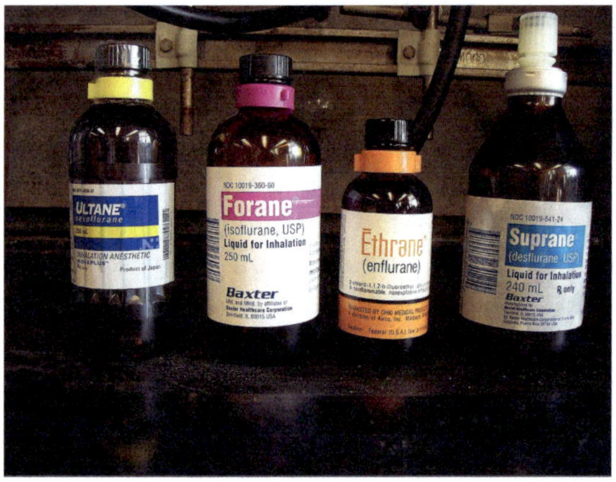

Figure 2.3. Importance of anesthetics in medical practice.

Source: By Diesel-50 (talk) - work (Original text: I created this work entirely by myself.), Public Domain, https://commons.wikimedia.org/w/index.php?curid=65246942.

2.1. Classification of Anesthetic Agents

Learning Outcome

1. Describe the general anesthetics and local anesthetics.
2. Discuss about adjunctive anesthetic agents.

Anesthesiology depends profoundly on how drugs are classified, and exceedingly often they get split between two huge categories: ones that put you out completely and just the ones that numb a specific area. In large operations, doctors routinely use general anesthetics that induce a reversible coma—consider inhaled like sevoflurane or intravenous like propofol, each of them doing their own unique thing. On the other hand, when only a small amount of area needs to be numbed for minor procedures, local anesthetics like lidocaine and bupivacaine step in, with the patient remaining largely awake. In most cases, knowing which of these to employ is not only a matter of choice—it also increases overall safety and the quality of the anesthesia care given (Shah et al., 2024). It also matters a great deal how these agents behave once they're in the body. You've got pharmacokinetics, the whole process of absorption, distribution, metabolism, and excretion, and then there's pharmacodynamics, which is more about how the drug actually does its thing at target sites. All in all, the speed of onset and the time which it stays active can be very unpredictable; for instance, the very dissimilar metabolic process of halothane as contrasted with a newer option like desflurane. All these changes—coupled with the range of side effects from mild reactions to severe issues—call for exact drug selection at the moment of surgery completely (Kawakami et al., 2022). Apart from these main options, there's also focus on the supporting agents that complement the primary anesthetics. Other drugs like muscle relaxants and painkillers play an important role in complementing the overall anesthesia and in making the patient comfortable thereafter. Neuromuscular blocking drugs such as succinylcholine, for example, may aid in intubation by helping in airway management, whereas opioid analgesics prefer to control pain after and during the procedure, occasionally even lowering the needed dose of the main anesthetic. It can be a bit complicated, but equating these adjuncts with the primary drugs—and modifying them for each patient's needs—is crucial in risk reduction and overall improvement in operations (Shah et al., 2024).

2.1.1. General Anesthetics

General anesthetics are not just knocking someone out; they also seem to alter the manner in which our brain cells talk to each other. Scientists now view these drugs as more than just mere sleep-inducing chemicals; they are implicated in bringing about changes like loss of memory and relief from pain during surgery. They work in most cases by targeting small protein channels, like those opening when a certain chemical attaches or ones that react to voltage changes. They keep the brain's chatty processes going, which help with thinking and memory. Modern critiques indicate that if we can pin down how these drugs interfere with synaptic signals, we can design safer, more predictable drugs with fewer side effects (Hao et al., 2020). Looking a bit further beneath the surface, anesthetics seem to disrupt the way brain areas generally talk to each other. Despite the fact that physicians have been administering them for more than a century, we're still only partially in the know about precisely how they knock out consciousness. Other studies suggest that these drugs also tend to break up the usual back-and-forth between cortical networks, perhaps an all-purpose trick leading to that familiar state of unawareness. Laboratory and clinical studies show that, regardless of what the specific molecular details may be, a variety of anesthetic drugs tend to dampen normal neurocommunication between different areas of the brain. Generally speaking, this steady indicator—that there is communication off balance—opens the door to more subtle investigation of these drugs' dynamics so that we can better grasp anesthesia and the very nature of consciousness (Voss et al., 2019). There is also pressure mounting to make these drugs more fine-tuned so they transmit the good stuff without the ghastly side effects. By addressing the very molecular targets, scientists are creating anesthetics that are still helpful to us in what we need—e.g., effective pain killing—yet less on risks such as suppressing the rate of breathing or affecting the heart. Targeting how these drugs respond at the synaptic level could eventually enable us to create more discriminant agents, opening up a window for further research. It almost feels as if every new finding nudges us a bit further along the path to closing gaps in our understanding of consciousness itself. As the science advances, increasingly close collaboration between pharmacologists, neuroscientists, and anesthesiologists seems to be the most significant factor for driving routine practice and cutting-edge research (Hao et al., 2020) (Figure 2.4).

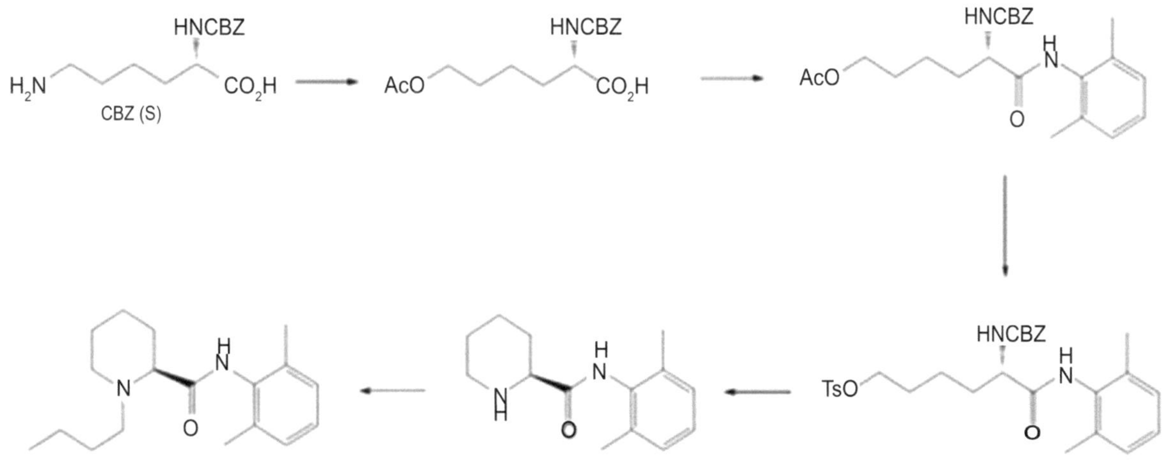

Figure 2.4. General anesthetics.

Source: By Adger, B. M., Dyer, U. C., Hutton, G., & Woods, M. doi:10.1016/0040-4039(96)01357-3, Public Domain, https://commons.wikimedia.org/w/index.php?curid=129786083.

2.1.2. Local Anesthetics

Local anesthetics are a standby in most offices now. They're used to keep pain away where you need it—no sweeping numbness from head to toe. Getting dental work or more extensive surgery; these medications quickly numb sensation by blocking nerve impulses within a field. They're fast-acting, whether used by infiltration, nerve block, or applied topically. Patients can even fine-tune their chemical structure, potency, and mode of delivery to optimize the effect. Otherwise, they are quite safe most of the time, but dosing and mode do matter—especially in sensitive populations such as children and the elderly (Kumar et al., 2015). New advances in local anesthetic formulations recently have led to new views on the action mechanism of these medications in us. Generally, they inhibit nerves from discharging by reversibly blocking sodium channels—this clever trick essentially breaks the action potentials. New delivery systems, including lipid-based carriers and some other adjuvants, play a role in prolonging the duration of numbness while keeping on the waiting time minimal before they act (Kumar et al., 2015). Patients might also be able to find specialized topical products that treat other medical conditions, showing the versatility of these medications. The use of eutectic mixtures—using multiple agents in combination—has allowed for their overall effectiveness to be amplified even further. Nothing is easy, however, and new studies have raised some eyebrows regarding the potential effects on neurodevelopment in children. Some studies suggest that exposure at periods of brain development can be linked to a heightened risk of learning difficulties in the future, especially if children are exposed repeatedly to anesthesia. This controversy requires doctors to be even more vigilant, weighing risk against reward for vulnerable patients, notably those under four years of age. Staying mindful of new findings—and employing these drugs judiciously—can presumably strike a better balance between effective pain relief and safeguard against possible side effects (Figure 2.5).

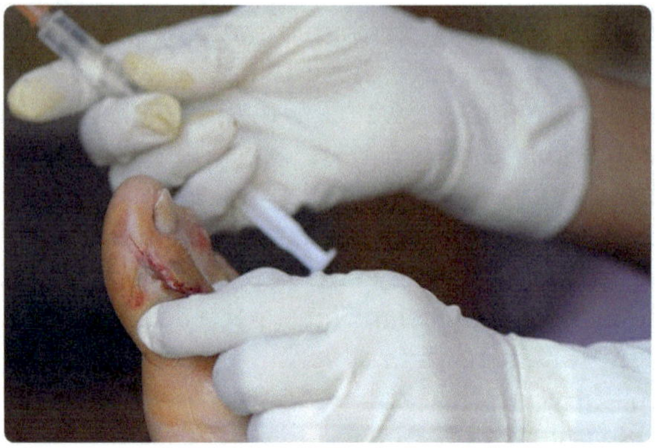

Figure 2.5. Laceration wound injecting local anesthetics.

Source: https://d2jx2rerrg6sh3.cloudfront.net/image-handler/picture/2017/8/shutterstock_563478487.jpg.

2.1.3. Adjunctive Anesthetic Agents

Adjunctive anesthetic medications are increasingly assuming a key function in optimizing outcomes in almost every clinical setting. They have a tendency to be complementary to primary anesthetics, supplementing relief of pain and sedation which seem to make a difference—especially with children's sensitive needs. Administer melatonin: its wide range of properties, from soothing sedation and analgesia to anti-inflammatory and even neuroprotection, is apt to make the perioperative course run smoothly and perhaps lower the threat of postoperative hiccups. In most cases, with improving techniques, using agents like melatonin is an advance toward anesthetic practices more finely directed toward safety and patient satisfaction (Subhadarshini et al., 2024). Management of acute pain remains an issue, with traditional methods sometimes not working for specific types of pain. In most instances, traditional anesthetic preparations don't quite reach all types of pain, leading to practitioners looking for other ancillary options.

Studies have also pinpointed that topical therapy available today for eye pain isn't sometimes quite adequate—providing a case for systemic interventions like opioids. Although progress in corneal pain management has been slow, some of the new treatments like the use of nonsteroidal anti-inflammatory drops and newer approaches targeting the endocannabinoid system appear to close the gap, indicating a general trend toward more immediate action against pain pathways (Lafreniere et al., 2023). Use of these other anesthetics not only augments the effect of the primary drugs but may also be used to reduce on unwanted side effects. When these drugs are applied synergistically, doctors are typically able to decrease the quantities of primary anesthetics, which itself diminishes the potential for overdose and lessens side effects. Take melatonin again—its use in pediatric patients has been encouraging in treating pain and diminishing dependence upon powerful drugs, a role which speaks volumes about its role in daily practice. This two-way benefit is the rationale behind adding such agents to standard regimens of anesthesia since not only does it add to better pain control but also seems to enhance recovery profiles. Ongoing studies, especially those investigating novel adjuncts and their mechanisms of action, will hopefully increase our understanding of these benefits and further improve the safety and efficacy of anesthetic management (Subhadarshini et al., 2024) (Figure 2.6).

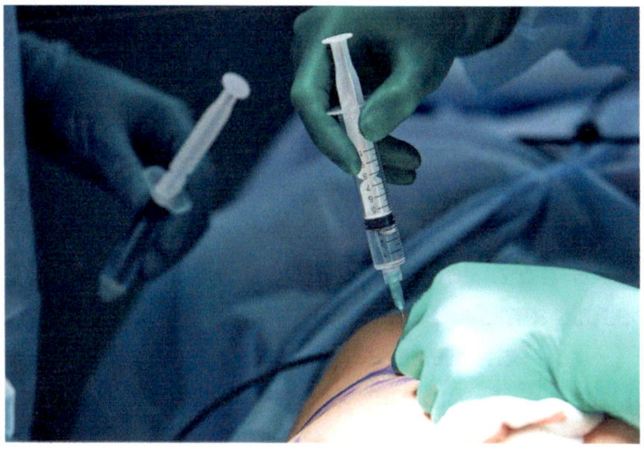

Figure 2.6. Adjunctive Anesthetic Agents.

Source: https://philadelphiaanesthesiaservices.com/wp-content/uploads/2024/11/fieldblock.jpg.

Test Your Knowledge

1. Discuss local anesthetics.
2. Describe the adjunctive anesthetic agents.

2.2. Mechanisms of Action

Learning Outcome

1. Discuss interaction with neurotransmitter systems.
2. Learn about the effects of anesthetic agents on ion channels.
3. Understand the influence on central nervous system activity.

Anesthesia works in idiosyncratic ways that mix up biochemical messages and brain circuits in unpredictable ways. Most of these drugs—think of propofol or barbiturates, for instance—modify alter the neurotransmitters like gamma-aminobutyric acid, γ-aminobutyric acid (GABA) and glutamate so that the brain settles down into unresponsiveness and pain relief. You notice that these intravenous medications tend to augment the effect of GABA, which, in very simple terms, makes inhibitory signals more compelling, resulting in sedation. Then there's ketamine—it operates under different rules. Instead, it blocks N-methyl-D-aspartate (NMDA) receptors, basically turning off excitatory chatter. In most cases, this shutting off of signals right away gives ketamine its rapid-acting anesthetic property, and, oddly enough, it's being looked at for having the potential to treat severe depression, which indicates a profile different from your run-of-the-mill anesthetics. Diving somewhat further into these drugs, one finds that their action isn't limited to that one receptor alone. Ketamine, for example, has a somewhat complicated approach—it doesn't merely blockade NMDA receptors, but also dances with AMPA receptors and even tweaks brain-derived neurotrophic factor (BDNF) pathways. For the most part, that second change is what is apt to provide it with its quick antidepressant boost, which differs from conventional anesthetics that will possess a more persistent action. Matveychuk et al. (2020) matter-of-factly states that ketamine turns on signaling pathways that involve synaptic plasticity, suggesting it is doing double duty as an anesthetic and a near-immediate antidepressant. This strange pairing of effects might in most cases give new insights on both enhancing anesthesia as well as studying add-on therapies for mental illness. Not all candidate agents are born in the lab; nature contributes as well. Beta (β)-caryophyllene(BCAR) shows some resort-like anesthetic properties by interacting with cannabinoid receptors, most notably CB2R, in a way that seems to yield both brain-protecting and pain-relieving benefits (Conceição Machado et al., 2018). This natural variant may well open up new possibilities for the use of nature-derived molecules in anesthesia practice, especially in patients who are managing pain linked to inflammation or neurodegenerative conditions. Additionally, its indirect effects upon the immune system indicate that it can potentially curb some of the unwanted side effects that come with the use of traditional anesthetic drugs. As ongoing research endeavors to peel away the layers of these complicated mechanisms, we might not only improve the efficacy of anesthesia but also see better recovery profiles in the middle of—and in the aftermath of—surgical procedures.

2.2.1. Interaction with Neurotransmitter Systems

Anesthetic drugs usually have activity in the undercurrent of our brain chemistry, playing with pain control and wakefulness in sometimes not-so-obvious ways. They work by influencing neurotransmitters in complicated, sometimes surprising ways. Certain drugs interact with systems that deal with amines and those dealing with cholinergic transmission, altering the manner in which chemicals like dopamine and norepinephrine are released. This tug-of-war in the brain can initiate new pathways for modulation of nerve impulses, and thereby affect an anesthetic's overall efficacy. Take propofol and sevoflurane, for example—they both seem to strengthen inhibitory signals through GABA in a different manner, a change that, in most cases, is crucial for sedation and analgesia. These fine points remind one that understanding the quirks of neurotransmitter activity is important in designing patient-specific anesthetic regimens. It's not simply GABA or the aminergic systems, though. Anesthetics also push the balance in serotonergic systems, which can confuse pain management plans. Numerous patients end up on multi-modal treatment schedules that involve the use of opioids in combination with antidepressants targeting serotonin—such a combination has the unfortunate side effect of heightening the risk for serotonin syndrome. Changes in serotonin levels following administration of an anesthetic can either augment the effectiveness of analgesics or, paradoxically, minimize their impact. Opioids, as an example, are seen to increase synaptic serotonin, at times creating side effects like increased sedation or even mood changes. All of which means that doctors have to pretty precisely consider how these drugs affect not just consciousness and pain, but the whole spectrum of emotional and sensory experience (Rastogi et al., 2011). Aside from this, when anesthetics interfere with the normal chatter among neurotransmitters, the body can retaliate in complex and adaptive ways that keep physicians on their toes. These drugs don't simply turn off the excitatory messages that keep you awake; they can also dampen cholinergic pathways, which just so happens to be a significant deal when you're performing surgery and acetylcholine is so vital to muscle function. During episodes of intense surgical stress, the sudden drop in cholinergic function may complicate recovery and even cause cognitive hiccups later on. Failing to comprehend these levels of interaction is critical to keeping debilitating side effects away and helping patients recover as smoothly as possible. In fact, the many ways in which anesthetic drugs engage with neural systems form the basis of modern anesthesiology, leading clinicians to monitor patients closely and make treatments responsive to individual cases (Talita et al., 2016) (Figure 2.7).

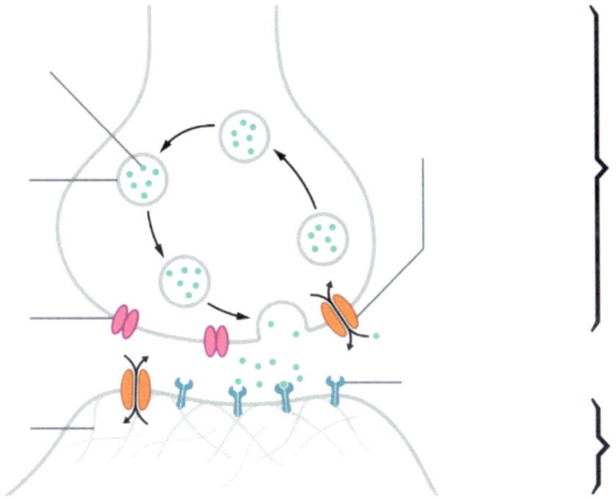

Figure 2.7. Interaction with neurotransmitter systems.

Source: By Thomas Splettstoesser (www.scistyle.com) - work, CC BY-SA 4.0, https://commons.wikimedia.org/w/index.php?curid=41349545.

2.2.2. Effects on Ion Channels

Anesthetics seem to wreak havoc on ion channels in ways that give surprising hints about their function. Many channels, especially those of the TRP family – including TRPC, TRPM, and TRPV – show clear responses to the application of such drugs. They are involved in the control of calcium signals, which are significant for nerve signaling and even for muscle contraction. In the majority of cases, altering these channels alters the way cells release and pass on signals along, indicating that anesthetics aren't simply shutting things down; they're engaging in a form of chemical push-and-pull with the channels. These channels, which act as detectors and messengers in the nervous system, ultimately generate effects far greater than the inhibition of neural activity (Blair et al., 2025). It's also fascinating how the effect on TRP channels seems to vary with the drug's concentration. Recent studies tend to uncover that some anesthetics can turn on or off TRPA1 channels – which can influence the way we feel pain – and may be the reason that some anesthetics also bring about pain relief during surgery. And then there are others, such as isoflurane and sevoflurane, which act to modulate TRPV channels, disrupting our sensitivity to temperature and touch in ways that we're only beginning to understand. All of these various interactions point to the complexity of the relationship between neurotransmitter release and ion channel activity, highlighting ion channels as being squarely at the focus of anesthesia's mechanism of action (Blair et al., 2025). From a therapeutic standpoint, knowing exactly how anesthetics work on these channels offers some new drug design and development possibilities. Researchers can, for instance, try matching single anesthetic agents with suitable TRP channels, with the aim of optimizing efficacy while reducing side effects. Such a targeted approach could even lead to new analgesics that specifically target certain channel subtypes, with the ultimate aim of better patient outcomes. In large part, as additional studies uncover such mechanisms—despite some twists and turns along the route—the promise of more effective, safer anesthetic compounds seems more within our grasp than ever (Blair et al., 2025) (Figure 2.8).

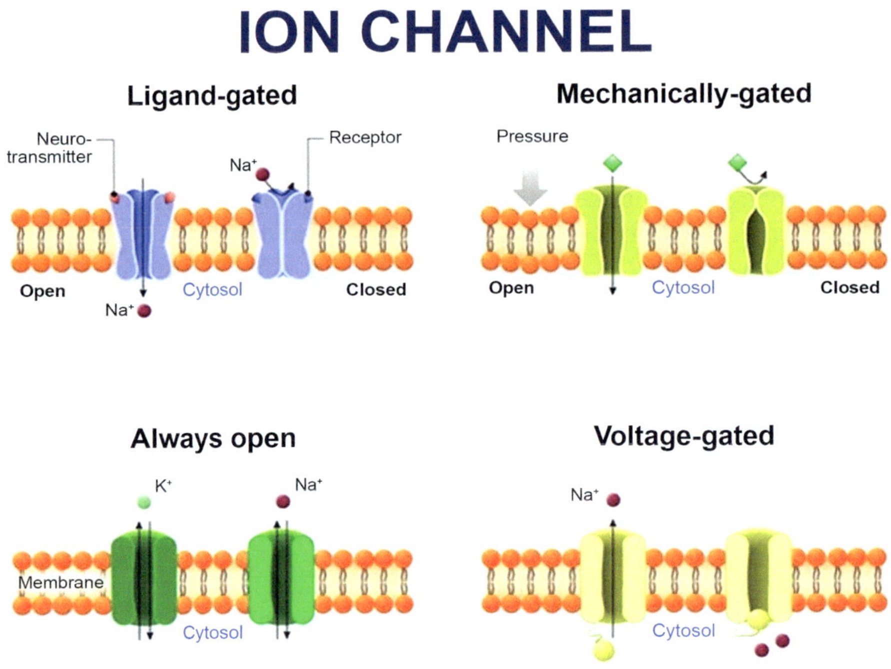

Figure 2.8. Importance of ion channels in the body.

Source: https://d2jx2rerrg6sh3.cloudfront.net/image-handler/picture/2018/10/shutterstock_480412786.jpg.

2.2.3. Influence on Central Nervous System Activity

Anesthetic drugs work by disrupting parts of the control system of the brain – they change how specific ion channels function, and of these, GABA receptors seem to be central. Researchers have shown, in most cases, that when these receptors are disrupted, it tends to drive a person into unconsciousness. There are several receptor subtypes spread all over the brain that are all part of this process, regulating the nerve impulses that keep us awake. Sometimes the organization in which these receptors show up on cell surfaces can be different in patients, which might explain why responses to anesthetics are not uniform. Pondering these facts in a sense not only maximizes the potential utility of anesthetics but also generates consideration for crafting new medicines that more optimally balance receptor stimulation—hence potentially improving surgical outcomes. With this understanding of such subtle electrical distinctions, so to speak, new thinking is introduced regarding crafting safer regimens of anesthesia for a wide range of individuals (Speigel et al., 2017). Potassium channels – the little gatekeepers that help decide a neuron's level of excitement – also have huge control over how potent an anesthetic can be. They help keep the resting state of the nerve cell stable and regulate when a cell releases signals, a system that becomes very important with outbursts of nerve activity in most disorders. Studies in general have found that when such channels move into a heightened state of activity, they can more readily excite neurons, a move anesthetic agents can manipulate to reach the desired degree of sedation. There is even some evidence pointing to potassium channel openers as advantageous in shutting off pain signals, showing their promise in limiting anesthesia. With some particular potassium channels being targeted, the pain can be controlled more effectively and undesirable side effects minimized, opening the door for new pain management approaches and finer control of the brain activity (Tsantoulas et al., 2014). The overlap between anesthetic medicines and the extensive system of neural signals is another complicated issue that needs to be unraveled. These drugs do not only put you into deep sleep but also remap how nerve cells talk to each other—something that, effectively, alters the way in which the brain works in general. Leveling out the excitatory as well as inhibitory signals, anesthetics create a good environment for not only deep muscle relaxation but also effective pain relief, an effect dual on which surgeons count in surgeries. At the same time, there is a concern that these drugs can leave an indelible mark on the functioning of neural circuits well into the future following the procedure—raising important questions about long-term recovery and brain function. In every instance except one, as the evidence shows, an intimate familiarity with these neural ripple effects is crucial to the development of anesthetic protocols that protect patients while moving the multiple pieces of the central nervous system into harmony (Speigel et al., 2017).

Test Your Knowledge

1. Describe the effects of anesthetic agents on ion channels.
2. Discuss the influence of anesthetic drugs on central nervous system activity.

2.3. Pharmacokinetics of Anesthetic Agents

Learning Outcome

1. Understand the absorption and distribution of anesthetic drugs.
2. Discuss metabolism and elimination of anesthetic drugs.
3. Learn about factors affecting pharmacokinetics.

Administering anesthetic drugs isn't really a cinch—it depends on what happens once the drug is in the body. The manner in which a drug acts, from quick entry into the circulation to roaming about all of these tissues, plays a large part. What the agent is absorbed and then distributed, metabolized, and eventually excreted all intertwined to create its safety and efficacy in surgery. By the time that the drug has arrived at its location, factors like body build or blood circulation can distort the equation. The agent's idiosyncrasies, e.g., solubility or molecular size, also determine the speed of its action. Such reasons exist as to why dosing must be so carefully so with groups like children who will inevitably respond differently (Coté et al., 2019). Digging yourself a little deeper, you find that the balancing act of providing sufficient sedation while not taking unnecessary risks is achieved. Metabolism becomes involved pretty frequently here; in general, the quicker the liver metabolizes the drug, the quicker its effects are lost as compared to mostly released unaltered. For the most part, doctors need to be cognizant of these breakdown mechanisms in order to adjust the way in which they dispense the medications, particularly in cases where other medical conditions complicate liver processes.

It's a game of balance—understanding how one medication is metabolized offers insight on avoiding toxic mixes or overdoing it (Ingrande, 2015). Tracking these drug highs is necessary, especially as medical procedures change with the years. Watching the behavior of anesthetic medications becomes even more necessary with sensitive subjects like children, whose responses can stray far from adult norms. Age, weight, and even the well-being of one's organs add their complicating features, so simple dosing rules simply aren't universal to every case. Small errors in dosing are hazardous, so conservative, sometimes lopsided methods of monitoring these factors act as a safeguard against errors. In total, a well-understood grasp of these processes of drugs enables practitioners to alter their practice in an attempt to reduce hazards in the direction of ultimate patient safety (Coté et al., 2019) (Figure 2.9).

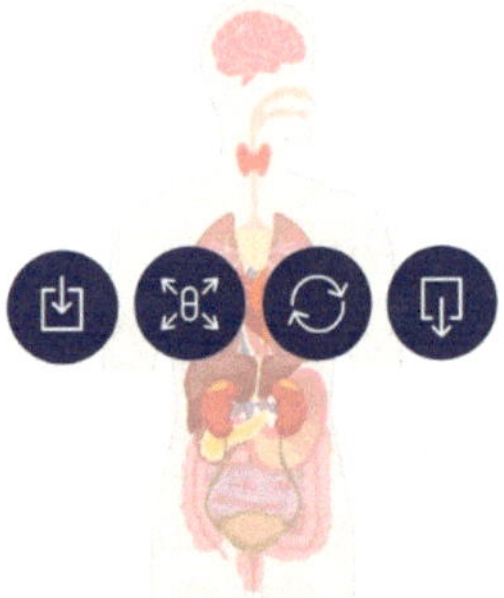

Figure 2.9. Pharmacokinetics.

Source: https://www.pharmaceuticalpress.com/wp-content/uploads/2024/05/What-is-pharmacokinetics-2.png.

2.3.1. Absorption and Distribution

Anesthetic drugs work primarily upon how they absorb and circulate throughout the body after having them. Once drugs are administered, they will follow a number of different paths—depending on whether it's a vein shot, muscle injection, or targeting one specific area—that eventually dictates how quickly it reaches your bloodstream. For example, an IV anesthetic quickly gets absorbed into the bloodstream so that you get drowsy quickly, while local anesthetics, which depend on how greasy they are and their pKa, can absorb unevenly in different tissues.

In most cases, knowing these tricks and secrets is really important so that you can make sure the drug acts the way it should and isn't creating too many side effects. How the drug pass through the body is not entirely about its chemistry; patient-related features play a big part in the process too. Well-perfused tissues like brain, heart, and lungs will trap more of the drug right after it's given, so the effects are more quickly noticed. The "volume of distribution" gives us an overall impression of how much of the drug goes into different areas of the body—a factor which also comes into a particularly important issue in operations involving strict control.

And if the anaesthetic is supposed only to act in one place, such as with fascial plane blocks, how a drug moves through tissue matters, as it is determined by small issues such as how tight those layers of fascia are and how proximity there is to blood vessels. Past trauma or surgery can interfere with this whole game of balance, as well. The absorption kinetics of each anesthetic brings about its unique personality. Take ketamine, for instance—it's infamous for getting absorbed and distributed almost immediately, with its dissociative effect coming seemingly out of nowhere after an IV injection.

Its metabolites, like norketamine, come into play as well, implying that there is more than the parent drug at work. For the majority of cases, the manner in which these metabolites impact different receptors not only tells us the length of time the anesthetic relief will last but its intensity, all dependent on how effectively they travel throughout the system. All in all, the interaction between distribution and absorption is an important determinant of the extent to which these anesthetics operate safely and effectively under a variety of clinical conditions (Figure 2.10).

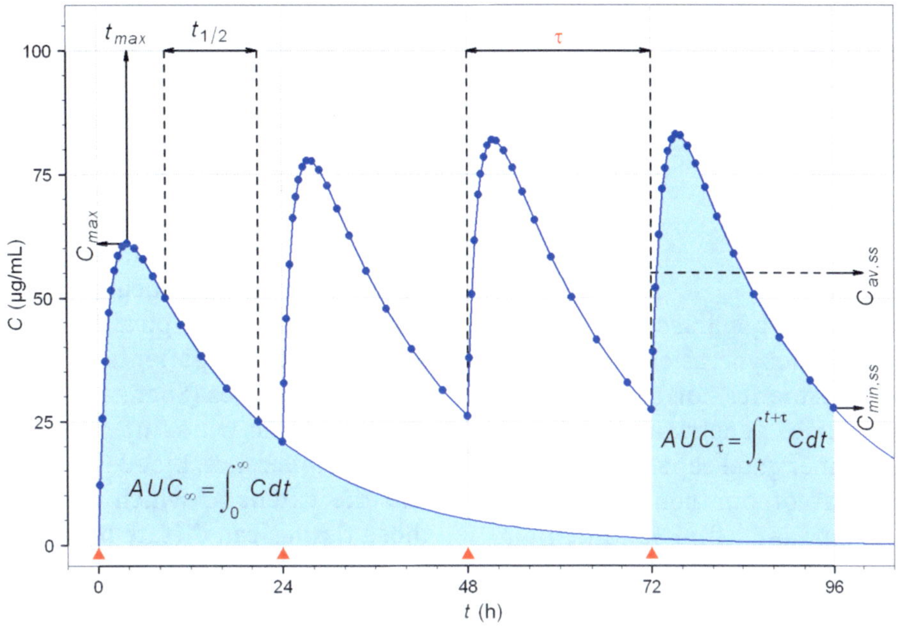

Figure 2.10. Pharmacokinetics (absorption, distribution, metabolism, and elimination).

Source: By Alfie↑↓© (Helmut Schütz) - work, CC BY 3.0, https://commons.wikimedia.org/w/index.php?curid=14784996.

2.3.2. Metabolism and Elimination

Metabolism and removal of the anesthetic drugs are most central to the way in which the drugs work and how safe they actually are when put to use. The body metabolizes them in unexpected ways—liver and kidney processes, and the random drug clash here and there, can change their direction considerably. Use propofol as an example here; this intravenous drug is cleared rapidly, due to an abbreviated half-life and high clearance rate, while sevoflurane mainly exits the body through the lungs with minimal liver use (Alves et al., 2024). Physicians find that they can make anesthetic plans more tailored by possessing knowledge of these idiosyncrasies, especially in high-risk surgeries like cardiac surgery. It's not just the rate of clearance; metabolism can also induce drug interactions. Most of the anesthetics share the same liver enzymes, and therefore, when co-administered, there will be plasma level changes that affect the efficacy and safety profiles of the medications. For instance, midazolam—cleaved by cytochrome P450 enzymes—can suddenly boost its sedative effect when administered with other medications (Cristofoletti et al., 2023). By using predictive models such as physiologically based pharmacokinetic (PBPK) modeling, doctors are able to have a better, though not necessarily perfect, idea of these drug-drug interactions and usually make more logical dosing choices. New developments in quantitative modeling have, for the most part, helped increase our knowledge of how different patients eliminate these drugs. Instead of relying on mean laboratory values only, newer methods combine *in vitro–in vivo* extrapolation (IVIVE) with PBPK methods to address interindividual variation related to genetics, physiology and even the environment (Cristofoletti et al., 2023). This shift is not merely cognitive—it ushers in anesthetic care that tailoring suits each patient's unique makeup, improving the potential for successful and safe treatment in a wider range of operating environments (Alves et al., 2024).

2.3.3. Factors Affecting Pharmacokinetics

Pharmacokinetics is a dirty phrase—it's affected by so many natural idiosyncrasies and outside influences. Take anesthetics, for example; they have trouble sometimes penetrating the blood-brain barrier, that inner gatekeeper which keeps most chemicals out of our central nervous system. Some compounds find it difficult to penetrate, which can roll straight into their overall effectiveness. A study on elimusertib, a blocker of the ATR kinase, for instance, showed that when a drug vanishes from the circulation too quickly, it leaves behind too much of none to effectively act within the brain. Such an understanding may force us to redesign the way we produce or give the medication, ensuring that it acts well when accuracy is literally a question of life and death when operating (Rathi et al., 2024). Another huge piece of the puzzle is how our bodies metabolize these agents. Liver enzymes and other drug interactions—are they even what we have to eat—can make things more complicated. Routine compounds present in our foods like curcumin and sulforaphane seem to interfere with our enzymes, sometimes accelerating or decelerating the metabolism of anesthetics. In most cases, this means the effects of these drugs will eventually become stronger or weaker than expected, perhaps why patient response can be unpredictable during and after surgery. Identifying such minute differences is essential, and this typically means dosing must be modified for patients with individualized metabolic profiles (Shannar et al., 2025). Where the anesthetic winds up within the body also makes a difference. Blood flow to various tissues and the extent to which a drug binds within those tissues can dictate how soon it arrives at its destination. Some drugs dissolve better in fats—so they directly travel into fatty tissues—while others that dissolve nicely within water remain longer within the blood, affecting both how rapidly they take effect and for how long they take effect. Research into such distribution patterns goes toward shedding light on ways of improving the efficacy and safety of anesthetic techniques. More insight into these trips of drugs can ultimately lead us to follow a road that heads toward better anesthesiology methods and better patient care (Shannar et al., 2025).

Test Your Knowledge

1. Describe the absorption and distribution of anesthetic drugs.
2. Explain the metabolism and elimination of anesthetic drugs.

2.4. Clinical Applications

Learning Outcome

1. Describe the surgical procedures.
2. Understand the pain management.
3. Learn about emergency medicine.

Anesthetic medications have come a long way—no longer are we merely arguing over how they act on the molecular level, but how they're actually being utilized on the ward. Ketamine, for example, was once largely only renowned as a dissociative anesthetic; now it's being recognized for its role to induce pain relief and sedation in all types of patients. To a large extent, its use in chronic pain treatment—prevalent among some 11–40% of adult Americans—is more and more considered an attractive option. Traditional analgesics like opioids and NSAIDs are probably going to have attendant side effects of dependence and tolerance, so there is increasingly a demand for alternatives such as ketamine, whether used singly or in combination as part of an overall pain-management strategy. This emphasizes the complex but resilient nature of its pharmacology in clinical practice (Fontanella, 2025). For children who are to be operated on, the discourse is somewhat different. In pediatric anesthesia, there has been more focus on agents corresponding to the particular nature of young patients. Take melatonin—it's not just a sleep aid; it's hope-inducing because its analgesic and sedative properties appear to calm nerves and mitigate post-op complications. Surprisingly, its application is not limited to tranquilizing children prior to surgery. Melatonin has also been researched as a supporting complement to other anesthetic techniques and even as a postoperative pain reliever. This adaptability shows it could help make pediatric medicine safer, reducing reliance on more traditional anesthetics that might lead to more serious side effects. This way, ongoing research into melatonin might even revolutionize pediatric anesthesia practice and improve outcomes (Subhadarshini et al., 2024). The whole method of anesthetic care is transforming in ways that challenge what we used to think was traditional. With the changing healthcare environment, there's greater focus on individualizing the anesthesia for each patient—again, not just the procedure being performed but overall health as well. The integration of agents such as ketamine and melatonin into practice indicates a broader trend in personalized medicine within the field. Continuing research continues to unpick layers of the agents' pharmacology, often uncovering new potential that drives advances in method and patient management. With the drug pharmacopeia continuing to expand, these emerging applications could well redefine what we might expect from anesthesia and be a giant step forward (Fontanella, 2025; Subhadarshini et al., 2024) (Figure 2.11).

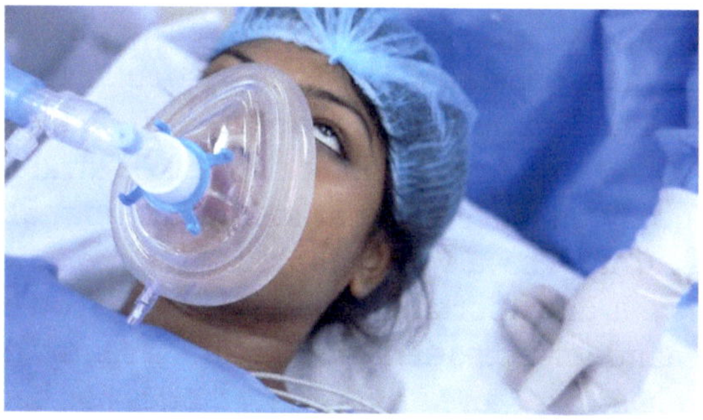

Figure 2.11. Anesthetic medications.

Source: https://i.ytimg.com/vi/am8ge0vjkqY/hq720.jpg?sqp=-oaymwEhCK4FEIIDSFryq4qpAxMIARUAAAAAGAElAADIQj0AgKJD&rs=AOn4CLBvFUBBGlLZV5gpOoU_C5vSlqxxng.

2.4.1. Surgical Procedures

Surgery itself has come a long, long way with most of the credit going to pharmacological advancements – more specifically to those pain-numbing agents. Back in the good old days, people utilized mainly natural plant compounds to put the hurt away for surgical procedures. A classic example is cocaine from Erythroxylon coca; it revolutionized eye surgeries by offering effective numbing agents. That shift, moving from clunky, early methods to more refined techniques, clearly shows just how intertwined drug research and surgery can be. In exploring what nature offers, we've unlocked better ways to operate and help patients, and, as (Pinheiro et al., 2018) reminds us, current research into these natural compounds generally holds plenty of promise for future developments in surgical anesthesia. Nowadays, pain relief during outpatient procedures is not nearly as black-and-white a matter. Multimodal analgesia – a sort of switch-and-match therapy for pain – has emerged as an undisputed first choice when older methods just don't work. Physicians now match up various painkillers that act in different ways to maximize the relief with a minimum of fuss and side effects. For instance, pairing nonsteroidal anti-inflammatory drugs (NSAIDs) and acetaminophen with regional anesthesia (RA) has provided a more tailored regimen of pain management, one that is particular to the individual patient and procedure. Usually, as Young et al. (2011) note, this kind of strategy not only enhances patient satisfaction but also speeds up recovery and reduces discharge times, which is an important benefit given the growing demand for outpatient treatment. Recently, the whole atmosphere around anesthetics has been evolving in intriguing ways. There has been a steady move towards new drug forms and delivery techniques that give physicians cleaner, more exact control over the operating room setting. New drugs that act quickly and then dissipate more quickly offer new opportunities to fine-tune anesthesia, especially when things get complicated out or incredibly painful. And with ongoing concerns regarding opioid abuse and usage, the search for safer alternate agents never abates. By embracing a comprehensive and up-to-date approach to pain management – typically one based on the most advanced anesthetic technology – surgeons today are much better equipped to produce superb results and genuinely enhance the patient experience both in and out of the operating theater (Figure 2.12).

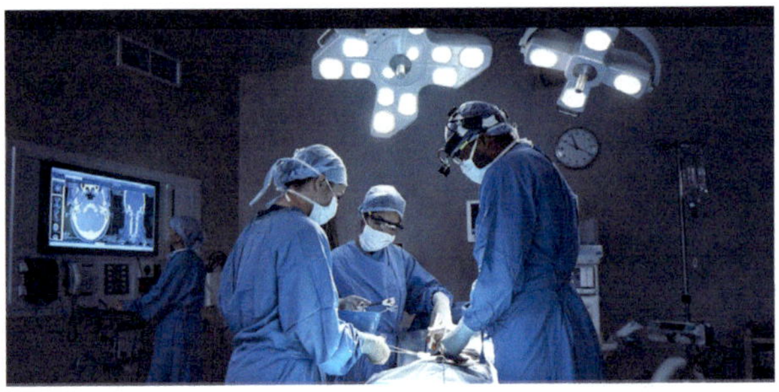

Figure 2.12. Surgical procedures.

Source: https://www.hopkinsmedicine.org/-/media/images/health/2_-treatment/surgical-care/common-surgical-hero.jpg?h=500&iar=0&mh=500&mw=1300&w=1297&hash=FD277EB2AEE62E1B53537767AEE778CE.

2.4.2. Pain Management

Pain management is a sensitive issue – especially when the standard therapies just aren't effective. Physicians usually start with opioids, but as the doses escalate, side effects begin to complicate and negate the whole plan. Recently, however, alternative choices have become available: like small pumps disbursing medication into the spinal fluid. This approach allows you to take lower doses that target the source of pain without inducing the widespread effects with which higher doses are associated. However, no method is flawless; these pumps require precise dosing and can behave badly or even get infected. That's why some clinicians are also exploring tunneled epidural catheters, which permit continuous local anesthetic drip that might prevent pain from worsening without some of the problems faced with intrathecal therapies (Young et al., 2024). In dentistry, managing pain takes a whole different turn. Dentists often have to deal with orofacial pain and turn to local anesthetics to anesthetize the area to be treated. As anesthetic techniques improve, there is increasingly sophisticated equipment to select from. New local anesthetics, in some cases combined with NSAIDs, are enhancing the control of pain during procedures. The goal is not very complicated – keep discomfort to a minimum so patients can depart feeling as good as possible. With more research going into even more effective pain relief methods, dental professionals are continually working to develop their approach to delivering care to patients (Rout et al., 2024). If the cancer has reached its terminal phases, it becomes even harder to manage pain. Remaining with the traditional opioid-based methods at this point no longer becomes effective, so innovative concepts are needed. Topical approaches, like tunneled epidural catheters, offer a new alternative. In one case, a patient with intractable pelvic and abdominal pain was administered continuous local anesthetic infusions through epidural catheter, which benefited them without having to increase their opioid dose.

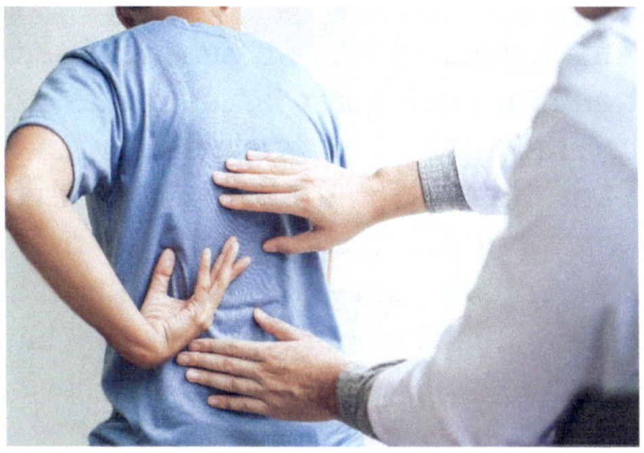

Figure 2.13. Pain management.

Source: https://cdn.ketteringhealth.org/wp-content/uploads/2021/05/Pain-Management-iStock-1007757616.jpg.optimal.jpg?resize=292,292.

That situation illustrates how tailoring treatment to fit the individual needs of a patient can make a drastic difference. With further research, these tailored choices can provide access to enhanced pain management in difficult oncologic cases, ultimately enhancing the comfort and overall quality of life of patients (Young et al., 2024) (Figure 2.13).

2.4.3. Emergency Medicine

Emergency room procedure sedation is not as easy as it seems. You have to know your drugs and your patients at the same time. In the ED, having painful procedures done with as little pain as possible is largely a question of using sedatives and pain medication – propofol, ketamine, midazolam – in exactly the right mixture. Even more recently, however, there's been a trend toward an even more individualized strategy, especially in children and the elderly who react in slightly dissimilar manners to the others. The way in which these drugs function within the body—their speed, strength, and duration—is quite basic when trying to sedate effectively without elevating risks too much. Even a narrative review concluded that, in most cases, the choice of the proper sedative on the basis of individual patient data does make a difference for safety and outcomes, particularly in pressurized emergencies (Piccini et al., 2024). Proper screening of patients before any procedure is equally important. An effective pre-procedure assessment detects risk factors that can affect sedation outcomes, especially in those at greater risk. Take neonates, for instance—these pose a totally different set of issues because their bodies are still playing catchup and their organs are still immature. That means planning on anesthesia for these little human beings is essential to reduce the chances of something happening adversely. Continuing education, in conjunction with sticking to clinical practice guidelines, helps the clinician keep in mind these unique requirements. In the vast majority of cases, keeping up to date with what the latest research says about practice is essential in the interests of better emergency care (Caliskan et al., 2017). Emergency medicine itself is ever-changing, and along with it, sedation methods and equipment are always changing. New anesthetic agents and new techniques for sedation are invented daily, pushing care teams to change direction at a moment's notice. Sometimes, mixing a dash of innovation with old-fashioned approaches not only reduces a patient's anguish during difficult procedures but also plays nice with current, evidence-based guidelines. It might sound strange to think about, but how technology complements back-to-the-future pharmacy gives practitioners more options for balancing both pain and anxiety. Overall, an open-minded attitude towards anesthetic drugs in emergency treatment is the means to find improved results and create a standard that is truly patient-oriented (Cappellini et al., 2024) (Figure 2.14).

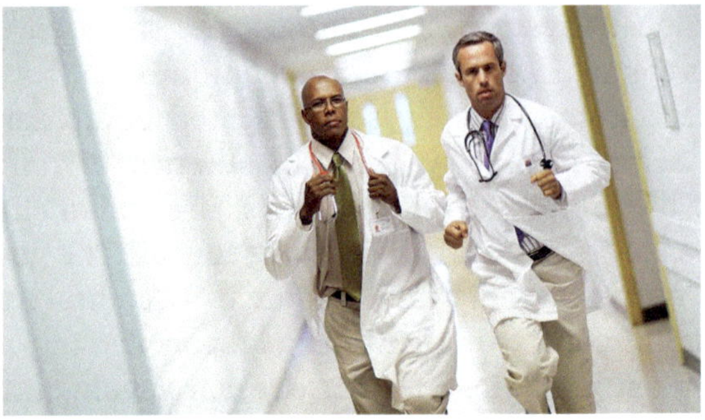

Figure 2.14. Emergency medicine.

Source: https://m.media-amazon.com/images/S/pv-target-images/bf434fad4020d9c78bdbacc27b 48bdb062d46de77ff4396bf371691c271dccd1._SX1080_FMjpg_.jpg.

Test Your Knowledge

1. Explain the surgical procedures.
2. What is emergency medicine?

2.5. Side Effects and Complications

Learning Outcome

1. Understand the common side effects of anesthetic drugs.
2. Describe the serious adverse reactions.
3. Describe the risk factors for complications.

Anesthetic medications also have patient recovery effects that are difficult to predict—a cluster of side effects may arise unexpectedly. Dexmedetomidine (DEX) is one such example; this ever-present sedative can abate coughing on extubation and ease the wake-up, but when the doses drift upward, it sometimes triggers bradycardia and hypotension, which upsets cardiovascular stability. For the most part, this balancing act of a beneficial sedative effect and possible heart issues makes it clear that carefully dosing is actually essential when using anesthesia (Salim et al., 2019). Another issue that still keeps coming back is the issue of postoperative pain—it's something that far too many patients undergoing surgery have to suffer through when pain isn't kept in check. Improper management at this point has been linked with higher rates of morbidity and even extended recovery period, contributing to healthcare costs in turn. While routine opioids are most commonly the default in pain management, their susceptibility to side effects complicates achieving the correct dose every time. More recent approaches that couple local anesthetics with nonopioid methods are also proving helpful. As an example, oliceridine acts by selectively engaging with the μ-receptor pathway and, in most cases, seems to allow for satisfactory pain control with less side effects than traditional opioids—a major advance in postoperative care (Gan, 2017). Side effects are not just a temporary problem; they can persist and have an effect on long-term recovery, too. If acute postoperative pain is not properly treated, it can actually set the stage for chronic pain syndromes that hinder rehabilitation. An effective perioperative pain control plan is important not only for relief during the immediate phase but also for preventing late pain issues. This relationship between early pain and later complications underscores the need to maximize anesthetic regimens. The combination of tried-and-true methods and innovative, newer techniques might just be the answer to enhancing patient outcomes and reducing complications, finally giving the in-depth analysis of anesthetic management pharmacology (Gan, 2017) (Figure 2.15).

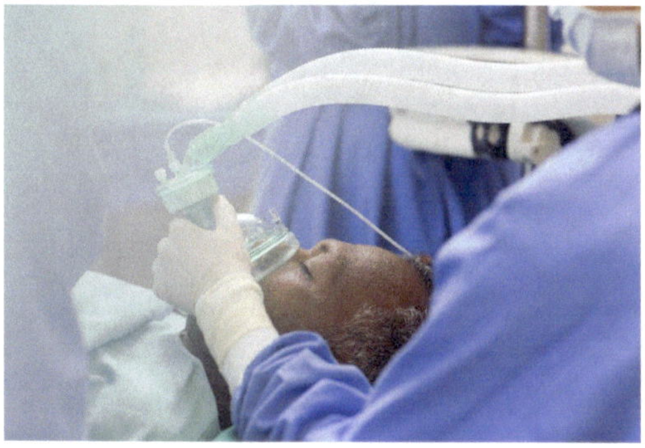

Figure 2.15. Anesthesia side effects and complications.

Source: https://www.verywellhealth.com/thmb/1sgK_zP22ZAs9d33MltnB3L4EkY=/1500x0/filters:no_upscale():max_bytes(150000):strip_icc()/GettyImages-530685559-9444100d86fc46bca7ca030523b230c0.jpg.

2.5.1. Common Side Effects

Anesthetic drugs not only serve their basic purpose; they also come with a range of side effects that can occur before, during, or after the drug. For example, opioids are very effective in terms of pain suppression but are often associated with nasty issues like nausea, vomiting, and even depressed breathing. Usually, such side effects necessitate that care teams closely watch patients and integrate other therapies or alter pain treatment in an effort to establish a balance between safety and efficacy—especially with cases like managing cancer pain (Young et al., 2024). Local anesthetics usually manage to get by with causing general problems, though they're not completely hiccup-free. They can cause local responses such as swelling, redness, or brief, odd nerve sensations that will interfere with the process of recovery. More often than not, when these agents are used in regional applications, it becomes even more difficult for patients with existing issues or sensitivities. Doctors need to, in general, make patients aware of these potential bumps well in advance so that everyone's on the same page. Also, ongoing modifications of drug formulations are striving to close that gap—reducing side effects while improving pain relief, which is relatively crucial in acute and chronic pain. Another growing concern is the impact of drug combinations when patients take more than one drug at the same time. Combination therapy can typically exacerbate side effects that would otherwise be less severe if each medication were taken individually. Interaction effects may, for instance, increase sedation or change the way anesthetic drugs react in the body. As clinicians work through this complex puzzle, they are relying more and more on a general approach—informing patients, using more sensitive monitoring methods, and carefully assessing every patient's drug history before giving anesthetics. This rigorous checking is not only key to short-term improvement but also plays a significant role in longer-term success, as recent work has emphasized (Jangwan et al., 2024).

2.5.2. Serious Adverse Reactions

Anesthetic pharmacology is no walk in the park. For the most part, dealing with the drugs given during surgery – from those that bring on anesthesia to muscle relaxants and analgesics – is a juggling act, as each, though necessary to make surgery proceed more easily, may also have some unwanted side effects. It is not just the drugs themselves but also how they interact with one another, the patient's history, and even their genetic quirks that are taken into account, making it even more complex if you are not attentive. Sometimes complications happen in unexpected ways, from bizarre blood issues to catastrophic allergic eruptions, which further complicate the whole perioperative regime. Thus, anesthesiologists find themselves having to balance the clear benefit of proper sedation against the potential for harmful effects, opting for a prudent balance of drug choice and careful monitoring (Jiang et al., 2025). Elderly patients, for example, have even greater challenge. They typically face a higher risk of serious reactions from polypharmacy and the natural changes that occur with aging. Evidence generally suggests that the elderly can become more vulnerable to toxic drugs and dangerous drug–drug interactions, which increases the risk of severe adverse effects during anesthesia. For instance, medications like usual antibiotics and NSAIDs can interact and result in gastrointestinal issues, especially in patients who are battling other conditions. Findings like these highlight the need for reconceptualization and strengthening of medication management by healthcare teams with the aim of reducing these perilous pitfalls for such a susceptible population (Jiang et al., 2025). The identification and avoidance of the most risky medications are paramount to ensuring patient safety is kept above all else. As you go through the long list of medications utilized during the perioperative and postoperative courses, identifying those that can trigger severe side effects remains one of the cornerstones of anesthetic practice. Evidence suggests that, in the majority of cases, drugs like neuromuscular blockers and certain antibiotics are always implicated in severe adverse effects, so it is valuable to be extremely cautious when administering them. And then there are the emerging challenges, such as the recent news of teicoplanin issues, which only go to highlight quite how dynamic and constantly changing drug reactions are. And there is the tricky task of distinguishing true allergic reactions from those that just look like them. As understanding of genetic risk slowly unfolds, anesthetists are increasingly taking this into their decision-making—even if that can sometimes make things feel just a bit more complicated. Overall, adopting patient-centered care with personalized drug therapies goes a long way in reducing the risk for serious side effects (Baldo, 2023) (Figure 2.16).

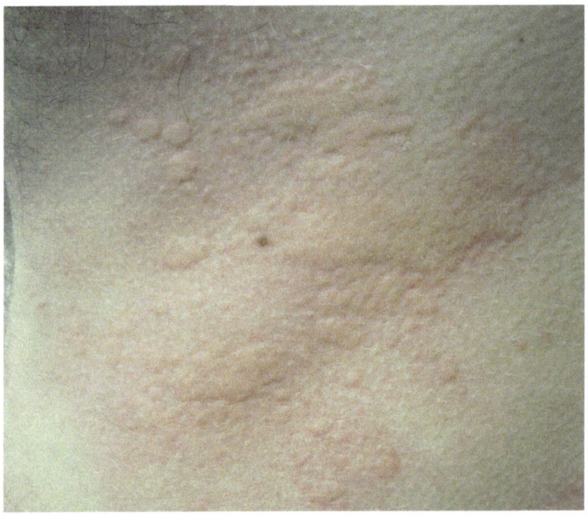

Figure 2.16. Allergic bursts.

Source: By James Heilman, MD - work, CC BY-SA 3.0, https://commons.wikimedia.org/w/index.php?curid=11508979.

2.5.3. Risk Factors for Complications

Surgery is complex; there's so much more at stake than the procedure itself—there are complications possible both under and after anesthesia. Patient factors, for one, are a leading consideration. Older patients or those already vulnerable with heart or lung disease are more likely to have higher risks of serious complications like heart attack and respiratory complications, which, in most cases, equate to higher rates of complications overall. The type of surgery performed, particularly if it's deeply invasive, increases the risk even more. Often, in a given situation, the approach to anesthesia must be as individualized as the patient themselves. Anesthetic options, also, are a significant consideration. Some medications, due to what they do in your body, are trouble makers—particularly if there is a person with liver problems or other metabolic idiosyncrasies. For example, drugs mostly broken down by the liver can be riskier for those with hepatic impairments. Also, whether the anesthesia is served via a regional block or given generally might alter outcomes more than you'd expect; the surgical setting and the individual's overall health can change things up. In general, it makes sense to take all of these into close consideration so that risks are kept to a minimum but potential advantage is maximized. Observation of the patients over the period around the date of the surgery is also important. Monitoring policies, which at times strictly follow guidelines like those in (Connolly et al., 2012), allow for patients to receive the extra careful attention that they might need. Risk assessment tools will also come into play, helping teams to determine who might need a little extra attention or an alternative plan altogether. Blended pain management strategies—using a combination of drugs to reduce the amount of opioids used—have been found to be effective, and all these interventions in combination help to respond to the many potential risk factors involved. When it's all done proactively, the risk of complication will often greatly diminish.

Test Your Knowledge

1. Describe the common side effects of anesthetic drugs.
2. What is considered a serious adverse reaction?

2.6. Advances in Anesthetic Pharmacology

Learning Outcome

1. Explain the development of new anesthetic agents.
2. Understand the innovations in delivery methods.
3. Describe the research on personalized anesthesia.

Recently, we've seen some quite considerable changes to anesthetic drugs—especially if you consider that the time shortly before and shortly after surgery is a very critical period when it comes to the way patients do recover in reality. We now find that rapid reactions from the body during surgery play a big role in recovery and long-term survival, and cancer patients are showing this all too readily. Anesthetic medications, although mainly used to relieve pain and keep patients sedated, also tamper with the immune system in a way that slows down or, in some instances, even hastens the development of tumors. Such duplicity explains that both drug-based and other types of intervention have a role to play at such critical points, something that, in most cases, transforms our whole understanding of what these drugs are doing. In many cases, their impact on immunity turns out to be as relevant as their pain-relieving potential (Bezu et al., 2024). Local anesthetic systemic toxicity, or LAST as it's also known, has recently been in the headlines, making usual RA use a priority once again. LAST can present with issues in the brain or heart, typically taking fairly uncomplicated procedures and making them somewhat more complicated than they otherwise would have been. With local anesthetics being used more extensively in a range of settings, determining exactly why and how LAST arises is something that healthcare providers cannot take seriously enough. Advanced imaging equipment like ultrasound (which, by the way, target injections more precisely) has reduced the risks somewhat, decreasing the chances of causing inadvertent toxicity. To this, new evidence—paired with a dash of real-world practice—suggests initial treatments like lipid emulsion therapy and speeded seizure management as being pivotal to keeping adverse events in check (El-Boghdaddly et al., 2018). There is also growing enthusiasm for customizing anesthesia to fit each patient, promising that it's time to break free from the age-old one-size-fits-all approach. New findings show that our genes can dictate how we metabolize and react to different anesthetic drugs, leading us toward a more personalized, individualized method.

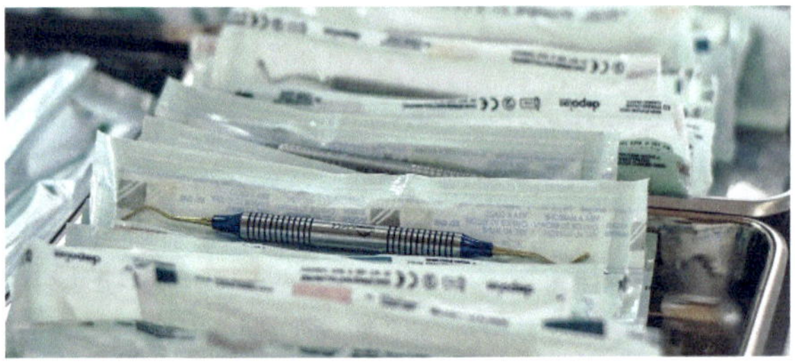

Figure 2.17. Anesthetic Pharmacology.

Source: https://sgrh.com/assets/img/uploads/16899366555.jpg.

This research in pharmacogenomics presents new opportunities for choosing the best drugs that will align with each person's metabolic peculiarities. That is, anesthetists will eventually have the option to select medicines that reduce side effects without losing potency in keeping patients on their journey for surgery. Overall, these developments paint a more comprehensive picture—not just sedating someone but tending to their overall health before, during, and after surgery. As studies gradually remove the veil from how these agents function, there is real hope that such knowledge could well revolutionize routine clinical practice for the better (Figure 2.17) (Bezu et al., 2024).

2.6.1. Development of New Anesthetic Agents

The development of anesthetic drugs has progressed a lot, always trying to advance safety and efficacy while concentrating on keeping patients comfortable. In the late 1990s, Glaxo Wellcome began a project to discover ester-type benzodiazepine derivatives—a project that unexpectedly led to remimazolam. The whole project hit a few speed bumps along the way (and ended up being bought by a smaller biopharma), but remimazolam besylate is distinctive for its quick metabolism and reduced impact on the heart as opposed to old-school drugs (Kilpatrick, 2021). It's pretty clear that moving towards sedatives that suit an array of clinical needs has been a constant drive in this field. And yet, concurrently, the quest for better anesthetics isn't simply a question of nailing down more favorable drug performance—it's also about what Mother Nature has to offer. Often, nature dishes up a cornucopia of active agents that can be the source of inspiration that generates new concepts. Even ancient morsels tell us that drugs like cocaine were first used in eye procedures, demonstrating that sometimes the most productive leads originate from plant and even animal sources. Research continues to indicate the different advantages of these natural products and challenge pharmaceutical groups to investigate such materials, especially for specialty areas like eye work (Pinheiro et al., 2018). Meanwhile, new developments are not just a question of enhancing efficacy but also minimizing the downsides of the previous agents. Take remimazolam, for example—it has less potential to induce respiratory depression and injection discomfort, both of which are significant to patients feeling good afterward.

Its quick metabolism to inactive metabolites enables people to get better faster, an important factor in outpatients and short cases. This kind of combination—mixing new ideas with consideration of what is beneficial for patients—seems to be the way forward for tailoring anesthetic practice to differing needs. Generally, the anesthetic care of the future is set to merge trailblazing innovations with precision-honed refinements to continue placing patient safety and satisfaction at its center (Kilpatrick, 2021).

2.6.2. Innovations in Delivery Methods

Anesthetic delivery has come a long way, much like other breakthroughs in healthcare that lean on nature's toolkit. We've seen that plant-based compounds often light the spark for modern medicines, a reminder—generally speaking—of how vital biodiversity remains in today's drug discoveries. Mixing old-school remedies with fresh, creative drug design not only points to nature as a great source for new anesthetics but also repeats a familiar story. Of course, sorting through these naturally occurring molecules has its set of issues: balancing high-quality, high-throughput screening protocols and keeping supplies at a constant can be problematic. Astonishingly enough, coordinating the activities of diverse specialists is mainly the solution to working out the kinks and eventually putting safer, effective anesthetic practices to use (Chaachouay et al., 2024). Wearable tech has become all the rage in recent years, transforming how we deliver treatments like anesthetics. Small, wearable sensors—many times electrochemical and non-invasive—are transforming the profession by tracking chemical indicators as you go about your day. Medical professionals can now, in real time, connect how a medication is being processed and the patient's response, then adjust on the fly if necessary. The real-time and non-invasive nature of these devices not only renders the patient's experience significantly less painful but also seems to reduce the risk of unwanted side effects. Overall, this interactive method of monitoring is preparing itself to redefine the standards of patient care, delivering more precise dosing and enhanced safety in surgeries (Teymourian et al., 2020). With future developments, new methods like nanotechnology have a great deal of potential for sending anesthetic delivery into a more advanced direction. Think of small particles that are tailored to encapsulate anesthetic drugs in a way so that they only fall where they are needed, and slowly release for hours or even days. That type of method can amp up the local effects of the anesthetic without adding on unnecessary exposure throughout the body. Most of the time, this would mean smaller doses, fewer irritating side effects, and overall, a smoother experience for the patients. By combining these newer, hi-tech methods with old-trusted techniques, clinicians might end up tailoring anesthesia to fit each patient more than ever before. With more research being conducted in these overlapping fields, the merging of these novel delivery systems with conventional agents could hold the solution to completely new approaches to the enhancement of care during the surgery course (Chaachouay et al., 2024) (Figure 2.18).

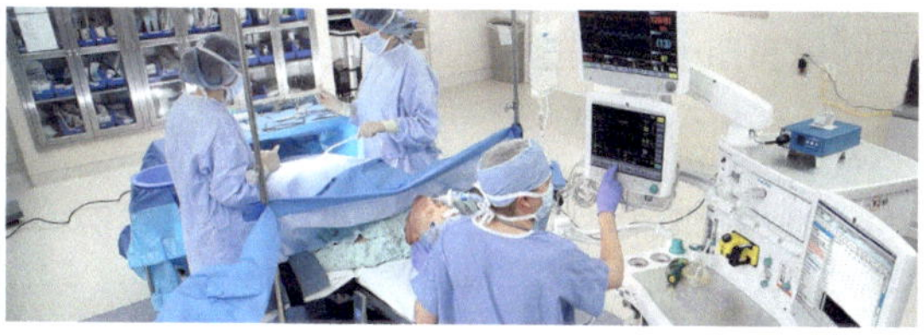

Figure 2.18. Innovations in anesthetic delivery.

Source: https://www.gehealthcare.com/en-my/-/jssmedia/widen/2018/01/25/0204/gehealthcarecom/migrated/2018/02/13/0542/nesthesia-delivery-general-home-page-carousel-images-anesthesia-delivery-carousel-0001_jpg.jpg?h=400&iar=0&w=1200&rev=-1&hash=ACE7CA76D2D360CB52ED093DBE314999.

2.6.3. Research on Personalized Anesthesia

Anesthetic method has been evolving in the past few years toward greater individualization and patient focus—a hypothesis that is now being underscored by many of the latest studies. There has been mounting evidence that not every patient reacts identically to anesthesia; genetic defects, environmental factors, and even normal physiology can play a part. When doctors take biomarkers or even hypotheses of genetic susceptibility into account, they can make better choices about what medicine to prescribe, how much to prescribe, and even adjust treatment on the fly. This smarter strategy not only goes to contribute to overall efficacy of treatments, but reduces side effects as well, smoothing out the recovery period thereafter. Generally speaking, all this work points to the need for a deeper look at each patient's unique makeup if we're going to refine anesthesia techniques to improve both surgical outcomes and hospital workflows. And then there's the role of enhanced recovery after surgery (ERAS) protocols, which have seriously contributed to this personalized vibe in anesthesia. These evidence-driven steps promote the use of a blend of methods to pain relief—a tactic that is increasingly important in a variety of surgical scenarios. With suitable anesthetic choice designed to meet an individual's needs, complications decrease and recoveries are less stressful. A combination of anesthesiologists, surgeons, and other medical professionals has become on board with utilizing ERAS steps alongside personalized anesthesia methods. It stresses the need for teamwork in the operating room. And when the likes of the Grading of Recommendations, Assessment, Development, and Evaluation (GRADE) framework come into the mix, they make sure that only the best evidence goes into guiding these practices (Debono et al., 2021). Advances in nanomedicine are giving rise to some intriguing possibilities in the years ahead. Researchers are trying out nanotech to develop novel drug-delivery systems capable of targeting individual cells or tissues with remarkable accuracy—ideas that have the potential to revolutionize anesthetic medications. These kinds of developments would deliver drugs more effectively and minimize undesirable side effects, making procedures safer and more manageable for patients. While more attention is being given to these high-tech strategies, so too is there a demand to respond in a thoughtful manner to the ethical, environmental, and health issues that come with them. In most cases, an even, standardized modus operandi will be necessary to ensure that the benefits of personalized anesthesia more than justify patient safety and overall healthcare goals (Malik et al., 2023). Overall, ongoing research with multifaceted dimensions is opening the door to an anesthesia era that's more personalized, streamlined—and honestly, a little more in tune with what patients need (Figure 2.19).

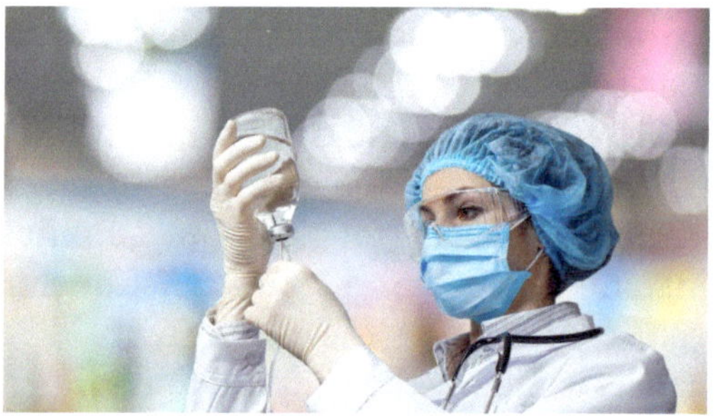

Figure 2.19. Personalized Anesthesia.

Source: https://actu.epfl.ch/image/104219/1108x622.jpg.

Test Your Knowledge

1. Describe the development of new anesthetic agents.
2. Discuss about innovations in anesthetic delivery methods.

SUMMARY

Anesthetic drug and our own body's reaction dance together in a somewhat complex waltz, which propels us toward more personalized techniques in surgery. Recent research in general suggests that anesthetics like isoflurane and sevoflurane trigger metabolic pathways—specifically by modulating plasma endocannabinoid levels throughout the process of anesthesia. A marked reduction of plasma anandamide after anesthesia indicates modified pain control and even nerve cell protection, perhaps. This new discovery calls for, in the majority of cases, an investigation of how varied anesthetics influence the endocannabinoid system and even could be smarter than before pain control during the surgical window (Chua et al., 2025).

The knowledge of how these drugs vary in terms of metabolism and how they function in the body is most essential, particularly when operations become complex, such as while working on the heart. A glance at recent studies will find all of the drugs like propofol, sevoflurane, and midazolam having some part to play in keeping circulatory conditions stable. For example, propofol has a quick onset and even delays nausea—which is why it's a number-one drug for quick maneuvers—and sevoflurane, with its low blood solubility, makes physicians able to alter doses instantly. These elements, when finely tuned, become central to customizing anesthesia for the unique patient, balancing surgical outcomes and reducing on any negatives that occur (Lacerda et al., 2024). Eventually, the lessons learned from ongoing anesthesia research can upend clinical practice. As we better understand the mechanisms of these agents, it is possible for anesthesiology to move towards ever more subtly calibrated practices that balance short-term effects and long-term impacts on patient health. A key function of co-ordination among researchers, clinicians, and educators is to knit these pieces together into strong anesthetic protocols. With our passion for learning, the practice improves—incrementally ensuring increased safety and effectiveness in the ever-evolving field of surgical care (Chua et al., 2025).

Drug administration and the brain's real needs are closely related. Studying anesthetic pharmacology is not just a matter of learning how a drug moves around in the body (its pharmacokinetics) or the strength of its effect (its pharmacodynamics); it's a matter of meeting the brain's need for oxygen and nutrients. Keeping cerebral blood flow (CBF) stable is crucial—if that balance is disrupted, you're asking for some serious neurologic issues. For the most part, learning anesthetics is looking at every component, from their alteration of nerve cells' excitability to their regulation of blood vessel response, with each component fitting into the overall puzzle of creating procedures safer and more efficient (Claassen et al., 2021). Pain management isn't quite as straightforward, either. Working with chronic pain—especially with the type that affects the bones and muscles—the approach has to be multi-dimensional. Rather than relying on anesthetics solely, doctors usually use a mix of both medicine and other, non-medicinal practices. All things considered, this method reduces the application of more intensive medication and, more often than not, overall improves quality of life, by offering solutions that treat each patient's individual pain experience (Salah et al., 2021).

The shifting face of anesthetic science certainly requires ongoing research. With the development of new anesthetics, it becomes more important to understand what they are actually doing and how they will react to other agents. Anesthetists, in general, are encouraged to keep up to date with the latest evidence-based practice so that anesthesia can continue to work efficiently and safely despite new challenges emerging. In delving so deeply into anesthetic behavior in the realm of pain control, clinicians do not merely better care for immediate patients but also bring new concepts to the larger science of anesthesiology—to provide assurance that new approaches remain solidly anchored in good scientific thinking.

KEY TERMS FROM THIS CHAPTER

Absorption
Anesthetic agents
Bupivacaine
Distribution
Lidocaine
Neurocommunication
Adjunctive anesthetic agents
Anesthetic science
Central nervous system
Excretion
Metabolism
Neuropathic pain

CRITICAL THINKING QUESTIONS

1. **Which of the following general anesthetics is known for its rapid induction and recovery due to low blood solubility?**
   a. Halothane
   b. Sevoflurane
   c. Nitrous Oxide
   d. Isoflurane
2. **Which IV anesthetic is commonly used for induction because of its rapid onset and antiemetic properties?**
   a. Thiopental
   b. Ketamine
   c. Propofol
   d. Etomidate
3. **Which inhalational anesthetic has the fastest onset and offset due to its low blood-gas partition coefficient?**
   a. Halothane
   b. Sevoflurane
   c. Nitrous oxide
   d. Desflurane
4. **Which of the following is a depolarizing neuromuscular blocker?**
   a. Rocuronium
   b. Vecuronium
   c. Atracurium
   d. Succinylcholine
5. **What is the primary mechanism of action of midazolam when used as an anesthetic adjunct?**
   a. GABA-A receptor agonism
   b. NMDA receptor antagonism
   c. Sodium channel blockade
   d. Alpha-2 adrenergic receptor agonism

Short Answer Questions

1. Define the anesthetic agents.
2. Why are anesthetics important in medical practice?
3. What are the three classifications of anesthetic agents?
4. What is the pharmacokinetics of anesthetic agents?
5. Describe the advances in anesthetic pharmacology.

Answers to Critical Thinking Questions

1. (c); 2. (c); 3. (d); 4. (d); 5. (a)

REFERENCES

1. AGS Faculty. (2015). The American Geriatrics Society/National Institute on Aging Bedside-to-Bench Conference: Research agenda on delirium in older adults. *Journal of the American Geriatrics Society, 63*, 843–852. https://doi.org/10.1111/jgs.13406.
2. Baldo, B. A. (2023). Allergic and other adverse reactions to drugs used in anesthesia and surgery. *Anesthesiology and Perioperative Science, 1*(2), 16. https://doi.org/10.1007/s44254-023-00018-2.
3. Bezu, L., Akçal Öksüz, D., Bell, M., Buggy, D. J., Díaz-Cambronero, Ó., Enlund, M., Forget, P., et al. (2024). Perioperative immunosuppressive factors during cancer surgery: An updated review. *Cancers, 16*(13), 2304. https://doi.org/10.3390/cancers16132304.
4. Black, N. D., Stecco, C., & Chan, V. W. S. (2021). Fascial plane blocks: More questions than answers? *Anesthesia and Analgesia, 132*(3), 899–905. https://doi.org/10.1213/ANE.0000000000005321.
5. Blair, N. T., Caceres, A. I., Carvacho, I., Chaudhuri, D., Clapham, D. E., De Clercq, K., Delling, M., Doerner, J. F., Fan, L., Grimm, C. M., Ha, K., Hu, M., Jabba, S. V., Jordt, S. E., Julius, D., Kahle, K. T., Liu, Q., Liu, B., McKemy, D., Nilius, B., Oancea, E., Owsianik, G., Riccio, A., Sah, R., Stotz, S. C., Tian, J., Tong, D., Vriens, J., Wu, L. J., Xu, H., Yang, F., Yang, W., Yue, L., & Zhu, M. X. (2025). Transient receptor potential channels (TRP) in GtoPdb v.2025.1. *IUPHAR/BPS Guide to Pharmacology*. https://doi.org/10.2218/gtopdb/F78/2025.1.
6. Caliskan, E. (2017). Neonatal care for anesthesiologists. https://core.ac.uk/download/322433592.pdf (accessed on 20 May 2025).
7. Cappellini, I., Bavestrello Piccini, G., Campagnola, L., Bochicchio, C., Carente, R., Lai, F., Magazzini, S., & Consales, G. (2024). Procedural sedation in emergency department: A narrative review. *Emergency Care and Medicine, 1*(2), 103–136. https://doi.org/10.3390/ecm1020014.
8. Chaachouay, N., & Zidane, L. (2024). Plant-derived natural products: A source for drug discovery and development. *Drugs and Drug Candidates, 3*(1), 184–207. https://doi.org/10.3390/ddc3010011.
9. Chua, A., McMichael, M. A., Jukier, T., Arnold, R. D., Hung, W. E., Harris, S., Zhang, C., & Bustamante, H. A. (2025). Premedication and general anesthetic agents decrease plasma concentration of the endocannabinoid anandamide in dogs. *American Journal of Veterinary Research*, 1–7. https://doi.org/10.2460/ajvr.24.11.0366.
10. Claassen, J. A. H. R., Thijssen, D. H. J., Panerai, R. B., & Faraci, F. M. (2021). Regulation of cerebral blood flow in humans: Physiology and clinical implications of autoregulation. *Physiological Reviews, 101*(4), 1487–1559. https://doi.org/10.1152/physrev.00022.2020.
11. Coderre, T. J. (2018). Topical drug therapeutics for neuropathic pain. *Expert Opinion on Pharmacotherapy, 19*(11), 1211–1220. https://doi.org/10.1080/14656566.2018.1501026.
12. Connolly, E. S., Rabinstein, A. A., Carhuapoma, J. R., Derdeyn, C. P., Dion, J. E., Higashida, R. T., Hoh, B. L., et al. (2012). Guidelines for the management of aneurysmal subarachnoid hemorrhage. *Stroke, 43*(8), 1711–1737. https://doi.org/10.1161/str.0b013e3182587839.
13. Coté, C. J., & Wilson, S. (2019). Guidelines for monitoring and management of pediatric patients before, during, and after sedation for diagnostic and therapeutic procedures. *Pediatrics, 143*. https://doi.org/10.1542/peds.2019-1000.

14. Cristofoletti, R., & Rostami-Hodjegan, A. (2023). Linking *in vitro–in vivo* extrapolations with physiologically based modeling to inform drug and formulation development. *Biopharmaceutics & Drug Disposition, 44*. https://www.semanticscholar.org/paper/29d0a6be0f55de2836932c70bb074727e731fd63 (accessed on 20 May 2025).

15. Debono, B., Wainwright, T. W., Wang, M. Y., Sigmundsson, F. G., Yang, M. M. H., Smid-Nanninga, H., Bonnal, A., Le Huec, J. C., Fawcett, W. J., Ljungqvist, O., Lonjon, G., & de Boer, H. D. (2021). Consensus statement for perioperative care in lumbar spinal fusion: Enhanced Recovery After Surgery (ERAS®) Society recommendations. *The Spine Journal, 21*(5), 729–752. https://doi.org/10.1016/j.spinee.2021.01.001.

16. Egan, T. D., & Svensén, C. (2018). Multimodal general anesthesia: A principled approach to producing the drug-induced, reversible coma of anesthesia. *Anesthesia & Analgesia, 127*(4), 1104–1106. https://doi.org/10.1213/ane.0000000000003743.

17. El-Boghdadly, K., Pawa, A., & Chin, K. J. (2018). Local anesthetic systemic toxicity: Current perspectives. *Local and Regional Anesthesia, 11*, 35–44. https://doi.org/10.2147/lra.s154512.

18. El-Tallawy, S. N., Nalamasu, R., Salem, G. I., LeQuang, J. A., Pergolizzi, J. V., & Christo, P. J. (2021). Management of musculoskeletal pain: An update with emphasis on chronic musculoskeletal pain. *Pain and Therapy, 10*(1), 181–209. https://doi.org/10.1007/s40122-021-00235-2.

19. Ferreira-Vieira, T. H., Olmo, I. G., Rodrigues da Silva, F., & Ribeiro, F. M. (2016). Alzheimer's disease: Targeting the cholinergic system. *Current Neuropharmacology, 14*(1), 101–115. https://doi.org/10.2174/1570159x13666150716165726.

20. Fontanella, N. (2025). Transdermal ketamine: A rising star in pain and inflammation. *Journal of Scrip Pharmacy*. https://doi.org/10.70390/YG6HB0ML.

21. Gan, J. T. (2017). Poorly controlled postoperative pain: Prevalence, consequences, and prevention. *Journal of Pain Research, 10*, 2287–2298. https://doi.org/10.2147/jpr.s144066.

22. Hao, X., Ou, M., Zhang, D., Zhao, W., Yang, Y., Liu, J., Yang, H., et al. (2020). The effects of general anesthetics on synaptic transmission. *Current Neuropharmacology, 18*(10), 936–965. https://doi.org/10.2174/1570159x18666200227125854.

23. Ingrande, J. (2015). Clinical pharmacology for anesthesiology. *Anesthesia & Analgesia, 121*(6), 1676–1677. https://doi.org/10.1213/ane.0000000000000954.

24. Jangwan, N. S., Khan, M., Das, R., Altwaijry, N., Sultan, A. M., Khan, R., Saleem, S., & Singh, M. F. (2024). From petals to healing: Consolidated network pharmacology and molecular docking investigations of the mechanisms underpinning *Rhododendron arboreum* flower's anti-NAFLD effects. *Frontiers in Pharmacology, 15*, 1366279. https://doi.org/10.3389/fphar.2024.1366279.

25. Jiang, H., Lin, Y., Ren, W., Lu, L., Tan, X., Lv, X., & Zhang, N. (2025). Potential inappropriate medications and drug-drug interactions in adverse drug reactions in the elderly: A retrospective study in a pharmacovigilance database. *Frontiers in Pharmacology, 16*, 1546012. https://doi.org/10.3389/fphar.2025.1546012.

26. Kawakami, H., Nishikawa, K., Shimokawa, T., Fujitani, K., Tamura, S., Endo, S., Kobayashi, M., Kawada, J., Kurokawa, Y., Tsuburaya, A., Yoshikawa, T., Sakamoto, J., Satoh, T., & On Behalf of the HERBIS-HERBIS-A and XParTS II Study Investigators. (2022). Histology classification highlights differences in efficacy of S-1 versus capecitabine, in combination with cisplatin, for HER2-negative unresectable advanced or recurrent gastric cancer with measurable disease. *Cancers, 14*(22), 5673. https://doi.org/10.3390/cancers14225673.

27. Kilpatrick, G. J. (2021). Remimazolam: Non-clinical and clinical profile of a new sedative/anesthetic agent. *Frontiers in Pharmacology, 12*, 690875. https://doi.org/10.3389/fphar.2021.690875.

28. Kooij, F. O., Schlack, W., Preckel, B., & Hollmann, M. W. (2014). Does regional analgesia for major surgery improve outcome? Focus on epidural analgesia. *Anesthesia & Analgesia, 119*(4), 740–744. https://doi.org/10.1213/ane.0000000000000245.

29. Kumar, M., Chawla, R., & Goyal, M. (2015). Topical anesthesia. *Journal of Anesthesiology Clinical Pharmacology, 31*(4), 450. https://doi.org/10.4103/0970-9185.169049.

30. Lacerda, D. A., Honorato, P. F., de Albuquerque, J. G. F., Rocha de Araujo, L. K. A., Rocha, F. G. A., Fernandes de Macêdo, M. G., Fragoso de Freitas Neto, V., et al. (2024). Pharmacology of general anesthetic agents in cardiac surgery: Pharmacokinetic and pharmacodynamic properties. *III Seven International Medical and Nursing Congress*. https://www.semanticscholar.org/paper/141a7009b0dc38a5296e2bc51f397a6482be2305 (accessed on 20 May 2025).

31. Lafreniere, J. D., Szczesniak, A. M., Courtney, E., Kelly, M. E. M., & Faktorovich, E. G. (2023). Topical analgesics for acute corneal pain: Current options and emerging therapeutics. *Journal of Cataract & Refractive Surgery, 49*, 1160–1167. https://www.semanticscholar.org/paper/ec1c074e5ccb92d428750a0b8910d4f01cf4e5f7 (accessed on 20 May 2025).

32. Machado, K. C., Islam, M. T., Ali, E. S., Rouf, R., Uddin, S. J., Dev, S., Shilpi, J. A., et al. (2018). A systematic review on the neuroprotective perspectives of beta-caryophyllene. *Phytotherapy Research, 32*(12), 2376–2388. https://doi.org/10.1002/ptr.6199.

33. Malik, S., Muhammad, K., & Waheed, Y. (2023). Emerging applications of nanotechnology in healthcare and medicine. *Molecules, 28*(16), 6624. https://doi.org/10.3390/molecules28186624.

34. Matveychuk, D., Thomas, R. K., Swainson, J., Khullar, A., MacKay, M. A., Baker, G. B., & Dursun, S. M. (2020). Ketamine as an antidepressant: Overview of its mechanisms of action and potential predictive biomarkers. *Therapeutic Advances in Psychopharmacology, 10*, 2045125320916657. https://doi.org/10.1177/2045125320916657.

35. Pinheiro, G. K. L. O., Araújo Filho, I., Araújo Neto, I., Rêgo, A. C. M., Azevedo, E. P., Pinheiro, F. I., & Lima Filho, A. A. S. (2018). Nature as a source of drugs for ophthalmology. *Arquivos Brasileiros de Oftalmologia, 81*(5), 443–454. https://doi.org/10.5935/0004-2749.20180086.

36. Rastogi, R., Swarm, R. A., Patel, T., & Riou, B. (2011). Case scenario: Opioid association with serotonin syndrome. *Anesthesiology, 115*(6), 1291–1298. https://doi.org/10.1097/aln.0b013e31823940c0.

37. Rathi, S., Mladek, A., Oh, J. H., Dragojevic, S., Burgenske, D. M., Zhang, W., Talele, S., et al. (2024). Factors influencing the central nervous system (CNS) distribution of the ATR inhibitor elimusertib (BAY1895344): Implications for the treatment of CNS tumors. *The Journal of Pharmacology and Experimental Therapeutics*. https://www.semanticscholar.org/paper/8e341855369076b3d69b7ee9649b4fb4860ae1ee (accessed on 20 May 2025).

38. Rout, M., Tomar, N., Kaushik, M., & Singh, S. (2024). Advances in local anesthesia and pain management for practicing dentists: A comprehensive review. *Journal of Drug Delivery and Therapeutics, 14*(5), 174–179. https://jddtonline.info/index.php/jddt/article/view/6572 (accessed on 20 May 2025).

39. Salim, B., Rashid, S., Ali, M. A., Raza, A., & Khan, F. A. (2019). Effect of pharmacological agents administered for attenuating the extubation response on the quality of extubation: A systematic review. *Cureus, 11*(12), e6427. https://doi.org/10.7759/cureus.6427.

40. Shah, A., & Pillai, A. (2024). Drug utilization study of pre-anesthetic, intraoperative, and post-operative medications use in various surgeries of orthopedic and surgery department of tertiary care teaching hospital. *National Journal of Physiology, Pharmacy and Pharmacology, 14*(8), 1592–1597. https://doi.org/10.5455/njppp.2024.14.12574202322022024.

41. Shannar, A., Chou, P. J., Peter, R., Dave, P. D., Patel, K., Pan, Y., Xu, J., Sarwar, M. S., & Kong, A. N. (2025). Pharmacodynamics (PD), pharmacokinetics (PK) and PK-PD modeling of NRF2 activating dietary phytochemicals in cancer prevention and in health. *Current Pharmacology Reports, 11*(1), 6. https://doi.org/10.1007/s40495-024-00388-6.

42. Speigel, I., Bichler, E. K., & García, P. S. (2017). The influence of regional distribution and pharmacologic specificity of GABAAR subtype expression on anesthesia and emergence. *Frontiers in Systems Neuroscience, 11*, 58. https://doi.org/10.3389/fnsys.2017.00058.

43. Subhadarshini, S., & Taksande, K. (2024). A comprehensive review on the role of melatonin's anesthetic applications in pediatric care. *Cureus, 16*. https://www.semanticscholar.org/paper/c353048f6c77a7e57297b63c58bceb6ba6153069 (accessed on 20 May 2025).

44. Taylor, K., Kim, W. T., Maharramova, M., Figueroa, V., Ramesh, S., & Lorenzo, A. (2016). Intraoperative management and early postoperative outcomes of pediatric renal transplants. *Pediatric Anesthesia, 26*(10), 987–991. https://doi.org/10.1111/pan.12979.

45. Teymourian, H., Parrilla, M., Sempionatto, J. R., Montiel, N. F., Barfidokht, A., Van Echelpoel, R., De Wael, K., et al. (2020). Wearable electrochemical sensors for the monitoring and screening of drugs. *ACS Sensors, 5*(9), 2679–2700. https://doi.org/10.1021/acssensors.0c01318.

46. Tsantoulas, C., & McMahon, S. B. (2014). Opening paths to novel analgesics: The role of potassium channels in chronic pain. *Trends in Neurosciences, 37*(3), 146–158. https://doi.org/10.1016/j.tins.2013.12.002.

47. Voss, L. J., García, P. S., Hentschke, H., & Banks, M. I. (2019). Understanding the effects of general anesthetics on cortical network activity using *ex vivo* preparations. *Anesthesiology, 130*(6), 1049–1063. https://doi.org/10.1097/ALN.0000000000002554.

48. Wilder, R. T., Flick, R. P., Šprung, J., Katusic, S. K., Barbaresi, W. J., Mickelson, C., Gleich, S. J., et al. (2009). Early exposure to anesthesia and learning disabilities in a population-based birth cohort. *Anesthesiology, 110*(4), 796–804. https://doi.org/10.1097/01.anes.0000344728.34332.5d.

49. Young, A., & Buvanendran, A. (2011). Multimodal systemic and intra-articular analgesics. *International Anesthesiology Clinics, 49*(4), 117–133. https://doi.org/10.1097/AIA.0b013e31821b7c20.

50. Young, J., Koh, A., & Martis, W. R. (2024). Successful management of opioid-refractory pelvic cancer pain using continuous local anesthetic infusion via a tunneled epidural. *Journal of Modern Medical Oncology, 4*. https://doi.org/10.53964/jmmo.2024002.

51. Zanos, P., Moaddel, R., Morris, P. J., Riggs, L. M., Highland, J. N., Georgiou, P., Pereira, E. F. R., et al. (2018). Ketamine and ketamine metabolite pharmacology: Insights into therapeutic mechanisms. *Pharmacological Reviews, 70*(3), 621–660. https://doi.org/10.1124/pr.117.015198.

ANATOMY AND PHYSIOLOGY RELEVANT TO ANESTHESIA

3

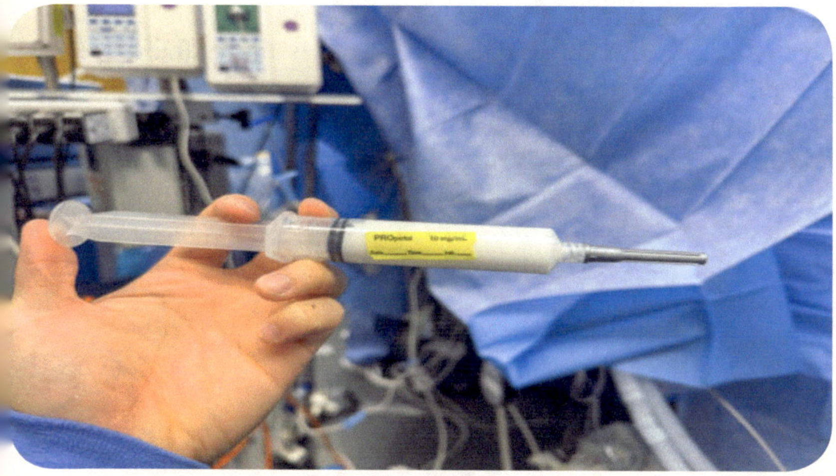

LEARNING OBJECTIVES

After studying this chapter, you will be able to:

1. Understand the basic anatomy of the human body.
2. Understand the physiology of the nervous system.
3. Describe the cardiovascular system and anesthesia.
4. Discuss about respiratory system considerations.
5. Learn about patient assessment and monitoring.

Introduction

Human body internal anatomical structure as well as how different internal organ;s function play a significant role in anesthesia. It is not simply pumping drugs in, it is understanding how each component of the body normally functions and how the surgery could alter the normal balance. Anesthetists rely on this sort of close-up anatomy knowledge in order to act on cue and manage complications. Take the airway, for example; knowing how it is laid out can be a life-saver when choosing intubation methods or managing difficult airways. That kind of applied expertise guarantees that emergencies due to natural variations are handled more effectively, and that, in most cases, patients are safer and surgical results are better. The response of the body to anesthetic medication is another variable added to the equation. These medications don't simply settle in; they interfere with the heart, lungs, and even nerves, and the alterations can be both subtle and profound. Vital signs, drug metabolism, and even how a patient responds as a whole can change — so anesthetists have to continually refine their strategy based on each patient's profile. A majority of clinics today include new technology, like 3D-printed models, in giving patients a better sense of what to expect (Marchetti et al., 2020). The old and new combined here mean that having a sense of both anatomy and body responses is key to a safe, successful surgery. Looking back, the creation of anesthesia was heavily driven by building on our understanding of human anatomy and physiology. General anesthesia (GA) itself rendered surgery formerly too risky feasible. In all but a few cases, this history shows why knowledge of basic body function still applies today. Current and future practitioners are likely to reflect on these lessons, as they continue to shape the practice of things. With methods changing all the time, there remains a need for continued anatomy and physiology training as anesthetists are kept appropriately skilled to handle the intricate nature of medicine today (Constantinoiu, 2018).

Definition of Anesthesia

Anesthesia is a vital component of modern medicine—especially when surgery is involved. It's not just a matter of sending d pain to sleep; it messes around with our senses and feelings so that the conditions can be rendered safer for treatment. In most cases, these drugs sedate and mess around with nerve conduction and blood vessel behavior. Their mechanism of action has to do with switching neurotransmitter function, which thereby blocks pain along with altering the way the body's overall stress response is processed. How their effects come to pass is significant since the subtle structure of the nervous system is directly proportional to how these agents operate. Additionally, the need of the brain to counterbalance oxygen and nutrient delivery with increased metabolic demand underscores the need to keep cerebral blood flow (CBF) within parameters during procedures, as outlined by (Claassen et al., 2021). Proper administration of anesthesia, in most cases, entails having a general idea of the inner structure of the human body. It impacts regions in the brain used to stay awake and make us feel, and the brain itself, which many consider a sprawling, multiscale dynamical system, is comprised of a variety of neural networks that help us think and communicate. When anesthetics disrupt these networks, even slight misalignments are problematic. In short, both physical responses and anatomical pathways need to be considered to keep risks limited. Growing knowledge of how brain function evolves over time is more and more affecting more tailored anesthetic practices—a notion highlighted in the new science of dynamic functional connectivity, noted by (Lurie et al., 2019). Anesthesia is not simply the delivery of drugs; it's more like an intricate dance of various body systems that must be closely monitored.

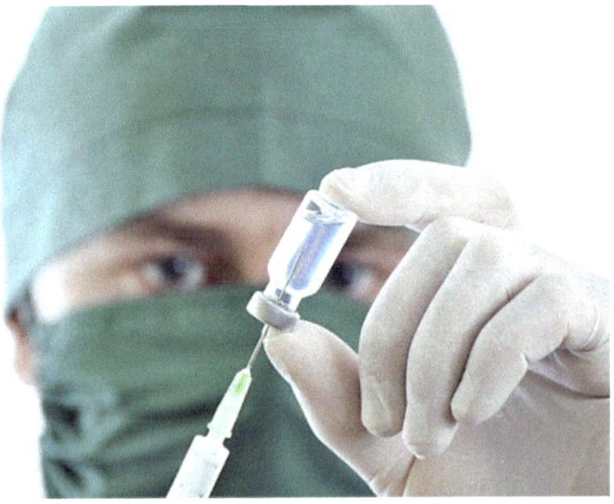

Figure 3.1. Anesthesia.

Source: https://domf5oio6qrcr.cloudfront.net/medialibrary/3795/conversions/w0615e16207252200938-thumb.jpg

Monitoring is critical during the process of a procedure because heart rate, blood pressure, and oxygen levels can give clues about the body's response to such substances. Practitioners will assess these signs along with individual anatomical features—like those in the cardiovascular and respiratory systems—to decide on the best approach. New technology has certainly enhanced our ability to monitor things, making the whole procedure less dangerous. As our understanding of these physiological reactions evolves, so do the methods used. Last but not least, anesthesia includes not only the pharmacology but also the intricate, sometimes paradoxical, interaction between different body systems, showing how closely anatomy and physiology are linked, even when it sometimes gets somewhat messy (Figure 3.1).

3.1. Basic Anatomy of the Human Body

Learning Outcome

1. Learn about major organ systems involved in anesthesia.
2. Describe the anatomical landmarks relevant to anesthesia administration.
3. Understand the variations in anatomy among patients.

The human body plan has an enormous amount to do with how anesthesia is achieved. At the very center of it all is the nervous system—that is, the brain and spinal cord—that controls just about every function and reacts to any message it receives. Anesthetic medications can disturb the applecart by changing our state of awareness and also altering pain sensitivity. Anesthesiologists make most decisions based on knowing how these nerve signals travel in order to figure out what drugs to give and in what amounts since each person can respond differently. As surgical techniques continue to evolve, even an approximate guide to our anatomy enables doctors to customize treatments, reduce risks, and have patients recovering more easily—all of this revealing just how intertwined our body's structure and the practice of anesthesia are. You also cannot overlook the significance of the musculoskeletal system. Not only does this system provide the body with shape and allow us to move, but it also protects major organs. The balance of muscle tone and proper depth of anesthesia is precarious at best, particularly in procedures in which muscle relaxation is of the utmost importance. Since anesthetic medications can disturb the way nerves communicate with muscles, both the direct impact of the medications and the recovery afterwards are affected. More frequently than not, this likewise implies that one size fits all simply won't do—individualized patient determinants like body mass index and where muscles are situated turn into significant details.

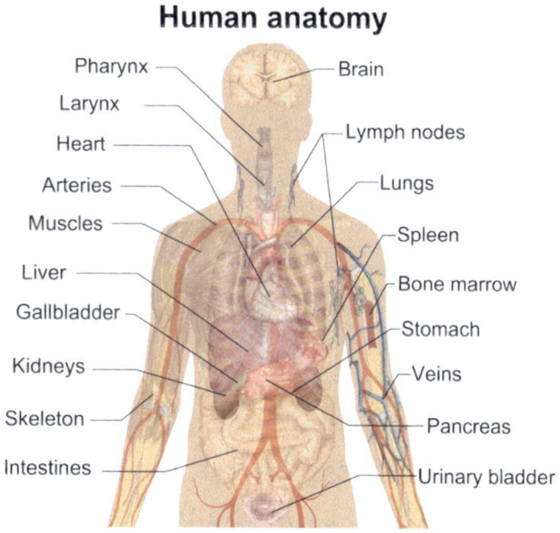

Figure 3.2. Anatomy of the human body.

Source: https://en.wikipedia.org/wiki/File:Man_shadow_anatomy.png.

Those sorts of things get double-checked and triple-checked to ensure the anesthetic plan is individualized and addresses complications more effectively. And then there is the circulatory system, which is responsible for distributing the anesthetic. The heart and its extensive network of arteries and veins deliver these medications to all parts of the body. Considering how the blood vessels are structured, along with factors like blood volume and heart output, can be a lifesaver for anesthesiologists. Without taking into account individual variations or pre-existing heart issues, unforeseen cardiovascular complications can develop. New technology—like 3D printing individualized anatomical models—

highlights how much precise anatomical maps are worth for preoperative planning and tailoring treatments (Aimar et al., 2019). Overall, a solid grasp of basic anatomy is crucial for anesthesiologists who wish to administer safe, effective anesthesia that is adapted to the unique physiological structure of each patient (Stout et al., 2018) (Figure 3.2).

3.1.1. Major organ Systems Involved in Anesthesia

Anesthesia works by acting together with our major organ systems, preparing the body for surgery and regulating its response in the meantime. The brain, being a component of the central nervous system, generally gets most of the drugs' attention—knocking you unconscious and anesthetizing pain. For the most part, the way the brain orchestrates sensory input gets a bit unhinged under anesthesia, and both your voluntary and automatic responses tend to shut down. And then there's the spinal cord; it tends to conduct pain messages, but local anesthetics can be of assistance by blocking those pathways exactly where needed.

It is still very important to monitor the brain activity in order to get a reading of consciousness levels and keep the patient safe from start to finish. The heart and blood vessels aren't immune to these changes either. Anesthetic medications tend to illicit a mixed bag of responses: sometimes your heartbeat is different, blood pressure is altered, and circulation in general goes off on its own little tangent. What happens is a form of vasodilation—, the vessels expand, which can reduce the blood pressure enough to be problematic, especially when there are other heart issues already involved. It also occurs that it is necessary to monitor the heart's rhythm and how well blood is being circulated in order to maintain stability. All in all, the way these drugs interact with the cardiovascular system underlines why understanding these twists and turns matters when trying to avoid risks. Breathing is another big piece of the puzzle. With many anesthetic agents, there's a natural dampening of the urge to breathe, so doctors step in with controlled ventilation to make sure you're still getting enough air. The whole idea is to keep oxygen levels stable and prevent problems like airway blockages—nothing too serious, but still important. And these drugs can mess around with how our lungs move air and exchange gases. Monitoring things like respiratory rate, tidal volume, and even arterial blood gases keeps any hiccups from getting out of control. Briefly, a sense of how lung function and anesthetics combine is the most important thing for ensuring surgical results are as optimal as possible (Figure 3.3).

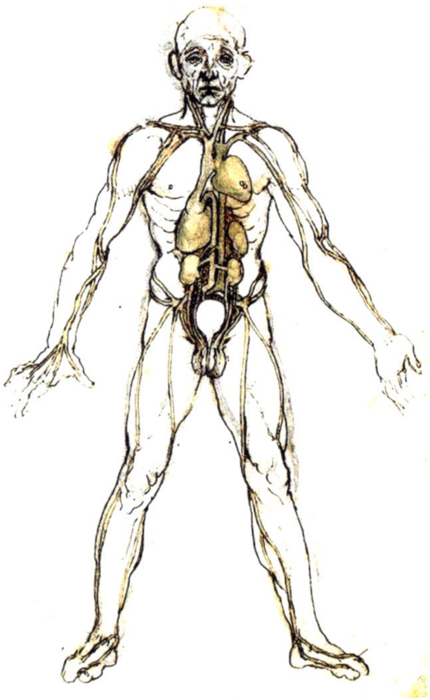

Figure 3.3. Organ systems in humans.

Source: By Leonardo da Vinci - https://www.metmuseum.org/special/Leonardo_Master_Draftsman/tour_gallery4.htm, Public Domain, https://commons.wikimedia.org/w/index.php?curid=1744423.

3.1.2. Anatomical Landmarks Relevant to Anesthesia Administration

Anesthesia hinges on knowing the body's landmarks. Medical professionals get a boost when they understand where key points lie, which helps them deliver regional anesthesia (RA) in a safe and effective way. Take Bennetts wallabies, for instance—experts have altered traditional anesthesia methods for these macropods using detailed anatomical observations. Dental blocks like the infraorbital and maxillary ones borrow ideas from old-school techniques used in domestic animals, proving that a good grasp of anatomy can open doors to treating different species. This all shows that having precise markers boosts pain management and post-op care in veterinary work, playing a crucial role in administering anesthesia (Walker et al., 2023). Spinal anesthesia (SA) in people works on the same principle. It depends a lot on finding the right anatomical landmarks for placing needles accurately and reducing on risks. In most cases, whether the approach is intrathecal or epidural, it all comes down to knowing the twists and turns of the spinal canal—especially since the end of the spinal cord can vary from one person to the next. Even though high-tech imaging helps reveal these nuances, the classic landmarks still matter. Familiarity with vertebral levels for common procedures is key to dodging serious issues like nerve damage (Imbelloni et al., 2023). In the end, a solid anatomical knowledge remains vital in both human and animal anesthesia. Kids and older patients add another layer of complexity. In younger ones, the size and layout of body structures can be quite different from adults, so adjustments in RA are a must. Even among seniors, natural changes—such as stiffer spines or altered vertebral shapes—mean that careful landmark mapping is essential before any procedure. Generally speaking, when practitioners mind these variations and lean on anatomical landmarks, they can make anesthesia safer and more efficient across different patient groups (Imbelloni et al., 2023).

3.1.3. Variations in Anatomy Among Patients

Patients show a lot of unique anatomical differences that can complicate anesthesia. Age, gender, ethnicity, and overall health all play a part, and it's not unusual for the airway structure to surprise clinicians—sometimes making intubation a tricky affair. Arteries and veins, too, often stray from what one might expect, which in turn can disturb RA or make vascular access more challenging. In most cases, grasping these nuances is vital, because the proper delivery of oxygen and nutrients (and the removal of waste) hinges on how well these features align with blood flow and nerve function (Claassen et al., 2021). When it comes to RA, the individual quirks of a patient can lead to varied outcomes in both effectiveness and safety. For example, if the spaces between the vertebrae are a bit wider or the epidural area lies deeper than usual, the spread of anesthetic might not be as even, affecting pain control. Sometimes, congenital issues or spinal malformations call for a customized approach—this can complicate what would otherwise be a routine technique. Generally speaking, handling these cases demands not only technical skill but also a solid understanding of basic physiology, since a small error might result in poor anesthesia or other complications during surgery. Anesthesiologists, therefore, often turn to imaging studies and detailed textbooks to help them anticipate such variations (Vatansever et al., 2020). Anatomical quirks can throw a wrench into the smooth delivery of anesthesia and even increase the risk of surgery complications. Think about it: if the branching of arteries isn't quite standard, it may hamper how anesthetic drugs flow, altering both their distribution and metabolism. Likewise, if a patient's anatomy doesn't match expected norms, there's a higher chance of nerve injury during peripheral nerve blocks (PNBs)—

underscoring the need for careful technique. The way every patient responds to anesthesia often ties back to these differences, adding another layer of complexity to managing doses safely. By mixing detailed anatomical insights with personalized evaluations, clinicians can boost both effectiveness and safety. Ultimately, appreciating these natural variations helps bridge the gap between surgical goals and successful anesthesia outcomes, paving the way for better patient care (Claassen et al., 2021).

Test Your Knowledge

1. What are the major organ systems involved in anesthesia?
2. What are anatomical landmarks relevant to anesthesia administration?

3.2. Physiology of the Nervous System

Learning Outcome

1. Understand the role of the central nervous system in anesthesia.
2. Describe the peripheral nervous system and its significance.
3. Understand the mechanisms of pain perception and modulation.

Neural activity and blood flow share a bond that's pretty crucial for keeping the brain working at its best. CBF pushes oxygen and nutrients around while taking out the trash—in other words, the metabolic waste gets cleared away concurrently. The brain, being as delicate as it is, can suffer if that balance falters; even a small drop in blood supply might injure nerve cells and mess with cognition. In most cases, knowing how the brain's energy demands and blood circulation team up becomes vital in anesthesia since the drugs used can sometimes twist vessel behavior. Doctors often need to keep these bodily mechanisms in mind, especially during surgery, to dodge any harmful side effects. Different ways to manage CBF, like the ever-popular neurovascular coupling, even now remain a focal point in research trying to curb anesthesia complications. Another part of brain physiology that shouldn't be overlooked is the glymphatic system—it acts as the brain's very cleanup crew. Unlike the standard lymphatic pathways, this glial-dependent network uses cerebrospinal fluid to sweep away metabolic byproducts and other soluble waste. The discovery of this system has turned heads in understanding brain diseases, particularly because its cleaning efficiency seems to dip with age. This fact is especially important for anesthesiologists, as many anesthetic compounds can alter how cerebrospinal fluid moves, thereby affecting waste clearance. A system that isn't functioning at its peak may even hasten cognitive decline or other neurological set-backs, which only stresses the need to nurture its operation during anesthesia.

In many cases, further research into this area could reveal fresh strategies for keeping the brain's performance intact through better waste management. On top of all that, the body's reaction to anesthesia can spark some tangled neurovascular interactions. Anesthetics are known to change neurotransmitter levels and alter how blood vessels tighten or relax, which can upset the brain's built-in ability to regulate blood flow. For instance, some agents might trigger unexpected vasodilation or vasoconstriction, thereby shifting the supply of essential nutrients to neural tissues. Generally speaking, understanding these interactions is not just necessary to ensure the brain gets its fair share of blood—it also helps lower risks of nerve damage after surgery. Meanwhile, as new details about neurovascular coupling keep coming to light, anesthesiologists are slowly, but surely, incorporating these insights into day-to-day practice. All things considered, by paying proper attention to how anesthesia affects the nervous system, practitioners can better optimize outcomes even if, at times, the process might seem a bit unpredictable (Figure 3.4).

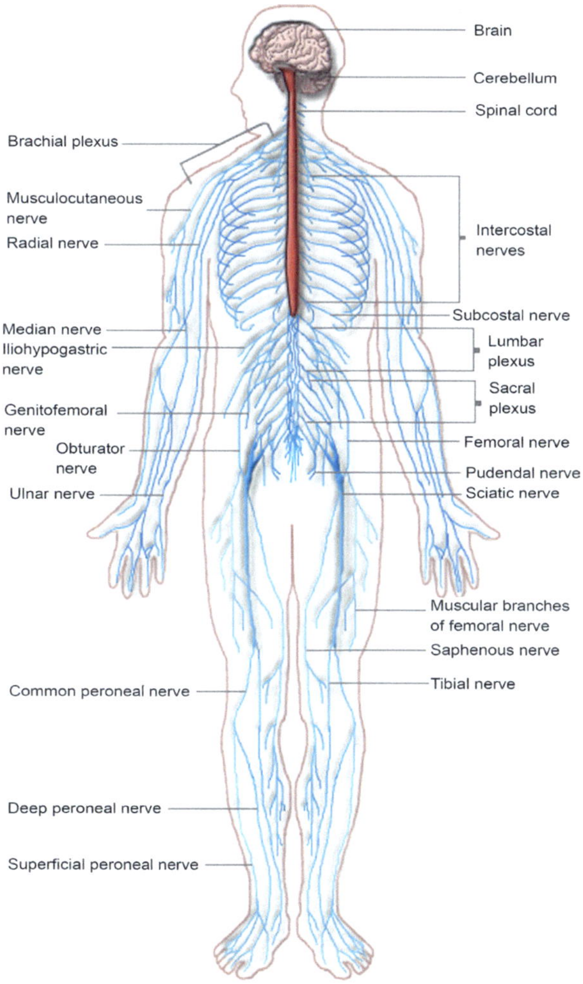

Figure 3.4. Nervous system.

Source: https://en.wikipedia.org/wiki/File:Nervous_system_diagram.png.

3.2.1. Role of the Central Nervous System in Anesthesia

Anesthesia's impact on our awareness ties back to how our central nervous system functions in an intricate way. The brain and spinal cord handle signals for both what we sense and how we move, which, in most cases, means our body responds naturally to what's happening around us. It's not hard to see that many anesthetics zero in on particular receptors and neurotransmitter systems – in fact, when the GABA receptors get activated, they tend to boost inhibitory signals and give rise to a sedative, almost numbing, effect. This kind of cascade not only shows us how these drugs pull us into unconsciousness but also nudges us to wonder about the basic physiological processes that keep this altered state going during procedures. There's another layer, too – the way the brain manages its blood flow. CBF is essential since it matches the brain's need for oxygen and nutrients, especially when consciousness is in flux. A little imbalance here can create problems like ischemia or other neurological hiccups.

So, anesthetics have to be dosed just right to keep brain metabolism stable, even as awareness changes. Without this delicate control, pushing someone into a state of GA might risk important functions, reminding anesthesiologists to stay sharp about how cerebral physiology works (Claassen et al., 2021). Taking a broader look, evolution also offers clues about how consciousness shows up in the CNS. Comparative research hints that the midbrain plays a key role by nearly "simulating" an integrated picture of the body's state in relation to its surroundings—a kind of baseline for what we experience subjectively. Remarkably, even simpler organisms sport similar structures, underscoring that our central nervous system has long been central to how consciousness develops. These insights raise some fascinating, if not challenging, questions about anesthesia's role in altering our subjective experience. They encourage healthcare pros to not only focus on the biochemical details but also consider the wider effects of altered awareness, a perspective that can ultimately refine patient care and surgical outcomes (Barron et al., 2016) (Figure 3.5).

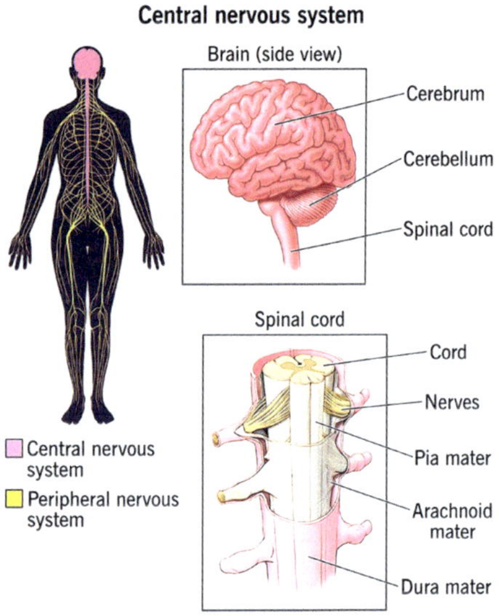

Figure 3.5. Central nervous system.

Source: https://my.clevelandclinic.org/-/scassets/images/org/health/articles/central-nervous-system.

3.2.2. Peripheral Nervous System and Its Significance

The peripheral nervous system's many parts shape how we sense the world and move around, which matters a lot in areas like anesthesia. It sends signals from the brain out to every corner of the body, making sure that reactions to touch or pain come in fast and in sync. In most cases, knowing just how these nerves carry pain and sensory clues helps doctors figure out the best way to put someone under. When anesthesiologists work out the twisty paths these nerves take, they can target specific spots to control pain and even improve how surgeries go. All in all, getting a solid grip on how the PNS is laid out is key to keeping patients safe and comfortable during operations. The PNS isn't just about carrying touch or movement messages—it also looks after those automatic body functions. Its branch that handles involuntary actions keeps things like the heartbeat, digestion, and even blood vessel widening in check. During an operation, it becomes pretty important to keep things balanced by watching over these automatic responses because even a small glitch can mess with heart or lung function. Sometimes, the drugs used can change that natural tone, so a careful understanding of this whole system helps avoid unexpected issues. In general, having a deep knowledge of these nerve pathways is crucial for delivering safe, reliable care when patients are anesthetized.

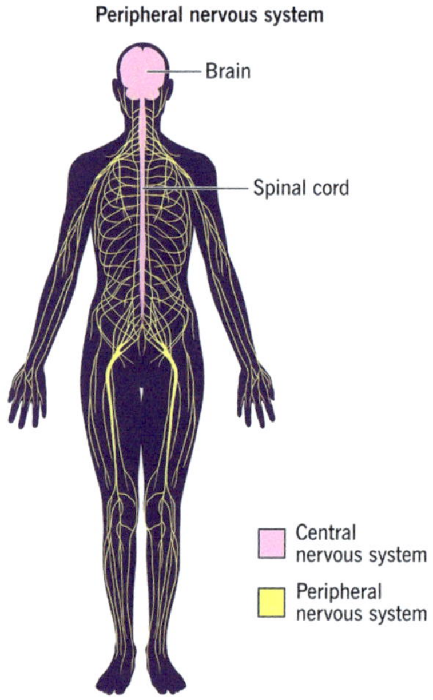

Figure 3.6. Peripheral nervous system.

Source: https://my.clevelandclinic.org/-/scassets/images/org/health/articles/23123-peripheral-nervous-system.

Recent practical studies have shown over and over how vital the PNS is in many clinical setups—anesthesia being a big one. For example, using animal models such as swine, which share many similarities with humans (as noted in comparative studies (Swindle et al., 2011), has given new insights that help refine anesthetic methods. These kinds of parallels let clinicians adjust techniques originally tested on animals for human treatments. As more research focuses on how peripheral nerves impact conditions like chronic pain, the role of the PNS in both everyday care and experimental work keeps growing. This emerging body of evidence generally underscores why weaving a strong understanding of the PNS into anesthesia protocols sparks innovative strategies that ultimately boost patient outcomes and overall care during surgery (Figure 3.6).

3.2.3. Mechanisms of Pain Perception and Modulation

Pain isn't just a simple signal—it's a messy conversation between our body and mind. Nerve routes known as nociceptive pathways carry messages right from our tissues up into the brain, but these signals don't travel in a vacuum. Instead, a mix of natural chemicals like neurotransmitters and neuropeptides—and sometimes a sprinkle of substance P together with calcitonin gene-related peptide—can crank these messages up or tone them down unexpectedly. When these agents trigger heightened sensitivity in the nerve cells, our experience of pain intensifies. In most cases, getting a handle on these messengers is especially important when it comes to anesthesia since a slight alter in the way pain is regulated might directly impact how patients recover after surgery. Clearly, the tug-of-war between peripheral signals and central processing underscores just how complicated managing pain can be. Hormones add another twist to the pain story, especially during pregnancy, when shifts in the body seem to throw curveballs at pain sensitivity. Researchers generally speaking have noticed that hormones like progesterone and oxytocin may actually help ease pain—observations often noted after a cesarean, for example. That said, the evidence isn't completely settled yet; there are still questions about exactly how these hormones alter the nerve signals, and why some individuals seem to benefit while others don't. This ongoing debate, with its occasional inconsistencies, opens the door for tailoring pain relief strategies specifically for obstetric care. In most cases, these hormonal effects offer a promising, if not entirely clear, opportunity to refine how we handle anesthesia during pregnancy. There's more complexity when you consider conditions such as Sickle Cell Disease (SCD), where long-term pain seems to dance to a different tune. Chronic pain in these patients can hinge on shifting CBF and changes in hemoglobin levels—two factors that might work together in unpredictable ways. Recent work suggests that differences in blood flow can drive alterations in pain perception, all while hemoglobin levels add another layer of variation. And don't forget the way genotypic differences among SCD patients can further complicate this picture—these small variations can change how pain is felt and managed. With so many moving parts, a deeper understanding of these intertwined factors might help medical professionals develop more personalized anesthesia and pain management approaches for people with SCD, ultimately leading to care that fits the individual a little better.

Test Your Knowledge

1. Describe the role of the central nervous system in anesthesia.
2. What is peripheral nervous system?

3.3. Cardiovascular System and Anesthesia

Learning Outcome

1. Describe the heart anatomy and its function during anesthesia.
2. Understand blood pressure regulation and its implications.
3. Describe the effects of anesthetic agents on cardiovascular dynamics.

The heart stands front and center during anesthesia—a fact that can't be ignored when surgeries are underway. Even though it might sound routine, those caring for patients need to know the ins and outs of the heart's layout and function, especially when conditions like tricuspid regurgitation (TR) show up. TR is pretty common in older folks and tends to overload the heart with extra volume, which in turn adds stress and complicates matters when it comes to managing anesthesia. Often, this means a closer look is needed before surgery, with extra checks on metabolism and cardiac function (Praz et al., 2021). In many cases, the way cardiovascular issues mix with anesthesia risks can catch even experienced providers off guard, making it crucial to keep an eye on fluid balances and overall heart stability to avoid bad outcomes. Anesthesia doesn't just put patients to sleep—it also deeply affects how blood flows through the body. The brain, for one, relies on a delicate mix of oxygen in and waste out, and a steady flow is key to keeping things running smoothly. When anesthetic agents are used, they can disrupt this balance, causing changes in what we call CBF that might even lead to some neurological hiccups after surgery (Claassen et al., 2021). In most cases, having a good grasp of how CBF is controlled gives anesthesiologists the tools they need to alter blood flow during procedures. By carefully adjusting the pressure and pace of blood circulation, doctors can lower the risk of brain issues, especially in those patients who already have heart problems. Teamwork in the operating room is another big piece of the puzzle. Often, it's not just the anesthesiologist but also cardiologists and surgeons who need to join forces to take on patients with heart complications. Recent developments—like transcatheter tricuspid valve interventions— show why a well-coordinated heart team consultation is needed before any procedure starts (Praz et al., 2021). This kind of joint effort, with everyone following a flexible but thoughtful screening process, helps anesthesiologists handle the tricky parts of cardiovascular abnormalities. In the end, bringing together different perspectives not only fine-tunes anesthetic care but also paves the way for better long-term outcomes, proving that understanding the heart in every detail is essential during anesthesia (Figure 3.7).

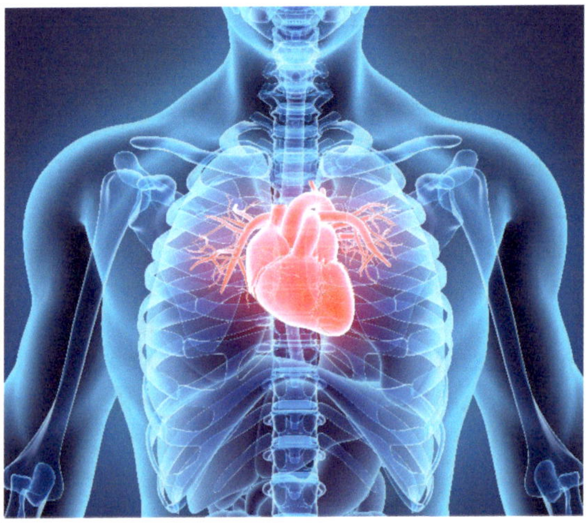

Figure 3.7. Cardiovascular system.

Source: https://img.livestrong.com/-/clsd/getty/edb7284fbbc14a3f83136d387d3183f1.

3.3.1. Heart Anatomy and Its Function During Anesthesia

The heart works in a surprisingly intricate way to keep our bodies steady when anesthesia is in play. Its chambers—both atria and ventricles—each have their part in moving blood, which in turn affects overall cardiac output and how well the body gets supplied with blood. For example, the right atrium picks up deoxygenated blood from the body via the superior and inferior vena cavae and then passes it to the right ventricle. Anesthesia can change blood volume and the tone of blood vessels, and these shifts may upset that flow, so monitoring the heart's function is crucial. The electrical system, which essentially conducts the heartbeat, might also act a bit differently under anesthetic drugs. Generally speaking, grasping how these dynamics work is key to preventing complications—especially in patients already dealing with heart issues—and it makes thorough preoperative checks necessary. As anesthesia deepens, various drugs start influencing both the heart's pace and the strength of its contractions. Some agents encourage vasodilation, allowing blood vessels to relax, while others push them towards vasoconstriction, mixing up the preload and afterload on the heart. For instance, many general anesthetics tend to drop systemic vascular resistance; this can lower blood pressure and might compromise the blood flow to key organs. This is especially worrisome for patients with preexisting issues like atrial fibrillation or heart failure. In most cases, managing such delicate situations requires a solid understanding of heart anatomy and its function. Monitors are typically used to keep a continuous check on cardiac performance, allowing clinicians to adjust anesthetic dosing on the fly to ensure organs receive enough blood and to reduce any risks during the perioperative phase. There's also the side of things dealing with certain anatomical details, such as valve performance and coronary circulation, which play a big role during anesthesia. Leaky valves or those narrowed by stenosis can create an imbalance that leads to instability during a procedure, forcing anesthetists to alter their methods accordingly. And then, those coronary arteries—delivering oxygen-rich blood to the myocardium—are vital; reduced blood flow can trigger cardiac ischemia, particularly in patients with atherosclerotic conditions. Understanding these heart details not only helps foresee potential issues but also guides which anesthetic techniques and medications to pick. Extra care in watching coronary blood flow and taking steps to prevent ischemia are central during anesthesia-driven procedures. In this context, the interplay of heart structure and function is a big deal, making a tailored anesthetic strategy essential for optimal outcomes (Hilscher et al., 2022; Joglar et al., 2023) (Figure 3.8).

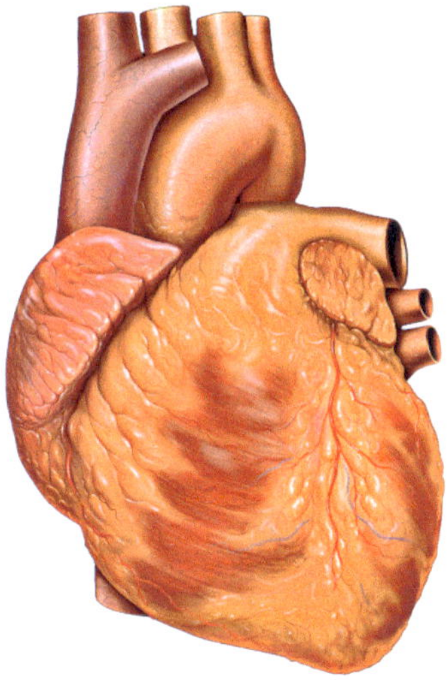

Figure 3.8. Heart anterior exterior view.

Source: https://upload.wikimedia.org/wikipedia/commons/1/1b/Heart_anterior_exterior_view.png.

3.3.2. Blood Pressure Regulation and Its Implications

Blood pressure regulation is a complex beast—a process that is crucial for keeping our circulation in check during anesthesia. The autonomic nervous system handles much of the heavy lifting here, mixing control over heart function and keeping our body temperature steady. When patients are under anesthesia, their bodies might not adjust to sudden shifts in blood pressure, especially when drugs that change blood vessel tone come into play. This lack of balance can lead to poor tissue perfusion and sometimes results in pretty serious issues during an operation. Older patients, in most cases, are even more vulnerable since their physiological reserves tend to wane, pushing complications over the edge. Recent studies even hint that blood pressure control and thermoregulation often share common ground (Giersch et al., 2024). Looking at the bigger picture, understanding how blood pressure is managed isn't just about handling the operating room drama; it goes far beyond that. Conditions like orthostatic hypotension are especially tricky, with patients on anesthesia sometimes suffering from a compromised autonomic response. Anesthesia can mess up the body's natural balancing act, causing instability when someone shifts position suddenly.

This risk, needless to say, is heightened among older folks who typically have a less robust reaction to gravitational changes. Some researchers now talk about various blood pressure profiles, including what's been dubbed orthostatic hypertension, which has become a real clinical concern (Owen et al., 2024). In most cases, grasping these bodily responses helps doctors predict and prevent potential hiccups during anesthesia. Then there's the whole matter of biological sex influencing blood pressure regulation—a factor that further complicates patient care when anesthesia enters the scene. Emerging work generally shows that our responses to stress, including fluctuations in blood pressure and temperature control, often differ between genders. This isn't a minor detail; it means that anesthetic plans sometimes need to be altered just a bit to fit individual needs. For example, women might react differently to heat exposure, which in turn can affect how they process anesthetic drugs and maintain cardiovascular stability. Such discoveries remind us that labeling one sex as having an advantage is an oversimplification; instead, a nuanced approach that considers the individual is key. Ultimately, knowing the ins and outs of blood pressure dynamics plays a major role in boosting surgical outcomes (Giersch et al., 2024) (Figure 3.9).

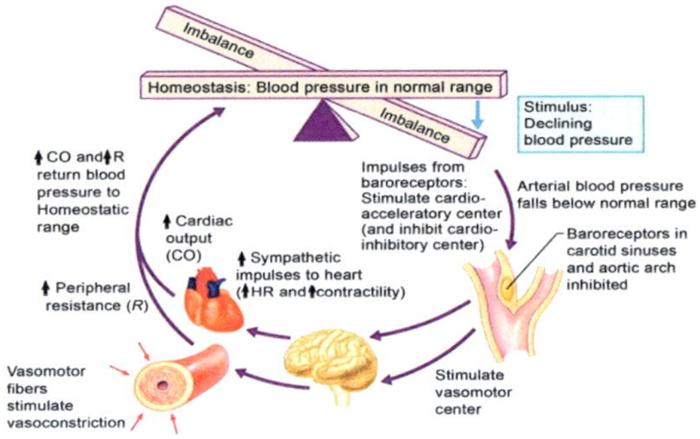

Figure 3.9. Regulation of blood pressure.

Source: https://i.ytimg.com/vi/anEyOM-EPDE/maxresdefault.jpg.

3.3.3. Effects of Anesthetic Agents on Cardiovascular Dynamics

Anesthetic agents have a strong impact on cardiovascular function – they change how the heart beats and how blood flows through the body. Take, for example, volatile drugs; when the dose goes up, these agents tend to relax the blood vessels, which drops blood pressure. This isn't just a neat scientific fact – in many cases, it means extra caution is needed, especially for older folks or those with already sensitive heart conditions. A full check-up before surgery and constant attention to blood pressure and heart signals are crucial, and tailoring the anesthesia plan to each patient's unique situation becomes key, as pointed out in recent reviews on perioperative care practices (Shaji et al., 2024). But there's more to it than just adjusting the flow. Beyond shifting blood dynamics (or hemodynamic behavior, which means how blood circulates), these agents also affect the heart's overall performance and even metabolic responses. Some drugs might nudge the heart's electrical patterns enough to trigger arrhythmias – that is, irregular heartbeats – and this risk is especially high for patients with conditions like ischemic heart disease or heart failure. In most cases, anesthesiologists have to know how these drugs travel through the body – how they distribute, break down, and exit – because each patient's physiology adds its twist to the story. Generally speaking, understanding this mix helps practitioners manage the tricky aspects of surgery more effectively (Alwahbi et al., 2024). The challenge ramps up further with burn injuries. Burn patients often face severe blood loss and unexpected shifts in how their blood vessels react, which can push the cardiovascular system into a state of crisis. In these situations, doctors must watch hemodynamic signs like heart rate and blood pressure especially carefully – and be ready to adjust fluid resuscitation tactics on the fly. Sometimes, the very anesthetic chosen could worsen a feeble heart or reduce the body's response to fluids, making things even riskier. All this means that anesthesiologists have to pine over the unique changes burns cause, selecting drugs and techniques that best match those specific needs. Teamwork across different specialties, and a careful, patient-focused approach, become vital to steer such cases safely (Alwahbi et al., 2024).

Test Your Knowledge

1. What is the function of the heart anatomy?
2. What are the regulations of blood pressure?

3.4. Respiratory System Considerations

Learning Outcome

1. Describe the anatomy of the respiratory tract relevant to intubation.
2. Describe the gas exchange processes and anesthetic implications.
3. Learn about the impact of anesthesia on respiratory function.

The breathing system is at the heart of anesthesia – it keeps oxygen flowing to our cells while clearing out carbon dioxide, which in most cases helps balance our body's acid-base levels. Oxygen fuels cell metabolism, and even a small disruption in how air moves or blood flows can trigger complications like hypoxia or breathing difficulties. Anesthesiologists need to keep in mind that the lungs handle a lot of work during procedures, especially when patients already have breathing issues. Variations in things like airway shape or lung mechanics only add another twist, guiding doctors to adjust their approach to airway care and ventilation. In most cases, knowing your respiratory physiology inside and out is what sets the stage for a smooth, successful anesthesia. Picking the right anesthetic drugs and techniques often comes down to how well the lungs can cope. For example, some agents that tend to depress breathing need to be used very carefully in patients with chronic lung problems or obesity – these drugs can sometimes further slow breathing down. Neuromuscular blocking agents are another tricky piece of the puzzle since they can dampen the work of key muscles like the diaphragm and intercostals, meaning that close (and sometimes inconsistent) monitoring of muscle signals is necessary. Before a procedure, assessing things like forced vital capacity and peak flow rates gives providers a clearer picture of lung function; these preoperative checks are repeated over and over to help predict complications such as atelectasis or infections. All told, weaving respiratory function assessments into the pre-surgery routine plays a huge part in guiding the best outcomes. After the procedure, keeping an eye on the breathing system remains critical during the recovery phase. It's not uncommon for early signs of airway blockage or slow breathing—sometimes even a bit of hypoventilation—to crop up, which can jeopardize recovery. Particularly for folks with pre-existing lung issues or who have undergone lengthy surgeries, respiratory failure becomes a serious risk. Steps like supplementing oxygen and employing physical therapy may ease these risks by boosting lung compliance and promoting better gas exchange. Moreover, protocols that encourage early movement and the use of incentive spirometry often help the lungs bounce back faster. In most cases, understanding how anesthetic techniques mesh with the quirks of respiratory physiology is key to post-op care and minimizing unwanted complications (Figure 3.10).

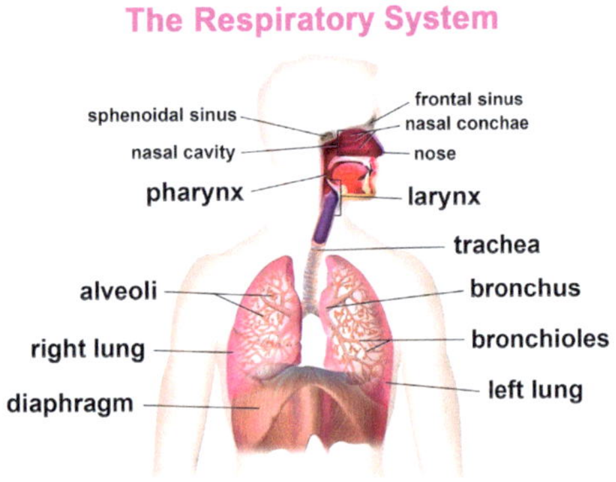

Figure 3.10. Respiratory system.

Source: https://i.ytimg.com/vi/ZB7uA5o0mS4/maxresdefault.jpg.

3.4.1. Anatomy of the Respiratory Tract Relevant to Intubation

The respiratory tract's detailed layout matters when it comes to intubation—small differences in anatomy can change the whole game. Typically, the route starts at the nostrils, winds through the throat and voice box (that's the larynx), then the trachea, and finally splits into the bronchi that lead to the lungs. The voice box itself is key since it acts like a gatekeeper, stopping food or other objects from slipping down the windpipe when swallowing. Knowing exactly how things are arranged around the larynx is important because even a bit of swelling or an unusual structure can throw off intubation. In many cases, landmarks like the anterior commissure and cricoid cartilage give a sort of natural guide, helping clinicians figure out the right angle toward the vocal cords while lowering the risk of accidental injury during this delicate task. Another twist in the whole process comes from differences in the size and position of structures like the epiglottis and the cricoid ring. The epiglottis, which looks a bit like a leaf tucked behind the tongue's root, can either open the way to the vocal cords or block it, all depending on its tilt and movement. Sometimes, a longer or even slightly swollen epiglottis can make things trickier, so anesthetists need to keep an eye out for those differences. Similarly, the cricoid ring plays an important part by acting as a marker during intubation, although its exact placement might vary. Then there's the trachea—a narrow, funnel-shaped tube—that adds another layer of challenge, meaning that understanding its form is generally crucial to performing intubation without harming nearby tissues. All in all, a solid grasp of these details usually helps to manage difficult airway scenarios much better. Before starting intubation, a careful check and some pre-planning are a must, especially when it comes to the nuances of airway anatomy. Imaging tools like 3D models of a patient's airway help in visualizing and even rehearsing the procedure ahead of time, which can reveal tricky variations that a simple exam might miss. Lately, simulation technology has upped the training game by creating realistic scenarios that mimic a variety of anatomical challenges. Generally speaking, this level of preparation is vital in critical care settings, where every moment and each decision count. By combining these visual aids and hands-on simulations with thorough planning, clinicians not only build confidence but also reduce risks linked to intubation, thereby boosting overall patient safety during anesthesia administration (Adams et al., 2018; Jarosław et al., 2022) (Figure 3.11).

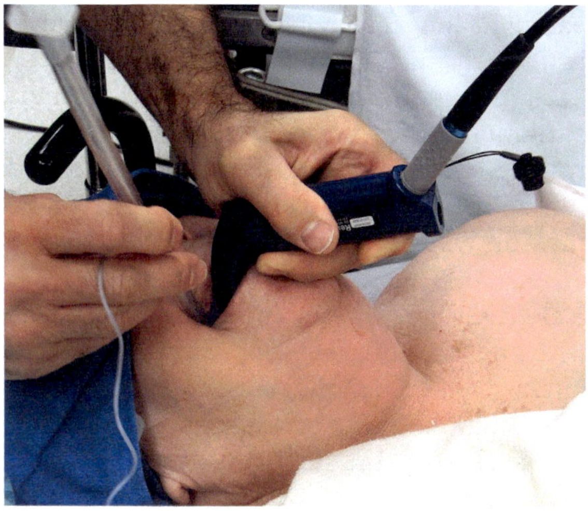

Figure 3.11. Understanding airway anatomy for intubation.

Source: By work by DiverDave (talk) (Transferred by PhilippN/Original uploaded by DiverDave) - I (DiverDave (talk)) created this work entirely by myself. (Original uploaded on en.wikipedia), CC BY 3.0, https://commons.wikimedia.org/w/index.php?curid=12052019.

3.4.2. Gas Exchange Processes and Anesthetic Implications

Gas exchange isn't just a textbook process—it's something anesthesiologists have to stay on top of, especially when patients bring their unique twists. The respiratory system just moves oxygen in and gets carbon dioxide out, a simple diffusion trick across the alveolar-capillary border. Yet, things can go awry during anesthesia, particularly with folks who already have breathing issues or when one-lung ventilation comes into play. Surgeries can shake up how lungs work; for instance, a thoracotomy might limit the lung's natural expansion and, as a consequence, upset the balance of ventilation and blood flow, ultimately affecting both anesthetic choices and outcomes (Murray-Torres et al., 2021). In most cases, it's a reminder that we shouldn't sweat the small stuff—often, these shifts in lung mechanics tell the bigger story of how surgery and respiratory physiology are tangled together. When it comes to anesthesia, patient details like obesity matter more than we sometimes think. Obese patients tend to have a lower functional reserve, which means oxygen levels can drop fast during induction. This quick plunge in saturation might even trigger complications like atelectasis if not managed just right. Because of this, tailored anesthetic plans are key—using non-invasive positive pressure ventilation during pre-oxygenation and, later on, alveolar recruitment maneuvers following intubation tend to help keep oxygen in a safer range. Several studies suggest that these interventions generally bring better oxygenation throughout surgery (Smith et al., 2017). So, it becomes clear that a layered, multifaceted approach is needed to tackle the risks that come with compromised gas exchange. The situation gets even more complex with different kinds of surgeries and specific patient conditions, as seen with children undergoing thoracic procedures. Kids naturally bring developmental differences in both anatomy and physiology, which makes the usual gas exchange process a bit trickier during anesthesia. Their lungs, being structured and functioning differently, leave them more prone to bouts of hypoxia during operations like mediastinoscopy or thoracoscopy. It's important—if not essential—for anesthesiologists to pick up on these nuances so that ventilation can be adjusted to ensure enough oxygen reaches where it's needed. Recognizing and working through these pediatric challenges ultimately helps clinicians tailor anesthetic plans that promote safety and work effectively during every stage of the perioperative period (Murray-Torres et al., 2021) (Figure 3.12).

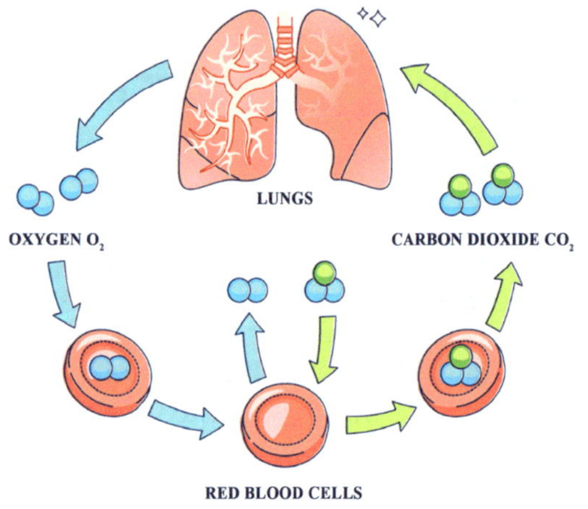

Figure 3.12. Gas exchange processes.

Source: https://www.respiratorytherapyzone.com/wp-content/uploads/2022/04/Gas-exchange-process-vector-illustration.png.

3.4.3. Impact of Anesthesia on Respiratory Function

GA tends to mess with how our body systems work together, especially the way we breathe. The drugs used to knock you out usually slow down the brain, which in turn scrambles the normal process of gas exchange. When your breathing rate and the depth of each breath drop, there's a risk that air won't move in and out as smoothly as it should. In some cases, this can even let oxygen levels fall while carbon dioxide piles up—issues that need close watching. It helps to have a good look at someone's lung function before the procedure since individual differences can change how things unfold. Adjusting the breathing support during surgery makes a big difference in keeping things on track, which may boost recovery down the line. At times, anesthesia pushes the body to rely on machines, because natural breathing might take a back seat. When patients can't breathe adequately on their, mechanical ventilation comes into play—and it can change the game for both heart and lung behavior. In certain scenarios, particularly during long surgeries under GA, alternative methods like apneustic anesthesia ventilation (AAV) have been tried with some promise. Generally speaking, these methods seem to raise arterial oxygen levels and reduce down on wasted air in the lungs compared to conventional ventilation techniques (Le-Bert et al., 2024). It's a reminder that sometimes switching up how we support breathing can matter, given the unique respiratory quirks each patient may have. The breathing challenges don't just vanish when the surgery is over. Anesthesia-induced respiratory slowdown can stick around, sometimes lengthening recovery or even leading to issues like atelectasis or pneumonia—especially among those already at risk. Keeping a close eye on how someone breathes from the start of anesthesia through recovery helps catch and manage any slip-ups along the way. With a bit of altering—whether it's adjusting pain relief or changing how a patient is positioned after surgery—many of these issues can be lessened. In most cases, having a solid understanding of the lung's routine and how anesthesia interferes with it is key to smoothing out patient care and speeding up the overall recovery process (Lotfollahi, 2024).

Test Your Knowledge

1. What are the processes of gas exchange?
2. What is the impact of anesthesia on respiratory function?

3.5. Patient Assessment and Monitoring

Learning Outcome

1. Discuss preoperative assessment of anatomy and physiology.
2. Understand the monitoring techniques during anesthesia.
3. Learn about postoperative considerations related to anatomy and physiology.

A careful look at a patient's background is key when preparing for anesthesia. You start by diving straight into their medical past, a basic physical check, and noting any extra health issues that might complicate things. In many cases, anesthesiologists keep an eye out for heart, lung, or brain problems because these can change how the medication works. Kids, in particular, can be a whole different story—their bodies sometimes react in ways that aren't seen in adults, which means the checkups need to be even more detailed. Blending these assessments with an understanding of the natural differences in body structure and function helps craft a personalized anesthesia plan that generally boosts both safety and performance. And it all ties back to having an open chat with the patient and their family, ensuring they understand and agree with what's planned. Watching over vital signs during the procedure is just as important. Sometimes, it isn't only about tracking the heart rate, breathing, blood pressure, and oxygen levels but also about using fancy monitors to gather real-time data, especially when the surgery is a bit complicated. With these tools in hand, any sudden change can be spotted quickly. For younger patients—whose unique anatomy may cause rapid shifts in circulation—the vigilance has to be extra sharp. This way not only protects the patient but also gives the anesthesiologist the chance to make quick, informed calls throughout the operation. Measurements like end-tidal CO_2 and intra-arterial pressure, for instance, offer helpful insights into respiratory and circulatory health, nudging overall safety a step further. Since sedation and anesthesia come with their risks, it makes sense to have a step-by-step method for monitoring. This means checking the patient before the procedure, staying alert during the operation, and following up carefully once the anesthesia wears off. High-quality monitoring protocols pave the way for timely actions, and they help spot issues—like airway blockages or unstable blood flow—before they escalate. In most cases, especially with pediatric patients, using the right training and equipment for airway management is crucial, given that their smaller structures can lead to breathing hiccups. Also, ensuring proper staffing and consistent checks on the patient's body signs creates an environment where safety naturally takes priority. In most instances, sticking to evidence-based guidelines helps smooth out the process, cutting risks and steering patient outcomes in the right direction (Coté et al., 2019; Guerguerian et al., 2021) (Figure 3.13).

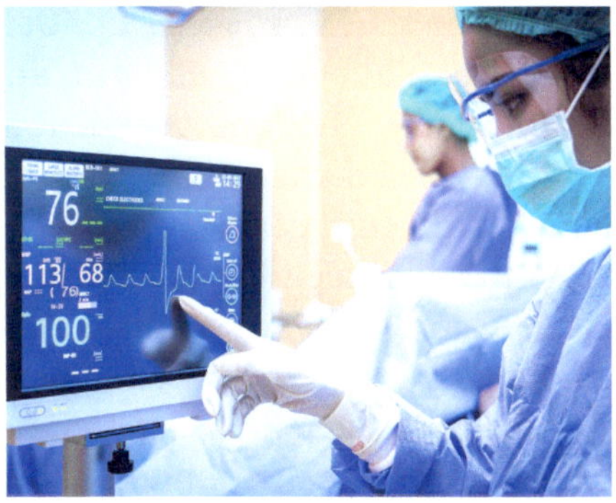

Figure 3.13. Anesthesia patient monitoring.

Source: https://www.apsf.org/wp-content/uploads/newsletters/2022/3701/anesthesia-patient-monitoring-featured.jpg.

3.5.1. Preoperative Assessment of Anatomy and Physiology

Before putting a patient under anesthesia, doctors take a deep look at both how the body is built and how it works. Checking the airway is one of those key spots – its little twists and variations can change how easy it is to secure breathing. Traditional ways of looking at the airway sometimes miss details, so ultrasound has come in as a neat, noninvasive alternative. It gives clinicians a live view of important bits like the epiglottis and vocal cords, and by measuring soft tissue thickness here and there, it can hint at when intubation might turn tricky. In many cases, this modern tool helps set the stage for safer outcomes and prompts a shift toward more flexible pre-operative routines (Zheng et al., 2019). The picture doesn't stop with the airway though. A patient's overall physiology also matters, especially for those with unique challenges like congenital heart defects. For example, individuals scheduled for procedures such as the Fontan operation—designed for those with a single ventricle—often battle elevated venous pressures and lower cardiac output. As survival rates improve, anesthesia providers find themselves juggling extra complexities from underlying heart issues, with complications like arrhythmias and ventricular dysfunction sometimes cropping up. Generally speaking, a detailed grasp of both anatomy and how the body functions goes a long way in fine-tuning anesthesia plans and curbing potential risks (Rychik et al., 2019). All of this also underlines the need for teamwork. When patients have more than one medical condition, anesthesiologists need to work hand-in-hand with other specialists to craft a plan that respects each limitation. For instance, understanding the subtle details of those who've had multiple heart interventions can steer choices in anesthetic techniques and monitoring. This blending of expertise often spots potential problems early—helping to keep complications at bay while supporting better overall recovery. In the end, a thoughtful pre-op evaluation that looks at both structure and function ensures that the diverse needs of patients are met with careful attention and a touch of flexibility.

3.5.2. Monitoring Techniques During Anesthesia

Anesthesia is complex, and when someone goes under, there's a lot to watch over to keep them safe. You've got heart rate, blood pressure, oxygen levels—in short, all those vital signs—and they're monitored almost non-stop to check on a patient's state. One tool that stands out here is end-tidal carbon dioxide ($ETCO_2$) monitoring, which offers immediate feedback on how well a patient is breathing and how their metabolism is doing. Fluctuations in $ETCO_2$ can sometimes signal ventilation slips or even heart issues, which, as many would say, calls for a swift reaction. These various checks not only help spot changes early on but also steer adjustments in anesthetic care throughout an operation; generally speaking, this underscores why modern anesthetic practice needs such all-around monitoring (Li et al., 2022). On a related note, beyond the standard measures, newer and advanced techniques have emerged—especially in complicated areas like neurosurgery. Take awake craniotomy (AC): when surgeons remove gliomas from critical brain regions, they might use either monitored anesthesia care (MAC) or what's sometimes called the asleep-awake-asleep (AAA) method. Each approach carries its unique set of bodily challenges. For example, blood gas readings and the chance of switching over to GA can differ quite a bit between them. In most cases, evidence hints that MAC might result in fewer post-surgery complications, which is one reason why many practitioners favor monitoring tailored to the specific surgical type and anesthetic strategy (Li et al., 2022). Mixing together various monitoring techniques further enhances patient care during anesthesia in surprising ways. Methods like cerebral cortical mapping and neuronavigation—tools you might think of as aiding surgery—also allow for close, real-time checks on neurological function, helping to reduce the risk of deficits after surgery. And then there are exciting tech boosts: wearable devices and even remote monitoring capabilities are slowly reshaping the field. There's even chatter about integrating artificial intelligence (AI) in the future, opening up new possibilities for even better oversight. All in all, these evolving strategies stress, yet again, how keeping up with technological advances is essential for safe and effective anesthetic care (Li et al., 2022) (Figure 3.14).

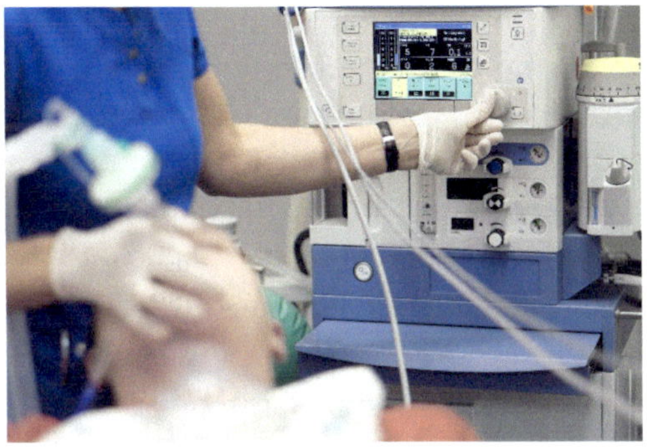

Figure 3.14. Monitoring techniques during anesthesia.

Source: https://cdn-assets.leister.com/pim/medias/17/04/77/170477.jpg.

3.5.3. Postoperative Considerations Related to Anatomy and Physiology

Understanding how our body's structure and functions intertwine with surgical outcomes is key to better recovery. After an operation, patients often notice shifts in how their bodies work, which can affect how fast or slow things get better. Take children, for instance – they sometimes have larger tonsils or other airway quirks that can make breathing trickier, meaning that the way airways are managed becomes a real concern. Because of these differences, a detailed check-up before surgery becomes a must, so any sedation or anesthesia risks are caught early, and the team is ready for any bumps along the way. Good recovery also leans on having staff who are comfortable with tools suited for different ages and sizes, showing how basic anatomy knowledge mixes with everyday clinical care to keep patients safe during their recovery (Coté et al., 2019). Not everybody reacts the same way after surgery—people's anatomical and physiological responses can vary surprisingly. Kids, especially, come with their challenges; since their systems are still growing, recovery times and complication rates don't always follow the usual script. Generally speaking, a higher rate of anesthesia-related issues in pediatrics pushes us to set up focused monitoring that can catch unexpected changes right away. Knowing these differences in depth helps clinicians decide on the right mix of pain relief, sedation, and the right moment to switch from close observation to sending someone home. This kind of deliberate, sometimes trial-and-error fine-tuning can lead to management strategies that put off complications and are likely to improve outcomes (Ferriero et al., 2019). Anesthetic choices don't exist in isolation—they connect with factors like hydration, electrolyte balance, and pain control, all of which tie back to a patient's basic anatomy and how their body functions. For example, noticing how the heart and lungs behave during recovery can prompt quick adjustments in fluid levels or pain meds, highlighting the value of close, ongoing monitoring. When surgical teams draw on a solid, sometimes even gut-level understanding of human anatomy, they're better at foreseeing potential issues and tailoring recovery plans accordingly. So, in most cases, bringing together both surgical and anesthesia insights into one team effort is key to achieving solid surgical results (Coté et al., 2019).

Test Your Knowledge

1. What are the different types of monitoring during anesthesia?
2. What are postoperative considerations related to anatomy and physiology?

SUMMARY

Understanding how our bodies are put together and how they operate together goes a long way towards making surgery safer, especially when an anesthetic is used. It's clear from the very start that having anesthesia right involves understanding your heart and lungs—the two sets of systems operating in equilibrium under the stress of drugs. Getting enough oxygen circulating and blood flowing is critical for safety; here, in most situations, even a minor mistake here can become a issue. Notably, Claassen et al. (2021) observe that one must monitor the brain's blood flow closely enough to satisfy its energy requirements—a subtlety that, if overlooked, could become a cause of neurological problems or postoperative complications. Taking this into account, the majority of practitioners of the healing art adjust their anesthetic practices to accommodate individual body idiosyncrasies, which often enough makes the whole process all the better. Recent advances in neuroimaging have taught us new things about just how busy the brain is, particularly through so-called default mode network. It is argued that experiments with brain scans (e.g., see Raichle, 2015) have shown that the brain functions in a far more intricate way than we used to believe. This has, in the majority of cases, led anesthesiologists to be able to better predict how different anesthetic medications might alter the patient's state of awareness and accelerate or slow d recovery. Knowing these trends—even when at times it's a question of the particulars being redundant—allows for more tailored anesthesia plans and reminds us that research must always seek further into brain function. In short, these knowledge bases ensure that while safety is at the forefront, cognitive ability is not neglected. Lastly, integrating anatomy and physiology knowledge with modern anesthetic techniques opens up new paths for better operating care. Overall, constant scrutiny of the interplay between variables like brain activity and blood flow with anesthetics not only further enhances the field but also facilitates a more aggressive form of patient caring. As more research continues to emerge, it will be necessary that doctors alter their styles to meet each patient's specific needs—a combination of safety and tailored care that defines modern practice. This kind of reflective, sometimes lovely, but hugely human thinking is what makes the importance of good anatomical and physiological know-how in determining the future of surgery and anesthesia so necessary.

Anesthesia relies on the complex interplay of our body structure and function. Think about it—anesthesiologists rely on understanding the nervous system's nooks and crannies, with all its idiosyncratic nuances, in order to reduce risks and keep patients safe in the OR. Being familiar with key body landmarks enables practitioners to get RA correct; they place the drug in the proper zone and leave neighboring zones relatively unaffected. Anatomical variations between individuals can, in most cases, alter the way anesthetic drugs work and even impact overall outcomes. The use of tools like ultrasound guidance is one such modern twist that weds old body knowledge to new technology, and one that is very necessary for procedures where every small thing counts. Also, familiarity with one's anatomical layout is a huge plus when navigating through possible complications and sidestepping unforeseen hazards (Mukherjee et al., 2022). Switching tracks, physiology's contribution to anesthesia is no less significant. Anesthetic drugs wreak havoc on bodily systems—heart rate, blood pressure, respiration, you name it—and a grasp of their underlying effect is crucial. For the most part, the interplay of these drugs with physiological processes offers a delicate balance: too light sedation won't calm the nerves, while too deep may slip into risky territories like respiratory depression or cardiac complications. Experiments often uncover that responses to anesthesia can vary, sometimes because of health conditions or even genetic quirks that subtly alter drug metabolism. Constant monitoring during the procedure offers a chance for anesthesiologists to modify their approach, maintaining the balance in check and the patient as safe as possible (Park et al., 2020). Finally, a synthesis of this intricate anatomical understanding and an awareness of how the body will react to these drugs constitutes a safeguard that allows anesthesia to be safer and more effective in general. Doctors like to gain a very thorough understanding of the patient's history, detecting all the way from unusual anatomical features to past surgeries, in an attempt to plan their approach. Preoperative consultations—replete with helpful information—help guide what drug to use and how best to utilize it on a case-by-case basis. Moreover, advancements in real-time monitoring devices strengthen this process by following the vital signs throughout the procedure, helping to keep everything in a stable condition. This combination of hard anatomy knowledge and real-time physiologic feedback has the immediate effect of reducing complications and enhancing patient outcomes, with safety always being top of mind for each procedure (Mukherjee et al., 2022).

KEY TERMS FROM THIS CHAPTER

- 3D printing
- Arteries
- Blood vessel
- Central nervous system
- Dynamical system
- Nervous system
- Peripheral nervous system
- Spinal canal
- Vital signs
- Anesthetic drugs
- Blood pressure
- Brain diseases
- Drug processing
- Heart rate
- Oxygen levels
- Spinal anesthesia
- Veins

CRITICAL THINKING QUESTIONS

1. **The narrowest part of the adult larynx is located at the:**
   a. Epiglottis
   b. Cricoid cartilage
   c. Rima glottidis (vocal cords)
   d. Arytenoid cartilages
2. **What is the primary muscle of inspiration?**
   a. Diaphragm
   b. Intercostal muscles
   c. Sternocleidomastoid
   d. Scalene muscles
3. **Cardiac output is determined by which two primary factors?**
   a. Heart rate and stroke volume
   b. Blood pressure and vascular resistance
   c. Stroke volume and preload
   d. Heart rate and afterload
4. **The epidural space lies between the:**
   a. Pia mater and dura mater
   b. Dura mater and ligamentum flavum
   c. Arachnoid mater and pia mater
   d. Subarachnoid space and dura mater
5. **Which neurotransmitter is released by preganglionic sympathetic fibers?**
   a. Norepinephrine
   b. Acetylcholine
   c. Dopamine
   d. Serotonin

Short Answer Questions

1. Define the anesthesia.
2. What is the basic anatomy of the human body?
3. What is the physiology of the nervous system?
4. How does anesthesia affect the cardiovascular system?
5. What is patient assessment and monitoring?

Answers to Critical Thinking Questions

1. (c); 2. (a); 3. (a); 4. (b); 5. (b)

REFERENCES

1. Aimar, A., Palermo, A., & Innocenti, B. (2019). The role of 3D printing in medical applications: A state of the art. *Journal of Healthcare Engineering, 2019*, Article 5340616, 1–10. https://doi.org/10.1155/2019/5340616.
2. Alwahbi, K. N., Alharbi, N. L. S., Almutairi, F. M. M., Alshammari, M. A., Alharbi, W. S., Aldhafeeri, M. M. M., Alharbi, Y. F. F., et al. (2024). Anesthesia for patients with burns: An updated review for anesthesiologists and nursing. *Journal of Eco Humanism*. https://www.semanticscholar.org/paper/c43bbec0139914157dbe4b1de2818ccbafc65deb (accessed on 20 May 2025).
3. Barron, A. B., & Klein, C. (2016). What insects can tell us about the origins of consciousness. *Proceedings of the National Academy of Sciences of the United States of America, 113*(18), 4900–4908. https://doi.org/10.1073/pnas.1520084113.
4. Bégay, V., Cirovic, B., Barker, A. J., Klopfleisch, R., Hart, D. W., Bennett, N., & Lewin, G. (2021). Immune competence and spleen size scale with colony status in the naked mole-rat. *Open Biology, 12*. https://www.semanticscholar.org/paper/0c49df2494e92f438a0cc2552e4d90f2f1765f28 (accessed on 20 May 2025).
5. Benveniste, H., Liu, X., Koundal, S., Sanggaard, S., Lee, H., & Wardlaw, J. M. (2018). The glymphatic system and waste clearance with brain aging: A review. *Gerontology, 65*, 106–119. https://doi.org/10.1159/000490349.
6. Chi, G., & Crowson, M. G. (2022). Anatomy and physiology of vestibular system. *DeckerMed Otolaryngology*. https://www.semanticscholar.org/paper/77735d4778294ccc6a9421a70fabb2c78f073a81 (accessed on 20 May 2025).
7. Claassen, J. A. H. R., Thijssen, D. H. J., Panerai, R. B., & Faraci, F. M. (2021). Regulation of cerebral blood flow in humans: Physiology and clinical implications of autoregulation. *Physiological Reviews, 101*, 1487–1559. https://doi.org/10.1152/physrev.00022.2020.
8. Constantinoiu, S. (2018). Esophageal surgery–past, present, future. *Chirurg, 113*, 7. https://www.semanticscholar.org/paper/9a678e8f3ec917abaef4f51a856e281cf6c4d8b3 (accessed on 20 May 2025).
9. Coté, C. J., Wilson, S., American Academy of Pediatrics, & American Academy of Pediatric Dentistry. (2019). Guidelines for monitoring and management of pediatric patients before, during, and after sedation for diagnostic and therapeutic procedures. *Pediatrics, 143*(6), e20191000. https://doi.org/10.1542/peds.2019-1000.
10. Ferriero, D. M., Fullerton, H. J., Bernard, T. J., Billinghurst, L., Daniels, S. R., DeBaun, M. R., deVeber, G., Ichord, R. N., Jordan, L. C., Massicotte, P., Meldau, J., Roach, E. S., Smith, E. R., & American Heart Association Stroke Council and Council on Cardiovascular and Stroke Nursing. (2019). Management of stroke in neonates and children: A scientific statement from the American Heart Association/American Stroke Association. *Stroke, 50*(3), e51–e96. https://doi.org/10.1161/STR.0000000000000183.
11. Giersch, G. E. W., & Charkoudian, N. (2025). Regulation of body temperature and blood pressure in women: Mechanisms and implications for heat illness risk. *Experimental Physiology, 110*(2), 196–199. https://doi.org/10.1113/EP091455.

12. Guerguerian, A. M., Sano, M., Todd, M., Honjo, O., Alexander, P., & Raman, L. (2021). Pediatric extracorporeal cardiopulmonary resuscitation ELSO guidelines. *ASAIO Journal, 67*(3), 229–237. https://doi.org/10.1097/mat.0000000000001345.

13. Hilscher, M., Wells, M., Venkatesh, S. K., Cetta, F., & Kamath, P. S. (2022). Fontan-associated liver disease. *Hepatology, 75*, 1300–1321. https://doi.org/10.1002/hep.32406.

14. Imbelloni, L. E., Gouveia, M. A., Neto, S. L., & Casali, T. A. A. (2023). Old anatomy and new anatomical concepts for single shot and continuous spinal anesthesia. *Journal of Anesthesia and Critical Care: Open Access*. https://www.semanticscholar.org/paper/b60ce5130e2f26c442529da18451a73c3721bed6 (accessed on 20 May 2025).

15. Joglar, J. A., Chung, M. K., Armbruster, A. L., Benjamin, E. J., Chyou, J. Y., Cronin, E. M., Deswal, A., et al. (2023). 2023 ACC/AHA/ACCP/HRS guideline for the diagnosis and management of atrial fibrillation: A report of the American College of Cardiology/American Heart Association joint committee on clinical practice guidelines. *Circulation, 149*. https://doi.org/10.1161/cir.0000000000001193.

16. Le-Bert, C., Bukoski, A., Downs, J., Hodgson, D. S., Thombs, L., Ridgway, S. H., & Bailey, J. (2024). Apneustic anesthesia ventilation improves pulmonary function in anesthetized bottlenose dolphins (*Tursiops truncatus*). *Frontiers in Veterinary Science, 11*. https://www.semanticscholar.org/paper/713f53c0940b9f0dfa97875a665e1ce9d8df26e4 (accessed on 20 May 2025).

17. Li, S. Z., Su, N., Wu, S., Fei, X. W., He, X., Zhang, J., Wang, X. H., et al. (2022). Monitored anesthesia care and asleep-awake-asleep techniques combined with multiple monitoring for resection of gliomas in eloquent brain areas: A retrospective analysis of 225 patients. *Chinese Neurosurgical Journal, 8*. https://www.semanticscholar.org/paper/48e351841130710b8c474829f9d1b9eaa38c9e6e (accessed on 20 May 2025).

18. Lotfollahi, Z. (2024). The anatomy, physiology and function of all skin layers and the impact of ageing on the skin. *Wound Practice and Research, 32*(1), 6–10.

19. Lurie, D. J., Kessler, D., Bassett, D. S., Betzel, R. F., Breakspear, M., Kheilholz, S., Kucyi, A., Liégeois, R., Lindquist, M. A., McIntosh, A. R., Poldrack, R. A., Shine, J. M., Thompson, W. H., Bielczyk, N. Z., Douw, L., Kraft, D., Miller, R. L., Muthuraman, M., Pasquini, L., Razi, A., & Calhoun, V. D. (2020). Questions and controversies in the study of time-varying functional connectivity in resting fMRI. *Network Neuroscience, 4*(1), 30–69. https://doi.org/10.1162/netn_a_00116.

20. Malviya, A. K., Gupta, A., Kumar, V., Gupta, J., Deepika, & Khanna, P. (2025). Effect of pregnancy hormones on pain perception in the peripartum period: A narrative review. *Journal of Anesthesiology Clinical Pharmacology*. https://doi.org/10.4103/joacp.joacp_174_24.

21. Marchetti, K., George, A., Wei, J. T., Ferrante, S., Hearn, J., Spratt, D., & Herrel, L. (2020). PD30-11: Initial patient-reported outcomes for men with prostate cancer undergoing rectal hydrogel spacer placement under local anesthesia. *Journal of Urology*. https://www.semanticscholar.org/paper/27c6cccc266ad5bef7150231c6f06e61ad1c7fb6 (accessed on 20 May 2025).

22. Meyer-Szary, J., Luis, M. S., Mikulski, S., Patel, A., Schulz, F., Tretiakow, D., Fercho, J., et al. (2022). The role of 3D printing in planning complex medical procedures and training of medical professionals—Cross-sectional multispecialty review. *International Journal of Environmental Research and Public Health, 19*, 3331. https://doi.org/10.3390/ijerph19063331.

23. Mukherjee, P., Roy, S., Ghosh, D., & Nandi, S. K. (2022). Role of animal models in biomedical research: A review. *Laboratory Animal Research, 38*. https://doi.org/10.1186/s42826-022-00128-1.

24. Murray-Torres, T. M., Naguib, A. N., Tobias, J. D., & Winch, et al. (2021). Anesthesia for thoracic surgery in infants and children. https://core.ac.uk/download/480389082.pdf (accessed on 20 May 2025).

25. Owen, C. M., Bacardit, J., Tan, M. P., Saedon, N., Goh, C. H., Newton, J. L., & Frith, J. (2024). Artificial intelligence driven clustering of blood pressure profiles reveals frailty in orthostatic hypertension. *Experimental Physiology, 110*, 230–247. https://www.semanticscholar.org/paper/ea9cec5b27c2edb57be4bbc927215238c8091efd (accessed on 20 May 2025).

26. Park, J., & Im, S. (2020). Of men in mice: The development and application of a humanized gnotobiotic mouse model for microbiome therapeutics. *Experimental & Molecular Medicine, 52*, 1383–1396. https://www.semanticscholar.org/paper/eb3ed84f73a8d70dd66da46c57cfb32ed0788214 (accessed on 20 May 2025).

27. Praz, F., Muraru, D., Kreidel, F., Lurz, P., Hahn, R. T., Delgado, V., Senni, M., et al. (2021). Transcatheter treatment for tricuspid valve disease. *Euro Intervention, 17*, 791–808. https://doi.org/10.4244/eij-d-21-00695.

28. Raichle, M. E. (2015). The brain's default mode network. *Annual Review of Neuroscience, 38*, 433–447. https://doi.org/10.1146/annurev-neuro-071013-014030.

29. Rychik, J., Atz, A. M., Celermajer, D. S., Deal, B. J., Gatzoulis, M. A., Gewillig, M., Hsia, T. Y., et al. (2019). Evaluation and management of the child and adult with Fontan circulation: A scientific statement from the American Heart Association. *Circulation, 140*. https://doi.org/10.1161/cir.0000000000000696.

30. Sacks, H. S., & Symonds, M. (2013). Anatomical locations of human brown adipose tissue. *Diabetes, 62*, 1783–1790. https://doi.org/10.2337/db12-1430.

31. Shaji, A., & Herakal, G. I. (2024). Evaluating the effects of anesthetic agents on geriatrics to enhance perioperative care practices: A narrative review. *International Journal of Scientific and Research Publications*. https://www.semanticscholar.org/paper/dc9e39c11d9a01ad523ef8509e296f3ca4d30225 (accessed on 20 May 2025).

32. Smith, J. (2017). *Non-Invasive Positive Pressure Ventilation in The Obese Patient Population: An Intervention to Enhance Oxygenation–A Quality Improvement Project*. Doctoral Projects, 69. https://core.ac.uk/download/301290078.pdf (accessed on 20 May 2025).

33. Sop, D. M., Zhang, Y. M., & Smith, W. R. (2024). Cerebral blood flow and pain perception in sickle cell disease: A mediation analysis. *Blood, 144*(Supplement 1), 5339. https://doi.org/10.1182/blood-2024-199307.

34. Sorby-Adams, A. J., Vink, R., & Turner, R. J. (2018). Large animal models of stroke and traumatic brain injury as translational tools. *American Journal of Physiology-Regulatory, Integrative and Comparative Physiology, 315*(2), R165–R190. https://doi.org/10.1152/ajpregu.00163.2017.

35. Stout, K., Daniels, C. J., Aboulhosn, J., Bozkurt, B., Broberg, C. S., Colman, J. M., Crumb, S. R., et al. (2018). 2018 AHA/ACC guideline for the management of adults with congenital heart disease: A report of the American College of Cardiology/American Heart Association Task Force on Clinical Practice Guidelines. *Circulation, 139*. https://doi.org/10.1161/cir.0000000000000603.

36. Swindle, M. M., Makin, A., Herron, A. J., Clubb, F. J., & Frazier, K. S. (2011). Swine as models in biomedical research and toxicology testing. *Veterinary Pathology, 49*, 344–356. https://doi.org/10.1177/0300985811402846.

37. Vatansever, S., Schlessinger, A., Wacker, D., Kanıskan, H. Ü., Jin, J., Zhou, M. M., & Zhang, B. (2020). Artificial intelligence and machine learning-aided drug discovery in central nervous system diseases: State-of-the-arts and future directions. *Medicinal Research Reviews, 41*, 1427–1473. https://doi.org/10.1002/med.21764.

38. Walker, B., Stone, A., Langan, J. N., Hostnik, E., & Alexander, A. B. (2023). Regional anesthesia of the dentition in Bennett's wallaby (*Macropus rufogriseus*): Anatomical landmarks and approaches assessed with computed tomography and gross dissection. *Journal of Veterinary Dentistry*. https://www.semanticscholar.org/paper/c7f4161ac1e20a43c6aec3fffdbcd5a88d82e582 (accessed on 20 May 2025).

39. Zheng, B., Zheng, H., & Lin, X. (2019). Ultrasound for predicting difficult airway in obstetric anesthesia. *Medicine, 98*(e17846), e17846. https://doi.org/10.1097/md.0000000000017846.

PREOPERATIVE ASSESSMENT AND PREPARATION

4

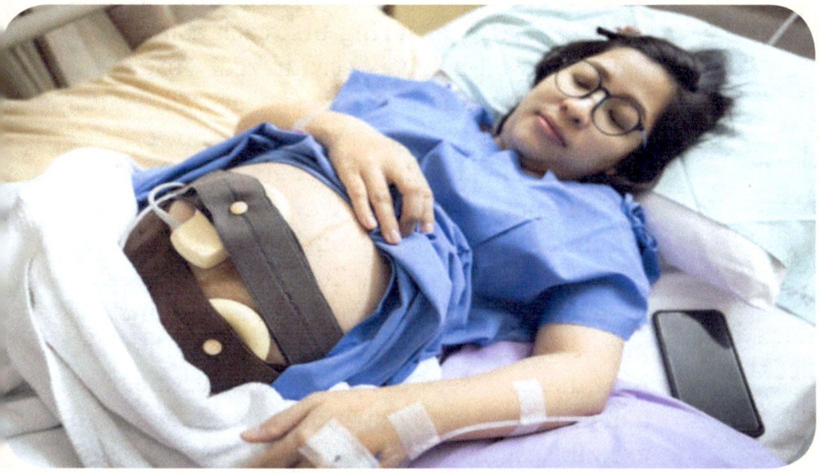

Introduction

Surgical care isn't merely about entering the operating room—it's about the painstaking groundwork established long before the incision. It starts with double-checking everything, which can truly impact the way a patient recovers. Sometimes problems like surgical-site infections somehow slip in and wreak havoc on recovery issues and added costs. A review, for instance, reported that patients were much less likely to develop these infections if they received oral antibiotics before surgery—especially if that was supplemented by intravenous antibiotics and bowel prep mechanically—instead of sticking with IV antibiotics alone. Together, in general, these pre-op strategies seem to enhance not just the success of the surgery but overall patient safety as well (McMahon et al., 2018). Anesthesia, though, adds another layer to the whole pre-surgery issue. CRNAs—Certified Registered Nurse Anesthetists—are the focal point of decision-making, and their street smarts (and what some call AUOs) give us a glimpse of how the care gets perfected long before scalpel ever touches skin. Learning from

LEARNING OBJECTIVES

After studying this chapter, you will be able to:

1. Understand the objectives of preoperative assessment.
2. Describe the components of preoperative assessment.
3. Understand the role of anesthesia in preoperative assessment.
4. Explain the multidisciplinary approach to preoperative preparation.
5. Describe the challenges in preoperative assessment.

their own experiences with models such as the Integrated Behavior Model (IBM) can assist in transforming the way anesthesia is provided so that it is tailored to each patient like a glove. In the majority of instances, this equates to pre-surgery screenings not merely being a checklist process; instead, they actually cross hands-on skills with actual-world judgment to address specific needs (Nosbisch et al., 2024). As far as enhancing the preoperative routine as a whole goes, it's not always a matter of keeping to the rules—it also has to do with engaging in empathy about how a patient feels. Surgeons, anesthetists, and nurses all must collaborate, not only taking into account a patient's physical readiness but also those psychosocial components that could affect recovery. A comprehensive, rigorous evaluation allows everyone to spot potential hiccups beforehand and thread all the pieces together in a more relaxed, more organic manner. Not only does this practical strategy reduce post-op complications, but also boosts patient satisfaction and refines overall healthcare performance. Each piece of the puzzle illustrates that it is critical to keep our preoperative practice current in order to achieve best outcomes for a wide variety of patients (Nosbisch et al., 2024; McMahon et al., 2018) (Figure 4.1).

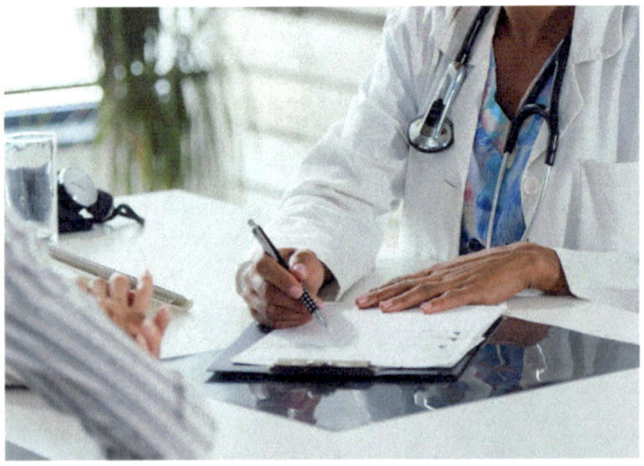

Figure 4.1. Preoperative Assessment and Preparation.

Source: https://drpulerammego.co.za/storage/2022/08/secondary-service-image-2.jpg.

Definition of Preoperative Assessment

Preparation for surgery reduces to taking a hard look at the preoperative assessment. Not so much a checklist, really, but rather a review of a patient's history, status, and individual risks for the planned procedure. It's more about signaling warnings concerning what may happen during or after surgery so that the care team may customize a response. Today, specialists from various disciplines donate their expertise, ensuring that each aspect of a patient's well-being is scrutinized. Through a closer examination of risk and overall health, teams will be able to create plans not only to ready patients for the procedure but to smooth out any potholes in the way back to recovery, potentially enhancing outcomes as well as costs (Neelakanta et al., 2025). A bit deeper in, preoperative workups range from a perfunctory physical exam to thorough lab work. They are intended to assess the patient's adjustment on a daily level, assess nutritional status, and even examine psychological well-being. An interesting aspect is the prehabilitation component—essentially, steps taken to enhance physical and mental preparedness before surgery, which creates a baseline to allow treatment plans to be tailored in a way that indeed enhances preparation. And, of course, individual idiosyncrasies—such as pre-existing conditions and differences in physical health—mean that no two tests are ever identical. This aspect of humanity helps sort patients by risk and keeps patients actively involved in the surgical process (Neelakanta et al., 2025). While surgical methodologies and patient care continue to accelerate at light speed, the old checklist system just doesn't cut it anymore. Preoperative assessment has developed today into a flexible model that combines patient-centered care with established, evidence-based practice. Overall, the aim is to have many different healthcare professionals work together so that tests and treatments cover all the bases. Focus continues on avoiding complications and facilitating recovery by using smart planning. Lastly, to what degree these assessments excel is dependent upon their ability to accommodate each patient's individual case and the requirements of different operations. Recent research even shows that greater testing of novel methods is needed to guarantee they are effective in the bigger picture of perioperative care (Englesbe, 2017) (Figure 4.2).

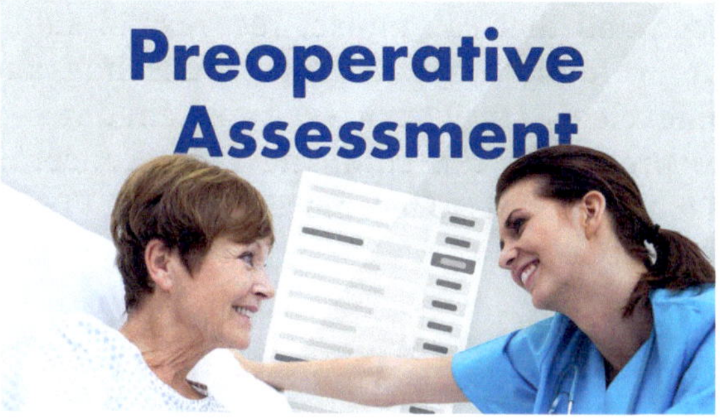

Figure 4.2. Preoperative assessment.

Source: https://ausmed-images.s3-ap-southeast-2.amazonaws.com/ausmed.com/ausmed-course/COURSE122_01v2.0.jpg.

Importance of Preoperative Preparation

Surgical preparation is essential in-patient outcomes; it doesn't just affect what happens right after surgery but also dictates how much an individual recovers in the long term. Screening patients thoroughly before surgery enables care teams to detect risks and come up with tailor-made strategies—something that has been seen time and time again. Many times, patients are asked to receive some sort of health baseline test in which issues like weight loss and other complications of the medical nature occur. Studies, for example, have pointed out that where the patients manage to lose about 8% of their weight before the surgery, the success of the surgery is much enhanced (PesoTrabalho et al., 2023). Generally speaking, possessing all the information required can calm patient anxiety, hence making the entire procedure less stressful even if sometimes things can get a bit crazy. Open, honest doctor-patient communication is yet another essential factor in this context. It's not necessarily a matter of the procedure details—discourse reaches as far as lifestyle changes, proper medication management, and even sometimes readjusting physical exercise levels. When patients are encouraged to feel as if they are included in the conversation, they will also comply with post-surgery instructions far more reliably. Secondly, certain clinics take advantage of indicators like the Thoracic Curve Correction Ratio (TCCR) (Landrum et al., 2022) to package up all of that pre-surgery data in a nice package. This approach, based primarily on numbers, provides some useful suggestions to minimize potential problems, even though it is not infallible each time.

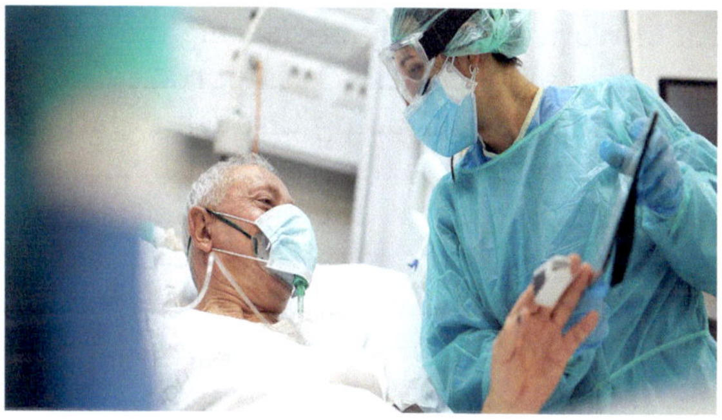

Figure 4.3. Importance of patient preoperative preparation.

Source: https://ntgic.com/wp-content/uploads/sites/278/facilities-scahealth-1254631619-550-e1657134017606.jpg.

Preparing for surgery also makes the process itself smoother. Through careful examination of patient health information and preparing both the staff and patients in advance, many surgical surprises are evaded. This progressive way of working has the effect of enhancing resource utilization, reducing the time that surgeries last, and avoiding complications. Being closely integrated with various specialists provides a broader perspective on what each patient requires, even though at times communication becomes a bit entangled. Since these early beginnings pave the way for positive results, ongoing variations in evaluation and preparation procedures still have the potential for better results in a wide range of fields (Figure 4.3).

4.1. Objectives of Preoperative Assessment

Learning Outcome

1. Identify patient risks.
2. Establish baseline health status.
3. Enhance surgical outcomes.

Detailed preoperative evaluation does a great deal of work in the way of clearing the road to better patient outcomes – its importance cannot be overemphasized. Going through a patient's past medical history, their current health, and the specific needs of the upcoming surgery enables any issues of concern to be brought to light. This careful examination enables doctors to individualize plans for anesthesia, postoperative care, and treatment overall to each patient's unique situation. In more complicated scenarios, i.e., in ovarian tissue cryopreservation cases, this kind of thorough check becomes all the more necessary to avoid hiccups and boost success rates (Turan et al., 2024). Fundamentally, the purpose of the preoperative evaluation is to stratify risks and ready patients for surgery. Generally speaking, it is not only a question of pinpointing existing health problems that can complicate surgery, but it also opens the door to making required changes ahead of time. For example, someone who has heart disease might need to have special precautions taken to stabilize their condition well before they undergo a major operation. It also helps guide the wise use of resources by focusing the clinicians on postoperative care trajectories that are in keeping with the predicted needs of the patient. In most instances, guideline recommendations from bodies like the European Society of Anesthesiology and Intensive Care Medicine have pushed preoperative care to more personalized and evidence-based practice (Lamperti et al., 2025). It's not simply a matter of crunching medical numbers, either – the evaluation also takes into account the patient's mental and emotional state. Patients can be anxious or uncertain about what's going to occur, and that can impact recovery in subtle but profound ways. A little counseling and some clear, straightforward explanations of the procedure can eliminate these concerns, enabling patients to feel more in control. (Turan et al., 2024).

4.1.1. Identifying Patient Risks

Understanding a patient's risk factors is what sets the stage for surgery to go well. Doctors explore more than a check-the-box evaluation of medical histories—they look at everyday choices, mood, and even tiny bits of social history that might increase the stakes. Instead of sticking to neat lists, clinicians like to meld their checks, looking for uninvited red flags like hidden illnesses or complications simmering in the background. This overall, sometimes disorganized, approach helps to hone surgery plans that are effective on an individual-by-individual basis and, in most cases, enhances overall safety and effective operations. Real-time case studies from trend-setting healthcare settings (Blumenthal et al., 2006) even suggest a less formulaic approach is better able to keep people safe. Taking a closer look at medicine routines is another component of the equation. Nowadays, with more opioid use among surgical patients, it can be complicated. It is no longer a question of using or not using pain medication; doctors need to assess how tolerance, dependence, and even withdrawal can make routine pain control harder. Patients often have some degree of opioid dependence that goes unnoticed until complications develop after surgery. When physicians identify these issues early in the game, they can adjust to better accommodate those with such hidden barriers. Protocols in most cases ask healthcare professionals to take additional care to watch for indications of opioid misuse (Coluzzi et al., 2017)—a fact that recognizes that each patient is as unique as they are. Apart from medication and behavior, mental health is a factor in determining surgery success for a patient. Mental health screenings are now as important as physical ones because anxiety and depression will prolong recovery times or even initiate complications, so the diagnosis is done a lot earlier. Rather than compartmentalizing, now teams incorporate mental well-being into the whole scenario, using day-to-day screening tools to identify early signs of distress. This sometimes means a little additional paperwork on one end or a quick referral on the other, but it all feeds into a more complete plan that nurtures both body and mind. In doing so, healthcare workers arrive at a care plan that's as adaptable and varied as the patients themselves—a strategy which in turn keeps the whole surgical process on track (Figure 4.4).

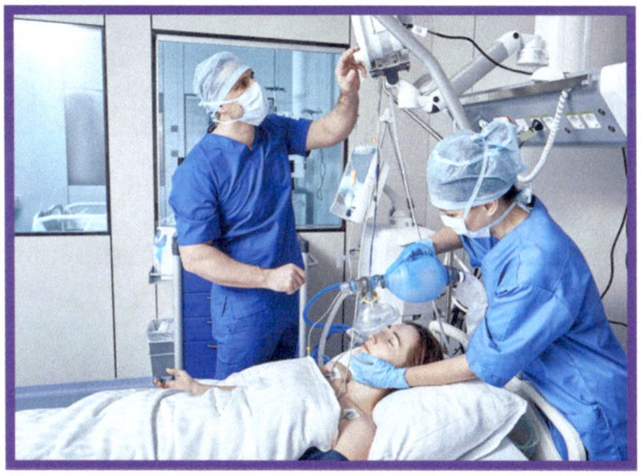

Figure 4.4. Patient safety risks.

Source: https://zaggocare.org/wp-content/uploads/2022/02/photo-of-doctors-taking-care-of-a-patient-in-the-ICU-canva-border-added.png.

4.1.2. Establishing Baseline Health Status

It is imperative to get a patient to a place of knowing where he is starting before any surgery is done. Doctors like to conduct rigorous check-ups beforehand so they can detect underlying issues that can complicate things in the future. This idea is not limited to long-stay surgery; it is just as viable for short visits and intricate operations. Following a clearly established routine not only helps to choose the appropriate individuals for surgery but also outlines what to expect in clear, down-to-earth language. For example, Dumfries & Galloway Royal Infirmary has installed its pre-assessment clinic, streamlines the assessment process, and speaks different teams more openly to each other (Bouamrane et al., 2014). With new technology intertwined with old-fashioned clinical procedure, the whole pre-surgery process has effectively been turned on its head—in a good way. Computer systems now make it much easier to collect and pass on patient data, so that anything that occurs to their health is picked up, nearly on time. With instant, real-time information aiding doctors in estimating risk, they have a clearer idea of what is happening with a patient and what more steps might be needed along the way. Overall, real-time data is mostly proof that when technology and medicine are harmonious, surgical care gets an authentic boost (Bouamrane et al., 2014). Second is the issue of reducing complications which include surgical site infections. A good pre-surgery evaluation can detect some important risk factors so that caregivers can change their approach to a specific patient. Take the case of streamlining skin preparation routines before surgery—it's been a winning strategy for lowering those infection rates. At one community hospital, data even revealed pre-op care gaps which, when plugged, kept everyone on track and avoided extra costs from infections. Finally, establishing a good baseline is less about safer surgery and more just one aspect of broader initiatives to enhance general surgical quality.

4.1.3. Enhancing Surgical Outcomes

Pre-surgery evaluations make a real difference. They don't just spot potential risks—they set up customized plans that can change how fast someone recovers. Sometimes, putting together a mix of experts—surgeons, anesthesiologists, a few other specialists—offers a broad glimpse into a patient's overall health. Working together, these folks can pick up on hidden issues, handle problems before they blow up, and choose the best anesthesia options. When patients get a clear idea of what's ahead and know the risks, their worry tends to drop, which helps everything run more smoothly in the operating room. And screening early for things like heart or lung concerns can steer those anesthesia choices in many cases, reducing complications later on. There's also a growing trend toward using targeted prehabilitation before surgery. Exercise programs, better nutrition, and even a bit of mental support are getting integrated into the whole process. Research generally shows that patients who dive into these routines end up leaving the hospital sooner and bouncing back with stronger function after surgery. Training the body and mind ahead of time means that healthcare teams can often see a smoother shift into recovery. For example, using specific nutritional alters—like immune-boost formulas—helps bolster a patient's reserves, making them better prepared for the challenges of invasive procedures. All of this underlines, in a very tangible way, just how critical solid preoperative prep is (Naranjo et al., 2017). Hospitals that stick with proven, evidence-based practices seem to nail better outcomes, too. Some institutions, drawing on successful case studies and a dash of trial and error, have shown that a methodical, patient-focused approach can improve safety in the surgical arena. The experiences shared by clinical teams—what they did, how it went—end up serving as a kind of roadmap for improving future strategies. Tips and recommendations flagged from these case studies help guide teams when they're fine-tuning their pre-surgery preparations. In most cases, this steady commitment to learning and adapting ties those meticulous pre-surgical checks directly to improved results, ultimately lifting the overall quality of healthcare delivery (Blumenthal et al., 2006) (Figure 4.5).

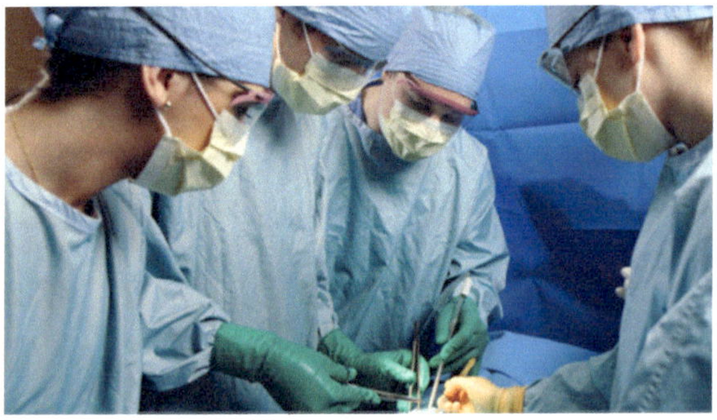

Figure 4.5. Surgical outcomes.

Source: https://www.mayo.edu/-/media/kcms/gbs/research/images/2014/05/13/14/31/shcd-surgical-outcomes-6col.jpg.

Test Your Knowledge

1. How are patient risks identified?
2. How to create a baseline health status?

4.2. Components of Preoperative Assessment

Learning Outcome

1. Evaluate the medical history.
2. Describe the physical examination.
3. Learn about laboratory and diagnostic tests.

Surgical procedures can be pretty complicated - a lot is going on that needs a closer look before the operation begins. Nutrition, for instance, turns out to be a key player. Research generally shows that when patients aren't getting enough to eat, the risks of things like infections and longer hospital stays tend to shoot up. In light of this, the Outpatient Nursing Nutritional Intervention (ONNI) was born to give both patients and nurses a boost. The idea is to figure out why these nutritional gaps exist, whip up custom care plans, and keep an eye on progress with regular check-ins. Nurses, who are often right at the heart of this process, sometimes miss out on understanding just how crucial good nutrition is—underscoring, in most cases, the need for more focused training programs (Noort et al., 2020). Then there's another part of the preoperative picture—evaluating both physical and psychological health as part of what's called a prehabilitation strategy., these activities check a patient's baseline functionality and spot any issues early so that healthcare providers can jump in with targeted fixes aimed at boosting both body and mind before surgery. This mixed approach involves everything from risk assessment to decision-making, blending different parts of care into one less structured, more ongoing conversation about readiness. In this vein, patients are simply encouraged to move, breathe, eat, and relax—a kind of four-step suggestion to foster a well-rounded state of readiness. Because people vary so much in their health and accompanying conditions, these personalized care plans naturally become indispensable in achieving real surgical success (Englesbe, 2017). When you put all these bits together, you build a solid foundation for both the surgery itself and the recovery afterward. By digging deeper into patients' nutritional and physical needs, caregivers can often nip potential setbacks in the bud. As studies continue to roll out new findings, it becomes clear that checking how well prehabilitation and nutrition strategies work is just as important for boosting fitness levels as it is for reducing post-surgery complications. The interplay between these factors is still a bit of a moving target, but any insights can easily be molded into practical, evidence-based actions. In the end, keeping a strong focus on a comprehensive preoperative look not only improves outcomes but also nurtures a patient-centered care culture—making sure that both the surgical team and the patients are as ready as they can possibly be for what comes next (Englesbe, 2017; Noort et al., 2020).

4.2.1. Medical History Evaluation

Before diving into surgery, it's crucial to dig into a patient's full health background—a step that isn't just a box to check. Gathering details about any past health issues, what medicines they're on, allergies, and previous operations isn't merely formal; it helps doctors catch potential hiccups, like diabetes or heart problems, that might interfere with anesthesia or how a person recovers afterward. Skipping even one important note here can lead to complications later on, so a careful, sometimes even redundant, review does make a difference. When we look at older patients, things tend to get even trickier. Aging is often mixed up with several chronic conditions and a body that might react in unexpected ways to surgery. Many believe that a detailed pre-surgical check is vital—in most cases, however, time constraints force rushed reviews (Lampugnale et al., 2017). Setting up a standard, everyday way to assess these patients could go a long way in easing treatment plans and helping them recover better, even if it means the process becomes less streamlined than we'd like. The mind, too, plays its part in how well someone does after an operation. Recent research has started to show that a history of mental health challenges can lower the starting line before surgery and dull the improvements afterward. Patients who have struggled mentally might not bounce back as dramatically, and adding a bit of psychological insight into the routine pre-op check-up could offer a broader view of what's needed. In doing so, clinicians get to tackle potential risks head-on, smoothing out the overall journey to recovery—even if the language ends up feeling a bit more conversational than strictly clinical (Langdown et al., 2018) (Figure 4.6).

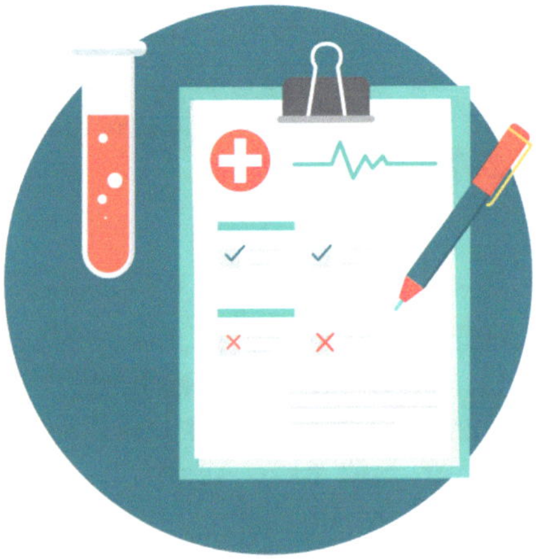

Figure 4.6. Medical history.

Source: https://cdn-icons-png.flaticon.com/512/387/387552.png.

4.2.2. Physical Examination

Preoperative preparation hinges on a hands-on physical check-up that, quite frankly, sets the stage for what happens later in the operating room. One can't ignore how this basic yet essential exam spots both the glaring and the sneaky health issues that might affect surgery. Usually, doctors look at vital signs, run through whole-body evaluations, and even zero in on neurological responses to gauge if someone is truly fit for the procedure. Generally speaking, recognizing how each person's unique body ticks—whether it's anatomical quirks or overall body function—is key, especially when dealing with complex surgeries like neurosurgery, where subtle differences in brain function can reshape the whole pre-surgery plan. This focused check-up not only guides anesthesia decisions but also molds strategies for what happens during and after surgery, boosting safety and recovery (Manninen et al., 2010). There's also a deeper side to the physical exam than just checking boxes. It reflects the clinician's knack for piecing together various clues to make smart surgical calls. Take, for instance, minimally invasive heart procedures, where evaluating a patient's past heart issues and organ performance isn't just routine—it's critical. A full-body screening can pick up on potential hiccups that might crop up while the surgery is underway, prompting plans for details like cannulation and safeguarding the heart muscle. In most cases, this proactive approach, based on subtle exam hints, tends to reduce complications and lead to better outcomes in the long run, underscoring just how central the exam is in patient care (Agnihotri et al., 2016). At its core, this practical exam ties the patient's overall health directly to surgical and anesthetic plans. Beyond simply spotting health concerns, it creates an atmosphere of personalized care, letting doctors design interventions that fit the patient's unique situation and improve surgical success. Especially where preexisting issues—picked up during the exam—might sway which surgical technique works best, every detail matters. In the end, weaving a thorough physical examination into the preoperative routine not only reinforces the integrity of the surgical process but also ensures, in most cases, that every patient-specific factor is carefully balanced in the drive toward the best possible outcomes (Agnihotri et al., 2016; Manninen et al., 2010) (Figure 4.7).

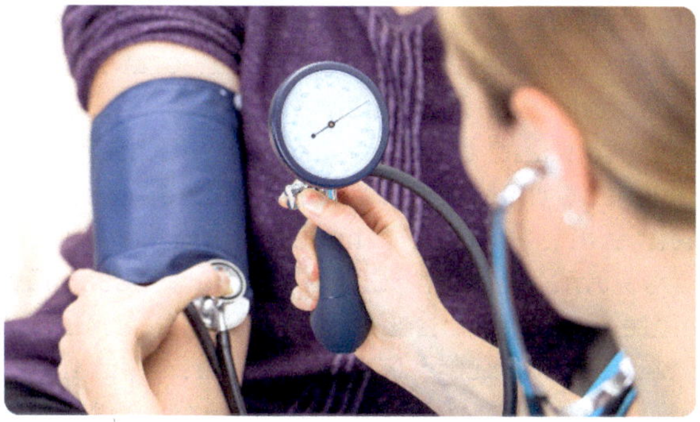

Figure 4.7. Physical examination.

Source: https://get.goreact.com/wp-content/uploads/2019/05/Physical-Examination-Methods_-Training-Your-Students.png.

4.2.3. Laboratory and Diagnostic Tests

Getting patients ready for surgery isn't just ticking boxes – it's about checking how things stand. Doctors dig into lab work and diagnostic tests well before the knife comes out, trying to spot hidden issues and catch any red flags in a patient's overall condition. A good look at these tests often means fewer last-minute cancellations—studies show that when screenings are done carefully, the number of avoidable surgery cancellations can drop dramatically. One clinic, for example, rethought its screening routine and saw cancellations tumble from roughly 15 a month down to only two over a few months (Flint et al., 2016). This drop points to how smart lab checks can keep the whole operation running smoothly. Sometimes, the evaluations include an odd mix of tests—complete blood counts, metabolic panels, even checks on how well blood clots—all picked to suit the kind of surgery planned. It isn't just about finding out what's wrong; it also means checking if the patient is ready for anesthesia and the surgery ahead. In neurosurgery, for instance, knowing about a patient's brain condition and how it might ripple through the body is key (Manninen et al., 2010). Different surgeries demand different checks, and leaning on the right tests can help reduce on risks related to anesthesia and post-op problems, generally leading to better overall outcomes. New technology also steps in here. Combining advanced diagnostic imaging—like MRIs or CT scans—with lab results gives doctors a fuller picture of what a patient's physically going through. These images often reveal important details about a person's anatomy and any underlying issues, details that can be easily overlooked otherwise. When these visual cues mix with lab findings, it feels like the puzzle is finally complete. As noted in the literature on preoperative workups (Flint et al., 2016), this more rounded, albeit sometimes messy, approach tends to make patients feel a bit more reassured and ready for what lies ahead. Overall, a committed, all-around preoperative check-up does a lot to boost surgical success and keep patients safer along the way (Figure 4.8).

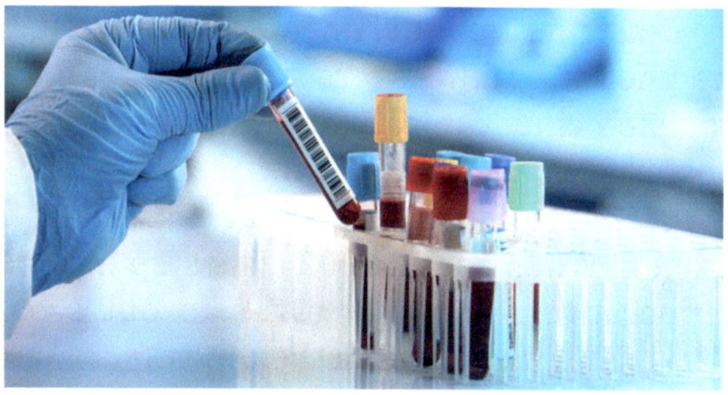

Figure 4.8. Laboratory and diagnostic tests.

Source: https://images.apollo247.in/pd-cms/cms/2023-10/Shutterstock_1114244621.jpg.

Test Your Knowledge

1. What is the medical history evaluation?
2. What is a laboratory and diagnostic test?

4.3. Role of Anesthesia in Preoperative Assessment

Learning Outcome

1. Understand the anesthesia consultation.
2. Assess anesthesia risks.
3. Learn about patient education regarding anesthesia.

Preoperative assessments get right into the heart of patient care, checking multiple angles to boost outcomes. Anesthesia, usually front and center in this process, isn't just about putting patients to sleep – it's also about sifting through their medical history, and current medications, and spotting potential issues that might show up during surgery. In many cases, doctors rely on solid, evidence-backed steps to connect the dots between individual patient details and any surgical risks; this approach helps shape a plan that's tailor-made for each person. Clear, sometimes even casual, chats among team members turn out to be key for carving out an anesthesia plan that not only keeps patients safe but also makes surgery go smoother, as hinted at by insights from Certified Registered Nurse Anesthetists (CRNAs) regarding anesthesia provision and clinical intentional behaviors (Nosbisch et al., 2024). Pain management is another piece of the puzzle that comes to light early on. When anesthesiologists step in at the preoperative stage, they can map out a pain relief plan stretching from before surgery until recovery kicks in. Unchecked pain after surgery can stir up trouble – it may lead to lingering, even chronic, pain and stretch out hospital stays. Generally speaking, knowing a patient's past pain experiences and how they handle opioids becomes especially crucial, particularly among folks who are already used to them; if things aren't handled just right, there's a risk of problems popping up from ever-higher doses (Wenzel et al., 2016). Addressing these matters right off the bat often helps boost patient satisfaction and sets the stage for a quicker, more predictable recovery. Behavioral insights are slowly weaving their way into anesthesia education and the pre-surgery routine too. It turns out that the way anesthesiologists see their work – something Certified Registered Nurse Anesthetist (CRNA) experiences have pointed out (Nosbisch et al., 2024) – can impact how they interact with patients during surgeries. They've noticed that when a patient feels jittery or anxious, it might throw off not just the prep work but even the healing process afterward. In most cases, altering communication styles and building a bit more trust goes a long way, helping patients understand their options and agree to the plan in a more informed way. This kind of thoughtful, sometimes slightly offbeat approach helps create an environment that can lead to better surgical outcomes and underscores the anesthesiologist's role as a vital, all-around team member committed to taking care of the whole person.

4.3.1. Anesthesia Consultation

Preoperative anesthesia consults set the stage for how well surgery goes. In many cases, starting off with a solid chat about anesthesia helps the team zero in on what each patient might need—they get a chance to spot unique risks and whip up a plan that isn't just cookie-cutter. Studies, in most cases, show that when folks in different roles don't exchange information clearly, it can delay things or even cancel surgeries. Bringing together input from the surgery crew, primary care providers, and anesthesiologists makes for a more rounded check-up before hitting the operating room. This kind of teamwork not only smooths out the preoperative experience but, generally speaking, also boosts both safety and patient satisfaction. Redesigning preoperative screening clinics (PSCs) has become a favorite trick for sharpening anesthesia consultations and cutting day-of-surgery cancellations. Some clinics, for instance, have shifted to an all-registered nurse staffing model – a alter that's reduce avoidable cancellations by a good margin. Many literature reviews and number-crunching point to the need for a more systematic approach to pre-op assessments, one that brings anesthesia into the mix in a smarter way. The data showed a dramatic drop in cancellations, affirming that tinkering with PSC operations keeps the whole surgical schedule on track. Plus, improvements like shorter wait times and increased patient throughput highlight how these changes can pay off for both patients and healthcare facilities (Flint et al., 2016). Good old communication between different teams is a must for nailing preoperative assessments in anesthesia consults. Checklists and set communication protocols seem to do a fine job reducing delays and smoothing out how decisions get made.

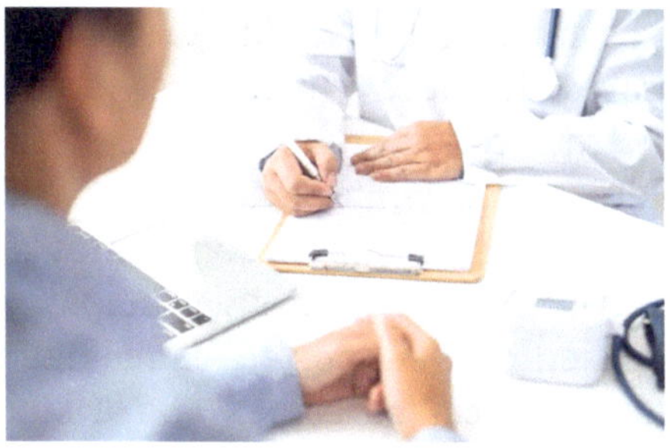

Figure 4.9. Anesthesia consultation.

Source: https://mariatsolakidou.com/wp-content/uploads/2023/05/ti-na-rotiseis-ton-anaisthisiologo.webp.

Using strategies like the Plan-Do-Study-Act (PDSA) model gives folks in pre-anesthesia clinics a chance to spot and fix issues that might slow down patient flow and affect safety. When providers chat more openly, patient assessments get better and the overall care feels more unified—even if things sometimes feel a bit fragmented in clinical settings. Empirical findings suggest that these collaborative efforts improve outcomes and lift the quality of care in pre-op environments, meaning that thorough anesthesia consultations are pretty crucial in making sure patients are truly ready for surgery (Perry et al., 2021) (Figure 4.9).

4.3.2. Assessment of Anesthesia Risks

Assessing anesthesia risks is crucial before surgery. You need to know the patient's overall health, the surgery's complexity, and that things might not always go as planned. A good check-up digs into the patient's medical history, current ailments, and past experiences with anesthesia. Research often shows that the opinions and beliefs of professionals like CRNAs can steer how these risks get handled. Their day-to-day experiences inform not only how they behave when giving anesthesia, but also how they plan and decide on strategies. Models—like the IBM—can be put to work here, offering a more workable framework to untangle these complex issues (Nosbisch et al., 2024). Thinking about individual risk factors isn't enough; the specific procedure matters too. The type and duration of a surgery can sway anesthesia plans and patient safety considerably. For instance, studies comparing methods in total knee arthroplasty—whether a tourniquet is used or not—show subtle shifts in things like pain levels and how much opioid medication is needed afterward (Kheir et al., 2018). These observations suggest that the surgical techniques and the anesthesia approach often mix in unexpected ways. This means every patient's unique situation might call for a custom strategy, one that keeps safety front and center while also addressing pain and discomfort after the operation. Good communication between the surgical team and patients is another key factor. Clear, sometimes even imperfect, conversations help patients understand what to expect and give them room to air their concerns about anesthesia. This back-and-forth can bring to light extra risk factors that might have slipped past at first. When providers listen to a patient's worries and preferences, they can alter the anesthesia plan a bit more effectively. Altogether, blending these open communication practices into preoperative checks not only builds teamwork but also paves the way for better outcomes and a more satisfying surgical experience (Figure 4.10).

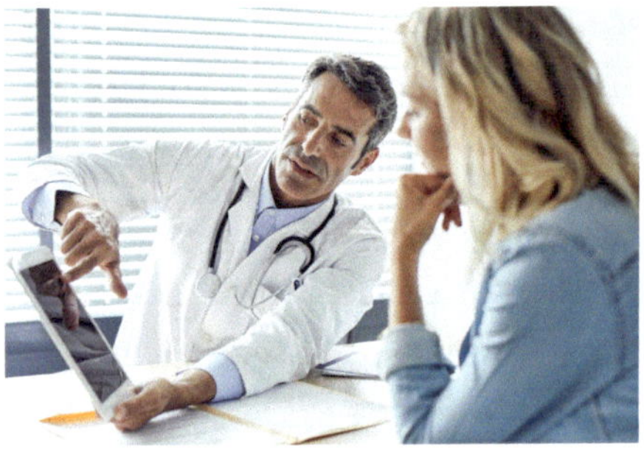

Figure 4.10. Anesthesia risk assessment.

Source: https://madeforthismoment.asahq.org/wp-content/uploads/2017/10/iStock-680482926-1024x683.jpg.

4.3.3. Patient Education Regarding Anesthesia

Patients often feel nerve-wracked before surgery, sometimes long before any actual procedure takes place. When they first learn about having an operation, a wave of anxiety hits unexpectedly, which can mess with both their recovery and how they feel about the care they receive. One study on total knee arthroplasty (TKA) showed that a mixed, team-based approach to educating patients—talking about everything from rehab exercises to what actually happens in surgery—can bring those nerves down. In many cases, as patients get a clearer picture of what anesthesia is like, their baseline stress seems to drop; this was clearly noticed (Yang et al., 2025). There's also a common mix-up about what anesthesiologists do, and that misunderstanding only adds to the worry. A descriptive study at Marmara University found that although many patients reported high satisfaction with anesthesia services, they still had little idea about the anesthesiologists' actual role. This gap in understanding suggests that a straightforward explanation of anesthesia can go a long way in easing preoperative nerves. When patients are given a clear rundown of what to expect and what the anesthesiologist's job entails, it helps build trust and comfort; in most cases, smoother communication leads to more positive overall experiences (Abdullayev et al., 2024). It turns out that not every patient reacts the same way to the same explanations, so tailoring the information is key. Research indicates that a one-size-fits-all educational approach might not cut it—especially for those dealing with high anxiety or other health challenges. For example, the TKA study mentioned earlier pointed out that patients with higher anxiety levels before surgery didn't benefit as much from standard sessions. This underscores the need for a more personalized plan, one that considers a patient's stress level and health status while laying out the details. Such a considerate, albeit sometimes slightly imperfect, communication style helps patients feel informed and supported—and that makes for better surgical outcomes and a smoother recovery overall (Yang et al., 2025) (Figure 4.11).

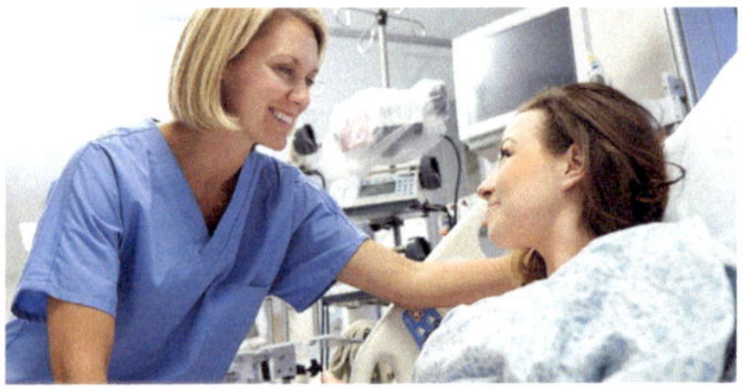

Figure 4.11. The importance of patient education in anesthesia.

Source: https://www.ccianesthesia.com/wp-content/uploads/2021/06/CCI_Patient_Edu.jpg.

Test Your Knowledge

1. What happens during anesthesia consultation?
2. What are the risks of anesthesia?

4.4. Multidisciplinary Approach to Preoperative Preparation

Learning Outcome

1. Describe the involvement of healthcare professionals.
2. Understand the coordination among surgical team members.
3. Understand the role of nursing in preoperative care.

Preoperative readiness depends on a mix of different medical experts working together—this kind of teamwork generally boosts patient safety and overall outcomes. A group that includes surgeons, anesthesiologists, nurses, and primary care providers all plays a key role here. Their knack for communicating without fuss covers so many angles of a patient's health, which in most cases cuts down on the chance of unexpected complications before surgery. For example, when teams put structured communication tools into play, workflow tends to improve, care doesn't get too fragmented, and patient evaluations before surgery come off as much more complete. All these collaborative moves tend to make patients better prepped for their procedures, leading to safer surgeries and smoother recoveries. Specialized know-how also fills in some crucial gaps within these mixed groups. Experts can, for instance, spot extra health issues, keep a close eye on medication routines, and gauge possible surgical risks through hands-on, tailored patient reviews. Generally speaking, having a set pathway helps get around the complexities usually tied to preoperative checks and brings different professionals closer together. In fact, a well-oiled preoperative anesthesia clinic often sees fewer cancellations and timelier surgeries, which underlines why a unified approach works. Plus, the constant back-and-forth among team members seems to spark ongoing improvements in care delivery and lift patient satisfaction in surgical settings. Keeping up with training and ongoing education is another vital piece of the puzzle in these multidisciplinary setups. Regular training sessions and collaborative workshops mean that team members can keep up with evolving practices and protocols that might affect surgical readiness, even if sometimes the updates feel a bit off-kilter. Some studies have pointed out that smoother communication across specialties not only reduces delays but also sharpens decision-making in the preoperative phase. Occasional cross-department sessions—even with their minor, natural typographical quirks—help bridge gaps in understanding and foster a more integrated approach to care. As surgical care continues to grow more complex, the blend of teamwork and consistent learning remains essential in fine-tuning how we assess and prepare for surgery (Giovanna et al., 2014; Perry et al., 2021).

4.4.1. Involvement of Healthcare Professionals

Healthcare professionals working together make a big difference when it comes to getting patients ready for surgery. Often, when surgical teams, nurses, and patients actually chat clearly, not only does the quality of care go up but the overall experience feels better too. A project at a Central Valley hospital, for example, mixed up a structured communication plan with everyday practice, and it helped unplanned surgical patients get better outcomes. They introduced an Add-On Communication Tool and brought back a strict pre-op checklist, eventually beating an initial target of 65%. This whole effort shows that when different providers share information openly, it can boost patient satisfaction and keep things on track in the perioperative stage (Vash et al., 2021). Taking it further, many facilities are now leaning into methods like the ISBAR(Identify, Situation, Background, Assessment and Recommendation) protocol to smooth out the handoffs at critical times. Generally speaking, this type of framework clears up the flow of information, cuts d on errors, and improves the overall preoperative process. One study with nursing students even found that practicing ISBAR using a desktop virtual reality app delivered learning benefits nearly as strong as the traditional methods. It seems that these innovative ways of training may actually get future healthcare professionals even more ready for the real world. This gradual change in training points out the need for ongoing alters in communication practices within the healthcare system (Andreasen et al., 2024). On top of that, having lots of different healthcare professionals involved in pre-op assessments makes sure that patient needs and risks don't get overlooked. When surgeons, anesthesiologists, nurses, and pharmacists put their heads together, they bring a mix of insights that leads to a fuller picture of a patient's health. This teamwork helps spot potential complications early and deal with them on time. Not only does this cooperative approach ramp up the safety of surgical procedures, but it also creates a kind of vibe where patient-focused care just thrives. Projects aimed at improving communication have shown that mixing knowledge from various professionals is key to building effective preoperative practices that, in the end, improve surgical results and patient satisfaction (Vash et al., 2021) (Figure 4.12).

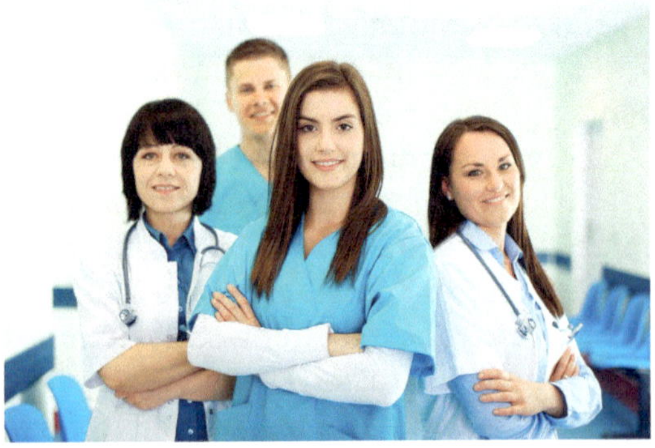

Figure 4.12. Healthcare professionals.

Source: https://medipharm.com.au/wp-content/uploads/2024/02/successful-medical-team.jpg.

4.4.2. Coordination Among Surgical Team Members

Team coordination in the operating room makes a difference in how patients do during surgery. Every person knowing what to do and being ready isn't just a nice-to-have—it smooths out the whole process. Clear, step-by-step communication and proper training seem to boost teamwork a lot; for example, when the VA rolled out its medical team training program, they not only saw fewer surgical deaths but also better quality care, quicker surgeries, and even happier staff overall (Chase et al., 2011). All this kind of proof points to the idea that when pre-op checks mix in good communication and team spirit, the chance of a safer surgery goes up. Before surgery kicks off, there's usually a chance for the crew to get together in a casual briefing—more than just ticking a box. These meetings help everyone feel responsible and get a jump on spotting any hiccups that might come up during the operation. Research in most cases shows that when every team member is part of the decision-making process around patient care, there's generally a clear drop in human-error-related mishaps (Barach et al., 2009). When people bounce ideas off each other and use what they do best, even the trickiest procedures seem less risky. Good coordination doesn't stop when the surgery ends; its benefits spill over into recovery and even affect how patients rate their overall care. When preoperative assessments clear the air and make sure key details get through, everything flows more naturally afterward. Hospitals that put such systems in place have seen fewer infections and other post-surgery problems, just as noted in several successful initiatives (Chase et al., 2011). In a way, raising the standard of care isn't just about credentials—it's a real pledge to patient safety, and it makes the whole surgical experience better. All in all, building solid teamwork from the start lays down the groundwork for smoother operations and better overall patient outcomes.

4.4.3. Role of Nursing in Preoperative Care

Nurses are front and center when it comes to getting patients ready for surgery. They check patients over in ways that go well beyond a basic exam, making sure that any hidden issues—like past surgeries or ongoing health problems—get noticed. A careful look at a patient's history can flag risks such as venous thromboembolism (VTE), especially when surgeries limit movement afterward. In most cases, these checks help shape follow-up care plans and actually reduce on the complications and even deaths that sometimes follow operations. By keeping patients as informed as possible and making sure they're physically set, nurses end up being a major factor in boosting surgical results and reducing on problems after the procedure. Taking care of how patients feel emotionally is another big part of what nurses handle before surgery. Anxiety and fear about the upcoming operation can throw a wrench in recovery, so nurses often use every day talk and even a bit of therapeutic communication to ease worries and explain what's ahead. This kind of support is particularly important for those facing tougher procedures—like setting up vascular access for patients with end-stage renal disease (ESRD). As many studies generally note, a good nurse doesn't just deal with physical prep; they also attend to the mental side of care, which in turn creates a smoother, more reassuring experience that builds confidence right before the surgery. Beyond prepping patients physically and emotionally, nurses also jump into risk management strategies that reduce surgery-related dangers. Spotting and sorting out VTE risks is key to crafting personalized preventative measures. Besides using drugs when needed, nurses also lean on other methods—like talking patients through the importance of staying active and keeping up with fluids after the operation—to help improve outcomes (Senem et al., 2025). This mixed approach shows just how crucial nursing work is, not solely for handling the surgery itself but for guiding patients toward a steady recovery afterward. In renal care, for example, careful handling of vascular access can lead to much better treatment results and a higher quality of life, reinforcing the idea that nurse-led care and patient education are indispensable, as outlined in (Wang, 2024) (Figure 4.13).

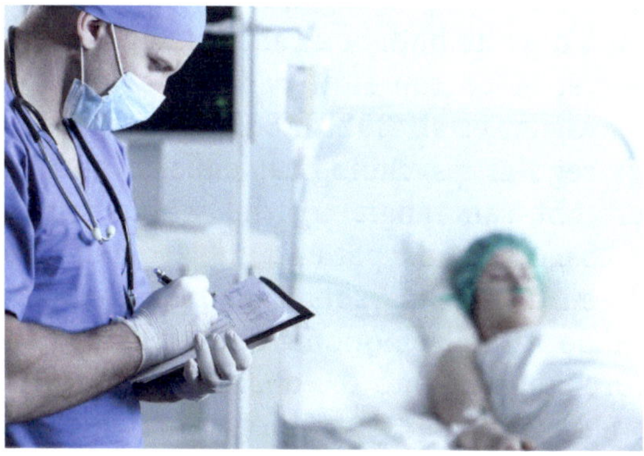

Figure 4.13. Role of nursing in preoperative care.

Source: https://www.verywellhealth.com/thmb/YbYKpd0JpktUmEycSd92qNhWjCQ=/1500x0/filters:no_upscale():max_bytes(150000):strip_icc()/iStock_72742951_XXLARGE-5764b8093df78ca6e42d0b8e.jpg.

Test Your Knowledge

1. What is the role of surgical team members?
2. What is the role of the nurse in preoperative care?

4.5. Challenges in Preoperative Assessment

Learning Outcome

1. Understand the patient-related challenges.
2. Describe the systemic and logistical challenges.
3. Understand the strategies to overcome challenges.

Getting ready for surgery isn't just about checking one's physical condition; it's a mixed bag of factors that often catch us off guard. Patients' reflections—feelings of stress, bouts of anxiety, and the overall emotional tone—end up weighing just as much as any physical sign. Generally speaking, a complete evaluation should dig into both body and mind since these inner stresses can slow recovery quite a bit (Vinayagam et al., 2023). Still, many practices skip regular psychological checks, and that oversight can tangle up the whole surgical process. Vulnerable patients, in particular, seem to need a more personalized plan that looks after both their emotional and physical needs before stepping into the operating room. Then there's the whole issue of logistics, which only adds to the challenge. Scheduling mishaps, the tricky business of lining up the right specialists, and getting various departments to actually coordinate can turn a routine check into a real headache. Some hospitals seem a bit too focused on speed and efficiency, often at the expense of a thoroughly planned evaluation—leading, for example, to rushed assessments or even last-minute cancellations (Vinayagam et al., 2023). This not only leaves patients feeling uncertain, but it may also affect the success of the surgery, especially when someone has a history of other medical complications. One can't overstate how important clear communication is in all this. Often, when details get lost between anesthesiologists and surgeons, the necessary information becomes scattered, and patient safety can end up in jeopardy. A collaborative atmosphere—even if it means a few extra conversations—is generally seen to smooth out the bumps in preoperative evaluations (Esplendori et al., 2016). Putting in place a set of shared guidelines for exchanging information, while allowing a little flexibility here and there, can help everyone stay on the same page. In the end, this mix of better coordination and attention to both emotional and physical details can boost surgical outcomes and overall patient satisfaction.

4.5.1. Patient-Related Challenges

Surgical procedures face a tangle of challenges that often begin long before the operating room door swings open. Patients can be gripped by anxiety – in fact, studies suggest about 30% wrestle with worries tied to anesthesia. That nervousness not only colors their whole experience but may also stir up problems during the operation and afterward, sometimes messing with pain relief and overall satisfaction. Doctors need to have solid tools and plans on hand to ease this mental load. In many cases, a clear grasp of these issues helps create a more relaxed, supportive setting before surgery (Bello et al., 2025). Other health concerns also add their twist to the pre-surgery mix. Conditions like high blood pressure, diabetes, and even obesity deserve careful attention because they can complicate how surgery goes and alter recovery. Generally speaking, a thorough check of these issues is crucial—tailoring anesthesia plans and sometimes even hinting at possible complications. It also means that healthcare teams should spend some time educating patients about how their current conditions might impact the results of surgery. Taking a proactive stance on managing these ailments can boost surgical safety and, in return, improve the overall patient experience (Qadrie et al., 2025). On top of that, getting patients fully on board with preoperative instructions can be a real struggle. Many folks misinterpret guidelines, whether it's skipping fasting rules or messing up medication adjustments, often due to simple miscommunication. This kind of slip-up not only risks the safety of the procedure but can also stretch out recovery times. Encouraging patients to take an active role—using clear language, one-on-one chats, or even casual info sessions—can go a long way toward better compliance. With a more relaxed and familiar approach, healthcare providers create a smoother transition into surgery, lowering complications and helping patients feel more prepared (Bello et al., 2025) (Figure 4.14).

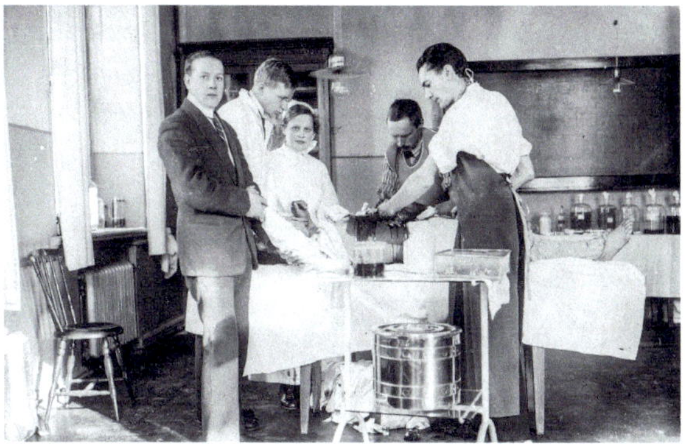

Figure 4.14. Surgery underway at the Red Cross Hospital in Tampere, Finland during the 1918 Finnish Civil War.

Source: By Museokeskus Vapriikki - Leikkaus Punaisen ristin sairaalassa Tampereella, Public Domain, https://commons.wikimedia.org/w/index.php?curid=49106016.

4.5.2. Systemic and Logistical Challenges

The preoperative phase is key to successful surgery but faces a range of system and logistical hurdles that can mess with proper patient evaluation and preparation. Getting everyone on the same page—surgeons, anesthesiologists, nurses, and even the administrative folks—often proves tricky as smooth communication isn't always there. When clear guidelines are missing, practices tend to vary, and these inconsistencies can complicate care. This is especially true for demanding procedures like pelvic exenteration, where teamwork is critical (Aalbers et al., 2021). In many cases, neglecting these underlying issues can end up compromising patient care quality, ultimately increasing the risk of surgical mishaps and prolonged recovery times. Logistical problems also play a huge role in the preoperative setup, sometimes altering how well patients are prepped for surgery. Scheduling can get messy; high demand for operating rooms leads to conflicts that might force delays, with cases being bumped or prioritized by urgency rather than pure clinical necessity. On top of that, limited staffing can stretch resources, reducing on vital interactions and follow-up during assessments. These challenges hit even harder in specialized units, where a dedicated team is supposed to manage complex cases. Variations in how facilities are used and how staff are allocated result in an uneven preoperative experience, highlighting the clear need for better, more efficient strategies to improve outcomes (Kontovounisios et al., 2020). Integrating preoperative assessments into one standardized protocol might just help ease some of these system and logistical snags. Setting out straightforward guidelines for patient selection, evaluation, and preparation—similar to the consensus on managing pelvic exenteration—could offer a solid routine. Not only does such a pathway build consistency, but it also boosts communication across the team, making it easier to spot potential problems early on. Plus, when there's broad agreement on the key parts of perioperative management, it leads to smarter resource use and better patient readiness, while reducing surgical risks (Aalbers et al., 2021). Given how the healthcare scene keeps changing, it's essential for institutions to seriously consider adopting comprehensive guidelines to tackle these challenges head-on.

4.5.3. Strategies to Overcome Challenges

Preparing for surgery isn't just about the scalpel—it's a mix of looking after both the body and the mind. Get a patient moving with some tailored prehabilitation, where exercise, good food, and even a bit of mental conditioning come into play. Patients often feel more in charge when they're part of this process, and it seems that less postoperative trouble follows. Sometimes, different healthcare folks end up working together in a more relaxed, almost improvised way, crafting a care plan that fits the individual like a glove. All of this, in most cases, leads to a smoother operation and quicker bounce-back (Zeppenfeld et al., 2022). There's also the mental side of things that can't be skipped over. It's common to feel nervous or even downright scared as surgery looms—nerves that might even affect recovery. Mixing in some cognitive-behavioral conversations and a few relaxation tips can help roll those jitters off. This kind of support gives patients a sense of control and builds some inner strength, you know, so they handle the stress better when the time comes. Occasionally, local support groups or informal workshops pop up, where sharing experiences helps ease the load. Doctors, therapists, and even peers sometimes chat over these issues, making sure that, besides being in good shape physically, someone's also a bit more emotionally ready before they head into the OR (Zeppenfeld et al., 2022). There's also the challenge of juggling any other health issues that might complicate surgery. Sometimes, a close look at everyday habits—think of cutting back on smoking or rethinking the diet—is needed to lower the risk. Often, a mix of specialists, including nutritionists and physiotherapists, gets involved to provide timely advice, even if their suggestions seem to come at different times. In most cases, checking on these lifestyle factors and doing a few capacity tests paves the way for a plan that's as unique as the patient's. Setting up simple referral paths to these experts not only fine-tunes the whole preoperative checkup but also builds a safety net that leads to better surgical outcomes and happier patients (Carli et al., 2021) (Figure 4.15).

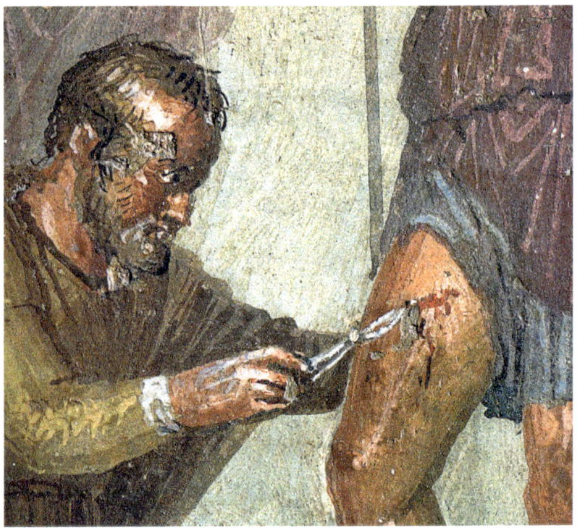

Figure 4.15. Iapyx removing an arrowhead from the thigh of Aeneas using a forcepts (Virgil Aeneid XII.383-440) Roman fresco from the Casa di Sirico in Pompeii.

Source: By WolfgangRieger - Filippo Coarelli (ed.): Pompeji. Hirmer, München 2002, ISBN 3-7774-9530-1, p. 218, Public Domain, https://commons.wikimedia.org/w/index.php?curid=6241903.

Test Your Knowledge

1. What are the systemic and logistical challenges?
2. What are the strategies to overcome challenges?

SUMMARY

Patient safety begins with an excellent pre-surgery examination that delves deeper than the body—it even covers mental and social well-being. Having a good going-over identifies risks early on, so physicians can balance and blend their strategy to minimize chances of complications. Consider Comprehensive Preoperative Assessment and Support (CPAS); most often, this technique is a miracle solution for elderly patients by being personalized to every individual. Targeted testing, research confirms, reduces surgical stress and hastens recovery, reminding us again that surgical oncology care needs to be as unique as the patient. It's all about having all the little things taken care of, time and again. Very advanced preservation methods make a big difference, too. Take ovarian tissue cryopreservation (OTC)—a technique that's gaining acceptance as more individuals want to save fertility prior to treatments that may disrupt reproductive function. Health professionals, more than ever, must drill deep with pre-procedure screening. The success of ovarian tissue transplantation (OTT) depends on a multitude of factors, like ensuring no perilous malignant cells make their way in during reimplantation and treating the ovarian tissues with care so as to leave as many follicles intact as possible. Generally, adhering to a formal preoperative protocol doesn't just improve fertility care, but it also fits the unique needs of different patients (Turan et al., 2024). Finally, anticipating problems before they happen is the hub of any good preoperative evaluation. Continual innovation in the field reminds us that training should stay in the loop among healthcare providers. By practicing on data-based approaches and an actual culture of safety, caregivers make significant leaps toward better outcomes in a range of surgical areas. CPAS findings even showed that personalized pre-op care decreases blood loss and decreases hospital stays—a clear push that shows rigorous examination is a concern. With surgery evolving and increasing, a sharp preoperative assessment remains at the center of quality care and ultimate success (Ushimaru et al., 2024).

Good surgery starts with getting patients well-prepared and well-checked up. It is not merely a case of ticking through a standard checklist—there is a need to look out for potential side effects of particular treatments like poly (ADP-ribose) polymerase (PARP) inhibitors. Sometimes things get complicated with blood issues or stomach issues needing to be watched. Physicians usually perform routine blood work to monitor for any hematological glitches, and if the standard remedies don't appear to be taking hold, a quick referral to a blood specialist is warranted. On the GI side, timing medications appropriately, modifying diet regimens, and addressing symptoms such as nausea or vomiting immediately are what make the difference. Mostly, this hands-on, inclusive approach enhances safety and paves the way for simpler recoveries (Carli et al., 2021). Obstructive sleep apnea (OSA) is found to be very common in surgical patients, making a thorough pre-op assessment even more important. Many patients, surprisingly, are not even aware that they have OSA—a factor that can bring added risks to a procedure. New guidelines from the Society of Anesthesia and Sleep Medicine (SASM) recommend that preoperative screening must do more than identify OSA, but also investigate individualized management plans. Generally speaking, awareness of the varied presentations and underlying forms of OSA dictates that treatment will need to move beyond the typical CPAP modality. This less overt appreciation of the condition enriches the overall preoperative picture, giving clinicians more room to minimize care and prevent complications (Madhusudan et al., 2017). Staying one step ahead of the potential side effects is worth it before surgery. Being proactive about risk and keeping a careful watch—sometimes even letting patients help monitor symptoms—can minimize problems during the pre-op period. This layered strategy is especially important when dealing with treatments like PARP inhibitors, which come with their own set of infamous difficulties. By collaborating in multidisciplinary teams (with some regular, human-type distractions along the way), clinicians more readily navigate the peaks and valleys of preoperative care. When thorough evaluations pair with tried-and-true protocols, patients end up better prepared—improving their chances for a smoother surgery and increasing overall satisfaction during that vulnerable perioperative period (Carli et al., 2021; Madhusudan et al., 2017).

KEY TERMS FROM THIS CHAPTER

- Anesthesia consultation
- Computer-driven systems
- Healthcare
- Medical history
- Physical examination
- Preoperative anesthesia
- Surgical care
- Surgical-site infections
- Antibiotics
- Diabetes
- Heart problems
- Nutrition
- Plan-Do-Study-Act
- Preoperative assessments
- Surgical procedures

CRITICAL THINKING QUESTIONS

1. **The primary goal of preoperative assessment is to:**
   a. Optimize the surgical procedure
   b. Identify and reduce patient risk factors
   c. Confirm the surgical site
   d. Select the type of anesthesia to be used
2. **The Mallampati classification is used to predict:**
   a. Risk of aspiration
   b. Risk of postoperative nausea
   c. Difficulty of intubation
   d. Respiratory complications
3. **Which of the following is a major risk factor for perioperative cardiac complications?**
   a. Controlled diabetes
   b. Previous myocardial infarction
   c. Mild hypertension
   d. Smoking history
4. **Routine preoperative laboratory tests are most appropriate for:**
   a. All patients scheduled for surgery
   b. Patients with specific clinical indications
   c. Patients younger than 50 years old
   d. Minor procedures under local anesthesia
5. **Informed consent for anesthesia must include:**
   a. Description of the surgical procedure
   b. The surgeon's credentials
   c. Risks and benefits of anesthesia options
   d. Laboratory test results

Short Answer Questions

1. Define the preoperative assessment.
2. Why is preoperative preparation important?
3. What are the objectives of preoperative assessment?
4. List the components of preoperative assessment.
5. Describe the role of anesthesia in preoperative assessment.

Answers to Critical Thinking Questions

1. (b); 2. (c); 3. (b); 4. (b); 5. (c)

REFERENCES

1. Aalbers, A. G. J., Abdul Aziz, N., Abecasis, N., Abraham-Nordling, M., Akiyoshi, T., Alberda, W., Albert, M., et al. (2021). Perioperative management and anaesthetic considerations in pelvic exenterations using Delphi methodology: Results from the PelvEx Collaborative. https://core.ac.uk/download/614047059.pdf (accessed on 20 May 2025).
2. Abdullayev, R., Ekinci, Ö., Taştan, M. E., Uluç, Ö. S., Hıdıroğlu, S., Zengin, M. B., Bakır Keser, N., et al. (2024). Preoperative patients' knowledge level regarding anesthesia procedures and anesthesiologist responsibilities. *Eurasian Journal of Anesthesiology and Intensive Care.* https://www.semanticscholar.org/paper/1f1d4b08e60656854bab168538b64d7bb50a3a6d (accessed on 20 May 2025).
3. Agnihotri, A. K., Ailawadi, G., Barnhart, G. R., Farivar, R., et al. (2016). *Minimally Invasive Mitral Valve Surgery I: Patient Selection, Evaluation, And Planning.* https://core.ac.uk/download/323076062.pdf.
4. Andreasen, E. M. (2024). *Interpersonal Communication During Preoperative Handover: Status of Current Practices and The Effect of a Desktop Virtual Reality Intervention for Learning Handover Skills in Nursing Education.* https://core.ac.uk/download/616581414.pdf (accessed on 20 May 2025).
5. Barach, P., Schraagen, J. M., Smit, M., Ven, H., et al. (2009). *Teams and Cardiac Surgery.* https://core.ac.uk/download/pdf/11476812.pdf.
6. Bello, C., Eisler, P., & Heidegger, T. (2025). Perioperative anxiety: Current status and future perspectives. *Journal of Clinical Medicine, 14.* https://www.semanticscholar.org/paper/43fbc64b35d71b04794d4be18fa15807ab0975d7 (accessed on 20 May 2025).
7. Blumenthal, D., & McCarthy, D. (2006). *Committed to Safety: Ten Case Studies on Reducing Harm to Patients.* https://core.ac.uk/download/71350251.pdf (accessed on 20 May 2025).
8. Bouamrane, M. M., & Mair, F. S. (2014). A study of clinical and information management processes in the surgical pre-assessment clinic. *BMC Medical Informatics and Decision Making, 14*, 22. https://doi.org/10.1186/1472-6947-14-22.
9. Carli, F., Awasthi, R., Gillis, C., Baldini, G., Bessissow, A., Liberman, A. S., & Minnella, E. M. (2021). Integrating prehabilitation in the preoperative clinic: A paradigm shift in perioperative care. *Anesthesia & Analgesia.* https://doi.org/10.1213/ane.0000000000005471.
10. Chase, D., & McCarthy, D. (2011). *Advancing Patient Safety in the U.S. Department of Veterans Affairs.* https://core.ac.uk/download/75777631.pdf (accessed on 20 May 2025).
11. Coluzzi, F., Bifulco, F., Cuomo, A., Dauri, M., Leonardi, C., Melotti, R. M., Natoli, S., Romualdi, P., Savoia, G., & Corcione, A. (2017). The challenge of perioperative pain management in opioid-tolerant patients. *Therapeutics and Clinical Risk Management, 13*, 1163–1173. https://doi.org/10.2147/TCRM.S141332.
12. Englesbe, M. J. (2017). We are doing it because they demanded it. *Annals of Surgery, 266*(6), e83–e84. https://doi.org/10.1097/SLA.0000000000001842.
13. Esplendori, G. F., Kobayashi, R. M., & Bianchi, E. R. (2016). Stress and coping strategies of women in preoperative period of valve surgery. *Journal of Nursing UFPE Online, 10*, 3537–3547. https://www.semanticscholar.org/paper/992ee227c70839a24cdc9c1beb315b4912a714a7 (accessed on 20 May 2025).

14. Flint, T. (2016). *Gaining Efficiency and Reducing Cost: The Re-Design of a Preoperative Screening Clinic.* http://deepblue.lib.umich.edu/bitstream/2027.42/137960/1/Flint2016.pdf (accessed on 20 May 2025).

15. Güneş Kara, S. (2025). The role of prophylaxis for preventing venous thromboembolism in major urological surgery and nursing management. *The New Journal of Urology.* https://www.semanticscholar.org/paper/527579517de257cea4776bb05decb164d1e5d66b (accessed on 20 May 2025).

16. Kheir, M. M., Ziemba-Davis, M., Dilley, J. E., Hood, M. J., Jr, & Meneghini, R. M. (2018). Tourniquetless total knee arthroplasty with modern perioperative protocols decreases pain and opioid consumption in women. *The Journal of Arthroplasty, 33*(11), 3455–3459. https://doi.org/10.1016/j.arth.2018.06.038.

17. Kontovounisios, C. (2020). Perioperative management and anesthetic considerations in pelvic exenterations using Delphi methodology: Results from the PelvEx Collaborative. https://core.ac.uk/download/363636236.pdf (accessed on 20 May 2025).

18. Lamperti, M., Romero, C. S., Guarracino, F., Cammarota, G., Vetrugno, L., Tufegdzic, B., Lozsan, F., et al. (2025). Preoperative assessment of adults undergoing elective noncardiac surgery: Updated guidelines from the European Society of Anesthesiology and Intensive Care. *European Journal of Anesthesiology, 42*(1), 1–35. https://doi.org/10.1097/EJA.0000000000002069.

19. Lampugnale, C. A. (2017). *Surgical Assessment of The Geriatric Oncology Patient* [Master's thesis, Boston University]. https://open.bu.edu/bitstream/2144/26707/5/Lampugnale_bu_0017N_13146.pdf.

20. Landrum, M. R., Milby, A., Yaszay, B., Parent, S., Nelson, S., Pahys, J., Samdani, A., et al. (2022). Thoracic curve correction ratio: An objective measure to guide against overcorrection of a main thoracic curve in the setting of a structural proximal thoracic curve. *Journal of Clinical Medicine, 11*, Article 1234. https://www.semanticscholar.org/paper/c3f19bbe9dab7be9e07531f52857a14d9d81a152 (accessed on 20 May 2025).

21. Lansdown, D. A., Ukwuani, G., Kuhns, B., Harris, J. D., & Nho, S. J. (2018). Self-reported mental disorders negatively influence surgical outcomes after arthroscopic treatment of femoroacetabular impingement. *Orthopedic Journal of Sports Medicine, 6*(5), 2325967118773312. https://doi.org/10.1177/2325967118773312.

22. Madhusudan, P., Wong, J., Prasad, A., Sadeghian, E., & Chung, F. (2017). An update on preoperative assessment and preparation of surgical patients with obstructive sleep apnea. *Current Opinion in Anesthesiology, 31*(1), 89–95. https://www.semanticscholar.org/paper/4cb8816bbabe9fa970ff5aaca50fdf82a710d6e6 (accessed on 20 May 2025).

23. Manninen, P., & Sivanaser, V. (2010). Preoperative assessment of adult patients for intracranial surgery. *Canadian Journal of Anesthesia.* https://core.ac.uk/download/207203745.pdf (accessed on 20 May 2025).

24. McMahon, A. J., McSorley, S. T., & Steele, C. W. (2018). Meta-analysis of oral antibiotics, in combination with preoperative intravenous antibiotics and mechanical bowel preparation the day before surgery, compared with intravenous antibiotics and mechanical bowel preparation alone to reduce surgical-site infections in elective colorectal surgery. *British Journal of Surgery.* https://core.ac.uk/download/159754946.pdf (accessed on 20 May 2025).

25. Naranjo, A., Isenring, E., & Teleni, L. (2017). Immune-enhancing formulas for patients with cancer undergoing esophagectomy: Systematic review protocol. *JMIR Research Protocols, 6*(11), e214. https://doi.org/10.2196/resprot.7688.

26. Neelakanta, A., Fitts, L., Fischer, K., Layell, J., Kester, S., Rajan, V., & Passaretti, C. (2025). P-376. Impact of a preoperative in-person assessment (PIPA) on hip and knee replacement surgical site infections (SSI). *Open Forum Infectious Diseases, 12*. https://www.semanticscholar.org/paper/27938bf004d9e7abcdff0fbfcb8909f24dd23833 (accessed on 20 May 2025).

27. Noort, H. J., Heinen, M., Asseldonk, M., Ettema, R., Vermeulen, H., Huisman-de Waal, G. H., & On behalf of the Grephepi group. (2020). Using intervention mapping to develop an outpatient nursing nutritional intervention to improve nutritional status in undernourished patients planned for surgery. *BMC Health Services Research, 20*, Article 202. https://www.semanticscholar.org/paper/67c7baec30891959f15e03b1e4bfaaf9b2f002bc (accessed on 20 May 2025).

28. Nosbisch, M. L. (2024). *Lived Experiences of Certified Registered Nurse Anesthetists Regarding Anesthesia Provision: A Heuristic Inquiry* (Doctoral dissertation, Walden University). https://core.ac.uk/download/639355835.pdf (accessed on 20 May 2025).

29. Paek, J. K. (2015). Preventing surgical site infections by utilizing CHG wipes for preoperative skin preparation (Master's thesis, University of San Francisco). *Master's Projects and Capstones, 154*. https://repository.usfca.edu/capstone/154 (accessed on 20 May 2025).

30. Perry, W., III. (2021). *Decreasing Same-Day Preoperative Delays and Cancellations: A Quality Improvement Project*. https://core.ac.uk/download/489832296.pdf (accessed on 20 May 2025).

31. Qadrie, Z., Maqbool, M., Dar, M. A., & Qadir, A. (2025). Navigating challenges and maximizing potential: Handling complications and constraints in minimally invasive surgery. *Open Health, 6*(1), 20250059. https://doi.org/10.1515/ohe-2025-0059.

32. Stephen, A., Giovanna, B., Bruce, D., & Kirkpatrick, P. (2014). Competencies and skills to enable effective care of severely obese patients undergoing bariatric surgery across a multidisciplinary healthcare perspective: A systematic review. *JBI Database of Systematic Reviews and Implementation Reports, 12*(9), 321–397. https://doi.org/10.11124/jbisrir-2014-1583.

33. Turan, V., & Oktem, O. (2024). Autologous ovarian tissue transplantation: Preoperative assessment and preparation of the patient. *Obstetrical & Gynecological Survey, 79*(11), 683–688. https://www.semanticscholar.org/paper/a89b65285cb63b3d751e90d87a38b6f672a89f1b (accessed on 20 May 2025).

34. Ushimaru, Y., Nagano, S., Kawabata, R., Nishikawa, K., Takeoka, T., Kitagawa, A., Ohara, N., et al. (2024). Enhancing surgical outcomes in elderly gastric cancer patients: The role of comprehensive preoperative assessment and support. *World Journal of Surgical Oncology, 22*. https://www.semanticscholar.org/paper/94e80ac1e32d2fbe1bdf73082f2439db58b8d209 (accessed on 20 May 2025).

35. Vash, S. L. (2021). *Closing communication gaps for unplanned surgical patients: One pre-op checklist at a time*. https://core.ac.uk/download/475631478.pdf (accessed on 20 May 2025).

36. Vinayagam, S., & Dhanger, S. (2023). Perioperative blood management: Current transfusion practices and challenges. *International Journal of Advanced Medical and Health Research, 10*(1), 4–11. https://www.semanticscholar.org/paper/315081ba59a98fc75cf49d8bca301d52cefd54b0 (accessed on 20 May 2025).

37. Wang, J. (2024). Comprehensive nursing care for vascular access in hemodialysis patients with end-stage renal disease. *International Journal of Public Health and Medical Research, 2*(1), 42–46. https://doi.org/10.62051/ijphmr.v2n1.05.

38. Wenzel, J. T., Schwenk, E. S., Baratta, J. L., & Viscusi, E. R. (2016). Managing opioid-tolerant patients in the perioperative surgical home. *Anesthesiology Clinics, 34*(2), 287–301. https://doi.org/10.1016/j.anclin.2016.01.005.

39. Yang, D. S., Jeon, Y., Kim, C. R., Kim, S. G., & Park, K. (2025). Severe preoperative pain, functional decline, and high anxiety levels hinder the efficacy of multidisciplinary interventions in patients who underwent primary total knee arthroplasty. *Journal of Orthopedic Surgery and Research, 20*. https://www.semanticscholar.org/paper/42af6ffb3d44c8c931ae5a095a3107e394ec97d8 (accessed on 20 May 2025).

40. Zeppenfeld, K., Tfelt-Hansen, J., Riva, M., Winkel, B. G., Behr, E. R., Blom, N. A., Charron, P., et al. (2022). 2022 ESC guidelines for the management of patients with ventricular arrhythmias and the prevention of sudden cardiac death. *European Heart Journal, 43*, 3997–4126. https://doi.org/10.1093/eurheartj/ehac262.

AIRWAY MANAGEMENT AND TECHNIQUES

5

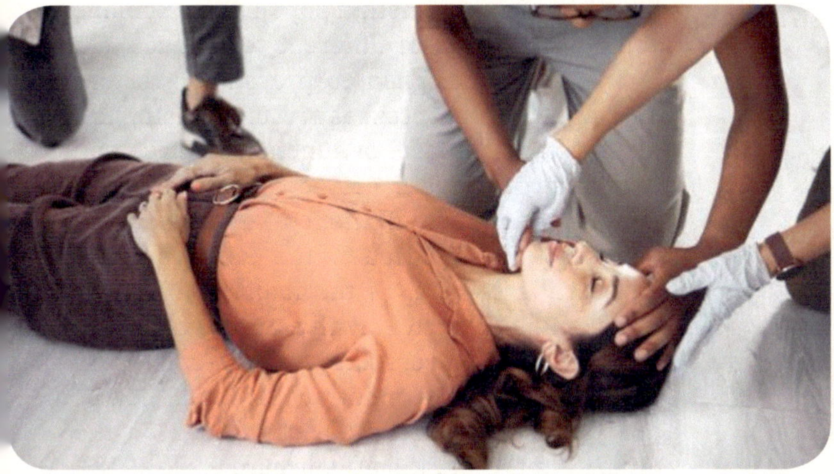

LEARNING OBJECTIVES

After studying this chapter, you will be able to:

1. Understand the anatomy of the airway.
2. Assess the airway patency.
3. Explain the basic airway management techniques.
4. Discuss about advanced airway management techniques.
5. Discuss about special considerations in airway management.

Introduction

Modern medicine today is teeming with life, and something that first occurs is the critical role of establishing a patient's airway. For simple procedures or a full-blown emergency, keeping that pathway open is what keeps anesthesia safe and enables good oxygenation when stakes are the greatest. More contemporary approaches—spawned by updated guidelines and emerging technologies—have illuminated the spotlight on this critical mission even as they introduce their own list of hurdles. It somehow feels as though with every step forward comes the directive to train firmly, constantly. It is by immersing oneself in the intricacy of airway anatomy, the response of the body, and proper procedures that therapists can minimize risks and enhance outcomes in everything from intricate operations to intensive care cases (Zhao et al., 2020). In a time of information becoming viral and technologies evolving, airway management has the double responsibility of staying abreast of two huge jobs: tapping into the complexities of new equipment and patient safety as its first priority. How ironic that the introduction of devices like the laryngoscope revolutionized anesthesia and turned it on its head, but those same problems continue to simmer beneath the surface. A lot of the time, when something doesn't go right, it is not so much a matter of screwing up some bit of kit—but rather, most frequently, of not fully getting the techniques right. This combination of human and technical issues urges us to prioritize more emphasis on continuous learning and putting the focus on people as much as on machines (Sorbello et al., 2018). Developing an effective strategy for airway management is not solely about mastering technical proficiency; it also involves a sense of knowing how decisions are made in an environment in which every second counts. Major authorities' recommendations serve as a sort of anchor, encouraging responsibility and a need for continuous improvement—though in most instances, no plan ever works out perfectly.

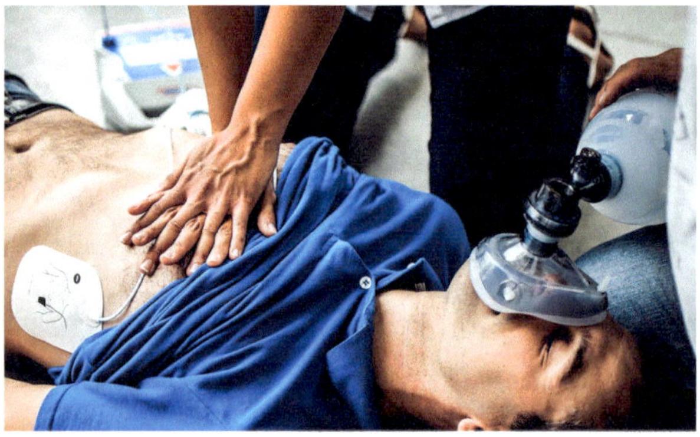

Figure 5.1. CPR patient airway management.

Source: https://www.pulsara.com/hubfs/blog-assets/CPR-patient-airway-management-1180x700.jpg.

The inclusion of simulations and even some cognitive aids into training sessions helps build the practical knowledge that is needed along with a setting in which teamwork and common understanding can grow. In the end, innovative devices are key, but making a world in which patient safety is the priority and mistakes are made rarely depends on understanding the human factor. It's this combination—and the occasional trial and error—that charts an airway management future where patient care and professional growth go hand-in-hand (Zhao et al., 2020) (Figure 5.1).

Definition of Airway Management

Management of the airway is essential for maintaining patients in a state of breathing and receiving adequate oxygen in many different clinical situations. Rather than being about literally keeping something open, the discipline combines a range of different techniques and interventions designed to prevent or restore blockage that could occur as a result of anatomical idiosyncrasy, disease, or function impairment. A clear protocol is necessary - not only does it specify what equipment and methods to use, but it differs based on the patient's status and setting of care. In the majority of cases, establishing the airway with accuracy can move from basic maneuvers like head-tilt–chin-lift to advanced steps like endotracheal intubation or the use of supraglottic devices, based on the urgency of the situation (Planchard et al., 2018). Airway management in medical emergencies is always between a necessity for an immediate response and a need for accuracy. Emergency doctors face many a challenge, whether that is trauma, acute respiratory distress, or change in mental status. Since an obstructed airway may become perilous very quickly, these experts tend to be trained to act promptly, they start with bag-mask ventilation very often and go on to more invasive techniques if that fails. Experience with paralytic drugs and sedatives also usually comes in handy, and routine practice with hands-on training and simulation protocols maintains those skills (Planchard et al., 2018). More than physically securing the airway, airway management involves a complete grasp of blockage effects on body functions and the risk that comes with them. Success in this setting is more than about guaranteeing oxygenation—it's also about balancing the patient's overall clinical picture and keeping an eye out for complications that may develop along the way. Contemporary practice is increasingly likely to involve calling upon experience from more than one specialty, and with advancing technology and technique, clinicians are encouraged to keep current on best practices and guidelines. Lastly, effective airway management continues to be a pillar of patient safety and quality of care within the emergency setting and beyond (Figure 5.2) (Counselman et al., 2017).

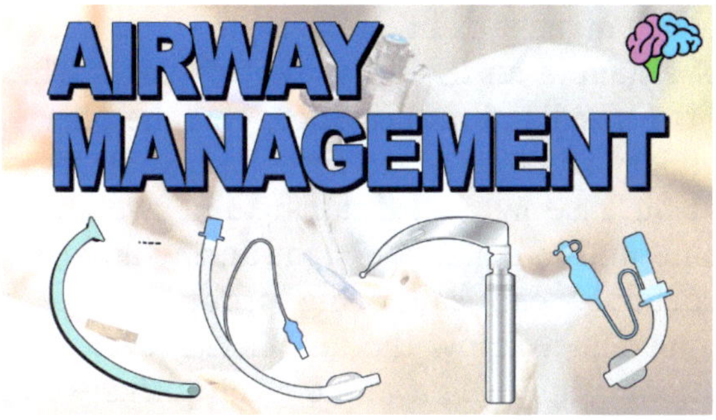

Figure 5.2. Airway management.

Source: https://i.ytimg.com/vi/Lurq9DroJag/maxresdefault.jpg.

Importance in Medical Practice

Health crises like COVID-19 have opened up airway management in ways we never expected. Today's medical teams meet patients with every kind of breathing problem imaginable, and knowing the ins and outs of airway management is not only helpful—it's necessary. You see, practice is what it takes to master procedures like tracheal intubation, and it has the possibility of exposing the care providers to the virus, a challenge that recent infection rates among healthcare workers have made impossible to ignore. Incorporating strict infection control practices in airway care not only safeguards the staff, but also ensures patients do not become worse off, especially where time is of the essence. It's not the physical aspect alone, either. The mental well-being of patients and clinicians during these processes is generally a neglected consideration. Intubation, for example, may heighten apprehension and disorientation, effects which can even influence treatment outcomes. Clear and direct communication—based on tested strategies—dissolves these tensions. At times, a few carefully thought-out infographics are the game-changer by d breaking down the most critical information in a more digestible form. In the pandemic of COVID-19, quick updates via social media kept everybody up to date with the latest protocols (Zhao et al., 2020). The situation isn't static either; as respiratory diseases evolve, so too must our methods of airway management. New research is still coming out, so healthcare providers are constantly having to adapt their procedures on the spot. Guideline updates on respiratory rehabilitation of COVID-19 patients, for example, are about customized therapy while maintaining effective airway management. These updates ensure that therapy is not only effective but also responsive to the unique needs of each patient and can speed up healing. In most cases, ongoing training in these techniques goes a long way to boosting public health outcomes, especially in the face of ever-changing pathogens and infection control challenges, as we've seen during this pandemic (Zhao et al., 2020).

5.1. Anatomy of the Airway

Learning Outcome

1. Describe the upper and lower airway structures.
2. Understand the physiological functions of the airway.

Knowing the anatomy of the airway is a big if you have to get it in order quickly in an emergency situation. Knowing how the midline glossoepiglottic fold (MVF) plays into the whole intubation story is one part of the equation. Most experts will say that having the laryngoscope up against the vallecula and subsequent engagement with the MVF can improve your glottic view.

But, in the majority of cases, training on the laryngeal inlet alone is inadequate for residents in emergency medicine. New simulation methods are dominating, offering practice with realistic airway anatomy—specifically the MVF—that helps to build hands-on skills and confidence (Tumminello et al., 2024). New technology is also transforming airway management. For example, point-of-care ultrasound provides a real-time view of the airway, and that can increase the chances of successful intubation in difficult situations. Distance from epiglottis to skin or hyomental gap provides hints regarding possible problem areas. And utilizing ultrasound to verify endotracheal tube placement can decrease on the likelihood of accidents. All things being equal, the marriage of close knowledge of airway anatomy and high-technology imaging tools is a recipe for safer, more effective interventions (Gottlieb et al., 2023).

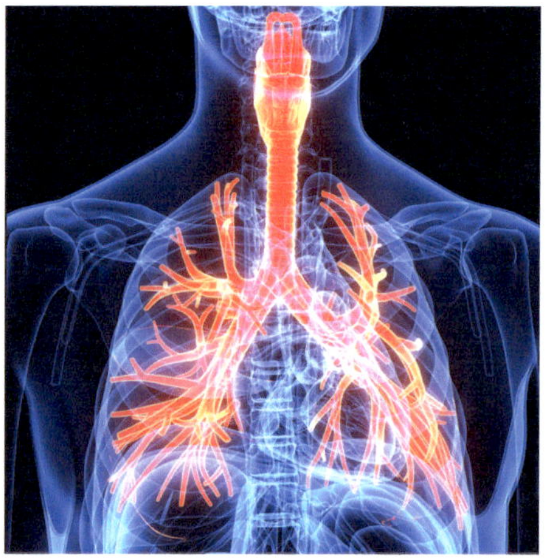

Figure 5.3. Anatomy of the airway.

Source: https://blog.sscor.com/hubfs/B%20264.jpg.

Simulation experience with airway anatomy in the hands is also highly successful. Most airway simulators today have components that enable you to touch and manipulate realistic-appearing anatomical structures—such as an open MVF—which makes practice more realistic. Such direct practice not only refines the skill of recognizing salient features but also creates extra confidence during real intubation attempts. In an overwhelming majority of cases, taking pains to follow a stepwise, anatomically based approach is possible with better clinical outcomes, as some of the recent studies have pointed out (Tumminello et al., 2024) (Figure 5.3).

5.1.1. Upper Airway Structures

Airway management isn't simple – you need to get a handle on the upper airway parts. Think of the nasal and oral cavities, plus the pharynx and larynx; these areas don't just let air in and out but also help with talking and swallowing. Sometimes a small oversight during an airway procedure can cause big problems, so it's important to know the landmarks, even when patients show slight anatomical quirks – from harmless variations to issues that border on serious. In many cases, being comfortable with these structures means a doctor can not only handle routine cases but also spot early signs that something's off, making it easier to intervene quickly. At the core of airway management is knowing which route to take for intubation or ventilation. The upper airway can be approached in a few ways – for example, some cases call for orotracheal intubation while others might be best managed with a nasotracheal route. When doctors expect a tough airway situation, techniques like awake fiberoptic intubation can make a difference – a controlled, sometimes lifesaving way to get through complex anatomy. NAP4, for instance, generally reminds us that leaving these options out, especially for high-risk patients, may lead to dangerous issues during induction. Having both the textbook knowledge and real, hands-on practice with these methods helps keep things balanced between technical know-how and patient safety. Changes in upper airway management practices keep challenging clinicians to stay on their toes. There's a noticeable shift towards using advanced tools such as video laryngoscopy –

these devices offer a clearer view compared to older, more conventional methods, particularly in the hardest cases. In emergency moments, having a rough idea of the procedural hierarchy becomes all the more critical since split-second decisions can be life or death. Protocols, therefore, need to weave together anatomy, technique, and technology in a way that isn't overly rigid but still keeps everything connected. Overall, these developments not only boost how effectively procedures are done but also build a culture that puts patient care first, as seen in the push for standardized airway setups in clinical settings (Chrimes et al., 2018; Wilson et al., 2018) (Figure 5.4).

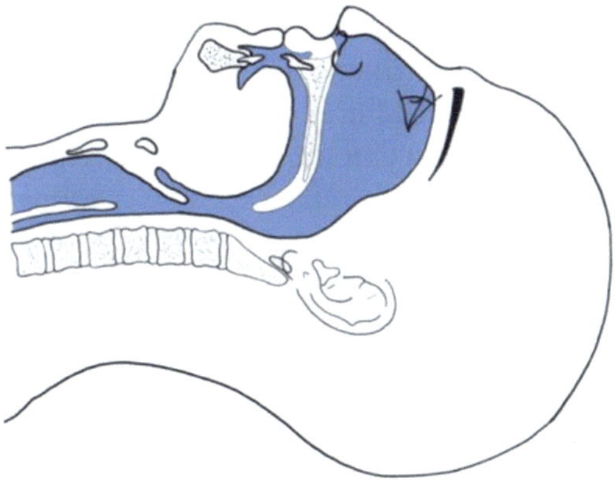

Figure 5.4. Functional upper airway.

Source: https://cdnintech.com/media/chapter/61712/1512345123/media/F1.png.

5.1.2. Lower Airway Structures

The human breathing system relies heavily on parts like the trachea, bronchi, and bronchioles—even if it might not sound too exciting at first glance. These parts work as simple passageways, moving air around so that gas exchange can happen in those tiny spots called alveoli. You see, the trachea acts like a sturdy tube supported by cartilage and then splits into a right and left bronchus, each feeding its lung. This split isn't just about moving air; it makes sure every lung section gets enough air for proper exchange. Overall, knowing how these channels fit together is key, especially when blockages or injuries can suddenly complicate breathing. Talking about troubles in these lower airways, conditions like bronchiolitis and asthma drive home just how important these structures are for keeping breathing on track. Inflammation in the lower passages can shift breathing off balance, making existing issues like asthma worse and even paving the way for long-term lung problems.

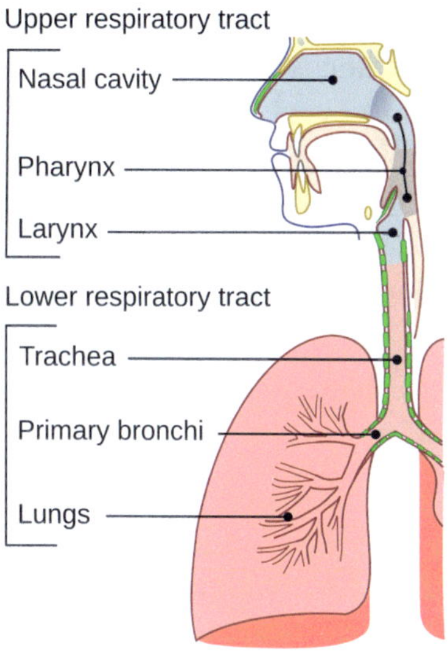

Figure 5.5. A diagram of the lower airway.

Source: By Lord Akryl, Jmarchn - Vectorized version of File:Illu conducting passages.jpg, which was in the public domain as a work of the US Government, Public Domain, https://commons.wikimedia.org/w/index.php?curid=112619332.

Research generally shows that viral infections—particularly those from respiratory syncytial virus (RSV) and rhinovirus (RV)—are closely linked to these disruptions, a fact that stands out, especially among kids. These infections may damage parts of the airway repeatedly, leading to chronic wheezing and sometimes even asthma. Recognizing this connection is crucial for healthcare providers as they develop strategies to lower the risks tied to these conditions (Jartti et al., 2017). When it comes to managing the airways themselves, a clear grasp of the lower structure's layout helps guide treatments like bronchodilation therapy and mechanical ventilation. For instance, giving bronchodilators can relax the smooth muscles in the bronchi and bronchioles, which in turn eases airflow and helps ease obstruction symptoms. In tough cases of respiratory failure, mechanical ventilation might step in to ensure enough oxygen is delivered, a process that underscores how important the integrity of these airways is. Recent advances, in most cases, show that a better look at how viral infections interact with airway structure has sparked new prevention and treatment methods. Keeping up with these changes remains essential for improving patient care (Rhodes et al., 2017) (Figure 5.5).

5.1.3. Physiological Functions of the Airway

Airway management starts with knowing how the airway works. A clear grasp of its basic functions is key—not simply for safe treatment but also because breathing hinges on getting oxygen in and pushing carbon dioxide out. Many factors, like resistance and how easily the airway stretches, affect this gas move; if it gets blocked—say, by swelling, unusual structures, or extra secretions—the whole process falters and can lead to low oxygen or too much carbon dioxide. In most cases, healthcare providers need to appreciate these points to keep the airway open and functioning, especially with patients in critical condition (Zhao et al., 2020). The airway isn't just a tunnel for air; it also helps shield the body from pathogens and pollutants. Think of the mucociliary escalator—a natural cleaning crew made of tiny hairs and mucus—that catches unwanted particles and pushes them back toward the throat, where they're either swallowed or coughed out. If this defense system gets affected by dehydration or smoking, patients (especially those with weakened immune systems or lung issues) might face infections like pneumonia or bronchitis. So, taking care of the airway means looking after this barrier too, ensuring nothing interferes with its job of clearing out contaminants (Segal et al., 2018). It's important to remember that the airway also has a lot to do with our voice and swallowing. The larynx, often just called the voice box, houses our vocal cords and lets us talk, while careful airway management helps prevent food or liquids from going down the wrong way—a mistake that can lead to aspiration pneumonia. Simple techniques, like making sure the patient is positioned correctly and checking how well they swallow, make a big difference. Overall, understanding the many roles of the airway helps clinicians take a broader approach to care that covers both urgent breathing needs and the patient's overall well-being (Zhao et al., 2020).

Test Your Knowledge

1. What is the upper airway composed of?
2. What are the parts of the lower airway?

5.2. Assessment of Airway Patency

Learning Outcome

1. Understand the signs of airway obstruction.
2. Discuss techniques for airway assessment.
3. Understand the importance of early recognition.

Checking whether the airway is clear isn't just a box to tick—it often shapes how well a patient does overall. In many critical cases, especially when folks are coming off mechanical ventilation, clinicians run things like spontaneous breathing trials (SBTs) and cuff leak tests to see if a patient's ready for extubation. They also check on things like neurological status and blood flow stability—details that are key before any intervention., these overlapping assessments help lower the chance of extubation problems and other issues, which is why careful prep and solid, evidence-based routines matter so much (Alqahtani et al., 2024). Sometimes, airway challenges get tricky during surgery; keeping the passage open can be a real puzzle. Patient might face extra hurdles in cases such as temporomandibular joint ankylosis, where both surgeons and anesthetists have to think on their feet. Fiberoptic intubation—now often seen as the gold standard because it gives doctors a direct view—has become a go-to option for safely navigating the airway. A look back at patient notes shows generally high success rates for intubation under GA, suggesting that when anesthesia plans are tailored to the situation, complications (like coughing or even a sore throat after extubation) can be kept well at bay (Saini et al., 2024). It isn't just about the immediate steps, though. After the breathing tube is out, patients often need ongoing support to keep their breathing steady. Tools like high-flow nasal cannula (HFNC) and non-invasive ventilation (NIV) frequently come into play, especially for those already dealing with lung issues. This sort of continued monitoring lets healthcare teams quickly catch signs of trouble—whether that's respiratory distress or even aspects of the patient's mental recovery, such as issues tied to post-intensive care syndrome (PICS). All in all, looking after the airway isn't merely ticking off a checklist; it's part of a broader, patient-centered plan that meshes immediate care with long-term rehabilitation (Alqahtani et al., 2024) (Figure 5.6).

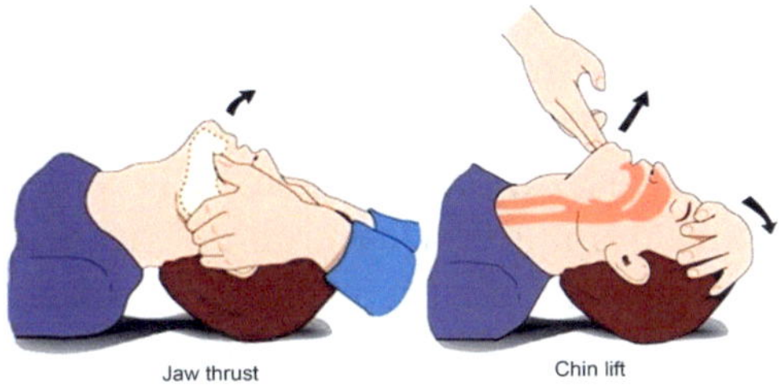

Figure 5.6. Airway patency.

Source: https://s3.us-east-2.amazonaws.com/medictests/app/public/ckeditor_assets/pictures/522/content_headtilt_chinlift.jpg.

5.2.1. Signs of Airway Obstruction

Spotting signs of a blocked airway is important, especially when it comes to managing breathing problems in kids who often get illnesses like bronchiolitis. One might first notice a high-pitched, almost whistling sound when the child exhales—what many call wheezing. But that's not all; sometimes the trouble shows up as longer-than-normal exhalations or obvious struggles with breathing. In many cases, such signs suggest that something is off with airflow and might hint at viral triggers like RSV or even RV (Jartti et al., 2017). Clinicians usually mention that these clues, when seen together with breathing difficulties, could eventually lead to chronic issues like asthma and more airway blockages. It's a reminder that being aware of these signs is key not just for quick fixes but also for thinking ahead about the patient's long-term lung health. Beyond that familiar wheeze, there are other hints that the airway is against itself. Alterations in how fast someone breathes—think rapid breaths or noticeable retractions where the muscles pull inward—often tell us the body is working extra hard to keep up with its need for oxygen. Often, doctors check for patterns like the use of extra muscles to breathe, and these moments call for a close look, especially if the patient turns bluish or seems a bit off mentally. In children, the connection between a viral bout and a blocked airway is even more worrisome since early-life wheezing generally points to recurring issues, sometimes even setting the stage for asthma (Vogelmeier et al., 2017). Long-term studies, generally speaking, show that nipping airway problems in the bud can change a child's respiratory journey. Kids who show signs of bronchial blockage almost always need that immediate help—which is only the start, since ongoing check-ups are pretty necessary to ward off chronic issues. Viruses like RSV and RV are known to do more than just cause a temporary setback; they can damage the airway over time, making it easier for more troubles to come later on (Jartti et al., 2017). So, using smart airway management techniques while keeping an eye on what a bad wheeze might mean matters. In most cases, catching these issues early and monitoring them can turn the tide on what might otherwise be a long-term problem, ultimately improving life quality for these young patients.

5.2.2. Techniques for Airway Assessment

Managing a patient's airway isn't something to take lightly, especially when risk levels run high. A good look at a patient's history can often hint at earlier challenges with intubation or reveal quirky anatomical details. Sometimes, a simple bedside check does the trick; for instance, tests like the Mallampati score—yes, that odd little measure comparing the tongue and oropharynx—can sometimes signal potential complications. In most cases, mixing what the patient shares with what's observed in a quick exam ends up forming the basic blueprint for anticipating trouble, even if things aren't always perfectly clear-cut. New tech breakthroughs have, generally speaking, turned airway assessment on its head. Computer-assisted reconstructions and even 3-D printing now let clinicians gaze at the airway's labyrinth in ways that used to seem almost futuristic—like having a detailed map in hand. Preoperative endoscopic checks give doctors a direct, sometimes surprisingly clear, look at airway structures, which can shift decision-making when things feel dicey. These modern methods, when combined with classic assessment techniques, end up allowing anesthesiologists to spot potential complications much sooner—readying them for when every second counts.

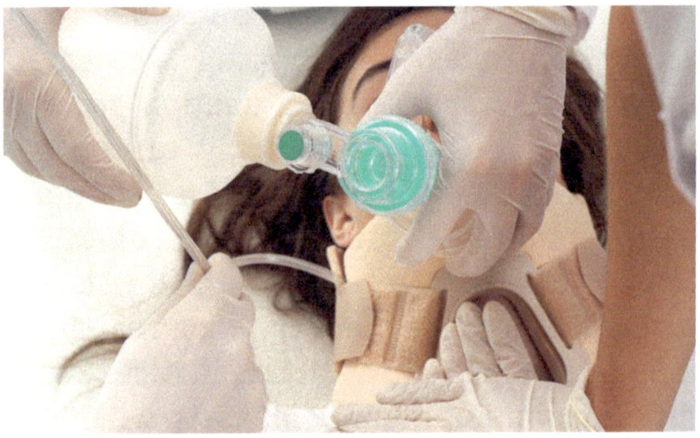

Figure 5.7. Techniques for airway assessment.

Source: https://www.cascadetraining.com/assets/images/blog/Advanced-ACLS_1000x600.png.

Then there's the whole growing role of artificial intelligence (AI) in this field. AI algorithms based on deep learning are being pressed into service to sift through imaging data, looking for subtle hints of a problematic airway. Rosa et al. (2024) point to machine-learning models that, in most cases, are sharpening predictions in real-time, while Chen et al. (2024) talk about various mathematical tricks that might streamline decision-making during anesthesia. As these digital tools keep evolving, clinicians are increasingly armed with fresh insights and unconventional strategies—even if the tech sometimes feels like a leap into the unknown. All in all, this mixing of classic checks with innovative tech seems set to take airway management to a safer and more effective new level (Figure 5.7).

5.2.3. Importance of Early Recognition

Airway management demands a hands-on mindset. Spotting trouble early—like during tracheal intubation or other airway maneuvers—can change the game. When issues pop up quickly, healthcare folks can alter their approach on the fly. Clinical guidelines emphasize that calling out problems without delay is a smart move. This kind of immediate attention kick-starts quick fixes and also builds a safety vibe among the team, where open chatter and shared problem-solving come naturally (Frerk et al., 2015). Early detection isn't just about jumping in at the last minute. It also sets the stage to prevent problems before they snowball. In a lot of cases, standard protocols call for a thorough pre-induction airway check—looking at everything from usual anatomy to the odd quirks that might complicate matters. These checks give clinicians the insights they need to pick the right tools and strategies. Plus, catching issues early can steer the choice of equipment, making it easier to shift over to alternatives such as supraglottic airways or even video-assisted intubation when normal methods stumble. This kind of pre-planning is pretty key to boosting patient outcomes and reducing on trauma during the procedure (Elliott et al., 2014). Not only does this early-warning approach help patients, it also sharpens the team's overall performance. When everyone is on the lookout for potential red flags, the responsibility to act gets shared more naturally. This collaborative spirit breaks down some of the mystique around airway management and creates an atmosphere where ongoing training and regular drills matter. Teams that run real-world rehearsals tend to handle surprises more confidently, reinforcing their readiness when things don't go as planned. In essence, noticing complications early empowers professionals to carry out airway interventions with genuine confidence, ultimately making the care provided both safer and more effective (Frerk et al., 2015) (Figure 5.8).

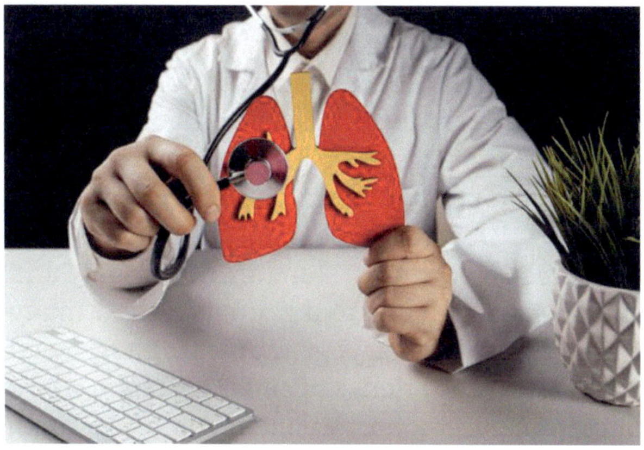

Figure 5.8. The importance of early detection recognizing signs of respiratory issues.

Source: https://www.geetanjalihospital.co.in/img/media/cache/blogs/02/825x408/1010/the-importance-of-early-detection-recognizing-signs-of-respiratory-issues.jpg.

Test Your Knowledge

1. What are the signs of airway obstruction?
2. What is the importance of early recognition?

5.3. Basic Airway Management Techniques

Learning Outcome

1. Understand the head tilt-chin lift maneuver
2. Understand the jaw thrust maneuver
3. Describe the use of oropharyngeal airways

Securing an open airway is crucial in many medical settings—think emergencies or times when anesthesia is needed. You quickly need to get the right patient position, clear out blockages, and sometimes even use extra tools when necessary. For example, placing someone on their back might work wonders for one patient, yet for another, a side-lying position can reduce the risk of aspiration. When secretions pile up, fast and decisive suctioning is key to getting breathing back on track; a small lapse here can easily lead to complications (Zhao et al., 2020). Extra techniques often bolster these basic moves. Bag-mask ventilation (BMV), for instance, steps in when a patient's breathing isn't cutting it. Despite its seeming simplicity, BMV demands a good understanding of anatomy and skillful hands to create a proper seal. In many cases, using oropharyngeal or nasopharyngeal airways can keep things open for someone who's unresponsive or has weakened muscle tone. These tools are not only critical during on-the-spot emergencies but also in pre-hospital care, where picking the right device—based on individual needs and the situation—can make all the difference (Vogelmeier et al., 2017). Airway management isn't a one-and-done deal either. Continuous learning is part of the picture, and in most cases, even mastering the basics means staying sharp for the complex instances. Take endotracheal intubation, which remains the gold standard in securing an airway during anesthesia or when respiratory failure hits. Knowing your equipment and protocols boosts a provider's confidence exactly when seconds matter, and even brief debrief sessions afterward can help refine techniques and set up better practices d the road. All of this—ongoing training, practical simulations, and occasional feedback— helps medical teams stay ready to deliver top-notch care under pressure (Zhao et al., 2020) (Figure 5.9).

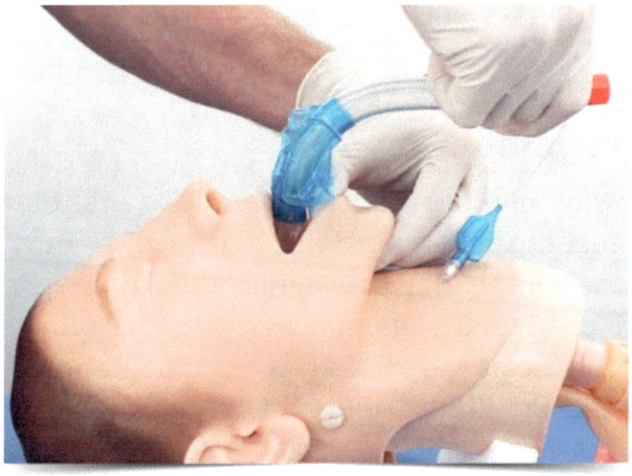

Figure 5.9. Basic airway management techniques.

Source: https://lh5.googleusercontent.com/proxy/v8WWAAj0-dANtEd_vozLCxO-soHfrwgGIHxm3TUauODI6oGDjVpkgzCs61nqcYXUMtRv1BUYH8tdsMn_6vRRy4j0OVDtsVZZwho.

5.3.1. Head Tilt-Chin Lift Maneuver

Airway management isn't always cut-and-dried—it often boils down to knowing a lot about how the body works and being aware of what could block airflow when things get urgent. A classic move, the head tilt-chin lift maneuver, pops up as a clear go-to for these moments. You simply tilt the patient's head back while lifting their chin at the same time; this moves nudges the tongue away from the back of the throat, reducing on any risk of it falling back and causing an obstruction. Because it doesn't require any invasive gear, this trick is especially handy for those who are unconscious or not fully aware, keeping the breathing passage open without extra help. When an airway seems on the verge of closing, the head tilt-chin lift maneuver can make all the difference—often acting fast enough to prevent serious issues like hypoxia. Its main aim is pretty much to get the airway open quickly, a step that's critical in trauma or severe breathing trouble. Of course, getting the positioning right is key; a tilt that's off can just make matters worse or even spike up neck injuries. That's why many healthcare providers train hard on this maneuver. In real-life emergencies, when high-tech airway devices aren't immediately at hand, a well-practiced head tilt-chin lift is a vital part of the skill set. Looking at the whole picture, airway management techniques—including this head tilt-chin lift—carry huge weight for patient outcomes. Poor airway care can lead to big problems, like aspiration pneumonia (Dziewas et al., 2021), and in cases such as Parkinson's disease where swallowing is already an issue (Umemoto et al., 2019), these techniques become even more critical. Recognizing when to use the maneuver and doing it correctly can reduce on the complications tied to inadequate airway protection. In most cases, mastering this simple but effective approach is a cornerstone of broader airway management strategies, ultimately boosting patient safety in a variety of clinical settings (Figure 5.10).

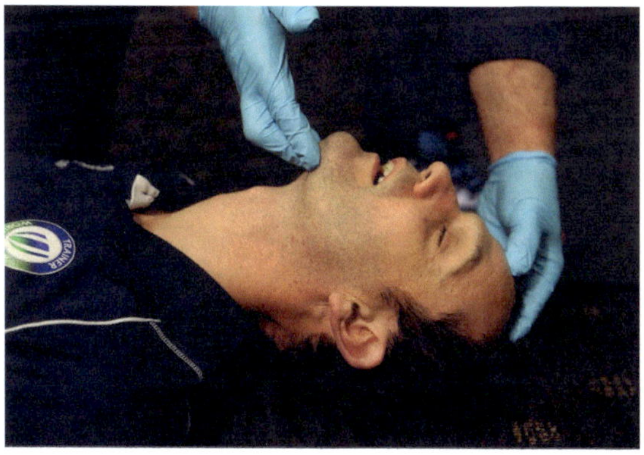

Figure 5.10. Head tilt-chin lift.

Source: https://passport.world.rugby/media/zfjnpx2q/chapter_4_head_tilt.jpg.

5.3.2. Jaw Thrust Maneuver

Airway management matters a lot, especially when patients aren't responsive. The jaw thrust maneuver is one trick that juggles the tongue out of harm's way so breathing isn't blocked. In cases where a neck injury might be lurking—generally speaking, when the cervical spine is a concern—this approach avoids stretching the neck too far, which in turn lessens the risk of more damage. It's often combined with other methods like bag-mask ventilation or the placement of more advanced airways, helping overall resuscitation efforts when standard options might just fall short (Law et al., 2021). Even though the jaw thrust seems pretty straightforward, it's not something you can just wing without practice. The clinician has to get hands-on—quite literally—by carefully gripping the patient's mandible and pushing upward. Keeping that jaw in place is crucial through the next steps. Sometimes, that means bringing in extra tools or even a helping hand to be sure nothing goes off track. At the same time, pairing this maneuver with supplemental oxygen is key, ensuring oxygen keeps flowing while other airway strategies are being worked on (Law et al., 2021). In emergencies, where every moment counts, nailing this technique can shift the outcome in a patient's favor. Nowadays, the role of the jaw thrust maneuver in airway management can't be overlooked. With guidelines steadily evolving, it's increasingly valued in scenarios where traditional intubation might run into trouble—like with patients who have suffered multiple traumas or who are less than fully conscious (Gács et al., 2017). In most cases, weaving the jaw thrust into both training routines and everyday practice reflects a solid commitment to improving patient safety and boosting the success of ventilation efforts. This small, yet essential, technique makes a difference when every second and every maneuver count (Figure 5.11).

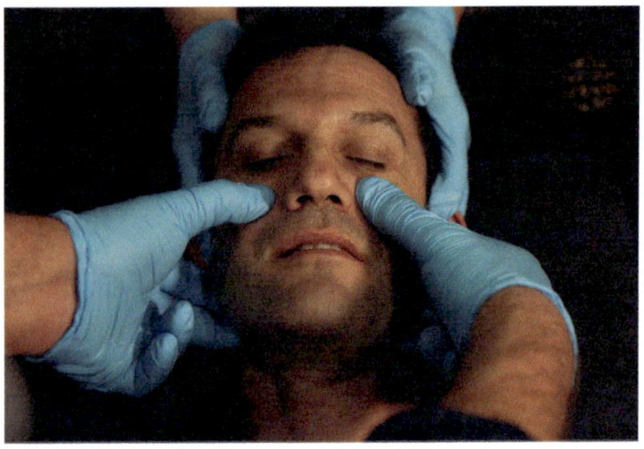

Figure 5.11. Jaw thrust.

Source: https://passport.world.rugby/media/5jsff0xl/chapter_4_inferior_approach_jaw_thrust.jpg.

5.3.3. Use of Oropharyngeal Airways (OPA)

Managing a patient's airway remains a top priority in medicine, whether during an emergency or while administering anesthesia. In many cases, a handy tool like the oropharyngeal airway (OPA) helps keep the throat open without invasive procedures—this is especially useful when a patient is unconscious. The design is simple: the OPA is slid into the oropharynx so that the tongue doesn't collapse into the airway, which is crucial when someone can no longer look after their breathing, as happens with sedation or trauma. Although the process appears straightforward, clinicians do need proper training—not only to know when to use it but also to select the right size, ensuring the technique works effectively and avoids complications. Using OPAs in everyday practice doesn't just improve how we manage airways; it also underscores the importance of hands-on training for healthcare providers. Without a thorough understanding of how and when to apply these devices, there's a risk of trouble, like airway blockage or even harm to the mouth, which, generally speaking, no one wants to see. Managing airways effectively means knowing a patient's unique anatomy and physiology, which helps decide if an OPA is the best choice. Also, having a good grasp of alternatives—like bag-valve masks or endotracheal tubes—lets practitioners pick the right tool for the job. All of these skills, when woven into training, build both confidence and competence over time. As technology in airway management steadily evolves, there's now a growing call for clear, standardized guidelines to help steer the use of OPAs along with other techniques. The sheer variety in patient conditions means that doctors need a detailed, if not sometimes flexible, understanding of how best to manage airways—especially for high-risk cases, such as patients on mechanical ventilation. Recent talks among clinical experts have generally pointed to the need for guidelines that tackle not just the mechanical side of things but also the subtler aspects of patient care and recovery. Collaborative efforts to create these consensus documents might well lead to better outcomes—say, smoother transport experiences with interventions like mechanical insufflation-exsufflation—highlighting how the field of airway management keeps evolving (Marchis et al., 2024) (Figure 5.12).

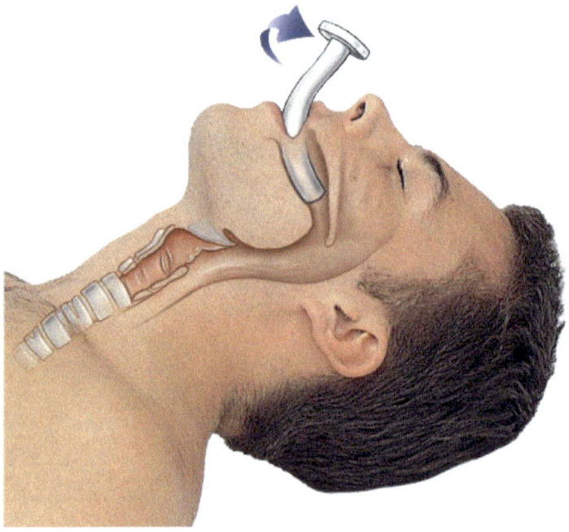

Figure 5.12. Use of oropharyngeal airways.

Source: https://clinical.stjohnwa.com.au/images/default-source/clinical-skill-images/airway/opa3.png?sfvrsn=6ff09c37_2.

Test Your Knowledge

1. What is the jaw-thrust maneuver used for?
2. What is the use of oropharyngeal airways?

5.4. Advanced Airway Management Techniques

Learning Outcome

1. Learn about endotracheal intubation and supraglottic airway devices.
2. Understand the surgical airway management.

Airway management has become a lot more challenging lately, and we're rethinking how to handle tough cases. The demand for quick, precise interventions before surgery has led to some surprising changes. Trans nasal endoscopy and even AI are no longer just buzzwords—they help spot potential airway issues by giving doctors a clearer look at the anatomy. These tools, mixed with ultrasound and 3D reconstruction technologies, offer fresh views on subtle differences in tissue structure. This extra insight is often vital, especially when patients have head and neck conditions that distort the usual airway layout (Marchis et al., 2024). Advanced techniques now play a huge role not only in scheduled operations but also in life-or-death emergencies. Effective ventilation is practically the foundation of any solid life support effort during CPR. Traditional methods can stumble during cardiac arrest, showing us the need for more innovative approaches. Automated transport ventilators (ATVs) have become popular because they keep volumes and pressures in check, especially when paired with strong chest compressions. And then there's chest compression synchronized ventilation (CCSV), a breakthrough designed for those critical moments when every second counts. Generally speaking, more research is needed to firm up these techniques as best practices in both out-of-hospital and in-hospital scenarios (Kill et al., 2024). Mixing modern technology with hands-on clinical know-how is the core of today's airway management, particularly as patient profiles and complications keep changing. Instead of sticking to one routine, experts from anesthesiology, emergency medicine, and critical care are teaming up. Getting used to new tricks like virtual endoscopy and advanced imaging is essential to help prepare teams for the real world. When specialists collaborate—even with a bit of overlap in technique—the chance to set up every day, standard protocols improves. Continuous learning and research boost skills and, frankly, lead to better outcomes for patients. In short, blending innovation with traditional care is the key to meeting the evolving needs of modern airway management (Figure 5.13).

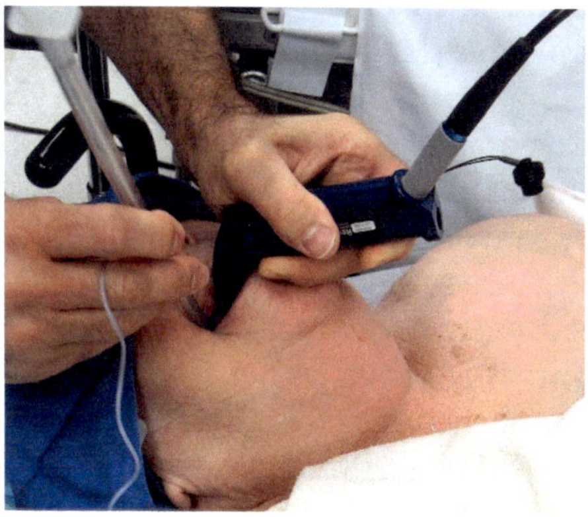

Figure 5.13. Advanced airway management techniques.

Source: https://upload.wikimedia.org/wikipedia/commons/3/36/Glidescope_02.JPG.

5.4.1. Endotracheal Intubation

Endotracheal intubation is vital, especially when time is short in emergency situations. In those critical moments, the ability to get a tube in place isn't just a technical move—it gives caregivers a secure airway so patients can breathe properly. This method comes into play during major trauma, respiratory breaks, and even when folks are put under general anesthesia (GA) for surgery. A well-done intubation even makes it easier to push inhaled anesthetics and other medications directly into the trachea, which often leads to better recoveries. Research shows that nailing this procedure requires a lot of fine skill and stresses the need for hands-on, comprehensive training in airway management. Modern medical practice, on the other hand, isn't resting on just traditional methods. New tech has jumped into the mix—imagine using advanced laryngoscopy gear (even ones originally made for studying small animals) to see more clearly and get that tube exactly where it's needed. Techniques like video laryngoscopy have switched things up, offering better views of the glottis and pushing success rates up, especially when the anatomy makes things tricky. Generally speaking, these high-tech tools not only boost safety but also reduce on risks like dental mishaps or accidentally intubating the esophagus (Molthen et al., 2006). As medical education keeps evolving, there's a growing emphasis on mastering these modern methods, which are increasingly seen as essential for everyone involved in managing airways. Yet, not all healthcare settings follow the same playbook when it comes to intubation—particularly outside the controlled environment of an operating room. In several urban trauma centers, policies meant for non-anesthesia providers don't always line up with the best practices found in current literature. This kind of inconsistency might lead to serious complications, especially if the staff isn't fully credentialed to use neuromuscular blocking agents during the procedure. There's now a pressing call to develop evidence-based guidelines so that training and protocols are standardized, ensuring every practitioner gets the skills needed for effective airway management. By gathering the available evidence and putting together solid recommendations, hospitals can ultimately boost the safety and success of emergency airway interventions, leading to better patient outcomes in critical care (Ridgway et al., 2022) (Figure 5.14).

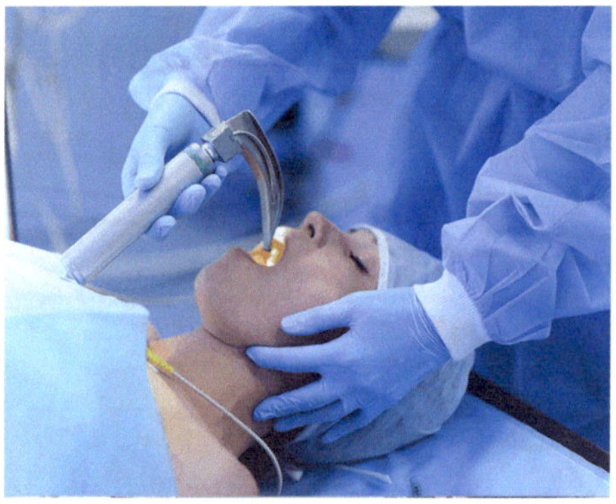

Figure 5.14. Endotracheal tube intubation procedure.

Source: https://www.apexhospitals.com/_next/image?url=https%3A%2F%2Fbed.apexhospitals.com%2Fuploads%2Fintubation_21a26521bb.png&w=1200&q=75.

5.4.2. Supraglottic Airway Devices

Supraglottic airway devices (SGAs) have grabbed attention lately in airway management. These devices mix the quick simplicity of bag-valve-mask techniques with a less invasive alternative to endotracheal intubation, often coming into play when intubation seems tricky—especially in emergency moments (Molthen et al., 2006). They're built for fast use and, in a lot of cases, not only offer a simple way to insert but also help keep patients oxygenated when their airways falter. Some prehospital and EMS studies hint that in situations like cardiac arrest or trauma, using SGAs can boost outcomes without adding extra risk, suggesting that this technology is a key part of today's airway toolbox (Carney et al., 2021). During the COVID-19 period, these devices gained even more prominence. Traditional airway techniques often raised concerns about viral spread, so SGAs sometimes became the go-to choice as they tend to generate fewer aerosols. In practice, that meant healthcare providers saw less exposure risk while patients were maintained with interim oxygenation until a more secure airway was sorted out. In most cases, this low-aerosol solution—if you think about it—had important implications for patient safety and clinical care during tough respiratory crises (Brown et al., 2020). Even with their growing popularity, SGAs aren't without issues. People still worry about whether everyone using them is skilled enough for proper placement or if the seal might sometimes fall short, leading to less effective ventilation. Continuous education and simulation training—even if a bit spotty at times—are pretty crucial for practitioners to nail their technique. While some studies indicate that SGAs can match or even surpass outcomes compared to bag-valve-mask ventilation or endotracheal intubation, more ongoing research remains essential to fine-tune best practices. All in all, as the overall field of airway management shifts, the role of SGAs will evolve too—making periodic review and adaptation in clinical protocols just as necessary (Carney et al., 2021) (Figure 5.15).

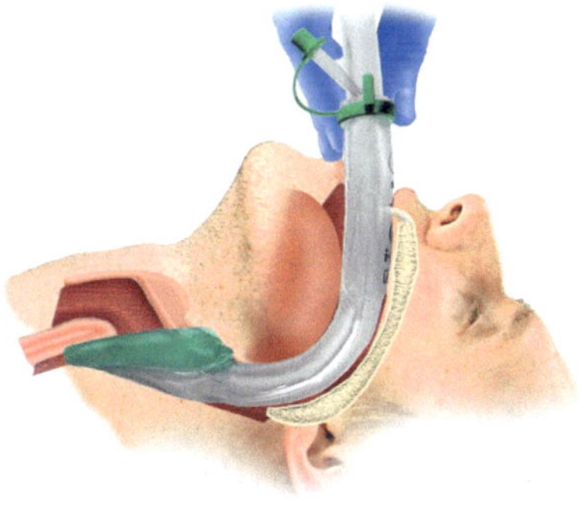

Figure 5.15. Supraglottic airway devices.

Source: https://www.jems.com/wp-content/uploads/2019/02/50087-1902JEMS-Holley.jpg.

5.4.3. Surgical Airway Management

Airway procedures sometimes hit a snag when regular intubation just won't cut it, forcing doctors to turn to surgical fixes. When standard methods fall short, there's a range of options—from urgent, emergency moves to planned, elective ones—that lean heavily on a solid grasp of anatomy. Think of it this way: procedures like tracheostomy or cricothyrotomy step in when placing a breathing tube isn't possible. For instance, a tracheostomy offers a steady airway route and lends a hand when long-term breathing support is needed, especially for patients with chronic lung issues. Knowing which approach fits best can change things up for patient recovery; in most cases, that extra edge in skill makes all the difference. The COVID-19 period added a whole new set of wrinkles. Suddenly, airway management had to work around the risk of aerosols — a real problem for everyone involved. Groups like PeDI-C, which mainly focuses on pediatric anesthesia, started recommending tools like video laryngoscopes and cuffed tracheal tubes to up safety during intubation. They even threw in the suggestion of using negative pressure rooms along with proper protective gear, a must when working with kids suspected of carrying the virus. These measures, generally speaking, shifted the whole approach, reminding us that sometimes routines have to evolve fast when clinical landscapes morph unexpectedly. There's also the twist brought by conditions like obstructive sleep apnea syndrome (OSAS). Research shows that adenotonsillectomy is usually the go-to remedy for kids with OSAS, and the outlook post-surgery is often positive. Still, when obesity plays a role, things can get messy — many patients, in fact, still experience OSAS despite surgery. This reality means doctors usually need to monitor patients a bit longer, sometimes even opting for an overnight stay to keep a close watch. It's a stark reminder that airway management isn't a one-size-fits-all deal; rather, it's a patchwork of strategies that wrestle with both immediate challenges and longer-term patient care, often requiring a flexible and thoughtful approach (Figure 5.16).

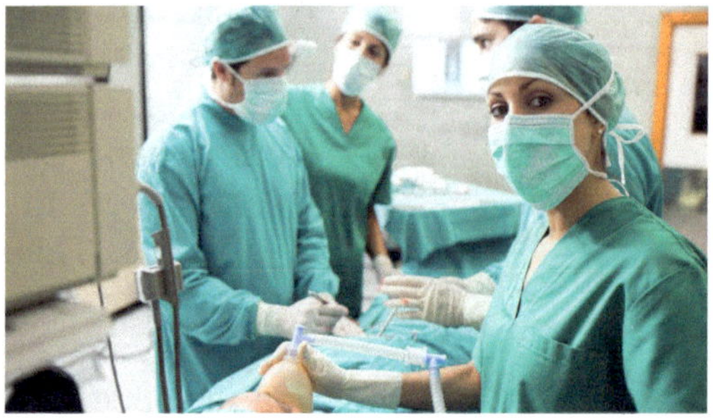

Figure 5.16. Surgical airway management.

Source: https://i0.wp.com/airwayjedi.com/wp-content/uploads/2025/01/nurse-and-MDs.jpg?resize=778%2C438&ssl=1.

Test Your Knowledge

1. What is endotracheal intubation used for?
2. What are the supraglottic airway devices?

5.5. Special Considerations in Airway Management

Learning Outcome

1. Understand pediatric airway management.
2. Know the airway management in trauma patients.
3. Understand the considerations for patients with obesity.

Airway management isn't as straightforward as it might seem—patient quirks can throw a wrench into both figuring out the problem and stepping in with a solution. Some patients show unexpected anatomical differences or have underlying health issues that make a standard routine fall short. This is especially evident in cases like ear, nose, and throat surgeries where even a slight variation in structure can mess up airway access. Lately, there's been a buzz around tools like the high-flow nasal cannula (HFNC), which gives a fresh spin on oxygen delivery for those needing non-intubated anesthesia. Experts have generally reached a consensus on how HFNC alters body functions, the best way to operate it, and when it's most useful—a step that many see as a big win for managing tricky airway situations. Pregnancy adds another twist to the whole picture. The changes that come with being expectant—think increased blood volume, shifting hormones, and altered lung mechanics—can mess with airway resistance and the way drugs are processed. These shifts often force a team-based approach; in most cases, the collective wisdom of obstetricians, anesthesiologists, and neonatologists is key. For instance, because gestational age can influence safety, regional anesthesia (RA) is usually favored over GA when it makes sense. In this setting, the care team works closely together to keep both mother and baby safe during procedures that demand careful airway management (Madkhali et al., 2024). Then there's the tech side of things, which isn't any simpler. Adapting non-invasive ventilation methods to fit the unique needs of different patients is a challenge on its. Techniques like HFNC, now wrapped up in a standardized consensus framework, bridge textbook theory with real-life practice. This approach proves especially vital after surgery, when patients face heightened risks—like airway blockage or insufficient oxygen levels. All in all, opting for an evidence-based strategy not only allows for care that's tailored to each individual but also helps reduce on risks in a variety of clinical settings, aiming to deliver the best possible outcomes for everyone involved.

5.5.1. Pediatric Airway Management

Managing a child's airway isn't simply a mini version of adult care—it's a whole different ball game. These airways are not just smaller; they're also more flexible, which tends to trip up the standard techniques. In infants, for example, having a bigger head compared to their body and a larynx positioned unusually means that obstructions are more likely to occur. In most cases, healthcare providers find themselves having to adjust their methods on the fly, staying extra alert and tailoring their approach to keep air passages open. Systematic reviews often point out that signs like visible secretions and sudden spikes in airway resistance call for prompt suctioning to maintain a clear passage (Blakeman et al., 2022). COVID-19, generally speaking, has another wrench in the works. Clinicians now face new protocols aimed at reducing contagion risks while ensuring that essential care isn't compromised. The Pediatric Difficult Intubation Collaborative (PeDI-C) even noted that minimizing aerosolized secretions—especially during procedures known to generate aerosols—is key to protecting staff. Recommendations now lean toward the use of video laryngoscopy and cuffed tracheal tubes, measures that not only boost patient safety but also streamline the process. And it goes without saying that proper personal protective equipment is critical in these times; such precautions highlight the need for evidence-based practices as our healthcare environment shifts in response to global crises (Matava et al., 2020). There's also a growing emphasis on using specialized techniques to reduce risks and improve outcomes. Effective suctioning plays a central role here. Recent studies suggest that both closed and open suction systems can work well if used correctly—with specific guidelines on catheter occlusion and suction pressure that change by age group. In most cases, a move toward doing suctioning only when needed, instead of on a fixed schedule, shows a more nuanced understanding of pediatric care. Following these recommendations not only hones clinical practice but also helps build a safer, more efficient care routine, underlining the importance of ongoing training and sticking with proven protocols in this critical area (Blakeman et al., 2022) (Figure 5.17).

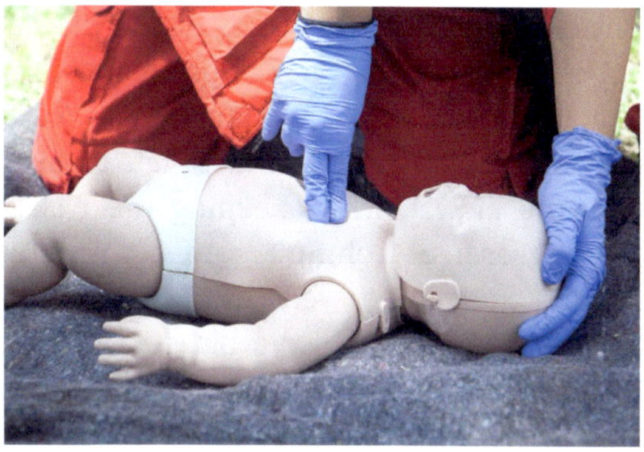

Figure 5.17. Pediatric airway management.

Source: https://blog.sscor.com/hubfs/B%20257.jpg.

5.5.2. Airway Management in Trauma Patients

A clear airway is key in trauma, and keeping it unobstructed can honestly save a life; it often means that medics have to work quickly and with real skill. Injuries to the face—maxillofacial damages and such—can complicate things, sometimes making regular intubation fail when broken bones block the usual path. In these moments, alternative ways to secure ventilation become necessary, and training in advanced airway strategies is a must. As Taljard et al. (2025) point out, basic airway know-how still carries a lot of weight even when newer, flashier techniques are introduced. Trauma care ends up relying on both innovative approaches and a solid grasp of fundamentals that form the bedrock of effective airway management. Picking the right method to manage the airway is crucial, especially when injuries in the midface throw a wrench into the works. Research shows that a mix of approaches—such as nasal, oral, or fiberoptic-guided intubation—can affect outcomes.

One retrospective study looking at cases from January 2017 to December 2019 found that nasal intubation was used in about 56% of incidents, while oral intubation got far less attention. This kind of split highlights the need to choose methods that fit the particular injury and anatomical hurdles (Alam et al., 2025). Using tailored strategies like these lets clinicians secure the airway while keeping the risks of more aggressive techniques to a minimum. Managing the airway well isn't just about the initial emergency; it's also a big deal for long-term recovery. The study mentioned earlier hints that less invasive techniques—fiberoptic-guided intubation, for example—offer a better look inside the airway without the need for heavy surgical steps like tracheostomy. Out of 150 patients, not one ended up needing such invasive measures, which kind of shows the strength of these nonsurgical options. By focusing on methods that enhance airway control and reduce complications, healthcare providers set a care standard that benefits trauma patients. Ultimately, blending tried-and-true basics with advanced techniques seems to be the key to improved outcomes (Alam et al., 2025) (Figure 5.18).

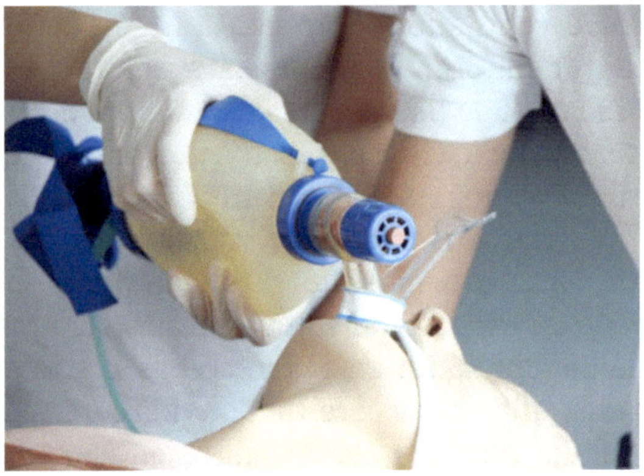

Figure 5.18. Strategies for airway management in trauma cases.

Source: https://hospitalprocedures.org/wp-content/uploads/2024/11/airway-management.jpg.

5.5.3. Considerations for Patients with Obesity

Airway management for obese patients can be quite a challenge. These patients often bring unexpected anatomical quirks—a thicker neck or a slightly altered jawline, for example—that make it harder to see the airway when intubating. Their high BMI often ties in with conditions like obstructive sleep apnea (OSA) and other health issues, which usually means more hurdles in getting the airway right. You might try positions like the Ramp Position to line things up better; after all, studies generally show that adjusting the approach to fit these unique challenges can reduce risk. New techniques, like video laryngoscopy, are showing promise by boosting first-pass intubation success. A meta-analysis even suggests that this method can increase the chances of getting it right on the first go—a big deal when patients might already have compromised breathing. Its ability to give a clearer view of the airway seems to lower the odds of complications, making it a smart alternative somewhere along the lines. In most cases, considering the extra risks during anesthesia with obese patients, integrating these advanced tools into everyday practice could seriously improve safety and overall outcomes (Chaudery et al., 2024). When you shift your focus to anesthetic management, dosing becomes another tricky area. Obese patients tend to handle drugs very differently, so relying on standard dosing guidelines might lead to overdosing; adjustments based on ideal rather than total body weight often work better. Plus, keeping a hawk's eye on intraoperative vital signs is crucial, given the heightened risk of cardiovascular complications. Research generally indicates that a thorough preoperative check and some careful planning go a long way. This might involve deliberate preoxygenation steps and measured doses of anesthetic agents to keep the right depth of anesthesia—even when post-intubation ventilation gets challenging. All in all, a multifaceted, individually tailored approach appears essential for managing these cases effectively (Bisri et al., 2024).

Test Your Knowledge

1. How to manage a child's airway?
2. How to maintain the airway in trauma patients?

SUMMARY

Airway management is not as simple as it appears – having actual-life strategies is a huge determining factor in keeping patients safe and having effective processes. Processes are still changing, especially when unexpected circumstances like the COVID-19 pandemic force us to revise our processes; this means that medical professionals need to make things interesting from time to time. Following core ideas like acting with urgency and protecting the team is key in building these strategies. Many studies remind us that protocols before, during, and after surgery must stay strict to reduce on exposure risks while aiming for the best surgical outcomes (Liang et al., 2020). Comparing various ways to intubate brings out how far we've come.

Research into methods—like SALAD (suction-assisted laryngoscopy and airway decontamination) and even intentional esophageal intubation (IEI)—teaches us that these competing strategies not only enhance airway protection but also augment the confidence of medical professionals in their skills. The results typically suggest that these modalities are just as effective in controlling aspiration, opening doors to future alters in difficult scenarios like extreme emesis (Fiore et al., 2019). It's clear that doctors, nurses, and others must keep themselves updated with these evolving techniques if they want to offer quick and effective treatment. Finally, the extremely close linkage between airway techniques and outcome of patients underscores so much the need for continuous learning and adaptability. New airway challenges – including infectious disease-related ones – entail doubling d on guidelines and trying new practices is called for. Various guidelines note that an alert, evidence-based approach will enhance patient and operating team safety, with medical professionals properly trained to manage the peaks and troughs of airway management, protect patient health, and business as usual (Liang et al., 2020).

Airway management isn't a one-size-fits-all deal. It means mixing many techniques that depend on each patient and what's going on at the time. Keeping the airway open and oxygen flowing isn't just a checklist item—it's crucial whether things are urgent or planned. You can use endotracheal intubation, try supraglottic devices, or rely on non-invasive ventilation; there are pros and cons to each, so doctors have to be reasonably adept at using them. New evidence and guidelines, in general, lead clinicians to revisit these modalities, especially when patient anatomy or lung status introduces unexpected kinks into the routine. Recent developments have some new concepts on the table as well. Take transbronchial lung cryobiopsy: now sometimes deemed a fair substitute for a surgical lung biopsy, all in the quest of making things less invasive and yet accomplishing a good diagnosis.

That tide of lesser severe procedures not only enhances safety but also diagnostic accuracy, even if it means rethinking old ways. Such conditions as progressive pulmonary fibrosis (PPF) have had their definitions altered, demonstrating how thoughtful observation can lead the way in decision-making when it comes to mechanical support or oxygen therapy. To a large degree, these developments are an extension of an already fluid picture, forcing the science to keep its feet moving in an evolving world of optimal approaches. Generally, airway management reaches a balance of traditional proven methods with a pinch of new, sometimes surprising, methods. Well-presented studies that give results in a straightforward way form a sound body of evidence, which in turn makes practitioners more comfortable to make decisions in the real world. Initiatives such as the revised ARRIVE guidelines remind everyone that research quality is equally important as possessing pragmatic skills and that staying current is equally as good for the patient. Doctors, by working together and ongoing assessments, continually improve their practice, balancing entrenched practice with fresher information so that end of day, they're always prepared for the numerous turns the practice takes their direction.

KEY TERMS FROM THIS CHAPTER

- Airway management
- Bronchioles
- Health crises
- Intubation
- Midline glossoepiglottic fold
- Paralytic drugs
- Respiratory rehabilitation
- Social media
- Trachea
- Upper airway
- Bronchi
- Endotracheal intubation
- Infection control
- Lower airway
- Oxygen flow
- Public health
- Rhinovirus
- Supraglottic devices
- Tracheal intubation
- Video laryngoscopy

CRITICAL THINKING QUESTIONS

1. **Which of the following is considered the first-line device for managing a difficult airway?**
   a. Supraglottic airway device (e.g., LMA)
   b. Fiber-optic bronchoscope
   c. Tracheostomy
   d. Rigid bronchoscope
2. **What is the most common cause of upper airway obstruction in unconscious patients?**
   a. Laryngospasm
   b. Foreign body aspiration
   c. Tongue falling back
   d. Epiglottitis
3. **Which of the following is considered a supraglottic airway device?**
   a. Endotracheal tube
   b. Laryngeal mask airway (LMA)
   c. Tracheostomy tube
   d. Nasopharyngeal airway
4. **The Mallampati classification predicts:**
   a. Risk of aspiration
   b. Difficulty of intubation
   c. Postoperative airway edema
   d. Presence of obstructive sleep apnea
5. **Fiber-optic intubation is most commonly indicated in:**
   a. Patients with a known difficult airway
   b. Routine airway management
   c. Trauma patients with facial injuries
   d. Emergency tracheostomy

Short Answer Questions

1. What is airway management?
2. Describe the anatomy of the airway.
3. How to assess for airway patency?
4. What are the basic airway management techniques?
5. What are the advanced airway management techniques?

Answers to Critical Thinking Questions

1. (b); 2. (c); 3. (b); 4. (b); 5. (a)

REFERENCES

1. Alam, M. B., Sultana, S. A., Alam, M. H., Tasnim, R., Shakil, M., Chowdhury, M. R., Arzoo, S., et al. (2025). Optimizing airway management and anesthetic techniques in maxillofacial procedures. *International Surgery Journal*. https://www.semanticscholar.org/paper/ece1605a635443e75229e0732c87549d4f9adfad (accessed on 20 May 2025).
2. Alqahtani, K. S., Alshamrani, R. A., Alanazi, S. O., AlJarbou, A. S., Alharthi, F. S., Alzahrani, M. M., Alromaihi, A. J., et al. (2024). Guidelines for safe extubation and respiratory rehabilitation in the intensive care unit. *International Journal of Community Medicine and Public Health*. https://www.semanticscholar.org/paper/752423322dc6aa859e20aed2cf26a454aa4e6363 (accessed on 20 May 2025).
3. Bevivino, A., Bacci, G., Dřevínek, P., Nelson, M. T., Hoffman, L. R., & Mengoni, A. (2019). Deciphering the ecology of cystic fibrosis bacterial communities: Towards systems-level integration. *Trends in Molecular Medicine, 25*, 1110–1122. https://doi.org/10.1016/j.molmed.2019.07.008.
4. Bisri, D., Maharani, M. I., & Bisri, T. (2024). Anesthesia for craniotomy tumor removal patient with morbid obesity. *Journal of Law and Sustainable Development*. https://www.semanticscholar.org/paper/c14c7100ace13a8e7917a2f2177c3fdabcd0cac0 (accessed on 10 May 2025).
5. Blakeman, T. C., Scott, J. B., Yoder, M., Capellari, E., & Strickland, S. L. (2022). AARC clinical practice guidelines: Artificial airway suctioning. *Respiratory Care, 67*, 258–271. https://doi.org/10.4187/respcare.09548.
6. Br, C. A., Mosier, J., Carlson, J. N., & Gibbs, M. (2020). Pragmatic recommendations for intubating critically ill patients with suspected COVID-19. *Journal of the American College of Emergency Physicians Open, 1*, 80–84. https://doi.org/10.1002/emp2.12063.
7. Carney, N., Totten, A. M., Cheney, T. P., Jungbauer, R., Neth, M. R., Weeks, C., Davis-O'Reilly, C., et al. (2021). Prehospital airway management: A systematic review. *Prehospital Emergency Care, 26*, 716–727. https://doi.org/10.1080/10903127.2021.1940400.
8. Chan, A. K. M., Nickson, C. P., Rudolph, J. W., Lee, A., & Joynt, G. M. (2020). Social media for rapid knowledge dissemination: Early experience from the COVID-19 pandemic. *Anesthesia, 75*, 1579–1582. https://doi.org/10.1111/anae.15057.
9. Chaudery, H., Hameed, H., Sharif, Z., Asinger, S., & McKechnie, A. (2024). Comparative efficacy of video laryngoscopy and direct laryngoscopy in patients living with obesity: A meta-analysis. *Cureus, 16*. https://www.semanticscholar.org/paper/831374e1511b105d1a93ca89a3079fc1bac458de (accessed on 20 May 2025).
10. Chen, H., Zheng, Y., Fu, Q., & Li, P. (2024). A review of the current status and progress in difficult airway assessment research. *European Journal of Medical Research, 29*. https://www.semanticscholar.org/paper/7d8bcfb7937503d1f86e67a25cbb9e4a33694410 (accessed on 20 May 2025).
11. Chrimes, N., Bradley, W. P., Gatward, J., & Weatherall, A. (2018). Human factors and the 'next generation' airway trolley. *Anesthesia, 74*, 427–433. https://doi.org/10.1111/anae.14543.
12. Counselman, F. L., Babu, K. M., Edens, M. A., Gorgas, D. L., Hobgood, C., Marco, C. A., Katz, E., et al. (2017). The 2016 model of the clinical practice of emergency medicine. *Journal of*

Emergency Medicine, 52, 846–849. https://doi.org/10.1016/j.jemermed.2017.01.040.

13. De Rosa, S., Bignami, E., Bellini, V., & Battaglini, D. (2024). The future of artificial intelligence using images and clinical assessment for difficult airway management. *Anesthesia and Analgesia, 140*, 317–325. https://www.semanticscholar.org/paper/2cd598171e4d7bfb20fccc81c57b7104c2932ff2 (accessed on 20 May 2025).
14. Dziewas, R., Allescher, H. D., Aroyo, I., Bartolome, G., Beilenhoff, U., Bohlender, J., Breitbach-Snowdon, H., et al. (2021). Diagnosis and treatment of neurogenic dysphagia–S1 guideline of the German Society of Neurology. *Neurological Research and Practice, 3*. https://doi.org/10.1186/s42466-021-00122-3.
15. Elliott, P., Anastasakis, A., Borger, M. A., Borggrefe, M., Cecchi, F., Charron, P., Hagège, A., et al. (2014). 2014 ESC Guidelines on diagnosis and management of hypertrophic cardiomyopathy. *European Heart Journal, 35*, 2733–2779. https://doi.org/10.1093/eurheartj/ehu284.
16. Fiore, M., Marmer, S., Steuerwald, M., Thompson, R., & Galgon, R. E. (2019). Three airway management techniques for airway decontamination in massive emesis: A manikin study. *Western Journal of Emergency Medicine, 20*, 784–790. https://doi.org/10.5811/westjem.2019.6.42222.
17. Frerk, C., Mitchell, V., McNarry, A. F., Mendonca, C., Bhagrath, R., Patel, A., O'Sullivan, E., et al. (2015). Difficult Airway Society 2015 guidelines for management of unanticipated difficult intubation in adults. *British Journal of Anesthesia, 115*, 827–848. https://doi.org/10.1093/bja/aev371.
18. Gottlieb, M., O'Brien, J. R., Ferrigno, N. W., & Sundaram, T. (2023). Point-of-care ultrasound for airway management in the emergency and critical care setting. *Clinical and Experimental Emergency Medicine, 11*, 22–32. https://www.semanticscholar.org/paper/aefaa09275d38b319059169a23c23645c502f928 (accessed on 20 May 2025).
19. Jartti, T., & Gern, J. E. (2017). Role of viral infections in the development and exacerbation of asthma in children. *Journal of Allergy and Clinical Immunology, 140*, 895–906. https://doi.org/10.1016/j.jaci.2017.08.003.
20. Kill, C., Manegold, R., Fistera, D., & Risse, J. (2024). Airway management and ventilation techniques in resuscitation during advanced life support: An update. *Journal of Anesthesia, Analgesia and Critical Care, 4*. https://www.semanticscholar.org/paper/966f85e1130f25bbc86d320522dddb428724fb2c (accessed on 20 May 2025).
21. Kovács, G., & Sowers, N. (2017). Airway management in trauma. *Emergency Medicine Clinics of North America, 36*, 61–84. https://doi.org/10.1016/j.emc.2017.08.006.
22. Law, J. A., Duggan, L. V., Asselin, M., Baker, P., Crosby, E. T., Downey, A., Hung, O., et al. (2021). Canadian Airway Focus Group updated consensus-based recommendations for management of the difficult airway: Part 1. Difficult airway management encountered in an unconscious patient. *Canadian Journal of Anesthesia/Journal Canadien D'Anesthésie, 68*, 1373–1404. https://doi.org/10.1007/s12630-021-02007-0.
23. Liang, Z., Chong, M., Sim, M. A., Lim, J., Castañeda, P., Green, D. W., Fisher, D., et al. (2020). Surgical considerations in patients with COVID-19. *Journal of Bone and Joint Surgery, 102*, e50. https://doi.org/10.2106/jbjs.20.00513.
24. Madkhali, N. A. M., Alsomali, M. D. Y., Al-Dosari, Y. N. M., ALHarbi, S. T. A., ALRUWAILI, S. T. F.,

Alahdal, A. A. M., Almutiri, G. H. D., et al. (2024). A comprehensive multidisciplinary strategy for the management of musculoskeletal fractures throughout pregnancy: Evaluation, treatment, and maternal-fetal considerations. *Journal of Eco Humanism*. https://www.semanticscholar.org/paper/1fadbcf125a68de23b44a434dd67281b5ece527b (accessed on 20 May 2025).

25. Marchis, I. F., Negruț, M., Blebea, C., Crihan, M., Alexa, A., & Breazu, C. (2024). Trends in preoperative airway assessment. *Diagnostics, 14*. https://www.semanticscholar.org/paper/0e88e1669983a08e83ee6a3a3a0f2452fffdbe19 (accessed on 20 May 2025).

26. Marcus, C. L., Brooks, L. J., Ward, S. D., Draper, K. A., Gozal, D., Halbower, A. C., Jones, J., et al. (2012). Diagnosis and management of childhood obstructive sleep apnea syndrome. *Pediatrics, 130*, e714–e755. https://doi.org/10.1542/peds.2012-1672.

27. Matava, C., Kovatsis, P. G., Lee, J. K., Castro, P., Denning, S., Yu, J., Park, R., et al. (2020). Pediatric airway management in COVID-19 patients: Consensus guidelines from the Society for Pediatric Anesthesia's Pediatric Difficult Intubation Collaborative and the Canadian Pediatric Anesthesia Society. *Anesthesia & Analgesia, 131*, 61–73. https://doi.org/10.1213/ANE.0000000000004872.

28. Medicine Chinese Society of Critical Care, Medicine Critical Care Medicine Branch of Beijing Associate, & Working Group of The Expert Recommendations on The. (2024). Expert recommendations on the clinical application of mechanical insufflation-exsufflation in mechanically ventilated patients. *Zhonghua Wei Zhong Bing Ji Jiu Yi Xue, 36*(8), 785–795. https://www.semanticscholar.org/paper/b4666ee310cd9adb4488198de07402c09affff6c (accessed on 20 May 2025).

29. Molthen, R. C. (2006). A simple, inexpensive, and effective light-carrying laryngoscopy blade for orotracheal intubation of rats. *Journal of the American Association for Laboratory Animal Science: JAALAS, 45*(1), 88–93.

30. Percie du Sert, N., Ahluwalia, A., Alam, S., Avey, M. T., Baker, M., Bre, W. J., Clark, A., et al. (2020). Reporting animal research: Explanation and elaboration for the ARRIVE guidelines 2.0. *PLOS Biology, 18*, e3000411. https://doi.org/10.1371/journal.pbio.3000411.

31. Planchard, D., Popat, S., Kerr, K. M., Novello, S., Smit, E. F., Faivre-Finn, C., Mok, T., et al. (2018). Metastatic non-small cell lung cancer: ESMO Clinical Practice Guidelines for diagnosis, treatment and follow-up. *Annals of Oncology, 29*, iv192–iv237. https://doi.org/10.1093/annonc/mdy275.

32. Raghu, G., Rémy-Jardin, M., Richeldi, L., Thomson, C. C., Inoue, Y., Johkoh, T., Kreuter, M., et al. (2022). Idiopathic pulmonary fibrosis (an update) and progressive pulmonary fibrosis in adults: An official ATS/ERS/JRS/ALAT clinical practice guideline. *American Journal of Respiratory and Critical Care Medicine, 205*, e18–e47. https://doi.org/10.1164/rccm.202202-0399ST.

33. Rhodes, A., Evans, L., Alhazzani, W., Levy, M. M., Antonelli, M., Ferrer, R., Kumar, A., et al. (2017). Surviving Sepsis Campaign: International guidelines for management of sepsis and septic shock: 2016. *Critical Care Medicine, 45*, 486–552. https://doi.org/10.1097/ccm.0000000000002255.

34. Ridgway, D. (2022). *Clinical Recommendations for Non-Anesthesia Healthcare Providers Performing Emergency Airway Management Outside the Operating Room*. https://core.ac.uk/download/519865988.pdf (accessed on 20 May 2025).

35. Saini, V. K., Saini, P., Soni, P., & Khandelwal, M. (2024). Retrospective comparative evaluation of airway management with different techniques of fiberoptic intubation in patients undergoing surgery for temporomandibular joint ankylosis. *Journal of Applied Pharmaceutical Research, 12*(1), 35–41. https://doi.org/10.18231/j.joapr.2024.12.1.25.41.

36. Segal, L. N., & Martínez, F. J. (2018). Chronic obstructive pulmonary disease subpopulations and phenotyping. *Journal of Allergy and Clinical Immunology, 141*, 1961–1971. https://doi.org/10.1016/j.jaci.2018.02.035.

37. Sorbello, M., Afshari, A., & De Hert, S. (2018). Device or target? A paradigm shift in airway management. *European Journal of Anesthesiology, 35*, 811–814. https://doi.org/10.1097/eja.0000000000000893.

38. Taljard, L. F., Müller, E., & Kemp, E. (2025). Airway management in patients with maxillofacial trauma—Part 2. https://www.semanticscholar.org/paper/e07fc6670395fe52839d5cbd3f67828152926d26 (accessed on 20 May 2025).

39. Tumminello, R., & Patino-Calle, D. (2024). Modification of an airway training mannequin to teach engagement of the hyoepiglottic ligament. *Journal of Education & Teaching in Emergency Medicine, 9*, I1–I6. https://www.semanticscholar.org/paper/bf7b52737c176d299f23ddb9b3cd2f60987a6c08 (accessed on 20 May 2025).

40. Umemoto, G., & Furuya, H. (2019). Management of dysphagia in patients with Parkinson's disease and related disorders. *Internal Medicine, 59*, 7–14. https://doi.org/10.2169/internalmedicine.2373-18.

41. Vogelmeier, C., Criner, G. J., Martínez, F. J., Anzueto, A., Barnes, P. J., Bourbeau, J., Celli, B. R., et al. (2017). Global strategy for the diagnosis, management, and prevention of chronic obstructive lung disease 2017 report: GOLD executive summary. *American Journal of Respiratory and Critical Care Medicine, 195*, 557–582. https://doi.org/10.1164/rccm.201701-0218PP.

42. Wilson, W., & Smith, A. F. (2018). The emerging role of awake video laryngoscopy in airway management. *Anesthesia, 73*, 1058–1061. https://doi.org/10.1111/anae.14324.

43. Zhao, L., Xie, Y. X., & Wang, C. (2020). Recommendations for respiratory rehabilitation in adults with coronavirus disease 2019. *Chinese Medical Journal, 133*, 1595–1602. https://doi.org/10.1097/cm9.0000000000000848.

GENERAL ANESTHESIA: INDUCTION AND MAINTENANCE

6

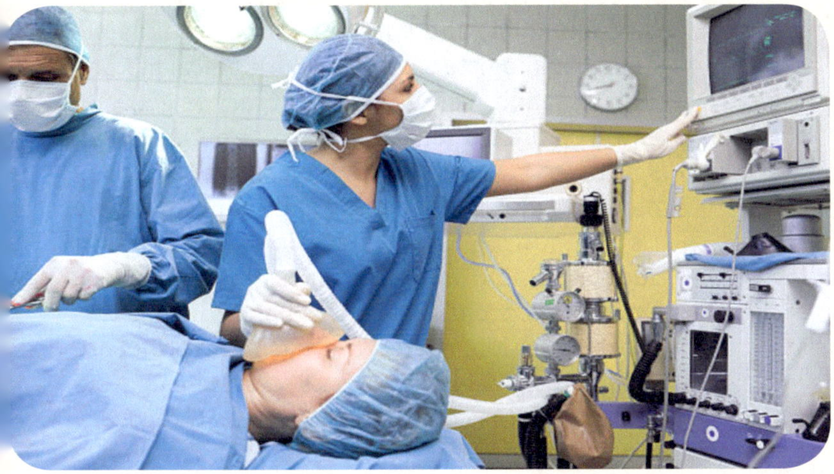

Introduction

Anesthetic practice has come a long way, transforming the conduct of surgery and making complex, hazardous operations much safer. General anesthesia (GA) today is a smart mix of medications and technology where doctors can cause and sustain unconsciousness. Much of the time, when clinicians realize how these drugs impact blood flow, they are able to customize their strategy to accommodate the individual's unique needs. Sophisticated monitoring equipment—including transesophageal echocardiography (TEE) and even cerebral oximetry—frequently play a key role in managing a patient's hemodynamics, ultimately improving overall safety for surgery (Ahmed et al., 2025). This blend of induction and maintenance is not static; it's a moving thing, constantly encouraged by new ideas. Increasing research is shedding light on the efforts being made to develop anesthetic drugs towards better patient outcome and experience. For example, ciprofol recently came into the picture as a potential drug for keeping patients under for a variety of procedures. Studies now compare

LEARNING OBJECTIVES

After studying this chapter, you will be able to:

1. Understand the mechanisms of action of general anesthesia.
2. Understand the induction of general anesthesia.
3. Learn about the maintenance of general anesthesia.
4. Learn about the risks and complications of general anesthesia.
5. Discuss advances in anesthesia technology.

ciprofol with the suspects such as propofol by tracking parameters such as recovery times and hemodynamic stability. This study is especially helpful in operations like thoracoscopic surgery, where the body response can be extremely unpredictable. Researchers are looking at factors like time to loss of consciousness (TLOC) and PACU stay to highlight the contrasts among techniques (Guo et al., 2024). Not only does it help in the reduction of clinical protocols but also helps us learn more about how new agents can be combined with the known techniques. Collectively, what we've learned about GA—from sparking unconsciousness to keeping it reliably maintained—shows a field driven by both necessity and creative problem-solving. As surgical procedures grow in complexity, the need for safer, more personalized anesthesia approaches becomes ever more urgent. Advances in both drugs and monitoring hint at a shift toward care tailored to individual patients, which is crucial in most cases. Ongoing research, generally weighing the advantages of the old against the new, keeps the end in mind: minimizing postoperative complications while speeding recovery. For the most part, sound knowledge of induction and maintenance strategies will remain key to improved patient outcomes and operating room safety (Ahmed et al., 2025; Guo et al., 2024) (Figure 6.1).

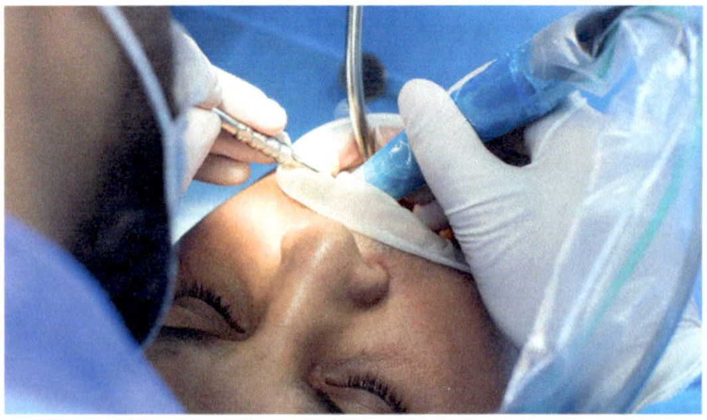

Figure 6.1. General Anaesthesia: A Professional Overview.

Source: https://www.evrenseldentalclinic.com/uploads/services_banner_2929724317.jpg.

Definition of General Anesthesia (GA)

Surgery is relatively high-tech—it's not just a matter of knocking you out. You need a state that not only renders you unconscious but also makes you not feel pain and relax your muscles; that is effectively general anesthesia (GA). This state is produced by carefully giving you different anesthetic drugs so that you don't know what's happening and don't feel pain while it happens. There's not only one way to do it, either; sometimes drugs enter your body through an IV, and sometimes they're inhaled. Anesthesiologists examine your medical history, allergies, and just what the surgery is going to entail before surgery even starts, creating a plan specific to you. Most of the time, this customized method helps ease the way and reduce possible risk. Following is the induction period – that sudden shift from wakefulness to anesthesia. Drugs like propofol are the norm during this short transition, but novel drugs like ciprofol are being tested as well. Current research suggests that ciprofol is capable of delivering a recovery similar to propofol (Shi et al., 2025). The choice at this point doesn't just determine the rate at which you lose consciousness; it also influences pain control later and how steady your blood pressure remains. In essence, gaining mastery over these early moments tweaks how anesthetic techniques are implemented in general. After induction has been gained, maintaining the anesthetic state in place takes top priority. During this time, drugs are constantly infused—either intravenously or inhaled—so that the essential body functions remain steady. Research identifies that while propofol is mostly favored based on the characteristic quick induction and rapid recovery, ciprofol has some desirable attributes regarding pain control and hemodynamic stability (Muhammad et al., 2024). Clinicians as a group need to stay on top of these evolving options so that they can balance effectiveness against safety for each patient throughout the entirety of the surgical experience (Figure 6.2).

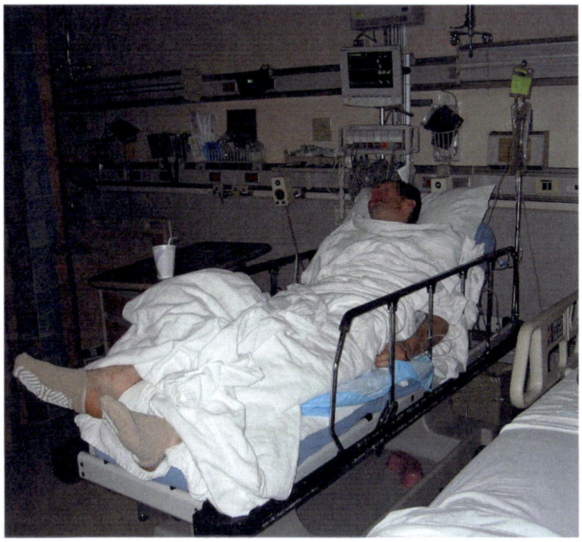

Figure 6.2. General anesthesia.

Source: By original author: Bobjgalindo - Own work, CC BY-SA 4.0, https://commons.wikimedia.org/w/index.php?curid=8042211.

Importance in Surgical Procedures

It is significant to know a patient's personal makeup when preparing for surgery—especially if they are going to receive GA. Those children with mitochondrial issues, for instance, have a variable reaction to anesthesia, and it can affect the outcome of the procedure. Researchers generally see that they need lower doses of sevoflurane to attain the correct level of sedation during induction, as proven via their BIS scores (Hsieh et al., 2021). This kind of personalization not only improves patient safety but also minimizes possible complications, improving the whole procedure, looking at a patient's individual conditions before surgery means an anesthetic plan that better controls sensitivity and, quite often, even speeds up recovery. Monitoring brain activity during anesthesia has also become very much at the center of keeping surgeries both safe and effective. Using evoked potentials from devices like ECoG and EThG in different states of sedation gives anesthesiologists an insight into the brain's control of sedation—and lets them conclude the depth of anesthesia. This kind of real-time monitoring, which tracks cerebral blood flow (CBF) and the activity of neurons, gives critical information for making real-time adjustments to anesthesia (Frasch et al., 2021). Picking up alterations in brain wave patterns enables anesthesiologists to rapidly adjust infusion rates to keep patients comfortably within their safe sedation range.

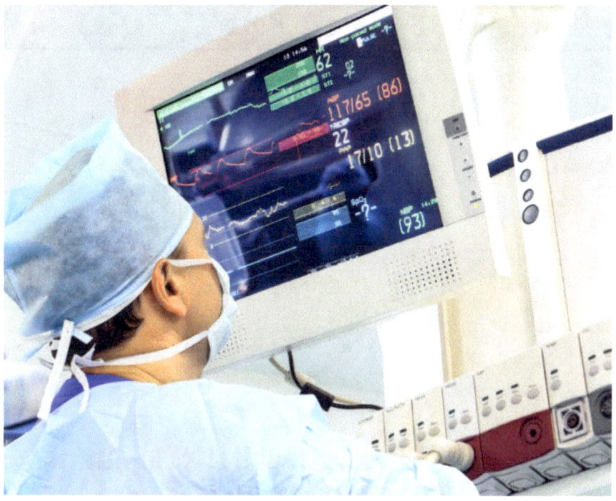

Figure 6.3. Importance of general anesthesia in surgical procedures.

Source: https://madeforthismoment.asahq.org/wp-content/uploads/2017/10/iStock-480733975-1024x797.jpg.

For most applications, these newer monitoring methods are indicative of the ways in which anesthetic practice is evolving to make surgery safer. Adequate coordination between the surgical team and the anesthesia team is something that you just cannot do without if you want safe results. Getting everyone on the same page as far as the patient's condition and specific anesthesia needs is critical—especially in difficult cases when the patient's history indicates other risk factors. When the team is working well, critical information like baseline vitals or deviation from anticipated changes is relayed with speed, and decisions to modify anesthesia happen promptly. Moreover, the knowledge of the minor quirks of each procedure helps anesthesiologists anticipate and handle any emergency situation (Frasch et al., 2021; Vincent et al., 2021). In summary, strong, sometimes imperfect, communication lies at the heart of good surgery and patient care throughout the entire procedure in the operating room (Figure 6.3).

6.1. Mechanisms of Action

Learning Outcome

1. Understand the pharmacodynamics of anesthetic agents.
2. Describe the effects of general anesthesia on the central nervous system.
3. Understand the role of neurotransmitters in anesthesia.

GA induces its effect through a combination of mechanisms that cumulatively block an individual from awakening. The inhaled agents, for example, influence the manner in which messages are communicated between brain cells—they increase the blocking activity of GABA, which, in most instances, decelerates brain activity and dampens response to external stimuli; at the same time, these drugs also typically deactivate segments of the stimulating circuits, thus communication in the brain as a whole collapses. This double action not only helps manage pain during surgery but also relaxes muscles (which is the most significant aspect of not developing complications in surgery). With these mechanisms active, knowing what occurs inside the brain enables clinicians to perfect their technique to achieve a balance between safety and efficiency (Drummond et al., 2023). Some recent studies have cast new light on the brain's wiring when it comes to how anesthesia operates—think drugs like sevoflurane. Researchers have been zeroing in on areas such as the paraventricular thalamus and how it relates to the bed nucleus of the stria terminalis, and, in general terms, these pathways seem to have a lot to do with turning the switch of consciousness on and off. Interestingly, when this connection is broken, patients wake up a lot more gradually. To illustrate, one study illustrated that chemo genetically inhibiting the glutamatergic neurons of these regions lengthened the emergence time considerably, indicating that these circuits are heavily associated with the manner in which we fall under and recover from anesthesia (Li et al., 2022a).

Merging molecular interactions with neural circuits captures nicely just how complicated maintaining someone under anesthesia is. It's not an issue of knocking someone out; it's more a question of keeping an eye on the depth of sedation, something that depends on how drugs move and dissolve d in the body. Anesthetic medications must hit the precise level to produce the desired effect, and new monitoring technology now enables practitioners to adjust dosages in real time. Several protocols have emerged to help anesthesiologists work through these challenges, holding patients in a balanced, safe space. With new medications and delivery devices still in the picture, ongoing research—grudgingly sometimes a bit patchy in its outcomes—will continue to guide best practices in safe, effective, responsive anesthetic care (Drummond et al., 2023).

6.1.1. Pharmacodynamics of Anesthetic Agents

Anesthetic drugs shape how safe and effective GA is during surgery. Clinicians need to know how these agents mix with the body's systems so they can adjust the plan to suit each patient's needs. Take propofol, for example—it's been the classic pick for starting anesthesia because it kicks in fast and wears off quickly, which works well for brief procedures and outpatient cases. Yet, some recent reports suggest that ciprofol—a newer option similar to propofol—might boost patient satisfaction and lead to fewer swings in blood pressure, especially in older or more frail patients. In many cases, the way these medicines interact with our biological processes directly impacts pain control and the success of starting anesthesia (Muhammad et al., 2024). Switching from the induction phase to keeping anesthesia steady shows how crucial these actions are. Keeping the proper depth of anesthesia is central to patient safety and comfort throughout surgery. The drugs' effects on nerve receptors and their ability to adjust neurotransmission essentially govern not just sedation but also pain relief. Interestingly, ciprofol seems to rival propofol's effectiveness during the maintenance stage while also causing less injection pain and fewer blood pressure ups and ds. This naturally suggests that choosing the right anesthetic can lower complications and help patients bounce back sooner (Wei et al., 2024).

Overall, a solid understanding of these dynamics is key for anesthesiologists who want to fine-tune patient care. Advances in how we understand these drug effects need to be brought into everyday practice to improve outcomes in GA. Evaluating the latest agents like ciprofol underscores why ongoing research matters in anesthesiology. Several studies comparing ciprofol and propofol have shown both can work well; however, ciprofol might lead to a lower incidence of injection pain and more steady blood pressure in vulnerable patients during the induction stage. These findings can, in most cases, reshape protocols and help practitioners pick agents that best suit both patient profiles and the demands of specific procedures. In this ever-changing field of anesthetic pharmacology, continuously reviewing how these drugs work gives clinicians the insight needed to make decisions that boost patient outcomes and satisfaction during both the start and continuation of GA (Muhammad et al., 2024) (Figure 6.4).

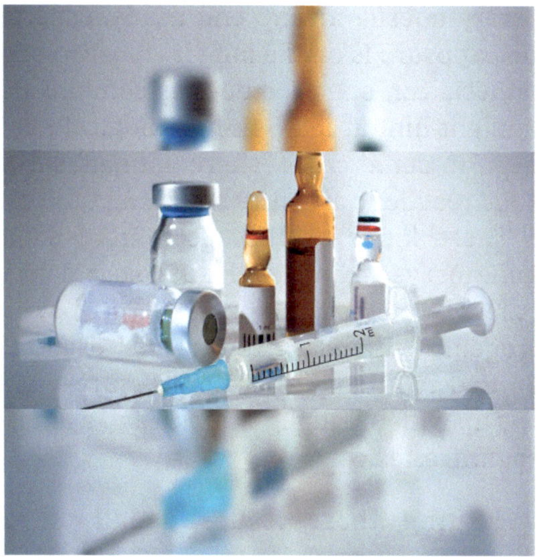

Figure 6.4. Anesthetic drugs.

Source: https://img.etimg.com/thumb/width-1200,height-1200,imgsize-126438,resizemode-75,msid-72534865/news/science/thee-most-important-functions-of-a-good-anesthetic-drug.jpg.

6.1.2. Effects on the Central Nervous System

GA shakes up the brain a lot—impacting both how we move and think. When these drugs knock you out, they also alter the nerve activity and the way signals bounce between your brain cells, which matters when trying to figure out the overall effects. For instance, during an anesthetic event, agents like isoflurane and halothane mix up the brain's electrical chatter, and you can actually catch these shifts with EEG recordings. You end up with different patterns that hint at just how deep under anesthesia someone might be, a sign of just how intricate our central nervous system can be. Still, while some of these shifts mark the right amount of brain suppression for a surgery, the sometimes-wacky EEG readings can be a puzzle—since folks can react in their unique ways to the same dose, underlining that our brains don't all behave uniformly. After the drugs wear off, the story doesn't always end neatly, especially when exposure is on the longer side. Prolonged anesthesia can open the door to complications that might hint at a dip in neurological health, as seen in some cases where animals showed strange reactions after the breathing tube came out. These kinds of findings remind us that keeping an eye on both vital life signs and mental alertness throughout the process is crucial. Take neurogenic pulmonary edema, for example—often tied to a jump in brain pressure—which shows up with breathing troubles and a faltering in cognitive tasks.

Treating these issues usually means throwing in extra medications to help sort out the symptoms, which brings into focus the link between how long you're anesthetized and what could go on in the brain. A careful look at these clues can help anesthesiologists get a jump on potential problems and, in most cases, keep things on track for better outcomes. On top of that, using quantitative EEG (qEEG) during anesthesia adds another layer of insight into how the brain's depth is managed. The raw EEG signals can be all over the place, and while some patterns tend to suggest a certain depth, they don't always fit every person—making it clear that a one-size-fits-all method just won't do.

For instance, alters in measures like the spectral edge frequency and median frequency for different anesthetic drugs can give practitioners hints about how these drugs alter the brain's excitability and silence certain nerve signals. Generally speaking, this kind of knowledge points to why ongoing research is so important in crafting monitoring methods that suit the messy reality of individual brain responses during surgery. All in all, digging deeper into these EEG patterns helps boost safety and effectiveness in the operating room, keeping patients both alert (in a monitoring sense) and stable while under anesthesia.

6.1.3. Role of Neurotransmitters in Anesthesia

General anesthetics mix with brain chemicals in ways that aren't straightforward. They don't just switch you off; they work on ion channels linked to nerve receptors, altering things on multiple levels. They boost channels that calm the brain—think GABAA and glycine receptors—and at the same time, they quiet d the ones that fire things up, like NMDA and nicotinic acetylcholine receptors. This kind of double action drops nerve activity significantly, so you lose consciousness and feel little pain during surgery. It's a subtle balancing act that shows just how complicated anesthetic effects can be (Guo et al., 2024).

Microglia—the brain's immune cells—are now getting some attention for their role in anesthesia. Recent findings suggest that when microglia numbers are reduced, animals lose and then recover their natural balance at different rates. In most cases, these cells seem to do more than just fight off infections; they tune how neurons respond to anesthetics. Genetic or drug-based alters aimed at microglial receptors tend to mess with the usual pace of anesthesia, pointing to a much bigger role for these cells than previously thought. This new twist means we might have to rethink what we know about anesthesia, as immune cells and neurotransmitter systems seem to team up during surgery (Guo et al., 2024). Lastly, the way neurotransmitters and their receptors interact—shown in several studies—backs up the main ideas of today's anesthesiology. Generally speaking, knowing how anesthetics adjust brain signals is key to refining techniques and keeping patients safe. Textbooks often note that understanding these processes gives practitioners the real-world tools to handle the bumps of anesthesia induction and maintenance. By merging insights about nerve signals and even the unexpected roles of microglia, doctors can alter their approach to fit each patient, boosting both safety and success. All of these factors combine to create a lively area of ongoing research that promises even more clinical breakthroughs in the future (Figure 6.5).

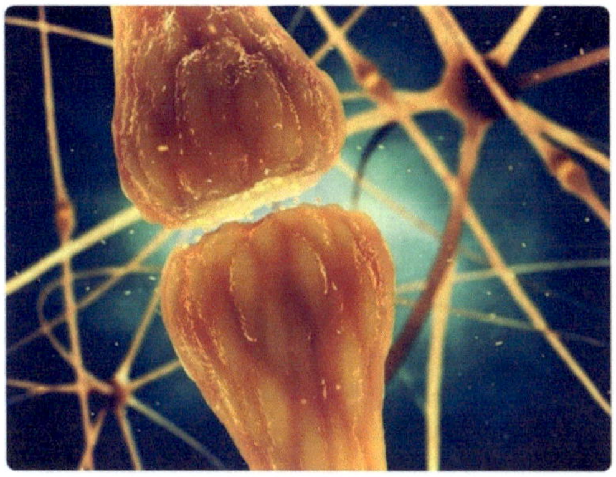

Figure 6.5. Synaptic transmission is the biological process by which neurotransmitters are released by a neuron and activate the receptors of another neuron.

Source: https://d2jx2rerrg6sh3.cloudfront.net/image-handler/ts/20200212122103/ri/673/picture/2020/2/%40shutterstock_567415408.jpg.

Test Your Knowledge

1. How does anesthesia affect the central nervous system?
2. Describe the role of neurotransmitters in anesthesia.

6.2. Induction of General Anesthesia (GA)

Learning Outcome

1. Describe the preoperative assessment and preparation.
2. Discuss about common induction agents.
3. Know the techniques for induction.

Switching a patient from being awake to falling into unconsciousness is a very delicate process—one that, in most cases, is all about keeping things safe and ensuring surgery runs smoothly. There's a whole mix of drugs used at this point, each doing its thing when it comes to affecting heart stability and how deep the anesthesia goes. Take a drug like propofol; many clinicians value it for its fast kick-in and that almost effortless smoothness when the patient is induced. Yet, one has to be cautious, especially if someone already has heart issues, because the wrong pick can mess up blood pressure and flow in ways no one wants. It's interesting, that ongoing research into new monitoring tools is letting doctors alter dosages almost on the fly so that each patient's heart gets just what it needs (Ahmed et al., 2025). Looking at newer options, there's been some buzz about agents like ciprofol that might be shifting the way induction is done these days. Early data generally points to ciprofol offering a few neat benefits—for example, it seems to keep the ups and ds in blood pressure and heart rate more under control when compared to the more traditional propofol regimen. For those high-risk patients, this gentler approach might just be the ticket, helping to smooth out potential complications during that tricky induction window. Some clinical trials even hint that ciprofol reduces the pain patient would normally feel from an injection and could lower the chance of problems after surgery, which is definitely an encouraging sign for future protocols (Guo et al., 2024). These days, the whole process doesn't stop at just getting the patient knocked out for surgery. Modern practice often wraps the induction phase into a broader strategy that looks closely at each individual's needs. Doctors are mixing in ideas like multimodal analgesia and fast-track recovery plans to reduce the overall toll anesthesia can take on the body. As the methods keep evolving, having the latest monitoring gadgets on hand means anesthesiologists can react more dynamically to how a patient is doing at that moment. Overall, the push to fold in newer drugs and smarter techniques shows a clear, ongoing commitment to making surgeries safer, more comfortable, and quicker in recovery, even if there's still a touch of unpredictability in the mix (Ahmed et al., 2025) (Figure 6.6).

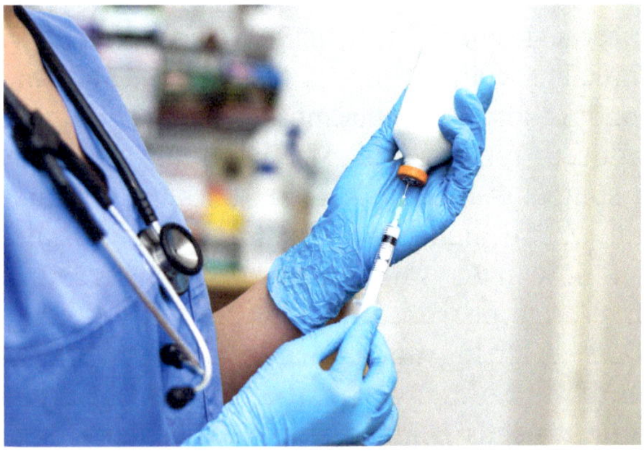

Figure 6.6. Propofol induction dose for general anesthesia.

Source: https://njanesthesiaservices.com/wp-content/uploads/2022/11/propofolinductiondose.jpeg.

6.2.1. Preoperative Assessment and Preparation

A careful check before surgery plays a key role in spotting issues that can show up during or after GA. Usually, it starts with digging into a patient's history—looking at any long-term conditions that might mean switching up the anesthesia plan. You examine aspects like heart and lung function, and even check the brain's stability, to see if everything's in order. It's also important to note hints such as a person's age or body mass, which can guide how anesthesia is adjusted. And when someone has a past with opioids, extra care is needed to spot tolerance, dependence, and potential withdrawal since these elements affect post-surgery pain strategies (Coluzzi et al., 2017). In most cases, getting these little details helps shape the anesthetic method and sets the stage for a smoother recovery. It isn't only about the physical side, though—what's going on in the mind matters too. Patients about to have surgery often feel anxious or scared, feelings that can even intensify physical symptoms and throw off cooperation during the whole process. A solid pre-surgery review usually includes a check on mental well-being to see if extra emotional support or a bit of counseling might be needed before the operation begins. Taking care of both body and mind not only makes folks feel more at ease but can also help ensure they follow post-op instructions. Plus, when someone has a long history of opioid use, the anesthesia team is often advised to cook up an all-around pain management plan—sometimes with input from addiction specialists—to cover all bases without upsetting the main anesthesia strategy (Coluzzi et al., 2017). This kind of layered planning helps build a solid foundation for the surgical process. Planning for anesthesia also means making sure that everyone on the team is in sync. The surgical crew, anesthetists, and nursing staff need to chatter and coordinate well so that every part of the patient's care comes together naturally. It's vital to go over the anesthesia plan with the patient ahead of time—clearly laying out the risks, and what to expect, and answering any lingering questions they might have. Good patient communication builds informed consent, boosts trust, and helps calm nerves. Keeping detailed notes on any identified risks also sets up backup plans in case something unexpected happens during surgery. For patients facing extra challenges—especially those with opioid histories—clear, sometimes repeated talks about alternative pain management options are key to keeping withdrawal symptoms in check. Altogether, this coordinated approach lays a strong groundwork for a safe surgical experience and better recovery afterward.

6.2.2. Common Induction Agents

Selecting the right induction agent matters a lot when starting GA safely and effectively. Propofol is a favorite in many cases – it kicks in fast and patients tend to wake up without a hitch. Its high lipid solubility means the drug quickly reaches the brain, leading to a rapid loss of consciousness. Also, its anti-nausea benefits help lower the chance of postoperative nausea and vomiting (PONV), which is especially important for procedures where that risk looms large. In pediatric cases, propofol remains the standard choice, proving both effective and safe across different age groups. Clearly, using propofol first underscores its practical advantages in a variety of surgical setups (Jamtsho et al., 2024). Another well-known option is sodium thiopentone, a drug that carries historical weight despite its reduced use today. This barbiturate knocks patients out fast by calming the central nervous system, making it handy for shorter procedures. That said, its use often comes with side effects like cardiovascular suppression and an increased risk of PONV; some studies suggest that certain groups – such as females or patients with a prior history of motion sickness – might be particularly vulnerable (Jamtsho et al., 2024). In many cases, this means that its administration requires a more careful look at patient risks and a coordinated effort by the anesthesia team to plan multimodal strategies that help minimize these sides. Beyond propofol and sodium thiopentone, alternatives like etomidate and ketamine have also found a place in clinical practice. Etomidate, generally speaking, is prized for keeping blood pressure steady, which benefits patients with cardiovascular concerns; meanwhile, ketamine stands out by offering both anesthetic and analgesic effects, serving dual roles during induction and postoperative pain care. This mix of features highlights the need to tailor anesthetic plans to the individual's specific health profile and surgical needs – an approach that often leads to better outcomes. Overall, these varied choices drive a more personalized practice in anesthesia, supporting optimal recovery in most cases (Sowbaraniya et al., 2023) (Figure 6.7).

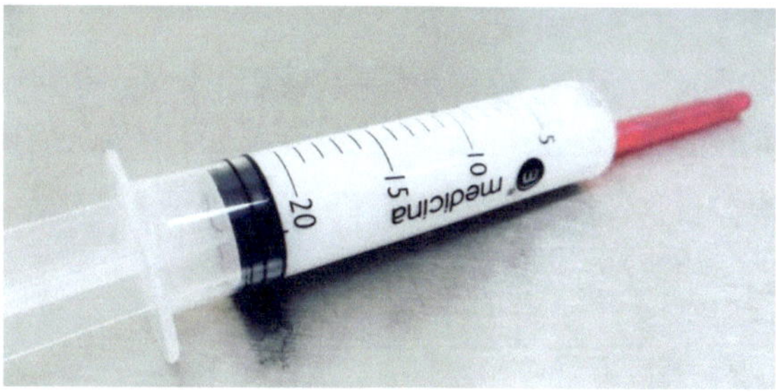

Figure 6.7. Induction agents.

Source: https://www.anaestheasier.com/content/images/2023/01/Screenshot-2023-01-03-11.58.24.png.

6.2.3. Techniques for Induction

Going from being awake to slipping under anesthesia is a crucial moment in surgery—a phase folks usually call induction. It all starts with choosing the right medications, and that choice is often shaped by a patient's unique health profile and what the surgery demands. For many, drugs like propofol and etomidate become the go-to picks because they kick in fast and behave predictably, which makes things smoother. The selection matters; you might say it not only sets how deep the anesthesia runs but also affects blood flow and heart stability. For instance, etomidate can be a smart move when dealing with heart issues, since its neutral effect on circulation tends to lower risk during this shift (Ahmed et al., 2025). In most cases, this careful balancing act helps ensure that the patient remains as safe as possible right from the start. Mixed in with these medications, keeping a close eye on the patient is vital. Tools like electrocardiography, pulse oximetry, and capnography provide snapshots of vital signs in real-time, so any hiccups can be spotted and handled quickly. Sometimes, especially in heart surgeries, TEE pops up as an extra resource—it gives doctors a look at the heart's function and blood flow dynamics during induction (Ahmed et al., 2025). Generally speaking, having these monitors in place means that even if things shift unexpectedly, a quick reaction is possible, which ultimately boosts overall safety and response. Then there's the broader picture of making sure that induction fits into a more comprehensive perioperative plan. A growing trend is to blend drug-based approaches with simple supportive measures to help patients recover faster and reduce on complications. For example, using warming devices during induction might lessen the chance of cooling too much, potentially speeding up recovery times without messing with the anesthesia's effectiveness. All this shows a shift toward a more patient-focused style of care—one that mixes advanced monitoring techniques and extra support steps to ease the journey into anesthesia and set up a smoother overall surgical experience.

Test Your Knowledge

1. What are the common induction agents?
2. What are the techniques for induction?

6.3. Maintenance of General Anesthesia

Learning Outcome

1. Monitor during surgery.
2. Know the maintenance agents and their administration.
3. Understand the adjustments based on patient response.

GA is a tricky undertaking that demands careful, almost hands-on attention to keep patients safe and surgeries on track. Induction kicks things off, getting the patient ready, but then comes the challenge of holding that anesthetic state throughout the whole procedure. Instead of complicated methods, doctors usually deliver the anesthetic continuously—often by having the patient breathe in a gas or using an IV drip—to gently adjust awareness and ease pain. Vital signs, like heart rate, blood pressure, and oxygen levels, are watched closely; they give clues about just how the patient is doing. This kind of watchfulness becomes even more critical when dealing with unusual cases, such as those small companion pigs, where natural differences can throw a wrench in standard approaches. In many cases, a few well-timed alters to the anesthetic plan help ward off risks such as hypothermia or low blood pressure (Smith et al., 2022). Keeping up the anesthetic state isn't just a matter of dosing drugs—it's also about keeping an eye on the body's many responses. During the procedure, the anesthesiologist checks out how well the drugs relax muscles, dull sensory responses, and affect automatic bodily processes. This kind of info, often essential for making adjustments in dosages or switching up the types of agents used, plays a big role. When you add advanced monitoring gadgets that peek at neuromuscular activity and brain signals, the control over anesthetic depth becomes much more precise. Such refined control is crucial to making sure the patient stays comfortably out of it and pain-free, without any unwanted moments of awareness. Recent studies, generally speaking, show that this kind of close monitoring can reduce on mishaps during surgery, highlighting the benefits of staying flexible with the anesthesia plan (Leonard et al., 2015). The process doesn't just vanish after surgery; it sort of stretches into the recovery phase too, and that transition can be just as delicate. Shifting a patient from being anesthetized into waking up again needs thoughtful titration of drugs and a look at how they're set to recover. Pain relievers and anti-nausea medications work together to ease post-operative discomfort and queasiness, making the bounce-back a bit smoother.

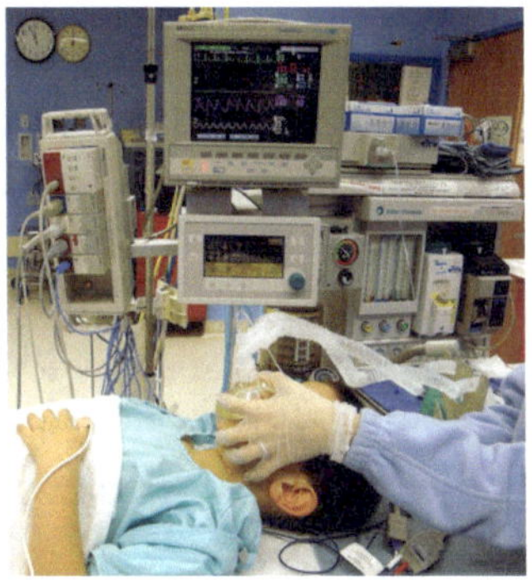

Figure 6.8. To maintain upper airway patency, the pediatric anesthesiologist holds the anesthesia mask snugly to the patient's face and performs the triple airway maneuver—neck extension, jaw thrust, and mouth opening—without applying pressure to the soft tissue or causing pain.

Source: https://aneskey.com/wp-content/uploads/2016/06/B9780323066129000134_f13-03-9780323066129.jpg.

Further, the duration and quality of the anesthetic maintenance may well affect longer-term outcomes like cognitive function and overall pain management. Some research even suggests that fine-tuning these steps not only improves immediate recovery but also boosts overall satisfaction and surgical success in the long run. In most cases, keeping a broad perspective on the whole process—right from the start until well after the surgery—is key to mastering anesthetic management principles (Smith et al., 2022) (Figure 6.8).

6.3.1. Monitoring During Surgery

Keeping a close watch during surgery is crucial to making sure anesthesia works safely and well. In most operations, the goal is simple – hold the right level of anesthesia so that patients don't end up feeling pain or even becoming aware mid-procedure. For example, one review found that around 34.8% of patients showed signs of connected consciousness when checked using the isolated forearm technique (IFT), with this happening more often during maintenance rather than during induction (Carron et al., 2018). These observations put our usual monitoring methods under some serious scrutiny and suggest we need to keep tabs on anesthesia depth throughout the procedure, especially when the risk of awareness seems higher. Technology keeps pushing forward, giving anesthesiologists more ways to gauge just how deep sedation is. Instead of merely watching for basic signs like changes in vital readings, modern practice now leans on more complex methods that tap into the brain's signals via electroencephalography. One method that's drawing attention uses multiscale entropy (MSE) – a tool that, broadly speaking, provides a layered look at brain activity over different time frames (Liu et al., 2015). This approach not only aims to boost the accuracy of our monitoring but also cuts d on the clutter of noise and other interference that can blur the picture. When these advanced algorithms come into play, clinicians often enjoy a more reliable reading of anesthesia depth, which can make a real difference to patient care. Monitoring isn't just about checking how deep the anesthesia is—it also covers keeping track of the patient's overall physical stability. Regularly measuring key signs like heart rate, blood pressure and oxygen levels is vital for spotting any adverse reactions to the drugs during surgery. A clear picture of the patient's hemodynamic state gives doctors the chance to adjust their protocols on the fly, acting as a kind of built-in safety net. Still, even with all these advances, some of our current methods fall short; a review of 34 anesthesia protocols even flagged significant gaps in practice (Carron et al., 2018). To summarize, striving for top-notch monitoring remains both a technical challenge and an essential part of anesthetic care, pointing to the ongoing need for fresh research and new techniques in the field (Figure 6.9).

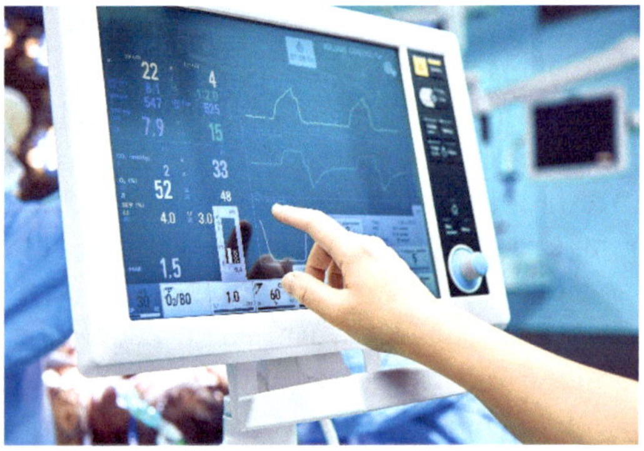

Figure 6.9. Monitoring during surgery.

Source: https://protrials.com/wp-content/uploads/2020/10/iStock-1130114408-Medical-device-scaled.jpg.

6.3.2. Maintenance Agents and Their Administration

GA is a tricky business that puts the spotlight on maintenance agents. They're the ones who keep patients safe and comfy during surgery. At some point, the anesthesiologist switches gears to keep the patient in a deep, steady sleep, all while juggling agents like isoflurane or halothane. These drugs, each with their quirks, seem to handle the job of suppressing awareness in different ways. One meta-analysis even showed that when inhalational agents are used, connected consciousness occurs less often than with intravenous ones (Carron et al., 2018). This kind of finding generally pushes practitioners to choose based on both the demands of the procedure and the unique patient characteristics. When you look closer at these agents, it's not just about a generic label, but rather how they work. Take isoflurane, for example. It's known to bring about burst suppression on EEG, hinting at heavy anesthesia. Yet, in most cases, its effect can vary enough to make monitoring rather challenging, especially since studies have noted varied EEG responses – even among equines (Aleman et al., 2015a). This variability means that anesthesiologists often rely on tools like anesthesia brain monitors (ABM) to quickly adjust and make sense of real-time patient feedback. There are, however, plenty of hurdles. Research has pointed out that methodological differences and quality issues have cropped up, with a good number of standard regimens falling short – clearly suggesting more work is needed (Carron et al., 2018). Factors like age and premedication can steer how these agents perform, making it clear that a one-size-fits-all approach just doesn't cut it. The need for personalized anesthetic plans is hard to ignore since these details can affect not only how effective anesthesia is but also the recovery process. In a nutshell, advancing training and technology remains vital for keeping anesthesia both precise and safe.

6.3.3. Adjustments Based on Patient Response

GA management isn't a one-size-fits-all process—it's a lively, ever-changing routine, especially during induction when every twitch or shift in a patient's state tells you something. Usually, doctors start with propofol to get things rolling, but, as many have noticed, its tendency to drop blood pressure can be a real headache. In most cases, research suggests that tossing in about 100 micrograms of phenylephrine helps curb those low-pressure moments; one study even showed that patients on the propofol-phenylephrine combo kept their blood pressure steadier than those who got just propofol. This alter, which kind of highlights how dosing should be tailored to each individual, smooths the way into anesthesia and shows a pretty refined grasp of how the drugs interact (Imran et al., 2007). When it comes to kids, the game plan shifts a bit, too. In pediatric cases, the choice of induction agent can truly hinge on how the little ones respond. That is, while both intravenous propofol and inhalational sevoflurane work well to ease a laryngeal mask airway (LMA), there are small but telling differences; for example, variations in jaw relaxation and how smoothly the LMA fits can make all the difference. One particular study noted that propofol delivered slightly better jaw relaxation and improved ease of insertion compared to sevoflurane—even though ultimately both agents achieved acceptable outcomes. It underlines that keeping a close eye on patient reactions is key when picking anesthetic agents to balance out effectiveness and safety during those procedures (Bakshi et al., 2019). And then there's the whole matter of altering the anesthetic approach beyond just which drug to use. It goes deeper into airway management and overall strategy—anesthetists must stay on their toes, watching for any hint of distress or signs that the sedation isn't quite cutting it. For example, if there's trouble getting enough air through the LMA, a switch to an endotracheal tube might be the way to go, boosting airway protection and ventilation in the process. This kind of flexibility is crucial, especially in busy, unpredictable surgical settings where things can change faster than you expect. In many cases, this personalized, if sometimes slightly improvised, approach shows a commitment to patient safety while capturing the delicate balancing act that is GA, making sure every patient's unique reactions get the attention they deserve (Figure 6.10).

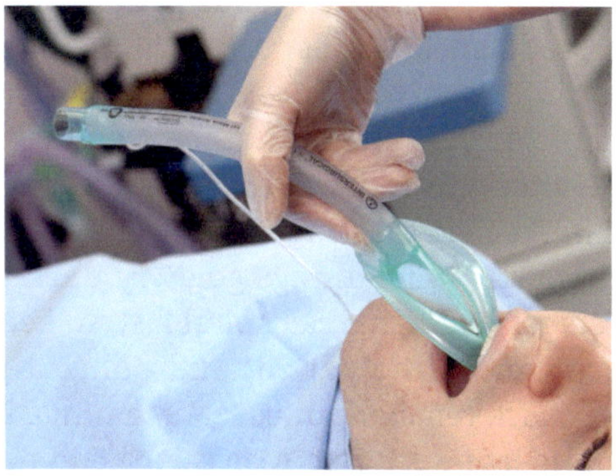

Figure 6.10. Laryngeal mask airway.

Source: https://marketresearchblog.org/wp-content/uploads/2023/11/Laryngeal-Mask-Market.jpg.

Test Your Knowledge

1. What are the 3 vital signs?
2. Describe the maintenance agents and their administration.

6.4. Risks and Complications

Learning Outcome

1. Know the common side effects of general anesthesia.
2. Understand the serious complications and their management.
3. Describe the risk factors influencing anesthesia safety.

GA is a tricky business—a mix of risks that both patients and providers have to handle. Breathing can get slowed down unexpectedly, sometimes right when the drugs kick in or later on. Propofol, which works quickly, is loved for its speed but sometimes sends patients into an overly sedated state, especially if their lungs already aren't at their best. Many still choose propofol for its reliable nature, yet the buzz around alternatives like ciprofol hints at ongoing alters in the field that might boost safety overall. And, honestly, when things go awry during the early stages, problems can spiral fast, so keeping a sharp eye on the patient and doing a good pre-op check remains a must (Muhammad et al., 2024). Heart issues also rear their head during GA. People with past cardiovascular problems tend to suffer more, and there's evidence to suggest that longer, more involved procedures might jack up the risks for serious heart complications. A study looking into endovascular aneurysm repair even found that patients under locoregional anesthesia had fewer heart attacks than those who went under GA (Li et al., 2024). Generally speaking, this points to the importance of tailoring anesthesia plans—factoring in a person's overall health and the specifics of the surgery—to help dodge potential cardiac mishaps. Then there's the matter of post-surgery brain fog and delirium—a worry especially for older adults. Some research shows that GA might increase the chances of cognitive slip-ups, affecting recovery and long-term quality of life. The exact reasons aren't totally sorted yet, but the effects, whether sudden or lingering, mean that choosing the right anesthesia doesn't come without its challenges. Adjusting how deep the anesthesia goes or even trying out different drugs is gaining ground as a way to reduce these risks. Doctors, for their part, must keep an extra watchful eye on neurological signs, ready to jump in and help smooth out recovery if needed (Muhammad et al., 2024).

6.4.1. Common Side Effects of General Anesthesia (GA)

GA does more than just put you to sleep; it kicks off a series of bodily changes that sometimes make the recovery process trickier than expected. One common twist is that blood pressure can drop to unexpectedly low levels—what many people call hypotension. You might see this happening more often when specific drugs are used during surgery. For example, one recent study pointed out that remimazolam, an ultra-short-acting benzodiazepine, needed less support with blood pressure compared to sevoflurane in laparoscopic procedures (Seong et al., 2024). This kind of data underlines the need to carefully choose an anesthetic plan, especially for patients already vulnerable to heart issues. There's also the curious case of how anesthesia can affect the brain. Patients sometimes experience what could loosely be called post-surgery brain fog—it might show up as a brief period of confusion or even longer-lasting cognitive hiccups, particularly among the older group. Researchers are still untangling exactly why the mind reacts this way, but it's clear that different agents have distinct impacts on blood flow and metabolism in the brain. Remimazolam tends to keep things on an even keel, while more traditional drugs like propofol can cause sharper drops in mean arterial pressure (MAP), which may, in many cases, worsen cognitive issues (Tsukimoto et al., 2024). Getting a handle on these differences helps clinicians steer their approach to better protect mental function, all while keeping surgical conditions optimal. Then there's the not-so-fun issue of post-operative nausea and vomiting—often abbreviated as PONV. This isn't just a one-size-fits-all reaction; the likelihood of someone feeling sick after surgery can depend on the length of the procedure, the type of anesthetic used, and even individual patient quirks. For instance, volatile anesthetics appear to push up the chances of nausea, whereas intravenous options like remimazolam might keep that risk lower. It's now common practice to give patients antiemetics before surgery to help fend off these unpleasant symptoms. In most cases, knowing these subtle differences is key to easing recovery and ensuring patients get through their procedures as comfortably as possible (Figure 6.11).

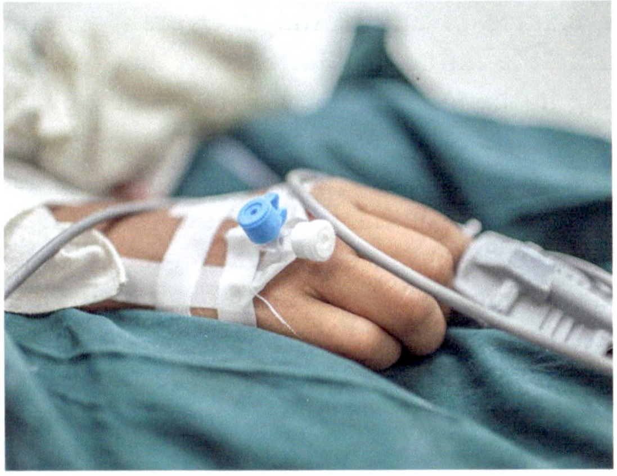

Figure 6.11. Side effects of general anesthesia.

Source: https://media.post.rvohealth.io/wp-content/uploads/2019/03/General_Anaesthesia-732x549-thumbnail.jpg.

6.4.2. Serious Complications and Their Management

Patients under GA can sometimes encounter sudden troubles – breathing issues tend to show up when you least expect them. In many cases, it's the respiratory problems that stir up worry, often linked to hidden underlying conditions. Kids with metabolic disorders like Pompe disease are especially at risk; extra glycogen in their muscles can cramp their breathing rhythm, and studies have noted that about 12.9% of these procedures see a drop in oxygen levels (Bosman et al., 2018). Doctors, particularly anesthesiologists, generally recognize that such challenges demand quick adjustments in monitoring, mixing careful checks with on-the-spot decisions. To summarize, the unpredictable nature of these events calls for a flexible, attentive approach. Then there's another serious snag – tension pneumothorax, which can suddenly emerge during a procedure when mechanical ventilation cranks up the working pressures. For instance, a 77-year-old patient having cervical laminoplasty experienced a rapid jump in inspiratory pressure that sent his cardiovascular system into chaos, eventually culminating in cardiac arrest (Lee et al., 2011). Incidents like that, where the situation flips in a heartbeat, drive home the importance of constant vigilance during surgery. Quick fixes, such as needle decompression and chest tube placement, often become the only way out when things escalate. These scenarios, with all their abrupt twists, remind the team that every moment counts and no precaution can be taken for granted. More than posing an immediate threat, such complications ripple into the broader planning of care. In most cases, thorough preoperative evaluations and detailed risk checks become essential, helping to spot vulnerable patients – whether it's someone with Pompe disease or those battling advanced respiratory issues. Recognizing these red flags lets anesthesiologists design a plan that's tailored to the individual, combining enhanced monitoring, specialized anesthetic tactics, and a collaborative team approach (Bosman et al., 2018; Lee et al., 2011). A mix of attentive observation and custom strategies is key to nipping potential problems in the bud. Ultimately, fine-tuning these protocols not only cuts down on complications but also boosts overall surgical success, underscoring just how vital foresight and preparedness are in modern medicine (Figure 6.12).

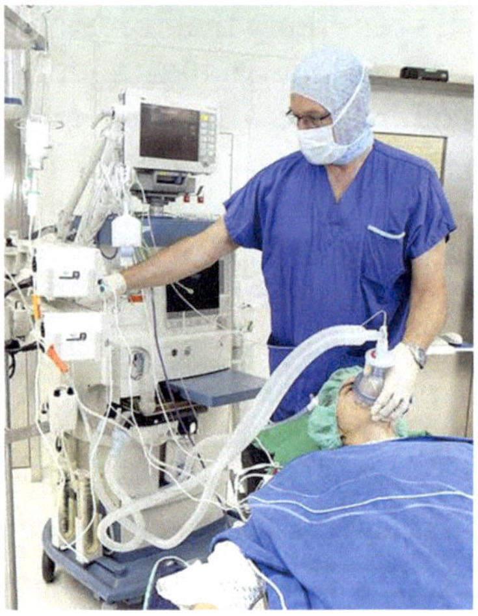

Figure 6.12. Complications of general anesthesia (GA).

Source: https://cdn.medizzy.com/UR5UIhuERrVj0pnBI_BMJ2WTV3g=/680x850/img/posts/65bcebb6-2e24-4313-bceb-b62e24e313be.

6.4.3. Risk Factors Influencing Anesthesia Safety

Administering anesthesia isn't straightforward – there are countless factors that, in most cases, affect patient safety in unexpected ways. Take pre-existing conditions, for example; someone with heart or lung issues often reacts differently to anesthetic drugs. In many situations, a patient with a weak heart needs a custom plan during both the start and maintenance stages, rather than a one-size-fits-all approach. The choice of drugs—whether it ends up being propofol or etomidate—must keep a close eye on the patient's blood flow and pressure to help avoid unpleasant surprises. Then there's the role of high-tech monitoring; tools like TEE, for instance, serve as extra safeguards for high-risk individuals. New developments in anesthetic pharmacology have, generally speaking, broadened the range of options available, aiming to boost safety and improve surgical results, as recent studies and clinical guidelines on cardiac surgery suggest (Ahmed et al., 2025). Safety during anesthesia isn't just about which drugs are used but also about how the procedure is monitored. Sometimes patients, against all expectations, may regain some awareness during GA—a condition known as awareness under general anesthesia (AAGA)—which can cause considerable psychological discomfort. Spotting those more likely to experience AAGA is key; for instance, using short-acting benzodiazepines right at the induction phase is one way to counter that risk (Khalil et al., 2023). Quantitative neuromuscular monitoring helps, too, by confirming that muscle function is recovering properly, thereby reducing the chance of any mishaps. Overall, whether during the initial drop of anesthesia or further along in the surgery, keeping levels of vigilance high and adapting as newer techniques emerge makes a difference in patient comfort and safety. Yet another essential piece of the puzzle is the experience of the anesthetist. Different skill levels and decision-making styles among practitioners can alter patient outcomes, often in profound ways. It isn't just about matching anesthetic drugs to a patient's physical profile, but also about considering how mentally prepared the patient might be for surgery. Regular, ongoing training in the latest methods and safety protocols is, in most cases, vital to reduce inherent risks. Plus, when the whole surgical team—surgeons, nurses, and anesthetists alike—chats openly and collaborates, it usually leads to smoother procedures and better outcomes. These combined efforts, even with the occasional little oversight, have steadily raised the bar for safety and effectiveness in anesthesia practice (Ahmed et al., 2025).

Test Your Knowledge

1. What are the most common side effects of general anesthesia?
2. What are the risk factors influencing anesthesia safety?

6.5. Advances in Anesthesia Technology

Learning Outcome

1. Understand the development of new anesthetic agents.
2. Know the innovations in monitoring equipment.
3. Discuss the future trends in anesthesia practice.

Advances in technology have reshaped medicine—and anesthesia gets its share of this change. Fancy monitors now let anesthesiologists keep a closer eye on patients' heartbeats and blood pressure during surgery. You might be surprised that TEE has become such a game changer; it ups the monitoring game and even lets teams check heart function in real-time, which is pretty crucial for cardiac cases. Generally speaking, this shift isn't just about new gadgets—it shows how clinical know-how and tech skills have to work together. Looking back at how cardiac anesthesia has evolved, one can see these innovations have even altered training and certification routes, steadily pushing patient care and safety forward (Tsai et al., 2023). New anesthetic agents and innovative delivery systems have turned the induction and upkeep of GA on its head. Modern inhalational anesthetics come in fast and fade away quickly, which means clinicians can adjust anesthesia depth almost on the fly—a huge benefit in constantly changing OR settings. Using targeted drug delivery, patients usually get doses that fit their unique needs; this precise approach cuts down side effects and often helps folks bounce back quicker. In most cases, such tailoring doesn't just lessen unwanted effects—it also contributes to better overall outcomes. In many ways, this focus on fine-tuning drug delivery marks an ongoing commitment to safety and effectiveness in anesthetic practice (Li et al., 2022a). The mix of anesthesiology with data science is opening up possibilities no one saw coming. AI and machine learning are now being wed into anesthesia management systems, sometimes throwing predictive insights into the mix to help with decision-making. By digging through huge datasets, these tools can spot patterns that a human eye might miss, nudging us toward evidence-based practices that boost patient safety. As GA continues to evolve, these innovations point to a shift meant to lower risks and improve outcomes—even if it sometimes feels a bit unpredictable. Research in this area keeps pushing the boundaries, ensuring that anesthesiology stays at the cutting edge of medical tech, drawing on emerging trends and fresh scientific insights (Tsai et al., 2023) (Figure 6.13).

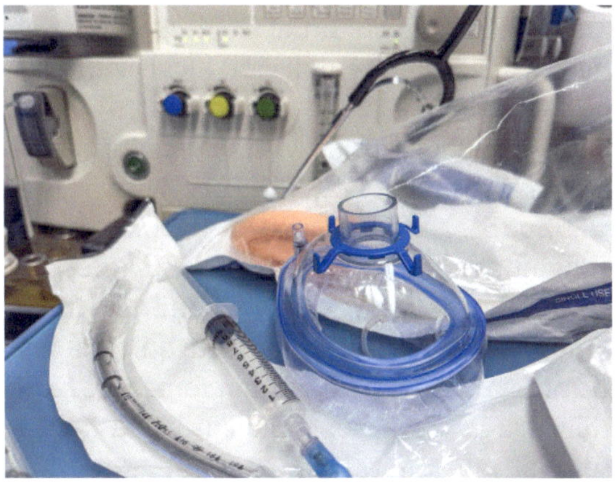

Figure 6.13. Technological advancements and emerging trends in anesthesia.

Source: https://world.skanray.com/wp-content/uploads/2023/09/anesthesia-mask-laryngoscope-represent-controlled-care-precise-intervention-hospital-airw-scaled.jpg.

6.5.1. Development of New Anesthetic Agents

The world of anesthetic agents has been shaken up over the last few years—doctors and researchers alike are chasing better outcomes, safer approaches, and more effective drugs. You now see new breakthroughs that speed up the start of anesthesia while also keeping things running smoothly during surgery. Some of these medicines seem especially tuned for patients with heart issues, offering extra protection for the heart during tough procedures. Recent articles even point out that when you mix advanced monitoring systems with these fresh anesthetic protocols, it tends to pave the way for a more patient-focused kind of care. Then, on top of that, drug formulations and delivery methods have also been given a makeover. Long-acting agents like alfaxalone, for example, have caught a lot of attention for use in both starting and maintaining anesthesia—sometimes even replacing the old inhaled techniques in certain situations (Ahmed et al., 2025). Generally speaking, there's a growing trend toward total intravenous anesthesia (TIVA) to reduce the cognitive side effects linked with some volatile drugs, which is a big help for more vulnerable groups like the elderly. This shift shows an improved grasp of how these agents move through the body and interact with it (Gise et al., 2025). And, we can't overlook how data management is being woven into anesthetic practice. Better record-keeping and the analysis of anesthesia events have shed quite a bit of light on overall trends and outcomes, revealing which drugs work best in real-world settings. For example, detailed logs of anesthesia protocols show varying levels of success across different drugs, and these insights both sharpen individual practices and add to our collective knowledge. In most cases, these findings are fueling ongoing research into new ways to use these developments safely and effectively for all kinds of patients (Ahmed et al., 2025).

6.5.2. Innovations in Monitoring Equipment

New monitoring gear has changed the game, making GA both safer and more effective. We used to only keep an eye on basic numbers, but now there's a whole host of devices that grab data live—even d to detailed checks of blood flow, muscle response, and just how deep the anesthesia actually is. These systems don't only log heart rate, blood pressure, and oxygen levels; they also offer insights into the patient's brain function (Burokiene et al., 2023). With this extra information, anesthesiologists can alter their approach on the fly, reducing on risks like patients partially waking during a procedure and other complications. Non-invasive devices have also stepped up the practice, giving patients more comfort along with better safety. Take tools like transcutaneous CO_2 monitors and advanced pulse oximeters—they feedback results in real time without the hassle of drawing arterial blood gases (Cappellini et al., 2024). This newer approach not only eases patient stress but also smooths out the overall surgical experience. Wireless monitors, for instance, let staff move around the OR freely instead of being stuck to fixed equipment, which in turn keeps the focus on patient care while reducing the feel of cumbersome machinery.

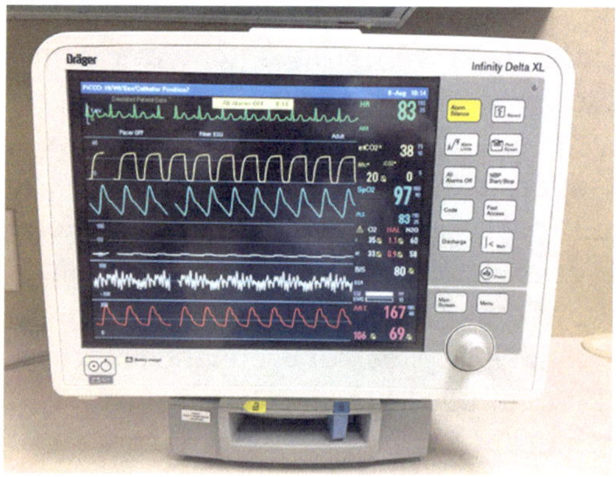

Figure 6.14. Anesthesia monitoring equipment.

Source: https://doctorsoxygenservice.com/application/files/8915/6529/4693/Infinity-Delta-and-Docking-Station.jpg.

The trend is clear: streamlined and accurate monitoring is pushing toward more patient-centered care. The push for smarter technology doesn't stop at making things less invasive. There's a growing role for predictive analytics and machine learning in anesthesiology. By crunching vast amounts of data, these tools can flag potential issues before they emerge. For example, some algorithms scan vital signs and response patterns to hint at the chance of intraoperative awareness, helping guide decisions along the way (Burokiene et al., 2023). As these predictive methods blend in with existing monitors, the landscape of GA is evolving quickly. Constant advances not only boost safety but also make surgeries run smoother, showing just how intertwined technology and anesthetic care have become (Figure 6.14).

6.5.3. Future Trends in Anesthesia Practice

Anesthesia is on the brink of big changes—breakthrough drugs and fresh technology are shaking things up. Instead of the old routine that leaned on just a handful of anesthetic drugs, there's now a push for safer, more effective options. New drugs, with simpler and more predictable behavior, promise quicker recoveries and fewer side effects. People are talking about how three parts—drugs, tech (both digital and mechanical), and the way we work as humans in healthcare—are starting to mix together, which could lead to procedures that are overall safer and smoother (Renxi et al., 2024). At the same time, fresh drug developments go hand in hand with the rising role of AI in handling pain during surgery. Traditional pain management has often wavered between too little or too much opioid dosing because real-time monitoring hasn't been on point. Recent research hints—generally speaking—that AI might offer more personalized, data-driven alters to pain control, adjusting treatments to fit each patient's needs. This kind of step-by-step, flexible approach could boost patient comfort and results. In addition, better education about the role of AI in keeping pain in check might slowly change how anesthesia providers view and use these emerging tools (Jacob et al., 2024). Looking ahead, it's clear that new tech will only work well if it fits with what patients and providers need. Understanding how healthcare systems either support or hinder these updates is key; even small misalignments can slow progress. Bringing together anesthesia experts and tech teams in more relaxed, cross-disciplinary talks might reveal practical ways to fold these advances into everyday practice. Sure, training programs might have a few hiccups along the way, but over time this adaptability could pay off. By gradually filling in the knowledge gaps and staying on top of new trends, the whole field of anesthesia can keep patient care first, aiming for safer, more effective results (Renxi et al., 2024) (Figure 6.15).

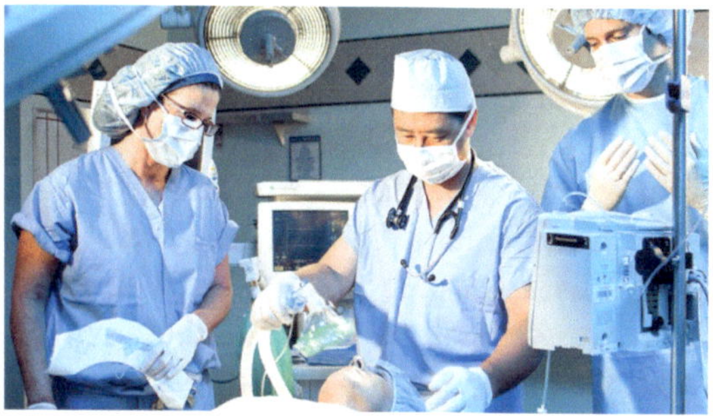

Figure 6.15. Future of Anesthesiology.

Source: https://www.teamhealth.com/wp-content/uploads/2019/01/TH-11586-December-Blog_Anes.jpg.

Test Your Knowledge

1. Explain the development of new anesthetic agents.
2. Describe the future trends in anesthesia practice.

SUMMARY

More recent monitoring modalities within anesthesia have quite a large impact on how care is provided, especially as we attempt to deal with the differing needs of populations of patients along the continuum. Recent studies point out that older patients, for instance, seem to be more vulnerable to cognitive blips after GA—generally, they're at greater risk. Instead of sticking with the old amplitude-based methods that sometimes fall short, researchers have started including processed EEG data. With the help of tools that analyze things like correlation dimension and even multiscale entropy while a patient is on the operating table, doctors are often able to reduce unwanted side effects and make the process safer—even if the methods aren't foolproof. All of this points to the need for anesthesia practice to shift gears and align itself with the unique way that an individual's body reacts, helping to improve recovery and brain function in vulnerable groups like the elderly (Drover et al., 2018). Shifting gears and lessening heavy reliance on opioids in anesthesia is another important development. In the past, most protocols were based on high opioid use, an approach that too often led to more pain after surgery and longer recoveries. Recently, though, pairing multiple techniques of pain relief—such as pairing regional anesthesia with multiple drug adjuvants—is expected to cut back on opioids without decreasing the degree of the pain control. This approach not only fits within broader public health efforts at combating the opioid epidemic but also has a tendency to afford patients a much better overall experience, whether for cardiac surgery or for other kinds of procedures. Clearly, the adoption of these opioid-sparing modalities is a key inflection point that offers the promise of more balanced, holistic patient care (Baez et al., 2022). At the end of the day, pushing on with novel strategies in getting and keeping GA up and running shows a strong commitment to patient safety and better outcomes. Tailoring protocols to fit particular populations—like the elderly or those at risk of opioid dependence—is coming to be regarded as essential (even if it means rewriting old ideas). As studies continue and healthcare providers continue to communicate and collaborate, this cooperation becomes critical to experiment with and develop new ideas of monitoring and pain management. There's a constantly growing body of evidence to back up the benefits of more complete monitoring and broader use of multimodal analgesia; not only does this validate current practice, but it also works to advance overall anesthesia safety and effectiveness in many diverse surgical contexts. Simply put, embracing these strategies will keep the field evolving in a way that maintains patient wellness as the priority, even in an ever-more complex healthcare landscape (Baez et al., 2022; Drover et al., 2018).

GA isn't really about giving a cocktail of drugs—it's something that unfolds in unexpected stages. Drugs such as propofol, sufentanil, and cis-atracurium first put the patient into a deep sleep, as if they were falling asleep innocently. Then, agents such as sevoflurane step in and keep things even-keel, not allowing any unwelcome wakefulness while the operation is performed. It's not so much about checking off boxes and more about controlling the body's response—modulating heart rate, suppressing pain, and bringing it just right. At the end of the day, a regimen that works for every patient is most desirable for an uneventful and safe surgical procedure. There was all the frenzy in recent times about newer anesthetic drugs, and remimazolam is one of those surprise participants. This ultra-short-acting benzodiazepine is known to effectively soothe hiccups after surgery, most notably emergence agitation (EA), which can complicate recovery. Some studies even propose that using remimazolam as operations conclude decreases EA rates markedly (Group R, 21% EA rate vs. Group C, 49% EA rate) (Lu et al., 2025). In addition, it seems to buffer changes in blood pressure and heart rate as patients come out of anesthesia—typically speaking, a measure that may simply contribute to overall comfort and results. Blending the new technique with tried-and-true methods supports the philosophy of keeping abrest of drug development is eventually worth it. Anesthesia complications are not limited to adult surgery; they extend to practices like cesarean, whose choice of medication determines the newborns significantly. Studies comparing Apgar scores and other parameters have shown that different anesthetic techniques may have varied impacts on the puppies, particularly in how their hearts work and in the distribution of blood to their limbs (Modrzewska et al., 2025). To put it in perspective, protocols integrating an epidural block into GA have been shown to keep newborns hemodynamically more stable, emphasizing a surprising correlation between what mom is administered and how her babies fare immediately after birth. All these facts remind us that the anesthetic plan is a balancing act in some way—something which has to protect not only the patient but new life entering the world as well, and it demonstrates how complex all of this must be.

KEY TERMS FROM THIS CHAPTER

- Anesthetic drugs
- Cerebral oximetry
- Excitatory circuits
- Glycine receptors
- Microglia
- Nicotinic acetylcholine receptors
- Post-anesthesia care unit
- Sevoflurane
- Brain cells
- Ciprofol
- General anesthesia
- Inhaled agents
- Neurological health
- Paraventricular thalamus
- Propofol
- Transesophageal echocardiography

CRITICAL THINKING QUESTIONS

1. **General anesthesia involves:**
   a. Only loss of consciousness
   b. Loss of consciousness and analgesia
   c. Loss of consciousness, analgesia, and muscle relaxation
   d. Only analgesia and muscle relaxation
2. **Which of the following agents is commonly used for induction of general anesthesia?**
   a. Sevoflurane
   b. Propofol
   c. Fentanyl
   d. Succinylcholine
3. **The least soluble inhalational anesthetic in blood, leading to rapid onset and recovery, is:**
   a. Isoflurane
   b. Sevoflurane
   c. Desflurane
   d. Nitrous oxide
4. **Which monitoring modality is essential during general anesthesia to detect apnea or hypoventilation?**
   a. Capnography
   b. Electrocardiogram (ECG)
   c. Non-invasive blood pressure
   d. Pulse oximetry
5. **Preoxygenation before induction of general anesthesia aims to:**
   a. Increase tissue oxygen stores
   b. Reduce the risk of aspiration
   c. Prevent hypoxemia during intubation
   d. Both a and c

Short Answer Questions

1. Define the general anesthesia.
2. Why is general anaesthesia important in surgical procedures?
3. What is the mechanism of action of general anaesthesia?
4. What is induction in general anesthesia?
5. Describe the maintenance of general anesthesia.

Answers to Critical Thinking Questions

1. (c); 2. (b); 3. (c); 4. (a); 5. (d)

REFERENCES

1. Ahmed, M. A. K., Bahurmuz, M. A., & Muthanna, F. M. S. (2025). General anesthesia in cardiac surgery: A narrative review for evolving techniques and patient-centered best practices. *Yemeni Journal for Medical Sciences.* https://www.semanticscholar.org/paper/b9f20626e344f524ee83d5ae25eff4809116ebe2 (accessed on 20 May 2025).
2. Aleman, M. R., Brosnan, R. J., Fletcher, D. J., & Holliday, T. A. (2015a). Electroencephalogram of healthy horses during inhaled anesthesia. https://core.ac.uk/download/323071267.pdf.
3. Aleman, M., Brosnan, R. J., Fletcher, D. J., & Holliday, T. A. (2015b). Qualitative and quantitative characteristics of the electroencephalogram in normal horses during administration of inhaled anesthesia. https://core.ac.uk/download/323068610.pdf.
4. Baez, D. E., Buscemi, C., & Valdes, J. A. (2022). Opioid-sparing anesthesia in cardiac surgery requiring cardiopulmonary bypass. https://core.ac.uk/download/548486067.pdf (accessed on 20 May 2025).
5. Bakshi, S. A., Bule, S. S., & Shingade, G. U. (2019). Comparative evaluation of induction with propofol vs induction with sevoflurane for insertion of laryngeal mask airway in children. https://core.ac.uk/download/543135804.pdf (accessed on 20 May 2025).
6. Bosman, L., Hoeks, S. E., González Candel, A., van den Hout, H. J. M., van der Ploeg, A. T., & Staals, L. M. (2018). Perioperative management of children with glycogen storage disease type II—Pompe disease. *Pediatric Anesthesia, 28*(5), 428–435. https://doi.org/10.1111/pan.13361.
7. Burokiene, V. Y. (2023). On the intraoperative awareness under general anesthesia. https://core.ac.uk/download/591386666.pdf (accessed on 20 May 2025).
8. Cappellini, I., Bavestrello Piccini, G., Campagnola, L., Bochicchio, C., Carente, R., Lai, F., Magazzini, S., & Consales, G. (2024). Procedural sedation in emergency department: A narrative review. *Emergency Care and Medicine, 1*(2), 103–136. https://doi.org/10.3390/ecm1020014.
9. Carron, M., Linassi, F., Ori, C., Tellaroli, et al. (2018). Isolated forearm technique: A meta-analysis of connected consciousness during different general anesthesia regimens. https://core.ac.uk/download/168406742.pdf (accessed on 20 May 2025).
10. Casoni, D., Giovannini, A. E. J., Precht, C. M., & Adami, C. (2016). A possible case of neurogenic pulmonary edema in a sheep following intracranial surgery. *Journal of Clinical Anesthesia and Management, 1*(3). http://dx.doi.org/10.16966/2470-9956.110.
11. Coluzzi, F., Bifulco, F., Cuomo, A., Dauri, M., Leonardi, C., Melotti, R. M., Natoli, S., Romualdi, P., Savoia, G., & Corcione, A. (2017). The challenge of perioperative pain management in opioid-tolerant patients. *Therapeutics and Clinical Risk Management, 13*, 1163–1173. https://doi.org/10.2147/TCRM.S141332.
12. Drover, C. M., Drover, D. R., Vaughn, D. A., MacIver, M. B., Cohen, M. S., et al. (2018). Do complexity measures of frontal EEG distinguish loss of consciousness in geriatric patients under anesthesia? https://core.ac.uk/download/323076544.pdf.
13. Drummond Júnior, D. G., Guimarães, A. C. C. M., Bezerra Neto, P. D., de Castro, C. T., & Santos, I. C. (2023). Advantages of using general anesthesia. *III SEVEN International Multidisciplinary Congress.* https://www.semanticscholar.org/paper/6313700b37ebe9f3541250f30dc9edd25bceb50c (accessed on 20 May 2025).

14. Frasch, M., Walter, B., Anders, C., & Bauer, R. (2021). Update on the multimodal pathophysiological dataset of gradual cerebral ischemia in a cohort of juvenile pigs: Auditory, sensory and high-frequency sensory evoked potentials. https://www.semanticscholar.org/paper/f504dafcb2548adc8b8e5a37d08e49ee0e920409 (accessed on 20 May 2025).
15. Gise, B. T., Thorbrogger, C. J., Rasys, A. M., Quandt, J. E., & Divers, S. J. (2025). Lizard anesthesia—A retrospective study of anesthetic protocol and monitoring quality of anesthetic episodes at a veterinary hospital over 23 years (2000–2023). *Journal of the American Veterinary Medical Association.* https://www.semanticscholar.org/paper/4ea3ce757760b9b4e99aa1c732035f33114bfc99 (accessed on 20 May 2025).
16. Guo, N., Cao, J., Duan, M., Zhou, F., Wang, W., Xu, L., Wei, C., et al. (2024). Effects of ciprofol infusion on hemodynamic during induction and maintenance of anesthesia and on postoperative recovery in patients undergoing thoracoscopic lobectomy: Study protocol for a randomized, controlled trial. *PLOS ONE, 19.* https://www.semanticscholar.org/paper/5c304a99ae42034c0679ded078896299a33bac57 (accessed on 20 May 2025).
17. Hsieh, V. C., Niezgoda, J., Sedensky, M., Hoppel, C., & Morgan, P. (2021). Anesthetic hypersensitivity in a case-controlled series of patients with mitochondrial disease. *Anesthesia & Analgesia, 133*, 924–932. https://www.semanticscholar.org/paper/573c05d1d6a04a86e63aec9552cde3054af53a4b (accessed on 20 May 2025).
18. Imran, M., Khan, F. H., & Khan, M. A. (2007). Attenuation of hypotension using phenylephrine during induction of anesthesia with propofol. *JPMA: The Journal of the Pakistan Medical Association, 57*(11), 543–547.
19. Jacob, C. B., & Diaz, V. J. (2024). Utilization of artificial intelligence algorithms in the perioperative management and reduction of pain: An evidence-based educational module. *Nicole Wertheim College of Nursing Student Projects, 199.* https://digitalcommons.fiu.edu/cnhs-studentprojects/199 (accessed on 20 May 2025).
20. Jamtsho, P., Dorjey, Y., Dorji, N., Tshering, S., Wangmo, K. P., Dorji, T., Wangchuk, T., et al. (2024). Factors associated with postoperative nausea and vomiting after laparoscopic cholecystectomy at the National Referral Hospital, Bhutan: A cross-sectional study. *BMC Anesthesiology, 24.* https://www.semanticscholar.org/paper/df8aa5001471170da0c4834fe36866fbf8edc0d8 (accessed on 20 May 2025).
21. Jense, R. J. (2017). Innovations in anesthesia: Past, present, and future. *International Journal of Anesthesiology & Research*, 1–2. https://core.ac.uk/download/pdf/144790137.pdf (accessed on 20 May 2025).
22. Lee, J. Y., Kim, J. U., An, E. H., Song, E., & Lee, Y. M. (2011). Bilateral tension pneumothorax caused by an abrupt increase in airway pressure during cervical spine surgery in the prone position: A case report. *Korean Journal of Anesthesiology, 60*(5), 373–376. https://doi.org/10.4097/kjae.2011.60.5.373.
23. Leonard, D. A., Powell, H., Albritton, A., Shanmugarajah, K., Mastroianni, M., Lofgren, S., & Cetrulo, C. L. (2015). Upper extremity transplantation in non-human primates: An orthotopic model for translational research. *Vascularized Composite Allotransplantation, 2*(1), 17–25. https://doi.org/10.1080/23723505.2015.1072261.
24. Li, J. Y., Gao, S. J., Li, R., Wang, W., Sun, J., Zhang, L., Wu, J. Y., et al. (2022a). A neural circuit from the paraventricular thalamus to the bed nucleus of the stria terminalis for the

regulation of states of consciousness during sevoflurane anesthesia in mice. *Anesthesiology, 136*, 709–731. https://www.semanticscholar.org/paper/69679589e1c0ad69730e91c54eef38f9cd6065ac (accessed on 20 May 2025).

25. Li, R., Sidawy, A. N., & Nguyen, B. N. (2024). Locoregional anesthesia has lower risks of cardiac complications than general anesthesia after prolonged endovascular repair of abdominal aortic aneurysms. *Journal of Cardiothoracic and Vascular Anesthesia*. https://www.semanticscholar.org/paper/732994acd5f2f74a65c8f718589fc49829090b32 (accessed on 20 May 2025).

26. Li, X., Yang, Y., Zhang, B., Lin, X., Fu, X., An, Y., Zou, Y., et al. (2022b). Lactate metabolism in human health and disease. *Signal Transduction and Targeted Therapy, 7*. https://doi.org/10.1038/s41392-022-01151-3.

27. Liu, Q., Chen, Y. F., Fan, S. Z., Abbod, M. F., & Shieh, J. S. (2015). EEG signals analysis using multiscale entropy for depth of anesthesia monitoring during surgery through artificial neural networks. *Computational and Mathematical Methods in Medicine, 2015*, 232381. https://doi.org/10.1155/2015/232381.

28. Lu, Y., Xu, Q., Dai, H., Wu, J., Ai, M., Lan, H., Dong, X., et al. (2025). Remimazolam for the prevention of emergence agitation in adults following nasal surgery under general anesthesia: A prospective randomized clinical controlled trial. *BMC Anesthesiology, 25*. https://www.semanticscholar.org/paper/28728f3fb2f94111aaf2ba05e8cd11c912184641 (accessed on 20 May 2025).

29. Modrzewska, A., Ochota, M., Kiełbowicz, Z., & Antończyk, A. (2025). Comparison of neonatal puppy vitality following elective cesarean section with different induction agents and epidural anesthesia. *Medycyna Weterynaryjna*. https://www.semanticscholar.org/paper/14d1e76d9b02acbc96c858c64ce6266be0fbeffa (accessed on 20 May 2025).

30. Muhammad, H., Hurais, M., Javeria, Z. S., Samra, R., Dhanushan, G., Shah, S. A. R., Fatima, S. N., et al. (2024). Efficacy and safety of ciprofol versus propofol for induction and maintenance of general anesthesia: A systematic review and meta-analysis. *Journal of Anesthesia, Analgesia and Critical Care, 4*. https://www.semanticscholar.org/paper/5e194dfabd2803ad878736580c060528ec2ce56a (accessed on 20 May 2025).

31. Ohiienko, M. M., Redko, S. I., Shyshchuk, V. D., Огиенко, et al. (2015). General questions of anaesthesiology. https://core.ac.uk/download/141448194.pdf (accessed on 20 May 2025).

32. Rastas, J. P., Zhao, Q., & Johnson, R. A. (2025). Comparison of two active warming techniques on body temperature in healthy, anesthetized dogs premedicated with acepromazine or dexmedetomidine: A pilot study. *PLOS ONE, 20*. https://www.semanticscholar.org/paper/3284d113443e7a4a66ad787a4870d7588206a896 (accessed on 20 May 2025).

33. Reda Khalil, A. M., Shaffik, A. M., & Mahmoud, Y. (2023). Updates in awareness under general anesthesia. *Benha Journal of Applied Sciences*. https://www.semanticscholar.org/paper/6390a21b54f7d6e6b1363d40f2d93b622987390e (accessed on 20 May 2025).

34. Seong, H., Cho, J. E., Yoon, S. Z., & Choi, S. U. (2024). Remimazolam reduces vasopressor use post-induction and during maintenance of general anesthesia in patients undergoing laparoscopic gynecology: A propensity score-matched analysis. *Journal of Clinical Medicine, 13*. https://www.semanticscholar.org/paper/7c91b3abe5a5da8079b01d1abb19cc935961d6bb (accessed on 20 May 2025).

35. Shi, S., Wu, J., Wu, Y., Han, X., Dai, H., Chen, X., Sun, Z., et al. (2025). Effects of ciprofol and propofol general anesthesia on postoperative recovery quality in patients undergoing ureteroscopy: A randomized, controlled, double-blind clinical trial. *Drug Design, Development and Therapy, 19*, 931–943. https://www.semanticscholar.org/paper/f1646ce5f3d9cfac434672d3452eb17bf7eff5e4 (accessed on 20 May 2025).

36. Smith, J. S., & Seddighi, R. (2022). Miniature companion pig sedation and anesthesia. *The Veterinary Clinics of North America: Exotic Animal Practice, 25*(1), 297–319. https://doi.org/10.1016/j.cvex.2021.08.007.

37. Sowbaraniya, S. M., & Govindaraju, L. (2023). Commonly used induction and maintenance drug for children treated under general anesthesia–A retrospective study. *Journal of Advanced Zoology, 44*(S7).

38. Tsai, A., Faloye, A. O., Bodmer, N. J., Madhok, J., Nunes, S., Shook, D. C., & Linganna, R. E. (2023). Preparing for the adult cardiac anesthesiology subspecialty certification: Recognition of expertise in cardiac anesthesiology. *Journal of Cardiothoracic and Vascular Anesthesia, 37*, 2405–2408. https://doi.org/10.1053/j.jvca.2023.08.152.

39. Tsukimoto, S., Kitaura, A., Yamamoto, R., Hirase, C., Nakao, S., Nakajima, Y., & Sanuki, T. (2024). Comparative analysis of the hemodynamic effects of remimazolam and propofol during general anesthesia: A retrospective study. *Cureus, 16*. https://www.semanticscholar.org/paper/0df1a02ac623a3cacb8032a07fef270fa911f8ec (accessed on 20 May 2025).

40. Wei, Y., Jia, L., Cheng, S., Ma, W., An, X., & Xu, Z. (2024). Efficacy and safety of ciprofol for general anesthesia induction in female patients with frailty: A prospective randomized controlled trial. *BMC Anesthesiology, 24*. https://www.semanticscholar.org/paper/d4ec57c85b7c16cc04918f78d56480ec2f98260e (accessed on 20 May 2025).

REGIONAL ANESTHESIA: SPINAL, EPIDURAL, AND PERIPHERAL NERVE BLOCKS

7

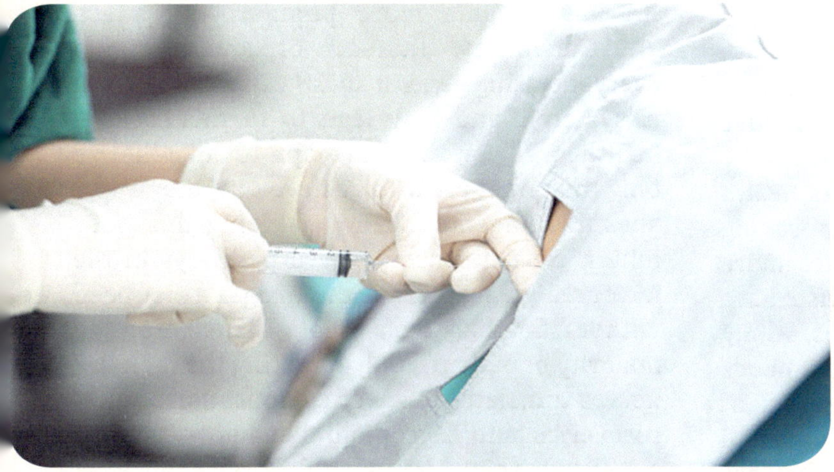

LEARNING OBJECTIVES

After studying this chapter, you will be able to:

1. Understand the mechanism of action of regional anesthesia.
2. Describe the spinal anesthesia and epidural anesthesia.
3. Describe the peripheral nerve blocks.
4. Learn about the complications and risks of regional anesthesia.

Introduction

Pain control during surgery has come a long way, motivated by the desire to reduce lower opioids and allow patients to recover more rapidly. Regional anesthesia (RA) is now front and center; spinal, epidural, and other nerve blocks are used more frequently. These interventions not only cut pain but seem to modulate the body's stress response to surgery, leading to better outcomes overall. There is much evidence, for instance, attesting to the idea that peripheral nerve blocks (PNBs) are effective as a pre-op pain protocol. There are some studies showing that these blocks can reduce on the necessity for further opioids and reduce their side effects, an aspect important for elderly patients (Dönmez et al., 2024). Briefly, knowing how these anesthesia techniques work, where and when they are most useful, and what they can achieve is vital for anyone who wants to raise the standard of surgical care. Employing RA methods, such as spinal and epidural blocks, has produced promising results in dealing with pain that persists long after surgery and even improving patient satisfaction. Studies cover a range of procedures—from those involving bone to chest procedures—and all report improvements both in short-term relief from pain and on the long term. Take thoracic paravertebral blocks, for example; they've been utilised to decrease the incidence of chronic pain after video-assisted thoracic surgery (Zhao et al., 2024). If one looks at the various approaches to nerve blocks, one gets an idea about the subtleties that lead to a case for customized anesthesia strategies depending on the patient and the specifics of the procedure. Such a targeted initiative enables practitioners to manage both the urgency of pain and the bigger picture of recovery. Integrating RA into clinical practice does pose challenges—training and resource limitations are the greatest hurdles. As health systems become more focused on improving care at the time of surgery, it becomes more and more important that anesthesiologists have hands-on training in these techniques. Along with this is continuous research. There needs to be refinement of the techniques, assessment of their impact on diverse patient groups, and even determination of whether or not they are cost-saving in a variety of diverse operating settings. New technology like ultrasound-guided methods has established a new standard of safety and accuracy with nerve blocks.

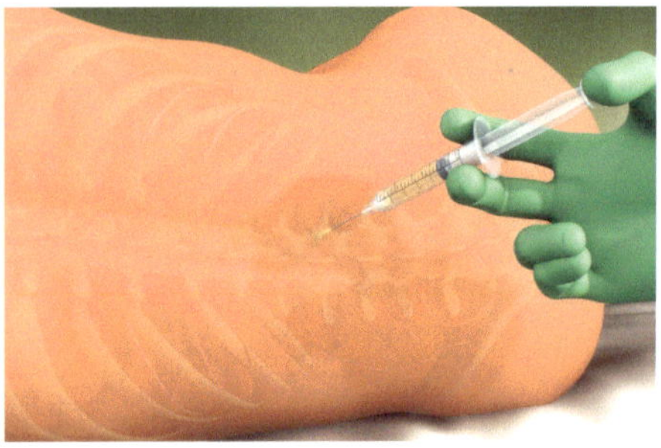

Figure 7.1. Understanding Regional Anesthesia.

Source: https://esaic.org/wp-content/uploads/2024/02/02-8-1260x808-1.png.

And while we continue to explore such methods—even if at times the research appears a bit scattered—there's truly potential for a revolution in pain management. That in turn suggests an authentic need for further education and receptiveness to shifting clinical practice as new evidence and techniques are developed (Dönmez et al., 2024; Zhao et al., 2024) (Figure 7.1).

Definition of Regional Anesthesia (RA)

RA has become more popular in modern anesthesiology. Instead of anesthetizing everyone using general anesthesia (GA)—which is systemic and may lead to further risks—healthcare workers now opt to anesthetize only the target area. To achieve this, they apply anesthetic agents locally; by doing this, they inhibit crucial sensory nerve pathways in the local area, giving patients the analgesia they need without flooding their whole system. For the majority of patients, only targeting the required nerves translates to fewer complications, faster recoveries, and less opioid demand (Wenzel et al., 2016). There are many flavors of this kind of approach. Consider spinal anesthesia (SA), for instance: the anesthetic is deposited into the cerebrospinal fluid in the lower back to create profound numbness for below-the-waist surgeries. Then there is epidural anesthesia, where the medication is placed in the space around the spinal cord, creating a more variable level of numbness—particularly helpful for labor or for after-surgery pain. And you have PNBs, which are aimed at specific nerves in an arm or a leg, enabling the patient to stay awake while alleviating pain in the limited area. These various approaches attest to the flexibility of RA and show its growing importance in improving outcomes both during and after surgeries (Diaz et al., 2022). Aside from the immediate benefits during surgery, RA also helps address wider public health problems—specifically, the problem of opioid overuse. Since opioid dependence is on the rise, particularly in the perioperative period, the use of regional techniques reduces the dependence on systemic opioids. This selective method, for the most part, eliminates the danger of both immediate complications and the long term of chronic pain that sometimes follows long-term opioid use. In this way, RA is not simply an issue of pain control for a surgery; it is a core element of a broader, patient-specific strategy for care that is moving the specialty of anesthesiology forward (Diaz et al., 2022; Wenzel et al., 2016) (Figure 7.2).

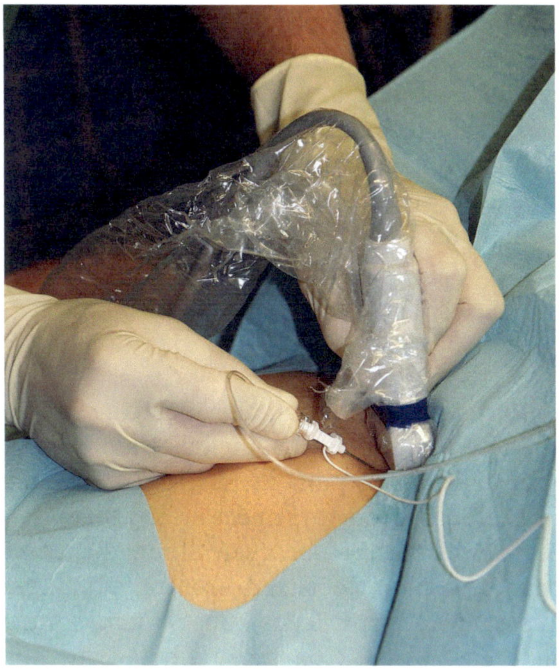

Figure 7.2. Regional anesthesia.

Source: By PhilippN - Own work, CC BY-SA 3.0, https://commons.wikimedia.org/w/index.php?curid=6995353.

Importance in Modern Medical Practice

RA has changed operations as they are done today. Spinal, epidural and even nerve blocks allow doctors to control pain relief without subjecting patients to full general anesthesia (GA). That approach means fewer drugs put patients at risk, and that tends to decrease risks and speed up recovery. Additional medicines mixed in at times give local anesthetics a kick, reducing normal side effects after surgery. Mostly, this custom-fit method tends to leave patients happier with their recuperation and treatment. Technology has contributed a great deal to the mix as well. There is a sudden burst of new devices that now help practitioners with accuracy in administering nerve blocks that were previously not possible. Ultrasound technology and neurostimulation, for example, work together quite like the unlikely marriage of old methods and modern technology, placing blocks accurately and reducing risk. Even sophisticated monitors and real-time information systems enable doctors to keep a watchful eye on patient safety during treatment—raising the stakes, so to speak, on care. Being comfortable with these technological innovations is quite important for anesthesiologists nowadays, who are required to be versatile as the world evolves. RA is not a trick for the OR either. Its uses have spread to trauma care and chronic pain management, proving its potential for many various sorts of patients.

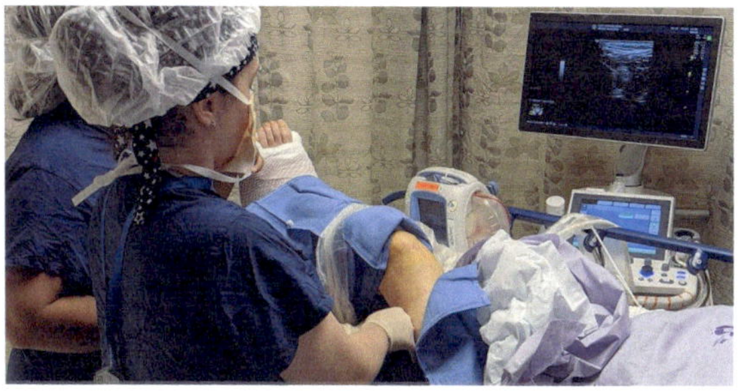

Figure 7.3. Importance of regional anesthesia in modern medical practice.

Source: https://www.upstate.edu/anesthesiology/images/headers/header-regional-anesthesiology.jpg.

Other recent research even suggests nerve blocks can be employed in treating acute pain in children and those with other medical conditions, inspiring a potential more integrated, multidisciplinary approach to treatment.

There is ongoing research into the potential applications of local anesthetics outside of conventional settings, and this has repercussions for promising future developments in pain management technique (Miščuks et al., 2008) (Figure 7.3).

7.1. Mechanism of Action

Learning Outcome

1. Explain how regional anesthesia works.
2. Differentiate between spinal, epidural, and peripheral nerve blocks.
3. Understand the pharmacological use of anesthetic agents.

RA is accomplished by inhibiting the nerve signals with local anesthetics. The drugs act on voltage-gated sodium channels on nerve membranes, stopping sodium ions from rushing in when a nerve has an electrical impulse. When that ion flow is inhibited, the nerve cannot fire normally and you lose sensation in the area. This type of block permits controlled pain relief for surgery while the rest of the body remains functional. But not all local anesthetics are the same; the degree of numbness, onset time, and duration can all differ with the drug being used—so doctors need to individualize their approach. The addition of other medications can augment the effect of local anesthetics. You can add things like opioids, alpha-2 agonists, or corticosteroids to augment the pain relief. For example, opioids have a tendency to work at mu-opioid receptors in the brain and spinal cord, which conveniently adds to the nerve-blocking action of the anesthetics. Research usually illustrates that the use of these agents together can extend pain relief and reduce the amount of opioids needed after surgery, addressing one of modern medicine's biggest challenges of managing postoperative pain while keeping opioid use to a minimum (Singhal et al., 2024). When clinicians are more aware of these interactions, they are able to adjust their RA plans to gain better outcomes. RA also has a huge role to play in postoperative recovery—this is seen especially in planned orthopedic surgeries. The evidence indicates that interventions like PNBs and epidural analgesia will lead to a decrease in the use of opioids in recovery. In a trial of tibial plateau fracture surgeries, patients who received RA consumed significantly less opioid medication throughout their hospitalization and even needed less after they were discharged for over three months. This reduction not only improves analgesia but also reduces opioid-related complication risks. For the most part, as we learn even more about how these mechanisms work, the integration of RA into a mix of pain control methods becomes increasingly essential to optimizing surgical care (Cunningham et al., 2022).

7.1.1. How Regional Anesthesia (RA) Works

RA works by sending numbing medicine straight to where the nerves pass signals—a move that essentially stops pain in its tracks. In many surgical setups, doctors inject these agents right into nerve clusters or even along the spine, creating a neat, localized area of numbness. This targeted approach boosts pain control while cutting back on those whole-body side affects you often see with GA. Zeroing in on the trouble spots helps keep post-op discomfort to a minimum and, in most cases, lessens the dependence on opioids—ultimately reducing opioid-related risks and leaving patients more at ease (Wenzel et al., 2016). It also messes with hemodynamics in ways that can be quite influential during surgery. Neuraxial methods, like spinal or epidural blocks, often alter arterial tone to help keep patients more stable throughout the procedure. Still, these effects aren't always predictable; adding extra nerve blocks doesn't necessarily mean arterial tone will drop further. For example, one study comparing combined spinal-epidural (CSE) with a lumbar plexus block found that while pain scores improved noticeably, the arterial tone hardly shifted—highlighting just how complex the body's response can be during big operations like total hip arthroplasty (Buschiazzo et al., 2016). RA isn't just about easing pain right after surgery—it's a key player in the overall plan for patient care. This technique lets anesthesiologists put together a multimodal strategy that kicks off even before the operation and carries through to discharge. Since managing acute pain is crucial to stopping it from becoming chronic, using these directed methods can enhance patient care. Better pain control in the recovery phase not only speeds up healing but also improves functional outcomes, underlining the vital role RA plays in contemporary anesthetic practices (Wenzel et al., 2016) (Figure 7.4).

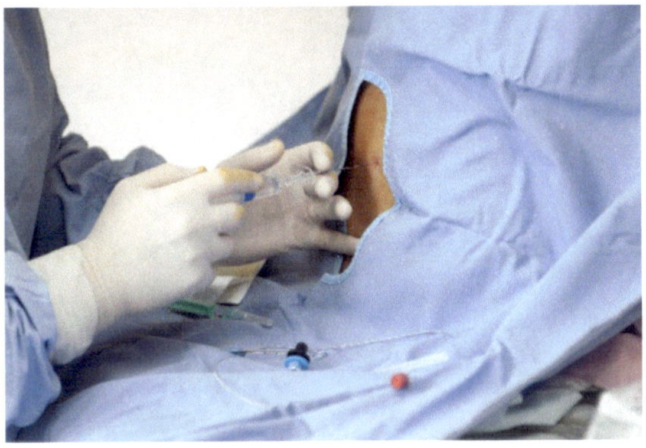

Figure 7.4. How Is Regional Anesthesia Used During Surgery?

Source: https://www.verywellhealth.com/thmb/YwoG7Rb7TaAEUUS1pxNEMCUEcvQ=/1500x0/filters:no_upscale():max_bytes(150000):strip_icc()/GettyImages-154725435-59a034a50d327a001006171b.jpg.

7.1.2. Differences in Mechanisms Among Spinal, Epidural, and Peripheral Nerve Blocks

RA comes in many different flavors that shape how well it works. Take SA, for instance – doctors inject the anesthetic straight into the cerebrospinal fluid. This direct hit tends to block both feeling and movement pretty fast because the agent latches onto sodium channels, which stops the nerves from firing action potentials. You get quick pain relief during surgery, yet sometimes patients also experience minor side effects – like brief, abnormal tingling sensations (transient paresthesia) that might appear after the procedure (Imbelloni and Gouveia, 2021).

Most often, knowing these details helps healthcare providers set realistic expectations and adjust anesthesia on the fly. Epidural blocks, on the other hand, follow a different route. Instead of jumping straight into the fluid, the anesthetic is delivered into the epidural space that envelopes the spinal cord. This method creates a more focused, even if less intense, sensory block compared to the spinal route. It's a common choice for childbirth or lower limb surgeries; however, the relief doesn't kick in as immediately, and the block can vary because it affects sensory and motor fibers unevenly. In many cases, doctors will mix in non-opioids or opioids to prolong and boost the overall effect (Mehta et al., 2020). This blend ends up giving a sort of personalized pain management strategy. PNBs show yet another twist, targeting specific nerves to ease pain without compromising movement too much. With the anesthetic placed close to the intended nerve, effective pain control can be achieved for limb surgeries—or even for chronic pain—without significant involvement of the central nervous system. Although the focused approach reduces the chance of widespread side effects, minor complications can still crop up. Often, pinpointing the best injection site relies on clear anatomical landmarks and increasingly on ultrasonographic guidance—a nod to how modern tech keeps pushing medicine forward. To summarize, the ways spinal, epidural, and peripheral methods each work their magic highlight unique roles in pain care, making it essential for clinicians to understand these nuances (Imbelloni and Gouveia, 2021; Mehta et al., 2020).

7.1.3. Pharmacology of Anesthetic Agents Used

Anesthetic agents play a huge role in RA because they help target pain where it matters most. Think about how common types—amide and ester local anesthetics—mess with sodium channels; by doing so, they block nerve signals. It's not just about dulling pain during procedures, but also about overall safety, and the drug you pick counts. Ropivacaine, for example, is generally seen as a step up from bupivacaine, thanks to how it differently affects sensory and motor nerves. This shift in drug options has led to better recovery outcomes after surgery and even less reliance on opioids, underscoring why those small chemical differences truly matter (Pooley et al., 2022). When it comes to kids, choosing the right anesthetic is even trickier because their bodies aren't just small versions of adults—they behave differently. Recent work shows that using a continuous catheter, like in a quadratus lumborum block, can be quite effective for relieving pain after colorectal surgery in children. In many cases, doctors alter the mix of ropivacaine and chloroprocaine, adjusting dosages to fit each child's needs. Looking at how pain scores line up with opioid use, it turns out that these focused techniques can lower risks such as respiratory problems and longer recovery times (Pooley et al., 2022). It's also worth noting that the nitty-gritty of pharmacodynamics influences how RA is managed., the way these local anesthetics interact with nerve tissues and receptors not only affects how quickly they kick in and how long they last, but also raises important safety and efficacy issues. Then there are the differences in pharmacokinetics—like absorption rates and protein binding—which can change the whole treatment picture. For example, anesthesiologists need to factor in the complex layout of the neuraxial space when administering drugs epidurally or intrathecally, since those routes can unexpectedly alter how the drug works. Ongoing research in these areas, generally speaking, is pretty important because it might lead to better practices and even spur the development of new agents more finely tuned for RA applications (Carness et al., 2019) (Figure 7.5).

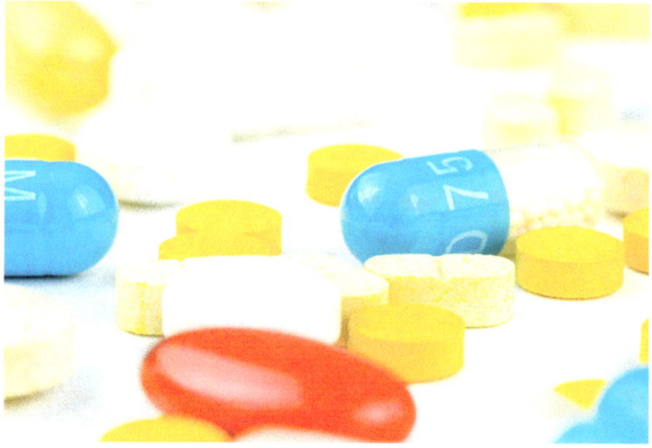

Figure 7.5. Anesthetic Drugs.

Source: https://mixlab.com/hubfs/assorted-colorful-pills.webp.

Test Your Knowledge

1. How does regional anesthesia work?
2. What are the differences in mechanisms among spinal, epidural, and peripheral nerve blocks?

7.2. Spinal Anesthesia (SA)

Learning Outcome

1. Understand the indications for spinal anesthesia.
2. Know the procedure and technique of spinal anesthesia.
3. Describe the advantages and disadvantages of spinal anesthesia.

SA has come a long way as a breakthrough for surgeries on the lower part of the body. It delivers strong pain relief—blocking sensation beneath the injection point while, in some cases, leaving some motor control intact. This rapid action is especially handy for procedures like cesarean sections or orthopedic work on the legs, reducing prep delays and boosting overall OR flow. Using local anesthetics in this way also means fewer systemic opioids, which many recent pain management studies point out as a key benefit (Wenzel et al., 2016). Every patient tends to wrestle with some level of pain after surgery, and if that pain isn't managed well, it can turn chronic. SA often stands at the heart of multimodal pain strategies, playing a central role by reducing opioid use after surgery, as noted in various studies (Warrit et al., 2022). When anesthesiologists mix this approach into a broader plan, they craft protocols that ease immediate discomfort and help stop acute pain from evolving into something longer-lasting. This kind of coordinated care, which fits nicely with enhanced recovery after surgery (ERAS) protocols, can up both patient satisfaction and long-term outcomes. Safety is another area where SA has improved a great deal—thanks largely to better techniques and newer equipment. For example, ultrasound guidance during needle placement generally increases accuracy and cuts down on problems like nerve damage or infections, and it can even help lower risks like hypotension or post-dural puncture headaches. Some reports suggest that careful patient selection and a thorough pre-operative check go a long way toward reducing these risks. Such ongoing improvements are making SA a more inviting option not only for traditional hospital stays but also for outpatient or same-day discharge scenarios. Overall, continuously fine-tuning these methods remains crucial for keeping patient care top-notch and in step with current evidence-based practices (Warrit et al., 2022; Wenzel et al., 2016) (Figure 7.6).

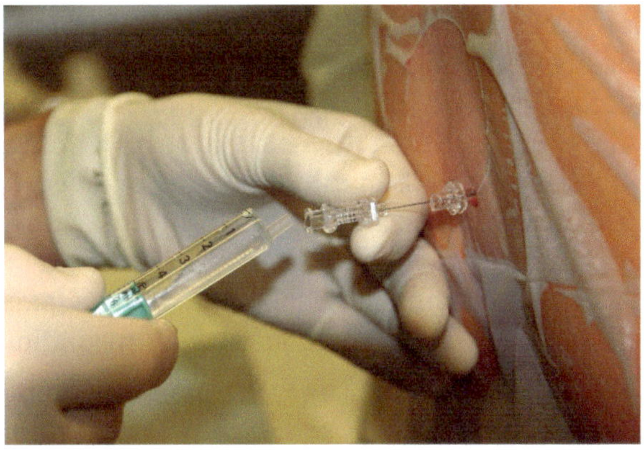

Figure 7.6. Spinal anesthesia.

Source: https://upload.wikimedia.org/wikipedia/commons/e/e5/Liquor_bei_Spinalanaesthesie.JPG.

7.2.1. Indications for Spinal Anesthesia (SA)

SA is getting a lot of use these days—especially in surgeries that target the lower abdomen, pelvis, and legs. It delivers strong pain relief and still lets patients stay responsive, which is why many surgeons lean on it for both planned and sudden procedures. Cesarean deliveries and orthopedic operations, for example, often call for this kind of focused numbing because controlling the anesthesia is key. It tends to kick in quickly and fits well with outpatient setups, helping patients bounce back faster. Overall, this method merges solid pain control with fewer body-wide side effects, generally leaving patients feeling more satisfied with their care. Some groups of patients, like younger individuals or those with conditions such as neuromuscular disorders, often have a tougher time with GA. In many cases, SA ends up being the better pick because it zeroes in on the pain while sidestepping the issues that come with systemic medications. Doctors even use tools like nerve stimulators and ultrasound to guide the process, which, to be fair, cuts down on complications in tricky operations. This hands-on approach lets healthcare providers adjust the technique to fit each patient's unique needs—reducing risks while boosting good outcomes. Then there are specific situations where GA just isn't the best match. Patients who struggle with breathing issues or need to be discharged quickly might do better with a spinal approach. In urgent surgeries, where time is of the essence, this technique manages pain without the usual problems tied to intubation and full-body anesthesia. Often, it's paired with extra techniques like ilioinguinal and rectus sheath blocks, a combo that generally improves pain management further. To summarize, this flexible method adapts to a wide range of clinical challenges, promoting patient safety and effective care (Hasani, 2015).

7.2.2. Procedure and Technique

Modern surgical care today owes a great deal to RA—techniques like spinal and epidural blocks that not only zero in on pain but also reduce on the need for heavy opioid use, which in turn dials back the risk of nasty complications. It's amazing how these procedures demand a kind of hard-earned know-how: the anesthesiologist has to navigate those lumbar and thoracic areas with care, picking an exact spot and method. A small misstep might lead to issues like infection or even spinal cord injury so that extra bit of attention does count. With so much chatter about multimodal pain strategies these days, ensuring safety and satisfaction in patients—even those tricky cases—is more about this careful, targeted approach than ever before. Beyond that, PNBs show just how flexible and effective RA can be. Targeting individual nerves not only boosts pain control in sync with surgical plans but also seems to help ease the recovery process. It's not just about knowing where everything is; it also takes a decent handle on tools like ultrasound to deliver the anesthetic with true precision. Reducing opioids has become a hot topic, and integrating these blocks before, during, and after surgery plays a pivotal role. With improvements in drugs and equipment, anesthesiologists are now altering these procedures to meet each patient's needs, opening the door to new techniques that jibe with modern pain management paradigms (Grabinsky et al., 2011). Stepping outside the confines of the operating room, RA is popping up in emergency and trauma care too. Take, for instance, using a femoral nerve block for lower extremity injuries—it not only eases acute pain but can also make a big difference in patient comfort during transport and the early stages of treatment.

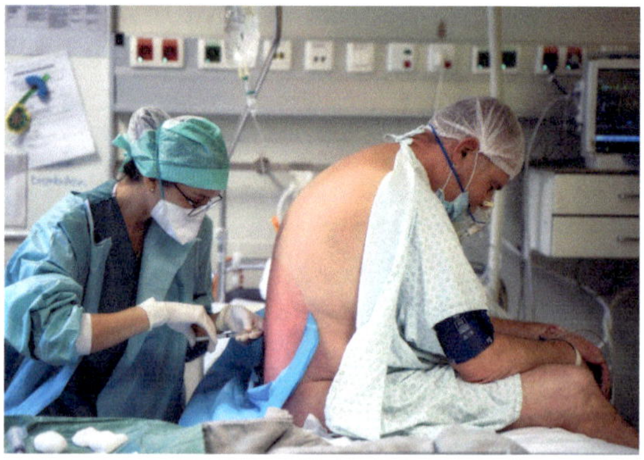

Figure 7.7. Procedure and technique of spinal anesthesia.

Source: https://www.nysora.com/wp-content/uploads/2025/01/spinal-anesthesia.jpg.

This shift, moving away from heavy reliance on systemic opioids towards more localized, subtle methods, marks a real change in emergency care. In most cases, the anesthesiologist's expertise becomes even more critical here, as these on-the-spot techniques ensure safety while still managing pain effectively, ultimately boosting both outcomes and patient satisfaction (Wenzel et al., 2016) (Figure 7.7).

7.2.3. Advantages and Disadvantages

RA has turned things around in surgeries like orthopedic procedures. Instead of relying on painkillers that affect the whole body, doctors often lean on methods such as spinal, epidural, or nerve blocks to knock down pain right where it hurts. This tactic cuts not only the discomfort during the operation but also reduces troubles like unexpected bleeding and infections afterward. Since it builds a sort of controlled pain zone, patients tend to recover faster and get moving sooner—stepping away from the risks that come with long bed rest. Older patients or those juggling other health issues especially seem to benefit, which makes regional techniques a pretty compelling option in many cases (Ibeanusi et al., 2018). That said, even though RA packs a lot of benefits, a few drawbacks still need a hard look. In most cases, complications like nerve injuries, bleeding, or even infections at the injection spot crop up only rarely, but they're there nonetheless. In situations involving patients with tricky airways or unusual anatomy, the success of these techniques can take a hit and calls for an anesthesiologist with solid, advanced skills. It's important to weigh in every detail of a patient's condition—overlooking a single variable might lead to issues later on. Practitioners need to plan ahead, preparing strategies to deal with any hiccups that could pop up during surgery, ensuring safety isn't ever an afterthought. So, while the upsides may boost recovery and comfort, the complexity and inherent risks shouldn't be brushed aside (Hasani et al., 2022). When looking at the broader field of anesthesia, weighing regional against GA becomes increasingly interesting. Research generally shows that regional techniques tend to bring about fewer perioperative complications, shorter hospital stays, and sometimes even lower costs—all of which make them an attractive choice in many surgical plans (Hasani et al., 2022). Still, it's important to balance these perks with the fact that there are scenarios where GA might still be the safer bet. Ultimately, tailoring anesthesia care to match each patient's unique needs and the specifics of the surgery is what counts. As the field continues to evolve, getting a balanced view of both the rewards and the risks of regional methods will be key to pushing patient care and overall surgical quality forward (Ibeanusi et al., 2018).

Test Your Knowledge

1. What are the indications of spinal anesthesia?
2. What are the advantages and disadvantages of spinal anesthesia?

7.3. Epidural Anesthesia

Learning Outcome

1. Understand the indications for epidural anesthesia.
2. Know the procedure and technique of epidural anesthesia.
3. Describe the advantages and disadvantages of epidural anesthesia.

Epidural anesthesia has flipped the script on pain management in surgery and childbirth. Its focused approach exactly targets the areas that hurt, giving patients noticeable relief both during procedures and afterward. This way of blocking pain helps to reduce on heavy opioid use—those meds often come with many extra side effects. In most cases, progress in local anesthetic drugs (Imbelloni and Gouveia, 2021) has upped safety and overall effectiveness, making it a solid choice. Plus, when extra medications are mixed in, the relief can last longer and be tuned to each patient's specific needs. In childbirth, the importance of an epidural stands out even more. Labor pain can be high and low unexpectedly, and having a steady way to ease that pain can change the whole experience. With the ability to continuously adjust the dose, the epidural adapts right along with the shifting pain levels during labor. Some studies (Wuest et al., 2005) point out that blending different pain relief methods—including epidurals—can ease pain better and may reduce on post-delivery complications. All these perks show why epidurals are a trusted option during labor. Of course, there are a few bumps along the way. Even though epidural blocks are generally safe, issues like infections, hematoma, or nerve complications mean that careful patient checks are a must. Research keeps reminding us that staying alert to these risks, well, is just as important as enjoying the benefits. Ongoing training for anesthesiologists helps them work through these challenges effectively. To summarize, the everchanging scene of RA—epidurals in particular—calls for a balanced view that blends historical progress with today's clinical practices (Figure 7.8).

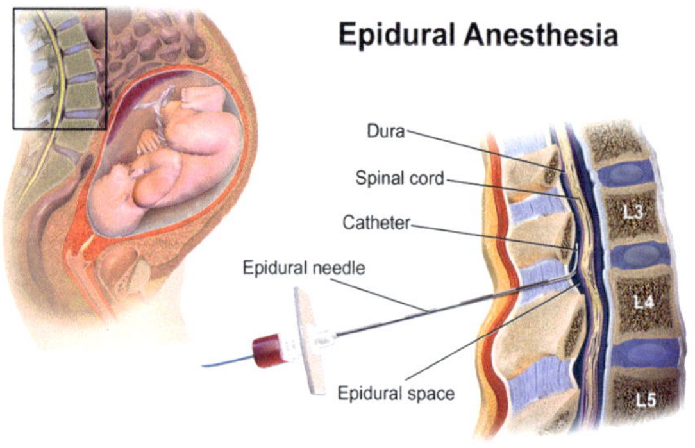

Figure 7.8. Epidural anesthesia.

Source: https://en.m.wikipedia.org/wiki/File:Epidural_Anesthesia.png.

7.3.1. Indications for Epidural Anesthesia

Epidural anesthesia often wins favor in the operating room because it helps with pain control. Surgeons use it a lot for procedures around the lower abdomen, pelvis, and legs—cases like C-sections or joint repairs where keeping a patient awake while zeroing in on pain works out well. It cuts down on the need for heavy systemic opioids, which, let's be honest, sometimes come with a baggage of unwanted side effects. In most cases, adding an epidural into one's anesthesia mix naturally eases discomfort and even sets the stage for a smoother recovery. It's also interesting to note that doctors sometimes mix other agents into the epidural cocktail to stretch out pain relief and boost patient satisfaction. With a dash of morphine or occasionally clonidine working alongside local anesthetics, the whole block becomes noticeably stronger—an effect that can help keep both sensation and movement in check for longer periods. Research even hints that these combinations not only soften postoperative pain but also reduce on the side effects often seen with high local anesthetic doses (Ukaj et al., 2024). To summarize, blending these extra components into the anesthetic plan often turns out to be a smart alter for better overall pain management. Taking a closer look at who's on the table is equally critical when choosing epidural anesthesia. Patients who've struggled with chronic pain or who are expected to need major pain care after surgery seem to do particularly well with this regional approach. Since sometimes acute pain that isn't well managed can linger and even evolve into a chronic issue starting off with a solid, effective analgesia strategy matters. This point becomes even more crucial for folks already used to opioids because typical narcotic solutions might just stir up additional complications. Increasingly, anesthesiologists are crafting all-encompassing plans that aim to maximize pain relief while keeping opioid fallout to a minimum, making the epidural a key player in today's pain management game (Wenzel et al., 2016).

7.3.2. Procedure and Technique

RA has become a common feature in many operating rooms these days. Doctors now often use techniques like spinal shots, epidural injections, or even pinpoint nerve blocks to boost patient comfort while sidestepping some of the broader effects you'd normally see with GA. Sometimes, they opt to inject the anesthetic right into the cerebrospinal fluid – a method that knocks out both feeling and movement pretty quickly, which is a big help for lower abdomen or leg surgeries. Other times, a more adjustable approach is taken by using an epidural; here, the anesthetic is placed in the area just outside the spinal canal, offering longer-lasting relief. Ultimately, the choice usually comes down to the specifics of the surgery and the individual patient, so it pays to know the little details of each method. Every method in RA carries its mix of advantages and possible hiccups. Take PNBs, for instance; they are meant to zero in on a particular nerve, so you get localized pain relief with the bonus of staying awake and alert. This adaptability makes them a popular option for outpatient procedures. Still, there's always a need for caution, since risks like nerve injury or an accidental vascular puncture can happen. In kids, the game changes a bit – variations in anatomy and the need to tailor the dose according to age and weight mean extra care is essential. Recent studies highlight that better safety measures and customized training are key if these innovative approaches are to work well for everyone, no matter their age or condition. Lately, more voices in the literature have been pointing out how RA needs to adapt to today's healthcare challenges.

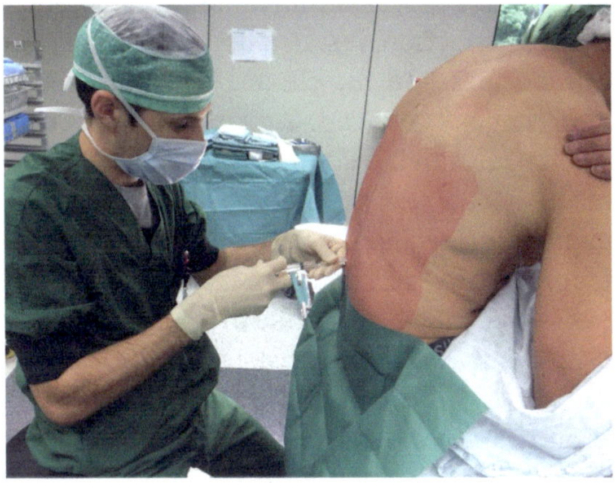

Figure 7.9. Anesthesiologist performing an epidural anesthesia injection.

Source: https://www.nysora.com/wp-content/uploads/2025/01/EPIDURAL-PXJX7837.jpg.

The COVID-19 pandemic, for example, pushed many to rethink safety protocols around anesthesia, especially for patients with respiratory issues. Since regional techniques usually aren't viewed as aerosol-generating, they've been embraced as a safer alternative in busy clinical settings. You can see a shift towards patient-focused assessments where preoperative checks take into account the individual circumstances of each person. Recent recommendations bring in guidelines that aim to reduce risks and amp up the success rates of these methods, ultimately opening the door to better outcomes in both every day and emergency surgeries (Berde et al., 2012; Mejía-Terrazas et al., 2021) (Figure 7.9).

7.3.3. Advantages and Disadvantages

RA has become quite the go-to in many surgical settings. Spinal, epidural, and even PNBs bring a host of benefits that sometimes get lost in the technical chatter. For example, patients tend to experience a noticeable drop in pain during and after procedures, which not only makes things more comfortable but also boosts overall satisfaction. It's also been seen to reduce on blood loss—so the chance of a problematic hemorrhage is reduced. On top of that, because patients get moving sooner, the risks that come with long bed rest aren't as pronounced. Sure, complications can happen, but these mishaps are pretty rare and usually manageable. In many cases, especially in areas like orthopedic surgery, the good outweighs the occasional bad (Ibeanusi et al., 2018). Still, it's important to keep an eye on the flip side. There are challenges with RA that shouldn't be ignored. Rare issues like nerve injury, bleeding, or even an infection near the injection spot need careful thought. Plus, how well these techniques work can depend a lot on individual differences—things like unusual anatomy or pre-existing health problems can throw a wrench in the works. For instance, patients with tricky airways or other comorbidities might need a more customized plan, which can complicate things further. So, anesthesiologists must stay alert and have a backup plan ready, especially for those high-risk cases. To summarize, weighing these risks against the rewards is key to keeping patients safe and making sure surgical outcomes are on target (Hasani et al., 2022). When you stack RA up against GA, regional methods often come out on top—especially for older folks or those saddled with multiple health issues. Some research generally speaking suggests that regional techniques lead to fewer complications during and after operations, making them not only efficient but also kinder on the budget. That's why a lot of healthcare professionals are leaning toward them, particularly as the push for less invasive, more patient-centered care grows. Still, let's not overstate things; the success of RA depends a great deal on the anesthesiologist's skill, and it's not a one-size-fits-all solution. Knowing both its striking benefits and its potential pitfalls is essential for getting the best results out of it (Hasani et al., 2022; Ibeanusi et al., 2018).

Test Your Knowledge

1. What are the indications of epidural anesthesia?
2. Describe the procedure and technique of epidural anesthesia.

7.4. Peripheral Nerve Blocks (PNBs)

Learning Outcome

1. Understand the indications for peripheral nerve blocks.
2. Describe the procedure and technique of peripheral nerve blocks.
3. Understand the advantages and disadvantages of peripheral nerve blocks.

Innovative new approaches in RA have shaken up how surgeries and pain treatments are done—especially with methods like PNBs. These nerve blocks deliver targeted, effective pain relief for a range of surgical procedures on the lower limbs, which means there's less need to rely on GA and deal with its risks. Ultrasound guidance has come into play in a big way, letting doctors see nerve structures in real time—a development that ups both accuracy and overall effectiveness. Recent studies generally point out that a solid grasp of the lumbar and sacral plexuses along with the best ways to perform these blocks is pretty key; having that anatomical know-how helps keep complications low and patient outcomes high, as several detailed reviews on lower extremity PNBs have noted (Tran et al., 2019). Many patients, after their surgery, end up dealing with considerable postoperative pain. When pain isn't managed just right, it can lead to extra complications. PNBs provide a multimodal route to analgesia by zeroing in on specific pain areas, which then cuts d the reliance on systemic opioids—which are notorious for coming with many side effects. Opioid toxicity risks are all too common because these drugs are used so often, fueling worries about dependence and even contributing to a wider public health crisis around opioid misuse. By using PNBs, anesthesiologists can carve out a balanced plan; this approach generally eases pain and also reduces the total opioid load needed both during and after surgery, a smart move that aligns with modern trends in pain management (Brown et al., 2018). Still, it's important to remember that even the best PNBs come with their set of potential complications. There's always a chance for nerve injuries, hematomas, or infections, which means that knowing the fine details of the technique and the underlying anatomy is essential. In most cases, anesthesiologists need to keep up with the latest recommendations and evidence so they can minimize these risks effectively—even using ultrasound-guided techniques can markedly lower the odds of adverse effects, boosting both patient safety and satisfaction. Ongoing research and continuous education in RA remain critical; they help fill in the knowledge gaps and improve patient outcomes overall. Being aware of these challenges and the strategies to offset them is vital for any doctor looking to provide top-notch care as part of a comprehensive anesthesia plan (Tran et al., 2019) (Figure 7.10).

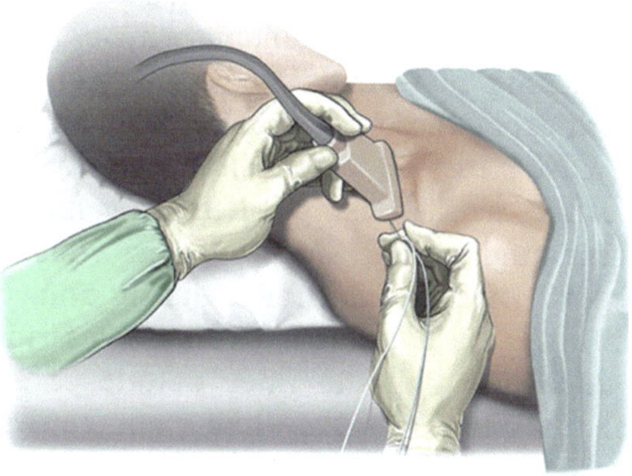

Figure 7.10. Peripheral nerve block (upper limb).

Source: https://media.healthdirect.org.au/images/inline/original/peripheral-nerve-block-upper-limb-1c12c3.png.

7.4.1. Indications for Peripheral Nerve Blocks (PNBs)

PNBs are gaining a lot of traction these days as an alternative way to achieve localized anesthesia, especially in surgeries on limbs and similar areas. Doctors now often use these blocks to avoid the pitfalls of systemic opioids—which might cause stuff like respiratory issues and postoperative nausea—even if it sometimes means a little extra planning. By numbing the nerve directly, patients usually notice less pain and can recover more quickly, often reducing on their hospital stays. You see, these techniques have shown their worth across a range of surgeries—from orthopedic and vascular procedures to even some abdominal operations—where the best choice of anesthesia depends on each patient's situation. Interestingly, ultrasound guidance has stepped in as a handy tool to help position the needle more precisely, which tends to boost both success and safety; this is becoming increasingly important as healthcare shifts toward more patient-centered care and multimodal pain management strategies (Zhang et al., 2022). Sometimes, it's particularly crucial to think about nerve blocks for patients with extra complications or risks tied to GA. For example, patients with pulmonary hypertension (PH) facing non-cardiac surgeries generally benefit from these regional techniques since they ease stress on the cardiovascular system. In other words, using PNBs can mean a patient might avoid GA altogether while still enjoying effective pain relief during and, yes, even after the operation. There's a lot riding on understanding the finer details of each patient's clinical status—like right ventricle performance and pulmonary artery pressures—to make the best call on anesthesia. Such careful assessments are vital, especially among high-risk groups where traditional approaches might worsen complications. A team effort among anesthesiologists, surgeons, and primary care providers, working closely together, makes a difference in managing these risks effectively (Zhang et al., 2022). It isn't just about getting through the surgery, though; nerve blocks are increasingly recognized as a key player in managing pain once the operation is over. Emerging research, in most cases, points to a multimodal use of these blocks that not only eases pain but also helps improve recovery and overall function. Take, for instance, techniques like the transversus abdominis plane block or even the quadratus lumborum plane block—they've proven to be solid alternatives when it comes to controlling abdominal pain post-surgery. This kind of shift toward RA is particularly useful when more traditional neuraxial or systemic methods just aren't the best fit or seem less effective. As our grasp of pain dynamics continues to grow, it seems likely that the role of PNBs will expand even more across various surgical fields, ultimately strengthening their place in today's anesthetic practices (Fernandes et al., 2021) (Figure 7.11).

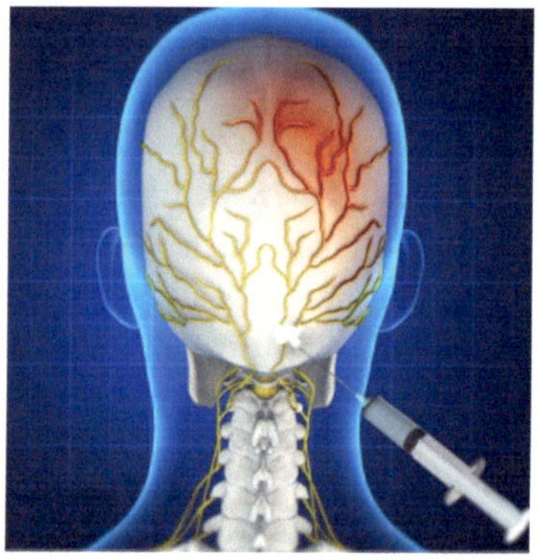

Figure 7.11. Peripheral nerve blocks.

Source: https://assets.yourpractice.online/2266/3d-images/occipital-peripheral-nerve-blocks.jpg.

7.4.2. Procedure and Technique

RA isn't what it used to be – it's now part of almost every surgical setup. Take SA, for example; it's a go-to method for many because it kicks in fast and drowns out pain pretty effectively. Usually, a lumbar puncture is performed, which means anesthetic is gently introduced into the fluid surrounding the spine. This method numbs the area from roughly the belly button downward – a huge plus when working on lower abdominal, pelvic, or leg surgeries. Of course, doctors have to watch out for issues like post-dural puncture headaches or occasional neurological problems. In most cases, the real strength of SA is not just the immediate pain relief but also its role in smoothing the recovery process after surgery. Knowing the ins and outs of this technique is crucial for better patient outcomes. Epidural anesthesia is another popular method that brings its set of advantages. Instead of a one-shot deal, a small tube—commonly known as a catheter—is positioned into the epidural space, letting practitioners drip anesthetic and other medications over time. This setup offers prolonged pain relief, which proves extremely useful in both surgical and labor scenarios.

It also keeps doing its job even after the operation, helping manage pain during the recovery phase. Still, there can be bumps along the way; for instance, the catheter might slip out of place, infections could occur locally, or the drugs might trigger side effects. Grabinsky et al. (2011) generally point out that having experienced anesthesiologists makes a big difference when using these advanced techniques, ensuring patient safety even in emergency settings. PNBs explore a different route by zeroing in on specific nerves or nerve plexuses for targeted pain relief. Using techniques such as ultrasound guidance and sometimes even nerve stimulation, these blocks help limit how much of the anesthetic spreads throughout the body. This focused approach can reduce risks compared to other methods; yet, as James et al. (2015) note potential hazards like minor trauma or nerve ischemia should still be kept in mind. These techniques are especially valued in orthopedic, plastic, and chronic pain surgeries, where early movement and rehabilitation count. With the growing trend toward less invasive, personalized medical care, PNBs are set to play an even larger role in tailoring anesthesia to individual patient needs (Figure 7.12).

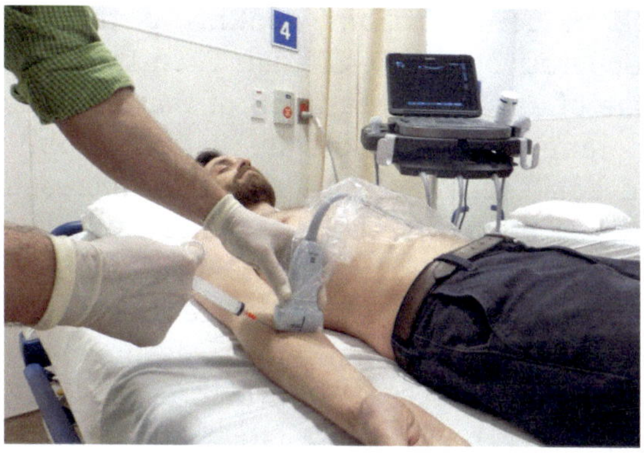

Figure 7.12. Procedure and technique of peripheral nerve blocks.

Source: https://www.bcpocus.ca/wp-content/uploads/2020/01/median-nerve-out-of-plane-scaled.jpg.

7.4.3. Advantages and Disadvantages

RA comes in many forms—think spinal, epidural, and even PNBs—and each brings its set of perks. It shines when it comes to dialing d postoperative pain, so patients feel less discomfort right after surgery, which, in most cases, smooths the recovery process. Cutting the use of systemic opioids is another bonus; by avoiding their common side effects like nausea and sedation, overall patient contentment tends to improve. People often get back on their feet sooner thanks to these methods, lowering risks such as deep vein thrombosis. There's a solid body of research showing that when these techniques are part of a broader pain-relief plan, outcomes get better (Zahn et al., 2017). In short, using these methods not only brings better pain control but also fits well with today's push for improved surgical care. Even with all these upsides, there are some notable drawbacks to keep in mind. A slip-in technique can sometimes lead to problems like nerve injury or even a hematoma, so careful handling matters a lot. Patient selection is a big deal—those with pre-existing conditions or unique anatomical quirks often run a higher risk of complications, making a thorough preoperative check essential. Then there's the issue of anesthesia duration; if the relief lasts too long, it might hold up patient mobility and delay recovery. Plus, while an increasing number of studies back the effectiveness of these methods across various surgeries, gaps remain—especially around understanding the finer anatomical details in cases like breast surgery anesthesia (Woodworth et al., 2017)., weighing the upsides against the potential pitfalls is critical for achieving the best patient outcomes. On a related note, new innovations in the field are reshaping how these techniques are used. For example, recent advances in local anesthetic formulations—like liposomal bupivacaine—promise to lengthen pain relief and reduce the need for frequent block re-dos. Improvements in imaging, especially with ultrasound guidance, have also made PNBs much more precise and safer, though there's always room for a small error here or there. With these changes, continuous education and training are indispensable for practitioners to stay on top of evolving practices. Clinicians, in most cases, need to keep a close watch on which approach best fits the surgical setting and individual patient needs. Addressing these challenges, even with a bit of trial and error, is what will ultimately steer the future of RA in everyday practice, further uplifting patient recovery (Zahn et al., 2017) (Figure 7.13).

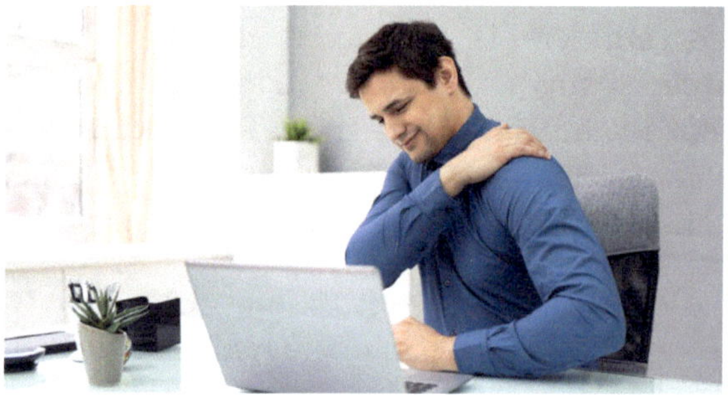

Figure 7.13. Pain.

Source: https://vispdocs.com/wp-content/uploads/2023/12/image.jpg.

Test Your Knowledge

1. What is the procedure and technique of peripheral nerve blocks?
2. Describe the advantages and disadvantages of peripheral nerve blocks.

7.5. Complications and Risks

Learning Outcome

1. Discuss common complications associated with regional anesthesia.
2. Describe the risk factors influencing complications.
3. Understand the management and prevention strategies of regional anesthesia.

RA is a great tool used in many surgeries, though it isn't without its hazards. Sometimes nerve injuries pop up—whether from drug toxicity, an accidental cut, or nerves being stretched too far during a procedure. These issues might show up as short-term numbness, motor weakness, or even stubborn nerve pain that hangs around, demanding extra care. Even if such events are pretty rare, they serve as a reminder to stick with careful, sometimes even cautious, techniques. The way an anesthesiologist picks the right method and watches the patient closely counts when these risks are in the mix. There's also the fact that RA can trigger body-wide effects that add another layer of concern. A drop in blood pressure is one of these, especially with spinal or epidural methods; blocking the sympathetic signals can reduce on blood returning to the heart. That fall in blood pressure—though it's usually manageable—can mean that important organs aren't getting enough blood if not monitored closely. Additionally, there's a chance of infection at the injection spot since any needle-based procedure can invite awkward microbial intruders. Still, the perks—like strong pain relief and less blood loss—often balance out the risks when proper steps are taken, as seen in fields like orthopedics (Ibeanusi et al., 2018). Looking even further ahead, the long-term side effects of RA, although uncommon, shouldn't be dismissed. Some patients end up with lingering pain or discomfort after a nerve gets injured, which can affect day-to-day life. At times, problems like nerve ischemia— not enough blood supply reaching a nerve—can happen if the block isn't done quite right or if nerves are under pressure for too long, leaving lasting issues. The real challenge is finding the right balance between effective anesthesia and avoiding these setbacks. It helps when both doctors and patients are well aware of potential complications before opting for spinal, epidural, or other nerve block methods. Getting this balance right is key for smooth surgeries while keeping future risks as low as possible (James et al., 2015).

7.5.1. Common Complications Associated with Regional Anesthesia (RA)

RA is often seen as safe, yet it comes with a mix of potential issues that deserve a closer look. Complications can pop up unexpectedly from both the way the procedure is done and how a patient reacts. In recent times, tracking these hiccups more closely has shown that the picture isn't as simple as we once thought. For example, one study noted that things can go wrong because of human slip-ups, equipment glitches, or even unique patient responses (Zunic et al., 2013). This messy interplay reminds us why staying alert and catching issues early is so important. Plus, using modern tools like ultrasound can lower the amount of local anesthetic needed, which in turn lowers the worry over toxicity—a big deal when doing these procedures. Beyond the risk of toxicity, physical issues are not unheard of with regional blocks. Needle insertions can sometimes cause rough trauma or stretch the nerves, leading to problems like neurological deficits, lingering pain, or brief changes in sensation (James et al., 2015). Even though monitoring suggests these events happen in only about 0.31% of cases, that small number still calls for careful handling. The slight chance of nerve ischemia and blunt injuries makes it clear that a careful technique and adherence to best practices are key. Looking closely at these risks helps practitioners be better prepared to spot and manage any unwanted outcomes.

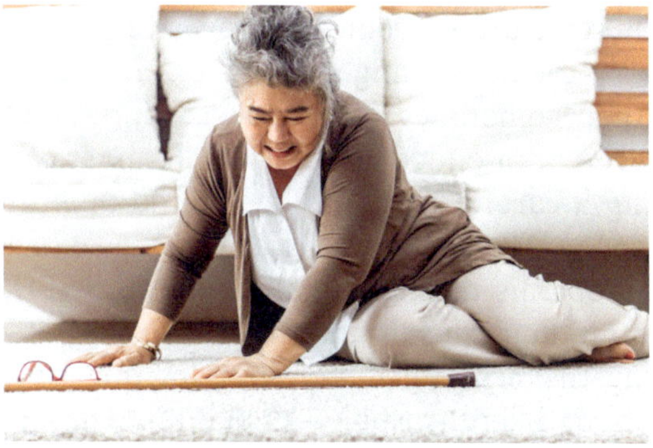

Figure 7.14. Complications of regional anesthesia.

Source: https://epmonthly.com/wp-content/uploads/2021/08/complications.jpg.

The trend of fewer complications in RA offers a hopeful outlook. Data generally show a noticeable drop in adverse events over the years thanks in part to rigorous monitoring, better teamwork in surgery, and steady upgrades in anesthetic methods (Zunic et al., 2013). As healthcare pros keep polishing their skills, it's wise to keep learning about possible risks—even if it means revisiting past mistakes. What we learn from those moments not only helps craft better prevention plans but also builds a care environment where patient safety comes first. To summarize, keeping an eye on outcomes and pushing for innovation remains crucial in reducing complications while still reaping the benefits of this effective pain management approach (Figure 7.14).

7.5.2. Risk Factors Influencing Complications

Risk with RA isn't just about one thing—it's tangled up with many factors that can make a big difference. Age, overall health, and even the way someone's body is built can tip the odds one way or another. Take, for instance, older individuals or folks with heart or lung issues; they often run a higher risk when these procedures are performed. And then there's body structure—if someone is overweight or has a curved spine, it might throw off the delivery method, sometimes leading to weaker pain relief or even unintended nerve harm. In most cases, doing a careful check-up before the operation to spot these issues is important for reducing on problems during spinal, epidural, or PNBs. The method chosen and, honestly, the person doing the procedure, matter a lot too. Newer methods like ultrasound-guided anesthesia let doctors see inside better, which usually helps dodge accidental hits to nerves or blood vessels. On top of that, using nerve stimulators alongside the other techniques can pinpoint nerves more precisely, so the block goes in just right. Still, even when everything seems to be done by the book, complications can pop up unexpectedly. Generally speaking, being on the lookout for potential snags and having a plan ready is a must for keeping things as safe as possible during surgery. It's not only about the technique or the operator—what kind of surgery is being done also plays a part. Different surgeries, especially in orthopedics, bring their unique challenges. Some operations that involve a lot of tissue handling might result in extra swelling around the area, which can make local anesthesia work less effectively and sometimes bump up the risk of complications. Plus, if the patient is already dealing with conditions like infections or blood clotting problems, these pre-existing issues could mess with a smooth anesthesia process. That's why anesthesiologists must check for such factors ahead of time. In most cases, though, the overall perks—like better pain management and a speedier recovery—tend to outweigh these risks, as several studies have shown (Hasani, 2015; Ibeanusi et al., 2018).

7.5.3. Management and Prevention Strategies

RA—think spinal, epidural, or nerve blocks—leans a lot on smart, sometimes even over-cautious, steps to cut back on post-surgery pain and other hiccups. Doctors often start with a good, in-depth check-up before any procedure; these pre-surgery evaluations help spot risk factors early and set the stage for personalized pain plans that blend safety with comfort. In many cases, such proactive moves not only add to overall satisfaction but also lower the chance that a nasty bout of acute pain sticks around and turns chronic, a challenge that's all too common in anesthesia practice and patient recovery (Wenzel et al., 2016). Lately, a mixed approach to pain relief—usually called multimodal analgesia—has been catching on., it's about pairing different drugs that each hit a different part of the pain pathway. Instead of relying on just one medication, clinicians combine non-opioid painkillers, anti-inflammatory agents, and other helper therapies in unpredictable, sometimes even quirky, ways that offer better overall relief while keeping side effects on the d-low. This adaptable method, tuned to match the specific needs of a surgery and the person undergoing it, often ends up significantly reducing the dependence on opioids (Schwenk et al., 2018). With the persistent opioid crisis nudging the field in new directions, anesthesiologists are being pressed to rethink traditional pain management. Emerging guidelines generally advocate for a move away from heavy opioid use towards a broader mix of analgesic options—an approach that, in most cases, manages to reduce on adverse events and the risk of long-term dependency. Of course, hurdles like drug shortages pop up, pushing healthcare professionals to get inventive with alternative agents. By boosting awareness and encouraging a bit of collaboration across the board, these efforts help ensure patients maintain steady access to essential pain relief, reinforcing just how crucial a comprehensive, versatile pain management plan can be alongside RA techniques (Schwenk et al., 2018) (Figure 7.15).

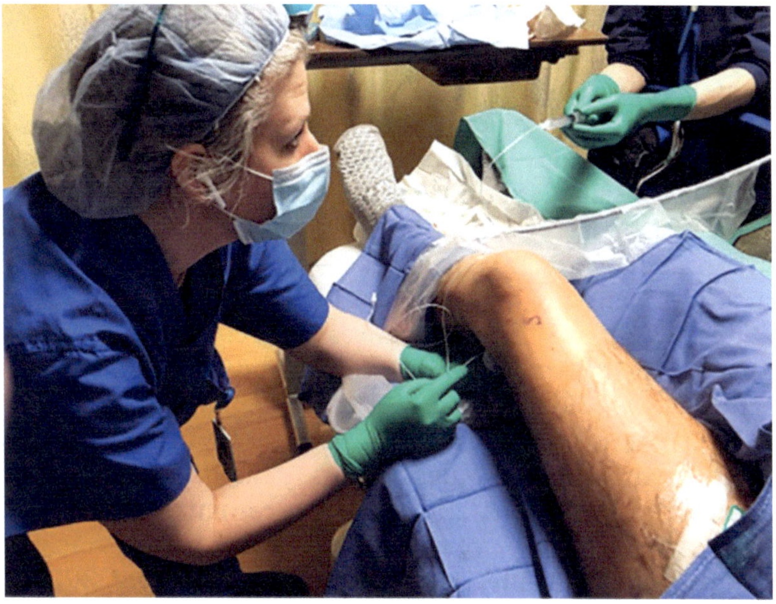

Figure 7.15. Peripheral nerve blocks allow providers to forgo, or at least lessen, the use of general anesthesia in surgical cases.

Source: https://www.aorn.org/images/default-source/aorn/osm/guides/pain-management/2021/images/18-hero.jpg?sfvrsn=47be9f07_0.

Test Your Knowledge

1. What are the common complications associated with regional anesthesia?
2. Describe the management and prevention strategies of regional anesthesia.

SUMMARY

RA, be it spinal, epidural, or PNB, has brought about some very significant advancements in the way patients are attended to under the knife. Recently, physicians have changed their strategy and often tend to adopt techniques that minimize the reliance on opioids, typically reducing side effects and the risk of drug addiction that was quite prevalent before. By integrating a number of pain management techniques, or multimodal techniques, as it happens, one can bring with them effective pain management and, at the same time, escape the issues of the older, more conventional approaches. An increasing body of evidence shows that the new methods, aside from coping with immediate surgery needs, also aid in smooth, longer-term recovery (Brown et al., 2018). Continuous PNBs have also become an increasingly viable option. They allow for extended pain relief after procedures, sometimes making it easier for patients to move and reducing overall discomfort. It is interesting to see how technologies like ultrasound-guided catheter placement have combined accuracy with simplicity, enhancing the accuracy of the block while reducing potential complications. The promising results of such interventions help to lay the groundwork for a patient-centered model of care; studies on when and how to implement them—and what complications might ensue—are giving clinicians practical guidance on how to optimize pain management regimens in a variety of clinical contexts (Ilfeld, 2016). In short, these advances in RA constitute an unambiguous revolution in the way surgical pain is managed. By tapping into innovative approaches and trusting good, evidence-based practice, anesthesiologists are not just improving perioperative results but also addressing the historic problems of opioid abuse. The push toward reducing adverse effects and enhancing post-operative function is well-demonstrating the discipline's growing focus on both patient safety and satisfaction overall. As more research continues to untangle and as clinicians learn and adapt, we can expect an even more sophisticated—and perhaps more effective—approach to managing RA in diverse surgical contexts (Emery et al., 2018; Ilfeld, 2016).

RA has proven to stand the test of time, and techniques like spinal, epidural, and PNBs have been backed by sufficient evidence as well as clinical experience. These techniques sound good alternatives to GA, especially when some patient status or contraindications make a whole-body technique risky. The American Society of Pain and Neuroscience (ASPN) dismissed a group of guidelines intended for interventional therapy for low back pain and wrote that we should utilize research when we are making clinic decisions. These guidelines help doctors sift through the literature for safety, effectiveness, and whether these pain management techniques cut the mustard, highlighting the need to have an official plan set in motion when using RA (Sayed et al., 2022). Far more frequently than not, the application of regional techniques ultimately enhances recovery and lessens d the need for opioids post-surgery. What is perhaps most interesting about these methods is how they work. Take spinal and epidural blocks. They act on specific nerve channels to offer pain relief directly where it's needed, thus freeing the body from the stresses of surgery. This local feature precludes cutting d on the broad side effects that GA would likely place, like mental confusion or slow recovery. The ASPN Back Guideline integrates a great deal of evidence to show that if properly done, these interventions have the potential to significantly improve patient outcomes by eradicating pain and minimizing the dangers associated with prolonged medication use (Sayed et al., 2022). As these techniques evolve, clinicians have to remain up to date on the latest improvements in order to offer patients the best possible care. A closer examination, RA is not merely about short-term pain relief—it also has long-term benefits that can change the recovery story of a patient. Pain control with excellent results using spinal, epidural, or PNBs can speed the process of one recovering, which on some occasions can mean shorter hospital stays and even lower healthcare costs. Entering into emerging technologies and new approaches in RA gives a broader understanding of how these approaches might be applied in different surgeries. Recent studies—skimming over advances in mechanical as well as neuro areas—suggest that it is most crucial for anesthesiologists and pain management professionals to stay updated on clinical guidelines and evidence-based practice. Simply put, continuous learning and accommodation to changing standards are very important in effectively making the most of RA techniques.

KEY TERMS FROM THIS CHAPTER

- Cerebrospinal fluid
- Epidural anesthesia
- Hemodynamics
- Infections
- Pain care
- Peripheral nerve blocks
- Pharmacokinetics
- Ropivacaine
- Chloroprocaine
- Headaches
- Hypotension
- Neuromuscular disorders
- Patient satisfaction
- Pharmacodynamics
- Regional anesthesia
- Spinal anesthesia

CRITICAL THINKING QUESTIONS

1. **Regional anesthesia involves:**
   a. Complete loss of sensation and consciousness
   b. Loss of sensation in a specific body region while maintaining consciousness
   c. Analgesia without muscle relaxation
   d. Sedation and muscle relaxation
2. **Which of the following is a type of regional anesthesia?**
   a. General anesthesia
   b. Spinal anesthesia
   c. Intravenous sedation
   d. Monitored anesthesia care
3. **The most common site for administering spinal anesthesia is:**
   a. L2-L3 interspace
   b. L4-L5 interspace
   c. T10-T11 interspace
   d. C7-T1 interspace
4. **Epidural anesthesia differs from spinal anesthesia because:**
   a. Epidural anesthesia has a faster onset
   b. Epidural anesthesia involves injecting anesthetic into the cerebrospinal fluid
   c. Epidural anesthesia allows for continuous infusion via a catheter
   d. Epidural anesthesia produces a denser motor block
5. **Which of the following local anesthetics is commonly used for regional blocks due to its long duration of action?**
   a. Lidocaine
   b. Bupivacaine
   c. Procaine
   d. Articaine

Short Answer Questions

1. Define the regional anesthesia.
2. Why is regional anesthesia important in modern medical practice?
3. What is the mechanism of action of regional anesthesia?
4. Why is spinal anesthesia preferred in lower part of the body?
5. What is epidural anesthesia?

Answers to Critical Thinking Questions

1. (b); 2. (b); 3. (b); 4. (c); 5. (b)

REFERENCES

1. Berde, C., & Greco, C. (2012). Pediatric regional anesthesia: Drawing inferences on safety from prospective registries and case reports. *Anesthesia & Analgesia, 115*(6), 1259–1262. https://www.semanticscholar.org/paper/5acbeb70ab321d8e44038c71040895a8a493398d (accessed on 20 May 2025).
2. Brown, E. N., Pavone, K. J., & Naranjo, M. (2018). Multimodal general anesthesia: Theory and practice. *Anesthesia & Analgesia, 127*, 1246–1258. https://doi.org/10.1213/ane.0000000000003668.
3. Buschiazzo, V., Goytizolo, E. A., Hurtado Rua, S. M., Marcello, et al. (2016). The effect of regional analgesia on vascular tone in hip arthroplasty patients. https://core.ac.uk/download/216952021.pdf (accessed on 20 May 2025).
4. Carness, J. M., & Lenart, M. J. (2019). Current local anesthetic applications in regional anesthesia. *Topics in Local Anesthetics*. https://www.semanticscholar.org/paper/b1674e59b5c219d04e5b4fb017aaeee6d0d5652d (accessed on 20 May 2025).
5. Cunningham, D., LaRose, M. A., Zhang, G. X., Patel, P., Paniagua, A. R., Gadsden, J., & Gage, M. J. (2022). Regional anesthesia associated with decreased inpatient and outpatient opioid demand in tibial plateau fracture surgery. *Anesthesia & Analgesia, 134*, 1072–1081. https://www.semanticscholar.org/paper/63eaf0801bf5c370384669a015112c016f1e0d81 (accessed on 20 May 2025).
6. Diaz, V. J., & Fukes, A. (2022). An educational module explaining the use of quadratus lumborum blockade to decrease opioid usage during colorectal surgery: A quality improvement project. https://core.ac.uk/download/548486127.pdf (accessed on 20 May 2025).
7. Dönmez, B., Vanhonacker, D., Lammens, R., & Bhutia, J. (2024). Role of peripheral nerve blocks in the preoperative pain management of hip fractures in the elderly: A narrative review. *Acta Anesthesiologic Belgica, 75*(4). https://www.semanticscholar.org/paper/122947fc0d40eea0536ca8adcd076eeaa1856eef (accessed on 20 May 2025).
8. Fernandes, H., Azevedo, A. S., Ferreira, T. C., Santos, S. A., Rocha-Filho, J. A., & Vieira, J. (2021). Ultrasound-guided peripheral abdominal wall blocks. *Clinics, 76*. https://www.semanticscholar.org/paper/3d373fb0792da83be52bcd9b6879efe0a473eb4b (accessed on 20 May 2025).
9. Grabinsky, A., Lollo, L., & Wu, J. J. (2011). Regional anesthesia in trauma medicine. https://core.ac.uk/download/pdf/8650416.pdf.
10. Hasani, A. (2015). Regional anesthesia in children: Indications and limitations. https://core.ac.uk/download/33280385.pdf (accessed on 20 May 2025).
11. Hasani, A. (2022). Regionalna anestezija u spinalnoj kirurgiji: može li to biti rješenje za teške intubacije? https://core.ac.uk/download/541038529.pdf.
12. Ibeanusi, S., & Obalum, D. (2018). The relevance of regional anesthesia in orthopedic surgery: Advantages, disadvantages and challenges. https://core.ac.uk/download/630469333.pdf (accessed on 20 May 2025).
13. Ilfeld, B. M. (2016). Continuous peripheral nerve blocks: An update of the published evidence and comparison with novel, alternative analgesic modalities. *Anesthesia & Analgesia, 124*, 308–335. https://doi.org/10.1213/ane.0000000000001581.

14. Imbelloni, L. E., & Gouveia, M. A. (n.d.). *Paresthesia*. InTech. https://core.ac.uk/download/478097875.pdf (accessed on 20 May 2025).

15. James, M. F. M. (2015). How safe are regional techniques? Evidence from large studies with big data. https://core.ac.uk/download/478367616.pdf (accessed on 20 May 2025).

16. Kabambi, F. K., Mumba, J. M., & Ngaka, C. T. (2017). Pharmacology of local anesthetics and commonly used recipes in clinical practice. https://core.ac.uk/download/322429789.pdf (accessed on 20 May 2025).

17. Mehta, N., & Qazi, S. A. N. (2020). Adjuvant drugs to local anesthetics. In *Topics in Local Anesthetics*. IntechOpen. http://dx.doi.org/10.5772/intechopen.91980.

18. Mejía-Terrazas, G. E., López-Muñoz, E., Vilchis-Rentería, J. S., Muñoz-García, A. J., & Alcántara-Muñoz, M. D. R. A. (2021). COVID-19: Regional anesthesia, benefits, and practical recommendations. *Asian Journal of Anesthesiology, 59*(3), 83–95. https://doi.org/10.6859/aja.202109_59(3).0002.

19. Miščuks, A., Vanags, I., & Vasilevskis, E. (2008). Special devices for regional anesthesia. https://core.ac.uk/download/480427274.pdf (accessed on 20 May 2025).

20. Pogatzki-Zahn, E., Segelcke, D., & Schug, S. A. (2017). Postoperative pain—from mechanisms to treatment. *PAIN Reports, 2*, e588. https://doi.org/10.1097/pr9.0000000000000588.

21. Pooley, R., Veneziano, G., Burrier, C., Tram, N. K., & Tobias, J. (2022). Preliminary experience with quadratus lumborum catheters for postoperative pain management in pediatric-aged patients with contraindications to epidural anesthesia. *Journal of Clinical Medicine Research, 14*, 425–431. https://www.semanticscholar.org/paper/8cd565cada34d078a6f94f50fb95dc0e19f40d22 (accessed on 20 May 2025).

22. Sayed, D., Grider, J. S., Strand, N., Hagedorn, J. M., Falowski, S., Lam, C., Tieppo Francio, V., et al. (2022). The American Society of Pain and Neuroscience (ASPN) evidence-based clinical guideline of interventional treatments for low back pain. *Journal of Pain Research, 15*, 3729–3832. https://doi.org/10.2147/jpr.s386879.

23. Schwenk, E. S., & Mariano, E. R. (2018). Designing the ideal perioperative pain management plan starts with multimodal analgesia. *Korean Journal of Anesthesiology, 71*(5), 345–352. https://doi.org/10.4097/kja.d.18.00217.

24. Siebner, H. R., Funke, K., Aberra, A. S., Antal, A., Bestmann, S., Chen, R., Claßen, J., et al. (2022). Transcranial magnetic stimulation of the brain: What is stimulated? –A consensus and critical position paper. *Clinical Neurophysiology, 140*, 59–97. https://doi.org/10.1016/j.clinph.2022.04.022.

25. Singhal, A., & Taksande, K. (2024). Role of adjuvants in enhancing the efficacy and duration of anesthesia blocks: A comprehensive review. *Cureus, 16*. https://www.semanticscholar.org/paper/8a49856bdc0392c804d329706d6503c28b043b9e (accessed on 20 May 2025).

26. Tran, D. Q. H., Salinas, F. V., Benzon, H. T., & Neal, J. M. (2019). Lower extremity regional anesthesia: Essentials of our current understanding. *Regional Anesthesia & Pain Medicine, 44*, 143–180. https://doi.org/10.1136/rapm-2018-000019.

27. Ukaj, A., & Ukaj, Z. (2024). The application of adjuvants in spinal and epidural anesthesia. *International Journal of Progressive Sciences and Technologies, 47*(2), 508–534. http://dx.doi.org/10.52155/ijpsat.v47.2.6761.

28. Warrit, K., Griffenhagen, G., Goh, C., & Boscan, P. (2019). Financial impact of ultrasound-guided lumbar plexus and sciatic nerve blocks with electrostimulation for tibial plateau leveling osteotomy surgery in dogs. *Veterinary Anesthesia and Analgesia, 46*(5), 682–688. https://doi.org/10.1016/j.vaa.2019.04.008.
29. Wenzel, J. T., Schwenk, E. S., Baratta, J. L., & Viscusi, E. R. (2016). Managing opioid-tolerant patients in the perioperative surgical home. *Anesthesiology Clinics, 34*(2), 287–301. https://doi.org/10.1016/j.anclin.2016.01.005.
30. Woodworth, G. E., Ivie, R., Nelson, S. M., Walker, C. M., & Maniker, R. B. (2017). Perioperative breast analgesia. *Regional Anesthesia & Pain Medicine, 42*, 609–631. https://doi.org/10.1097/aap.0000000000000641.
31. Wuest, M. A. (2005). Femoral nerve block in total knee arthroplasty: Utilization of technique by certified registered nurse anesthetists. https://core.ac.uk/download/352870452.pdf (accessed on 20 May 2025).
32. Zhang, A., De Gala, V., Lementowski, P. W., Cvetkovic, D., Xu, J. L., & Villion, A. (2022). Veno-arterial extracorporeal membrane oxygenation rescue in a patient with pulmonary hypertension presenting for revision total hip arthroplasty: A case report and narrative review. *Cureus, 14*. https://www.semanticscholar.org/paper/28b2fe8c9dbf36788556f2117b7ceacea0af6508 (accessed on 20 May 2025).
33. Zhao, Y., Guo, Y., Pan, X., Zhang, X., Yu, F., & Cao, X. (2024). The impact of different regional anesthesia techniques on the incidence of chronic post-surgical pain in patients undergoing video-assisted thoracoscopic surgery: A network meta-analysis. *Pain and Therapy, 13*, 1335–1350. https://www.semanticscholar.org/paper/49e28480499d563cc287a1cef526f42f8049dbcf (accessed on 20 May 2025).
34. Žunić, J., Belavić, M., & Lončarić-Katušin, M. (2013). Reducing the incidence of adverse events in anesthesia practice. https://core.ac.uk/download/14468892.pdf (accessed on 20 May 2025).

MONITORED ANESTHESIA CARE (MAC) AND SEDATION

8

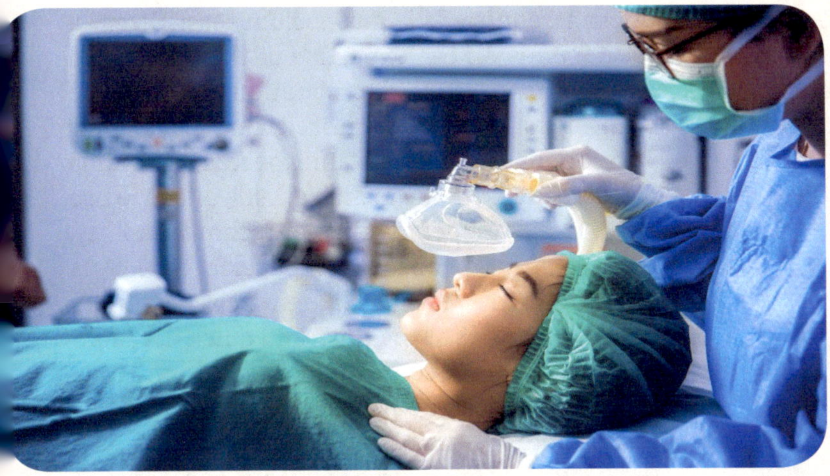

LEARNING OBJECTIVES

After studying this chapter, you will be able to:

1. Describe the types of sedation.
2. Know the indications for monitored anesthesia care.
3. Understand the benefits of monitored anesthesia care.
4. Describe the risks and complications of monitored anesthesia care and sedation.
5. Understand the role of anesthesia providers.

Introduction

Patient comfort remains a big problem in medicine today. Practitioners are relying mostly on a method called Monitored Anesthesia Care (MAC) – patients breathe on their own but receive adequate sedation and pain relief, which has worked well with such as burn dressing changes. It's being used in both a mix of outpatient and inpatient facilities, and overall, this approach seems to improve the overall experience and results. Even though MAC's use is widespread, however, the nitty-gritty—especially when it comes to dosing and how these kinds of anesthetic agents work—still needs a more in-depth look in the literature (Sayali et al., 2025). More recent studies have started to suggest several MAC's influences on patients after a procedure. In procedures like burn care, where the shots at pain control in the typical style may not quite be within reach of pain and anxiety, MAC appears to fill the gap quite easily. Patient, nurse, and even anesthesiologist feedback tends to be unanimous in reporting a common theme of reduced discomfort, and often, if satisfaction is measured on a standard scale, all three rate it highly (Fatma et al., 2024). It is interesting the manner in which such uniform positive reaction indicates MAC's value in reducing current distress under challenging procedures. The horizon for MAC could extend far beyond the treatment room. While its near-immediate returns are rewarding, there is still a strong need for further study on best practice—namely the impact of selection, combination, and timing of anesthetic medication on elements of hemodynamic stability and respiration. In the majority of cases, adjusting these details for each individual patient's particular conditions might not only increase individual safety but redefine standard anesthesia norms. Overall, more research in the subject area could pave the way for protocols rendering medicolegal processes safer and more comfortable (Sayali et al., 2025) (Figure 8.1).

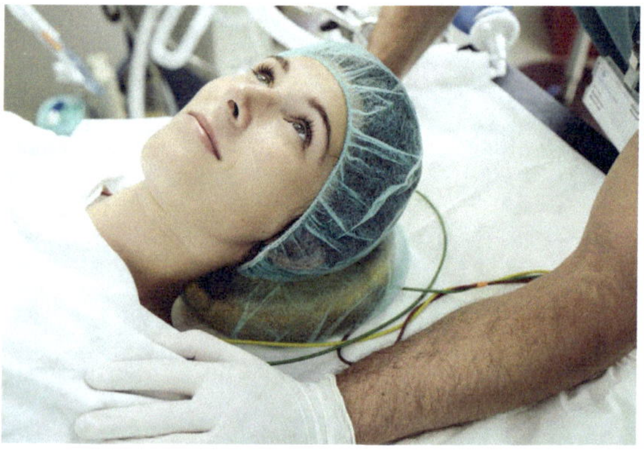

Figure 8.1. Understanding Monitored Anesthesia Care.

Source: https://www.verywellhealth.com/thmb/w-cV8ALONTgbp1rMdot1cKmRRjU=/1500x0/filters:no_upscale():max_bytes(150000):strip_icc()/operating-nurse-soothing-patient-on-table-in-operating-room-596435375-57ab2f223df78cf4597c4dc7.jpg.

Definition of Monitored Anesthesia Care (MAC)

When it involves anesthesia, having a general understanding of different methods can make all the difference in how patients are kept safe and procedures go smoothly. Take Monitored Anesthesia Care (MAC) for example – it's an extremely specialized technique that incorporates individualized sedation with continuous, watchful monitoring, and, overall, it's different from general anesthesia (GA). Instead of putting a patient fully out, MAC enables them to be comfortable and fairly alert, something which can be crucial when a procedure is going to be uncomfortable but doesn't require full unconsciousness. Often, a lot depends on the expertise of the anesthesia team, who must titrate sedation doses, keep vital signs closely monitored, and have their wits about them when unexpected problems occur. Aside from the technical skill, effective use of MAC also depends on non-technical ability. Accounts are prone to emphasize that it is essential to have skills like swift recognition, setting priorities at the time, and quick decision-making when events take a sudden turn during sedation. Being able to set a patient's status quickly—necessarily under stress—can radically alter the course of events. For instance, research into the task-management abilities of Student Registered Nurse Anesthetists (SRNAs) highlights, in the majority of instances, the necessity of rigorous education in such softer, yet no less essential, skills, particularly in high-pressure moments such as a sudden airway block in MAC anesthesia (Majewski et al., 2017). Seasoned practitioners feel more comfortable with their skill set, thereby promoting safer practice and improving patient outcomes as a whole. The art of anesthesia is progressive, and the progress introduces additional concerns for patient consent and standards of safety. Current studies have indicated that some patients, being administered what is supposed to be MAC, sometimes receive levels of sedation similar to GA (Jenna Lee 2014). The practitioners therefore have to be that much more careful when explaining the sedation process—clearly indicating the risks as well as the advantages. As MAC continues to find its place within a variety of operating room settings, its nuances must still be realized by not only medical personnel, but patients who are trying to make educated choices about their care (Figure 8.2).

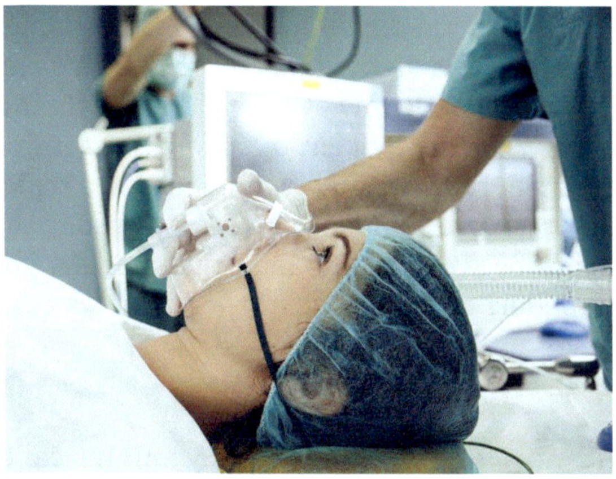

Figure 8.2. Monitored anesthesia care (MAC).

Source: https://media.post.rvohealth.io/wp-content/uploads/2021/04/surgery-anesthesia-732x549-thumbnail-732x549.jpg.

Importance of Sedation in Medical Procedures

Sedation is essential in the majority of medical procedures. Sedation quiets body and mind, enabling patients to meet challenging procedures with reduced anxiety. MAC sedates patients—to the point of drowsiness—so that they may better endure what would otherwise be an agonizing experience. It also preserves airway patency and minimizes side effects. Now, as procedures become more common in outpatient settings, the benefits of MAC become even clearer. Patients heal better, with a smoother recovery and greater satisfaction, when sedation is used, and it is thus a key element in modern anesthesia practice. In procedures where intense precision is required—dental surgery or endoscopies, for example—a deeper level of sedation may be required at times. This conservative approach not only seeks to prevent complications that are involved with airway issues but also renders patients motionless enough so that experts may work on them without distraction. Anesthesia providers, as a general principle, titrate the amount of sedation to meet the specific risk factors and needs of each patient, an endeavor guided by evidence-based guidelines and professional organization guidelines (Jeffrey et al., 2021).

Individualization reduces the risk of mistakes and makes every phase of the intervention as safe as possible. At the same time, sedation awareness entails understanding its hazards in the setting of an operating room. For instance, some malpractice case reviews state that MAC-based settings are at risk for fire due to electrocautery. An ignition source and the presence of supplemental oxygen—when uncontrolled to the perfect amount—can amplify a small error. This level of risk awareness, more broadly speaking, creates a safety culture where good communication and ongoing education are among healthcare professionals' priorities. Overall, responsible sedation use not only improves the patient experience but also improves overall efficacy and safety in most procedure types (Mehta et al., 2013) (Figure 8.3).

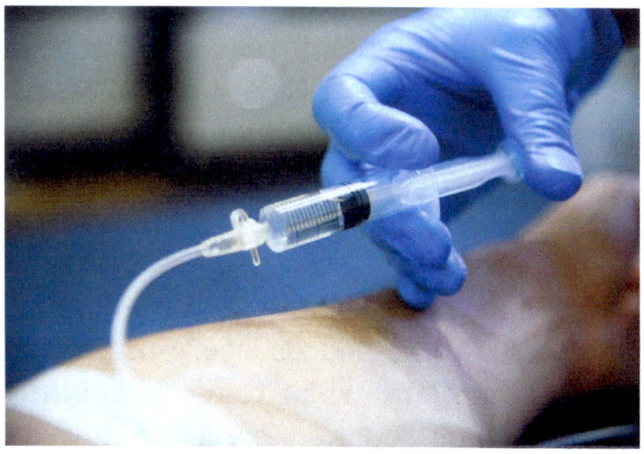

Figure 8.3. An Overview of Procedural Sedation.

Source: https://radiusohio.com/wp-content/uploads/2024/02/overviewproceduralsedation.jpeg.

8.1. Types of Sedation

Learning Outcome

1. Describe the minimal sedation and moderate sedation.
2. Define the deep sedation.

Sedation is not a solution for everyone; it's determining the appropriate method to the patient and to the process. Instead of rigid categories, think of it as a sliding scale. With minimal sedation, one can remain fully alert—to talk and respond, which is handy if cooperation is necessitated. Moderate sedation, in which individuals will still respond to questions but perhaps will not be quite as mentally quick or coordinated, is also an option. This level, for lack of a better term, is good for less complicated diagnostics or minor procedures—patients calm without crossing into harm. Naturally, every level has its requirement for close monitoring, particularly when the subject approaches deep sedation, something highlighted by a few recent studies (Cappellari et al., 2020). Deep sedation, however, is different. It brings patients to a state where they're barely aware or even lose consciousness outright. This degree of intensity in the majority of cases demands constant monitoring and frequently control of the airway—the risk of respiratory slowing is simply too immediate. Notably, other research comparing general anesthesia (GA) with a more conscious (alert) sedation shows that keeping someone just slightly more alert can reduce negative outcomes (Welter et al., 2016). In more complex cases, like neurosurgery or extensive orthopedic surgery when total immobility is the goal, nailing sedation precisely how deep it needs to be is the ticket to a successful operation. It's not only the surgery itself that dictates the choice of sedation—patient considerations mean a lot, too. For instance, with children's cases, there's a specific challenge: getting the right amount of sedation to calm fear without too much, given the special physical and emotional requirements of kids. Then with elderly patients, alterations in how their bodies process drugs translate into adjusting doses to prevent things like post-procedure confusion or falls. As medicine becomes increasingly tailored to the individual, the clinician's task is understanding how every sedation technique works with a patient's specific situation. Ultimately, regardless of whether it's on a typical MAC or a more sophisticated setup, striking that balance between safety and comfort is the goal (Cappellari et al., 2020).

8.1.1. Minimal Sedation

MAC now often rides on a technique called minimal sedation, which isn't just a lighter version of deep sedation—it's a way to keep patients comfortable yet responsive. In practice, patients stay at a moderate level of alertness, able to follow simple verbal cues but not plunged into full unconsciousness. Some studies, for instance, comparing self-administered propofol with sedation given by an anesthesiologist, show that those under minimal sedation tend to use less propofol and report high satisfaction rates (Mazanikov et al., 2013). This approach even cuts d on risks like respiratory depression that can pop up with heavier sedation methods. Minimal sedation also gets a boost in specific scenarios, especially in gastrointestinal procedures such as Endoscopic Retrograde Cholangiopancreatography (ERCP). Patient-controlled methods here let individuals feel more involved in their care; they're not just passive recipients but active participants in easing anxiety and discomfort. Research generally points out that patients undergoing ERCP with this gentler sedation recover faster and encounter fewer sedation-related mishaps compared to traditional approaches (Chaniotakis et al., 2018). That balance—enough sedation to ease the pain but also enough awareness to stay safe— underlines its potential benefits. Using minimal sedation within MAC isn't a one-size-fits-all deal, though—it calls for a careful pick of patients and close monitoring. Doctors need to check factors like medical history, possible medication interactions, and even how complicated the procedure is before dialing in the right sedation level. Keeping a steady watch on vital signs is key, particularly to stave off issues like hypoxemia and unexpected respiratory drop-offs. In most cases, altering sedation techniques to fit an individual's needs not only smooths the procedure but also reinforces minimal sedation as a smart, safe choice amid broader anesthetic care options (Mazanikov et al., 2013) (Figure 8.4).

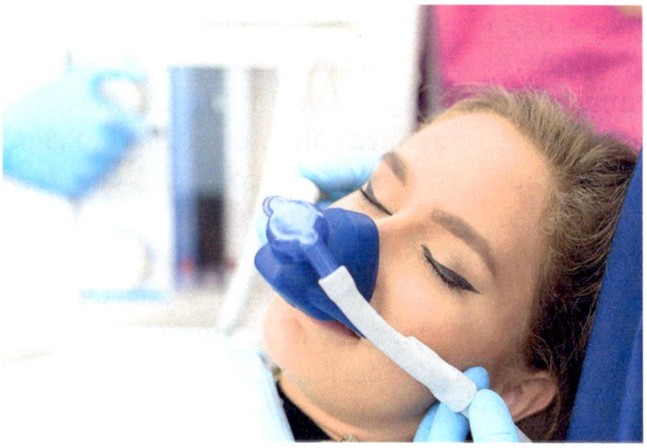

Figure 8.4. Minimal sedation.

Source: https://eastlakedentalexcellence.com/wp-content/uploads/2025/01/351377.jpg.

8.1.2. Moderate Sedation

Dental offices these days rely on knowing the ins and outs of sedation—not just for the sake of patient comfort but also to keep safety on point during treatments. Often, they use what's loosely called conscious or moderate sedation, where patients stay responsive while easing off some of the anxiety and discomfort of dental work. This method is pretty unique because it finds a middle ground: patients get relaxed enough to not be overwhelmed, yet they still keep their natural airway defenses intact. Keeping someone partially awake during a procedure lowers risks like airway blockages or accidental inhalation of fluids, which matter a lot in tougher, more intricate dental cases involving local numbing. It's all a bit muddled sometimes since many end up confusing moderate sedation with deep sedation—a mix-up that can open the door to complications (Cannesson, 2018).

When we step into the realm of MAC, moderate sedation takes on an even sharper role. Guidelines set out by groups like the American Society of Anesthesiologists generally spell out the differences between sedation levels, reminding practitioners to watch closely during the sedation process. Those handling moderate sedation need a good grasp of how sedative drugs work; for example, propofol can be very effective if used just right, but it also carries risks when it's not managed properly. Practitioners are expected to have enough know-how to spot and correct issues that pop up if sedation slips into a deeper state, ensuring patient safety remains front and center throughout the treatment (Cannesson, 2018). New technology is also shaking up the sedation scene in dentistry. There's been a move towards using physiological closed-loop systems, which are kind of like automated partners in delivering and keeping tabs on sedation. As these systems start showing up more frequently, anesthesiologists and the sedation teams have to adapt—they're not just following the old routine anymore, but also integrating these innovations without losing sight of safety. Sure, using these systems can boost the precision of dosing and monitoring, reducing some of the typical human guesswork. Still, making these devices work well means rigorous testing and real-world feedback from clinicians during their development. In the end, the success of these new approaches depends on a hands-on collaboration between engineers and anesthesia pros, reinforcing that ongoing learning and flexibility are crucial as MAC continues evolving (Cannesson, 2018) (Figure 8.5).

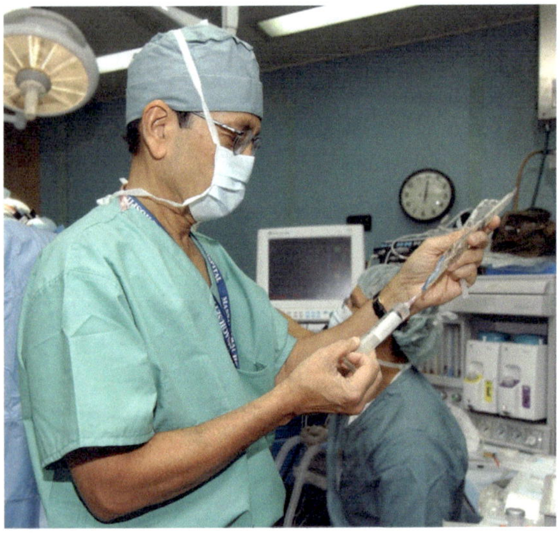

Figure 8.5. Moderate conscious sedation for dental anxiety.

Source: By US_Navy_050419-N-6665R-030_Dr._Akshay_Dalal_provides_medication_for_an_Indonesian_patient_as_the_medical_team_aboard_the_Military_Sealift_Command_(MSC)_hospital_ship_USNS_Mercy_(T-AH_19)_performs_surgery.jpg: U.S. Navy photo by Photographer's Mate 2nd Class Jeffrey Russellderivative work: Vearthy (talk) - US_Navy_050419-N-6665R-030_Dr._Akshay_Dalal_provides_medication_for_an_Indonesian_patient_as_the_medical_team_aboard_the_Military_Sealift_Command_(MSC)_hospital_ship_USNS_Mercy_(T-AH_19)_performs_surgery.jpg, Public Domain, https://commons.wikimedia.org/w/index.php?curid=12364806.

8.1.3. Deep Sedation

Deep sedation in MAC isn't always straightforward. In many clinical settings, finding the right balance between keeping someone sedated enough yet breathing steadily is a constant challenge, especially when dealing with painful procedures like burn dressing changes. Recent studies generally point out that a patient's background plays a role in judging both safety and how well the sedation technique works. Drugs such as propofol, midazolam, and ketamine tend to be used most often—they calm and relieve pain at the same time, but they can also lead to issues like apnea, reduced oxygen levels, or even hypotension, as was seen in several cases (Sayali et al., 2025). So, it becomes important not only to select the right medication but also to get the dosing just right. Another twist appears when you start looking at how various parties feel about the process. Research shows that satisfaction levels can vary widely among patients, burn nurses, and anesthesia providers, often depending on the quality of both sedation and pain management during the procedure. In most cases, patients end up giving deep sedation techniques a strong nod of approval, with average satisfaction scores running quite high. This point underscores that clear communication and setting the right expectations can be just as crucial as the drug choices themselves. When everyone—from the nurses and doctors to the patients—is on the same page about the sedation's success, the overall effectiveness of care naturally improves, leading to better experiences all around (Fatma et al., 2024). Keeping a close watch and being ready to adjust sedation levels is key to preventing side effects. Recent observations highlight that factors like blood pressure swings and oxygen saturation readings are directly tied to patient safety in MAC. Issues like apnea and hypotension might be manageable, yet they still prompt serious questions about the medication protocols and the need for constant oversight. Since deeper sedation carries inherent risks, continuous monitoring remains critical—multidisciplinary teams keeping an ongoing chat about sedation levels and patient responses help ensure that patients well-being stays top of mind. In most cases, additional research is needed to refine these best practices, always aiming to create the safest possible setting for patients undergoing painful procedures (Fatma et al., 2024) (Figure 8.6).

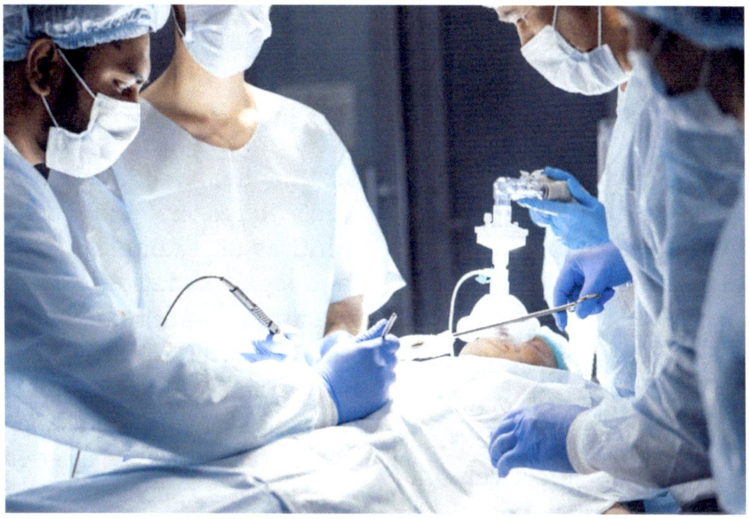

Figure 8.6. Deep sedation.

Source: https://smilescience.com/wp-content/uploads/2023/09/deep-sedation.jpg.

Test Your Knowledge

1. Define the minimal sedation.
2. What is a moderate sedation?

8.2. Indications for Monitored Anesthesia Care (MAC)

Learning Outcome

1. Understand the surgical procedures requiring sedation.
2. Explain the diagnostic procedures and interventions of monitored anesthesia care.
3. Describe the patient-specific factors influencing MAC use.

Anesthetic care that pays close attention to details can shape how well patients bounce back. In situations where procedures are less invasive and comfort matters – along with a speedy recovery –MAC often comes into play. Instead of going under full GA, MAC lets patients stay awake while easing them with sedatives. This approach not only keeps the body and mind at ease during surgery but also fits neatly into today's emphasis on Enhanced Recovery After Surgery (ERAS), which generally discourages heavy opioid use. Recent studies like (Soffin et al., 2019) even hint at lower opioid intake when techniques like opioid-free anesthesia (OFA) are used alongside MAC, proving that this method often cuts complications without sacrificing safety. MAC isn't just for routine, minimally invasive work. Sometimes operations call for a lighter anesthetic touch while still needing the patient's active feedback.

Take, for example, sacral neuromodulation (SNM) for urinary incontinence—here, a responsive patient is key, because their immediate reactions help tailor the treatment just right. In most cases, guidelines from groups like the International Continence Society push for anesthesia options that match individual needs; this makes MAC a natural fit. Unlike the old, one-size-fits-all methods, MAC shifts the focus to a more adaptive, patient-centered approach (Goldman et al., 2018).

Patient safety and comfort are, after all, top priorities, especially when treatments are done on an outpatient basis. MAC comes off as a smart choice because it provides sedation without dragging in the full effects of GA—helping manage pain and ease anxiety effectively. In procedures that might spark extra worry, such as endoscopies or even certain orthopedic interventions, being able to monitor vital signs closely means that any hiccups can be addressed quickly. This kind of real-time attention not only helps during the surgery but also builds trust and reassurance once the operation is over. Overall, MAC is about more than just efficiency—it's woven into a broader strategy for enhancing every stage of care while keeping patients both safe and genuinely cared for (Figure 8.7).

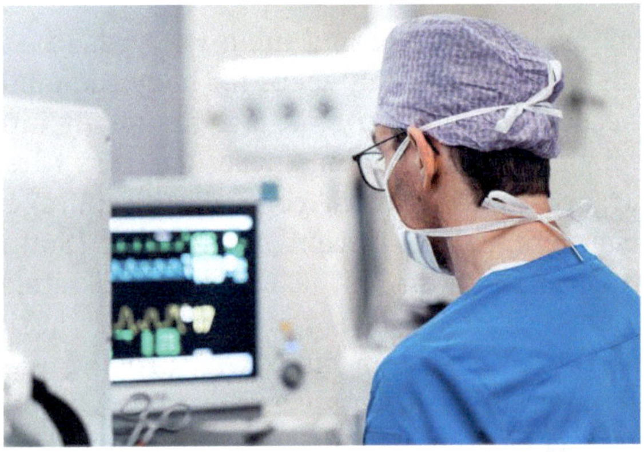

Figure 8.7. Indications for Monitored Anesthesia Care.

Source: https://lirp.cdn-website.com/7605998d/dms3rep/multi/opt/GettyImages-1215243447-640w.jpg.

8.2.1. Surgical Procedures Requiring Sedation

Surgical practices have come a long way. Nowadays, patient comfort and safety are at the heart of almost every decision, and techniques have shifted accordingly. Take MAC as an example—it lets patients slip into a deeper sedation yet keeps their natural breathing and reflexes alive. In most cases the American Society of Anesthesiologists has noted that MAC works for many diagnostic and treatment needs, which is why roughly 10–30% of surgeries these days rely on it (Zhan et al., 2021). This approach not only makes the whole experience easier for the patient but also helps speed up recovery—a definite plus for everyone involved. Look at orthopedic procedures, for instance. In the past, hip surgeries would usually call for full general or neuraxial anesthesia. Recently, though, there's been a move toward pairing a fascia iliaca compartment block (FICB) with MAC, and the results have been pretty promising. In a study with geriatric patients—each carrying their set of health challenges—hip operations were successfully carried out without the usual complications that come with GA (Zhan et al., 2021). A single injection, ultrasound-guided nerve block combined with light sedation managed to keep pain in check and blood pressure steady, showing MAC's ability to handle even tougher surgical needs. There's also a clear trend toward more personalized care. Sedation protocols are getting tailored to fit each patient's needs, which helps anesthetists tackle anxiety and pain directly; this usually makes for a more comfortable surgical experience (Das et al., 2015). With more folks becoming aware of these benefits, it looks like MAC is set to become even more widespread. This steady shift not only highlights ongoing innovation in anesthesia but also reaffirms that keeping patient well-being front and center remains a top priority—even if the approach sometimes winds up delightfully imperfect (Figure 8.8).

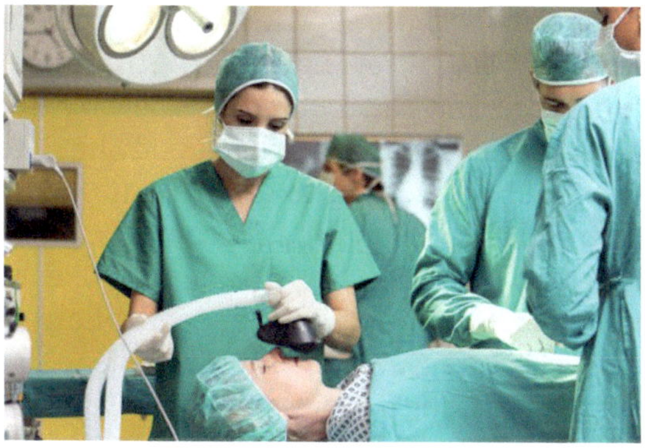

Figure 8.8. Surgical procedures requiring sedation.

Source: https://www.belolaw.com/wp-content/uploads/2019/08/Sedation-and-Anesthesia-Required-Preoperative-Checklist-for-Texas-Dentists.jpg.

8.2.2. Diagnostic Procedures and Interventions

MAC isn't just about following a checklist – you need to understand the signals that drive your decisions. BIS monitoring, for example, comes into play during elective procedures to tell how deep the sedation goes. I remember a study with colonoscopy patients where every participant eventually reached sedation levels similar to GA (Jenna Lee, 2014); results like this remind us that staying alert and ready to adjust isn't optional. Anesthesia providers have to use these real-time cues, and reading them carefully can make a big difference in how safe and effective MAC ends up being. When you dig into the observational data, it becomes clear that individual factors play a huge role in shaping anesthetic plans. Things like a patient's BMI and how long a procedure lasts can seriously affect sedation depth. For example, longer procedures often lead to deeper sedation—and sometimes the $ETCO_2$ waveform disappears, which is a sign tied to apnea. The research even hinted that quite a few patients might end up needing sedation levels that mirror GA, pointing to the need for better preoperative checks and more solid consent discussions. In most cases, matching the consent approach to a patient's unique profile can help reduce risks and keep them safer throughout sedation (Grey et al., 2014). Looking at MAC versus GA, some critical questions about consent and patient safety naturally arise. It turns out that many patients set up for MAC wind up with sedation levels that are no different from GA, a noteworthy point from both clinical and legal sides. And since every procedure brings its quirks, getting a handle on the nuances of these diagnostic evaluations is important. Looking forward, studies designed to fine-tune consent steps and use BIS monitoring to check anesthetic depth might offer insights that boost safety standards considerably. This isn't just academic chatter—it's likely to reshape how anesthesia providers handle sedation protocols, ensuring that patient care remains firmly rooted in robust, evidence-based practices (Jenna Lee et al., 2014) (Figure 8.9).

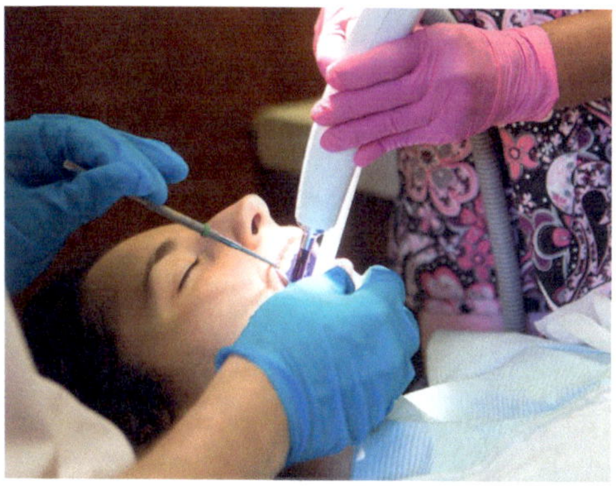

Figure 8.9. Diagnostic Procedures and Interventions.

Source: https://media.post.rvohealth.io/wp-content/uploads/2018/11/Woman_Getting_a_Filling-732x549-thumbnail.jpg.

8.2.3. Patient-Specific Factors Influencing MAC Use

Patient care is shifting in ways that make a difference, especially when we consider MAC.

These days, a mix of factors—like age, body weight, other health issues, and even a person's mental state—plays into how MAC is used. Older patients, for instance, often handle medications differently as their bodies change with age, so doctors generally tread more carefully with sedative doses. And when extra conditions come into play, like obesity or ongoing breathing troubles, the risks during sedation can creep up. Often, this means that healthcare teams end up doing a pretty thorough check before surgery to alter their anesthesia plans to fit each patient's profile—aiming for better safety and smoother results. Look closer at the drugs used for sedation and you'll see why this personal touch matters so much. Take dexmedetomidine (DEX), which stands out because its effect can vary a lot from one person to the next—factors like size, liver performance, or even heart output can change the game. As a result, anesthesiologists generally find themselves weighing its perks against any potential problems carefully. It's worth noting that, in most cases, DEX doesn't knock the wind out of someone's breathing, making it a pretty good option for patients with shaky respiratory function (Weerink et al., 2017). Still, doctors have to keep an eye on blood pressure or heart changes, especially if someone already has heart issues. In short, getting to know each patient's unique situation is key when it comes to making MAC work best. On top of all that, the way someone feels mentally is a big deal in how well MAC works. Often, anxiety or outright fear about surgery can change how a person responds to sedation, not to mention how they feel about the whole experience afterwards. Many times, a good pre-surgery chat can help calm those nerves, which might lead to a smoother, more natural induction of MAC. Some studies even suggest that patients who are better informed and more mentally prepared tend to need a bit less sedative overall, lowering the chance of going too far (Calkins et al., 2017). By taking these emotional factors into account along with the physical ones, healthcare providers are better able to adapt MAC approaches, making the whole process safer and more satisfying for patients.

Test Your Knowledge

1. Describe the surgical procedures of sedation.
2. What is the patient-specific factors influencing MAC use?

8.3. Benefits of Monitored Anesthesia Care (MAC)

Learning Outcome

1. Discuss on enhanced patient comfort and satisfaction.
2. Reduce recovery time compared to general anesthesia.
3. Know the flexibility in managing patient sedation levels.

Enhancing patient ease is one of MAC's big draws. Using remifentanil through a target-controlled infusion, doctors can often achieve outcomes that patients appreciate. One study, for example, looked at awake patients during fiberoptic bronchoscopy and found that around 78% said the experience was "comfortable or very comfortable" — and they didn't need any extra pain relief (Caron et al., 2021). This method lowers worry and typically speeds up recovery when compared to GA, sometimes letting patients head home sooner. In most cases, by keeping the focus on the patient's experience, MAC also tackles some of the psychological stress tied to surgery. MAC isn't just about making patients feel better; it also helps smooth out the everyday hustle in healthcare settings. The use of sedative techniques here often means that surgeons and anesthesiologists can concentrate on the specifics of the procedure without wrestling with the complications that come with GA. Fewer holdups, a quicker pace, and a more manageable schedule all tend to follow. Plus, fewer extended stays in recovery—typically seen with heavier anesthetic methods—translate into better bed availability for new patients (Rosenberg, 2021). Overall, these workflow improvements not only boost patient care but also push the efficiency of the entire system. On top of that, modern monitoring tools built into MAC ramp up safety by a good deal. Continuous checks on vital signs and patient responsiveness let clinicians alter sedation levels on the fly, ensuring safety throughout the process. Simulation-based training for anesthesiology teams, for instance, gives them a chance to practice handling emergencies — even if it means a few training mishaps along the way (Rosenberg, 2021). With a steady mix of real-time monitoring and practice drills, MAC helps keep procedural risks low while aiming high on patient satisfaction. To summarize, this well-rounded approach makes MAC a strong contender as a preferred choice in many surgical settings (Figure 8.10).

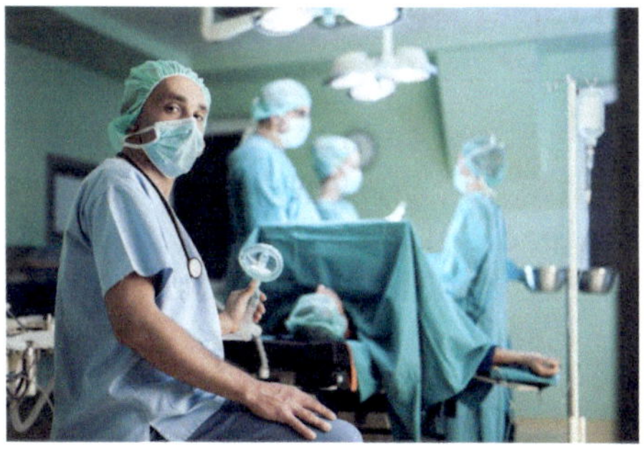

Figure 8.10. Benefits of monitored anesthesia care (MAC).

Source: https://radiusanesthesia.com/wp-content/uploads/2020/11/MAC-1024x684.jpg.

8.3.1. Enhanced Patient Comfort and Satisfaction

MAC has recently taken center stage as doctors try to make procedures that normally make people jittery feel a bit gentler. Many studies indicate that altering anesthetic plans lowers stress and improves how patients feel overall. One study, for example, looked at awake craniotomy sessions where they mixed in some adjustments to the ERAS protocol. Patients in those cases had fewer issues with anxiety and even showed slightly better cognitive responses afterward—even if the numbers weren't always statistically dramatic, this trend hints that MAC might ease the burden during tough surgeries (Azghadi et al., 2025). Sedation, on the other hand, isn't just about relaxing; it's also about treading that fine line between easing pain and quelling anxiety. Under MAC, anesthesiologists get to choose from a variety of meds, tailoring the mix to what each patient needs. I recall a study on burn dressing changes where the reported pain scores varied noticeably before and after the procedure. That kind of feedback underscores that a one-size-fits-all approach just doesn't cut it (Sayali et al., 2025). Being able to monitor and adjust pain relief in real time not only lifts satisfaction, but gives patients a real sense of being in safe hands—even if the adjustments happen on the fly. In the end, MAC's knack for boosting patient satisfaction seems to come from its flexible, patient-first mindset. Practitioners aim to build a setting where both physical and emotional comfort matter, which is key when it comes to sticking with recovery plans. From awake craniotomy sessions, patients have repeatedly stressed how important it is to feel safe and cared for throughout the operation (Azghadi et al., 2025). In burn care and beyond, similar experiences point to the fact that smart, adaptable anesthesia makes a meaningful difference. When patients feel looked after and at ease—even if there are little quirks here and there in how things are managed—it appears they tend to recover with a bit more confidence and better overall outcomes (Sayali et al., 2025) (Figure 8.11).

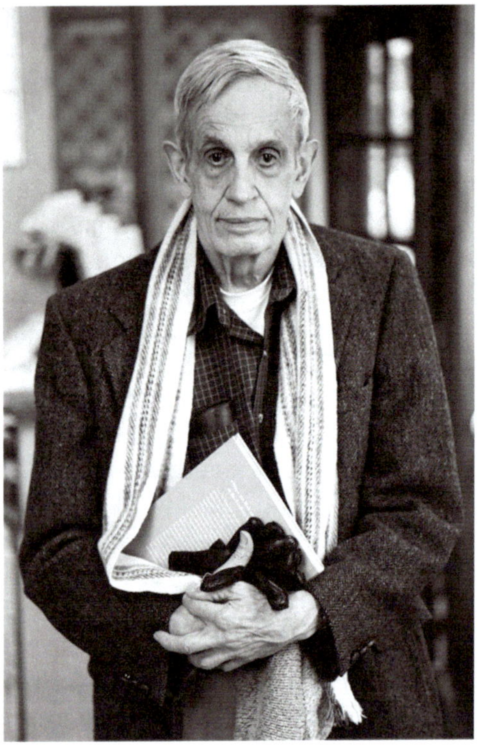

Figure 8.11. Patient comfort and satisfaction.

Source: By Peter Badge/ Typos1 - submission by way of Jimmy Wales, CC BY-SA 3.0, https://commons.wikimedia.org/w/index.php?curid=6977799.

8.3.2. Reduced Recovery Time Compared to General Anesthesia (GA)

Reduced recovery time plays a big role in the overall success of MAC in real-world practice. Patients receiving MAC tend to bounce back to their usual mental and physical state faster than those given GA—a fact that proves especially important in outpatient settings were getting back to everyday life quickly matters a lot. This speedier return not only boosts patient satisfaction and streamlines healthcare but also seems to reduce on the complications that often come with longer recoveries, helping to ease some of the risks tied to more advanced procedures. One major reason for this quicker bounce-back is how MAC weds personalized sedation with each patient's unique needs, generally speaking. By tailoring the sedation, MAC avoids the over-sedation pitfalls common with GA, so patients tend to keep more stable bodily functions and clearer cognitive skills afterward. The smooth shift from the operating room to full alertness also appears to reduce the chance of post-surgery delirium—especially among older adults, a group that's growing in surgical settings (Berger et al., 2018). Quick recoveries with MAC can do more than just help in the short run. Research indicates that the faster a patient recovers, the better their long-term cognitive health may be. It turns out that the way anesthesia affects brain function—particularly in older folks, where changes in blood flow can sometimes lead to unexpected cognitive hiccups (Claassen et al., 2021)—is less dramatic with MAC. In effect, less overall physiologic stress means fewer mental disturbances d the road. To summarize, choosing MAC protocols might not only promise a smoother immediate recovery but also serve as a smart strategy to enhance care quality over time, especially for those at risk for cognitive decline.

8.3.3. Flexibility in Managing Patient Sedation Levels

Managing patient sedation isn't a one-size-fits-all deal—it's more like fine-tuning an instrument based on each patient's quirks and what the moment calls for. Under MAC, being able to shift sedation levels on the fly is pretty crucial for keeping folks both safe and comfortable. In most cases, anesthetists keep a constant check on how patients are responding; sometimes, they need to dial up the sedation, sometimes ease it off, all based on what the patient shows. This kind of adaptability becomes especially key when things get unpredictable—when a patient's reaction isn't what you'd expect—and it's that swift response, despite occasional moments of uncertainty, that marks truly effective sedation management, blending both the art and science of anesthesia. Advancements in monitoring tech also play into this flexible approach. Take capnography, for example—it might sound all technical, but it's now a must-have tool that gives clinicians a real-time read on respiratory status and sedation depth. Generally speaking, these innovations let doctors make quick and informed calls thanks to clear physiological feedback. And when you factor in guidelines from the American Society of Anesthesiologists, which push for a tailored approach that considers each patient's individual traits and needs, you see how personalized care not only improves the overall experience but also lowers the risks of over- or under-sedation (Apfelbaum et al., 2021). Sometimes, a little extra monitoring goes a long way in making sure the patient stays safe—even if the process isn't perfectly smooth. There's also a constant evolution happening in how we monitor sedation. New guidelines lay out the bare minimum requirements during anesthesia and sedation, shedding light on that ever-important balance between keeping the patient comfortable and ensuring their safety (Klein et al., 2021). With a growing plunge into tools like processed EEG and neuromuscular monitoring, clinicians are moving toward more detailed, real-time checks. This extra layer of data lets them adjust sedation levels with more nuance—even if, on occasion, the punctuation in their notes isn't always spot on. To summarize, these advances give anesthetists the means to improve their clinical judgment and foster an environment that genuinely puts patient well-being first. Flexibility here isn't just a bonus; it's essential for handling the intricate challenges that come with administering MAC to a diverse group of patients (Figure 8.12).

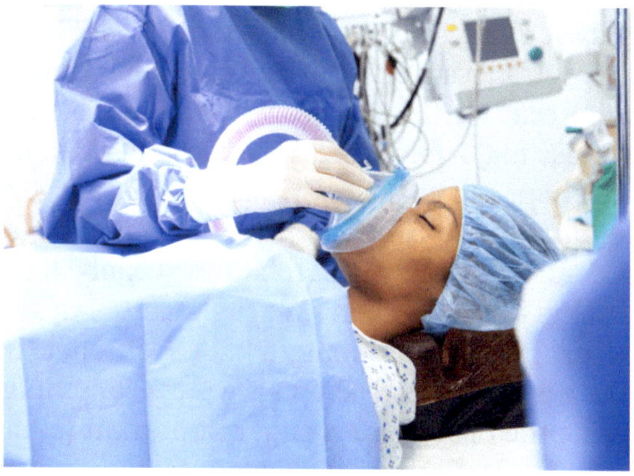

Figure 8.12. Managing patient sedation levels.

Source: https://hospitalprocedures.org/wp-content/uploads/2024/09/what-are-the-5-levels-of-sedation.png.

Test Your Knowledge

1. What are the enhance patient comfort and satisfaction?
2. What is the average recovery time from general anesthesia?

8.4. Risks and Complications

Learning Outcome

1. Know the potential adverse effects of sedation.
2. Understand the monitoring requirements during MAC.
3. Explain the strategies for minimizing risks.

MAC is seen as promising, but it isn't just about the good parts – there are hidden risks that can make a big difference in how patients do. A study looking at conscious sedation versus GA during transcatheter aortic valve replacement found that MAC had lower 30-day death rates and less major bleeding. Still, these perks don't cancel out the chance of troubles after surgery, like breathing problems or heart events, which tend to hit high-risk patients especially hard. Patients react in their unpredictable ways to the drugs used, so doing a thorough checkup before surgery and keeping an eye on things during the procedure is super important (Hung et al., 2023). Getting the balance right between reducing complications and giving enough sedation is at the heart of MAC. High-risk groups sometimes have their set of issues with MAC. For instance, older adults – often those over 80 with conditions like diabetes or chronic lung problems – more frequently end up on MAC rather than general or spinal anesthesia (SA). Even though MAC generally looks safe, some studies show it comes with a bump in major heart-related problems compared to GA (Ayoub et al., 2023). This is something that has to be considered carefully, and it usually means that anesthesiologists, surgeons, and primary doctors need to work together closely to figure out the best approach for each patient. Besides heart concerns, there's also the risk of things like airway blockages and aspiration, especially when the depth of sedation isn't watched closely enough. Such issues can turn into major problems later on – sometimes lengthening hospital stays or, in bad cases, even causing death. It helps a lot when anesthesiologists get the ins and outs of the drugs they're using. Looking at how safe and successful MAC is compared to GA, the takeaway seems to be that while risks are always there, careful use and extra vigilance during and after the procedure can make a big difference (Ayoub et al., 2023; Hung et al., 2023).

8.4.1. Potential Adverse Effects of Sedation

MAC isn't just about putting patients to sleep—it's about walking the fine line between getting sedation right and keeping people safe. Sometimes, sedation causes issues that show up as breathing troubles or unstable blood circulation. For example, one recent study found apnea in 84 of 118 administrations, while low oxygen levels appeared in 34 cases and blood pressure drops in 24 (Sayali et al., 2025). These breathing lapses, especially in patients with existing health challenges, can be pretty unsettling. When the sedation gets deeper than moderate, the risk of blocking the airway goes up, meaning caregivers have to keep a sharp watch and maybe step in. Even though MAC is supposed to let patients breathe on their, it demands constant vigilance—generally speaking, nothing here is left to chance. Beyond the breathing issues, sedation can mess with blood flow in unpredictable ways. Take, for instance, a case study of patients with hypertrophic obstructive cardiomyopathy (HOCM); these folks seem extra prone to sudden hemodynamic changes that can lead to serious complications (Cunningham et al., 2024). Different anesthetic agents—each with its quirks—can jostle a patient's blood pressure, heart rate, and overall vascular resistance, complicating the care before, during, and after a procedure. When you mix various sedatives, the whole picture gets even murkier, so understanding how these drugs work together becomes important. This all points to a need for approaches that are tailored to each patient's unique setup, rather than one-size-fits-all solutions. Then there's the aftereffect of sedation to consider. Studies suggest that the build-up of sedative effects can trigger complications after the procedure, sometimes leading to longer hospital stays, higher costs, and even lower patient satisfaction. A notable drop in mean arterial pressure (MAP)—a frequent observation during sedation—has been linked with tougher challenges later in managing pain (Sayali et al., 2025). Essentially, finding the sweet spot between effective sedation and avoiding side effects remains the heart of MAC's challenges. With this ever-present balancing act, it becomes clear that ongoing research and regularly rethinking sedation protocols are key to improving patient outcomes.

8.4.2. Monitoring Requirements During MAC

Patient safety and smooth procedures depend a lot on the right kind of monitoring during MAC. Constant checks—heart rate, blood pressure, oxygen levels, and breathing—tell us if a patient is handling sedation well. These numbers hint at the body's balance and reaction to the drugs. Take endoscopic sinus surgery, for example; patients may quickly shift in how they respond depending on how deep the sedation is. Keeping a close, sometimes imperfect watch lets us step in fast when things stray from normal, which seems to boost outcomes when comparing approaches like TIVA and MAC (Singla et al., 2024). Sedation levels under MAC can vary a good deal from one person to another, usually meaning that monitoring needs to be flexible. Patients needing moderate to deep sedation might bounce between different states of wakefulness, so extra caution is necessary. It's worth noting that factors like anxiety, previous health issues, and the complexity of the surgery mix into this unpredictable picture. Studies looking at procedures such as burn dressing changes show that these variations can impact how both institutions and practitioners feel about the process. Regular checks on sedation depth not only ease the minds of the team but also help patients feel safer and more comfortable throughout the procedure (Fatma et al., 2024). Working well under MAC calls for a team effort where anesthesiologists, surgeons, and nurses all keep an eye on the patient. Everyone tuning into the patient's condition makes it easier to adjust sedation on the fly if needed. Sticking to well-known monitoring routines might seem routine, but it lowers surprises and bumps in the road. Keeping a running log of a patient's responses—even if the notes aren't always perfect—helps shape better practices for next time. In most cases, when safety truly comes first, understanding all the little details behind MAC monitoring leads to better results overall and leaves patients feeling genuinely cared for (Fatma et al., 2024) (Figure 8.13).

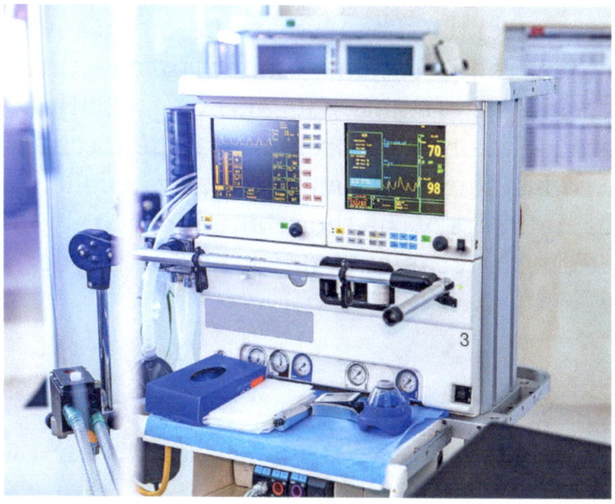

Figure 8.13. Monitoring requirements during MAC.

Source: https://www.apsf.org/wp-content/uploads/newsletters/2023/3802/anesthesia-monitor-featured.jpg.

8.4.3. Strategies for Minimizing Risks

Choosing the right anesthetic can be a real game-changer when it comes to successfully managing anesthesia care. Recent findings hint that remimazolam, for instance, performs about as well as DEX when it comes to recovery after procedures such as transcatheter aortic valve replacement (TAVR). Patients given remimazolam often end up needing fewer postoperative vasopressors and temporary pacemakers - a clue, perhaps, to a steadier blood pressure during recovery. It's interesting how a careful pick of an anesthetic not only cuts down potential complications but also seems to speed up the overall recovery process. In most cases, leaning toward agents with fewer side effects helps reduce the inherent risks of MAC, underscoring the value of making decisions based on evidence rather than guesswork (Kim et al., 2024). Before any procedure, taking time to dig into a patient's history can seriously pay off. A thorough preoperative assessment—which means checking out their medical background, any existing conditions, medication use, and doing essential diagnostic tests—often reveals hidden complications related to anesthesia. Consider, for example, patients living with HOCM; because their blood pressure can be incredibly sensitive, this group may face extra challenges during surgery. In those situations, regional anesthesia techniques might just be the better bet to keep things steady while still offering good pain relief. This kind of tailored approach not only bumps up safety but can also lead to better satisfaction and recovery rates. Generally speaking, addressing potential risks early on with comprehensive assessments and custom strategies does help providers lower the odds of unexpected events during MAC (Cunningham et al., 2024). After a procedure, keeping a close watch on patients is equally crucial. Continuous or round-the-clock monitoring of vital signs, coupled with an attentive look at how responsive a patient is, lays the groundwork for handling issues as soon as they show up. When the surgical team spots a problem early, it gives anesthesiologists the chance to jump in right away. Take TAVR patients, for example—they often need particularly careful observation because their hemodynamic status can fluctuate unexpectedly. Recent studies suggest that by using structured protocols in the recovery phase, not only do recovery outcomes improve, but the complications tied to anesthesia also drop noticeably. Streamlining these postoperative practices helps ensure patient safety while highlighting how MAC can truly help pave the way for successful recoveries (Kim et al., 2024).

Test Your Knowledge

1. What are the potential adverse effects of sedation?
2. Describe the strategies for minimizing risks.

8.5. Role of Anesthesia Providers

Learning Outcome

1. Describe the responsibilities of anesthesiologists and nurse anesthetists.
2. Understand the importance of preoperative assessments.
3. Focus on postoperative care and monitoring.

Anesthesia providers do a lot more than just administer sedative drugs during surgeries. They get into the nitty-gritty of a patient's background – checking their past health records, current meds, and even any allergies – which then helps decide whether a MAC or another sedation approach fits best. This pre-surgery check isn't merely a formality; it shapes the entire care process and sparks better chats between the anesthesia crew and the surgical team, making overall patient safety better. You can see how these assessments play a big role, especially now when new monitoring tech is constantly evolving to boost procedure outcomes and keep patients comfortable (Miyasaka et al., 2021). During an operation, providers lean on a range of monitoring techniques to keep things safe and, frankly, as comfortable as possible. Take capnography – it's become a go-to tool for checking if a patient's ventilation is on point by providing live data on their breathing. Updated guidelines even stress that effective monitoring doesn't stop once the surgery ends; it carries over into recovery too (Klein et al., 2021). By quickly making sense of these data points, anesthesia providers can nip potential problems in the bud, reducing sedation risks. This nonstop, dynamic monitoring calls for continual learning, which makes it necessary for providers to stay current with emerging tech so they can keep patient outcomes on track. Teamwork is another huge part of what anesthesia providers do. They often huddle with surgeons, nurses, and other healthcare folks to hash out tailor-made care plans for patients undergoing procedures that involve MAC. When everyone's on the same wavelength—even if sometimes the discussions get a little messy—the whole process of sedation and monitoring works smoother and safer. This collaborative approach is especially crucial in those tricky situations where other health issues might throw a wrench into the works. As medical advances keep rolling in, the growing expectations on anesthesia providers only highlight how vital their role is, pushing them to keep learning and adjust to new challenges (Klein et al., 2021; Miyasaka et al., 2021) (Figure 8.14).

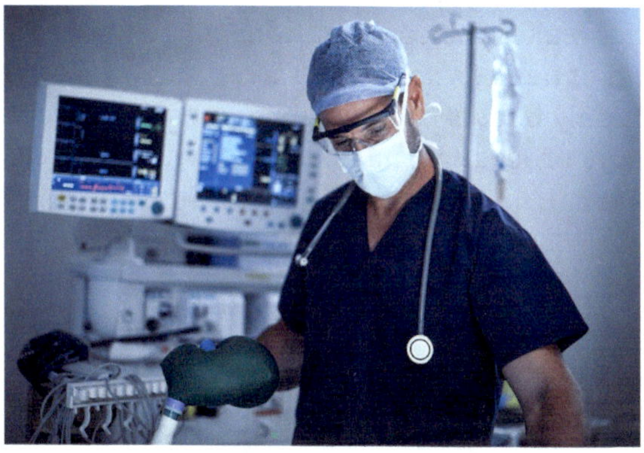

Figure 8.14. Role of anesthesia providers.

Source: https://www.summithealth.com/sites/default/files/2022-04/Anesthesiology_iStock-592648028.jpg.

8.5.1. Responsibilities of Anesthesiologists and Nurse Anesthetists

Anesthesiology isn't a straight-line field—it demands you get patient care during sedation and MAC. Anesthesiologists and nurse anesthetists, for one, mix the technical with the personal; they keep patients both safe and as comfortable as possible. They start by looking into a patient's history, spotting red flags for sedation risks, and they don't stop at just the physical side—sometimes, a patient's mood or stress levels matter too. They monitor vitals continuously, sometimes relying on a word here or a subtle gesture there; this constant watchfulness is usually what helps stop problems before they crop up, all while keeping the sedation level just right for a smooth procedure. Teamwork stands front and center in anesthesiology. Generally speaking, these professionals don't work in silos—they chat and coordinate with surgeons, nurses, and other healthcare folks to match anesthetic plans with the ups and ds of the surgical process. They might explain their plans in a laid-back yet clear way, answering questions on the fly and even repeating key points when needed. Sometimes the back-and-forth is a bit unpolished, but that's what makes the conversation feel genuine. This kind of flexible, sometimes irregular, interaction not only boosts patient safety but also helps the whole procedure run its course without a hitch.

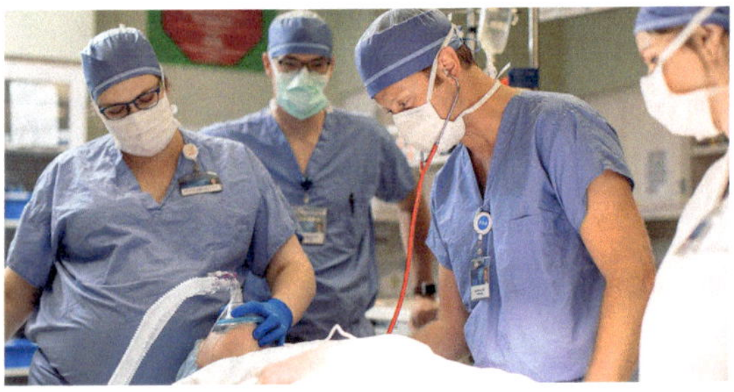

Figure 8.15. Responsibilities of nurse anesthetists.

Source: https://college.mayo.edu/media/mccms/content-assets/academics/explore-health-care-careers/nurse-anesthesia-career-3647383-0026-hero-tablet.jpg.

There's more to the job than just handling the procedure. In most cases, anesthesiologists and nurse anesthetists also carry a broader duty when it comes to the environment and workplace safety. Inhaled anesthetics, long a part of the routine, are now under the spotlight because of their greenhouse gas impact—leading many to wonder if it's time to switch things up (Gaya da Costa et al., 2021). They're increasingly exploring newer technologies and pushing for alternatives like local-regional or total intravenous anesthesia when it makes sense. Sure, balancing patient care and sustainability isn't simple, but this responsibility stretches across healthcare, urging everyone to take a few extra steps toward a greener practice overall (Figure 8.15).

8.5.2. Importance of Preoperative Assessments

When it comes to MAC sedation, checking a patient's unique health background is a must. Getting a pre-op look into each person's history not only paves the way for a custom anesthesia plan but also helps sidestep unexpected issues during the procedure. Take, for example, someone with heart or breathing problems—a thorough review can often point out exactly which type of sedation works best. In most cases a full preoperative check-up gives care providers a rounded picture of the patient's overall state, letting them decide more wisely and alter treatments to boost both safety and effectiveness. It's not just the physical side that counts; patients' mental readiness is equally critical, even if it sometimes slips under the radar. Anxiety and worry have a way of altering outcomes and even dampening how satisfied a patient feels about their care. A bit of casual pre-op counseling or simply keeping lines of communication open can make a big difference, easing those nerves and laying the groundwork for smoother recovery—especially in high-volume surgeries like transurethral resection of bladder tumor (TURBT) (Cho et al., 2025). Sometimes, a little extra reassurance is all it takes to level the field before things get serious. Then there are special cases that demand extra care. Certain groups, such as folks with HOCM, call for an eye for detail during the pre-op run-through. Recognizing these unique traits early means the team can try alternative approaches—perhaps leaning toward regional blocks or targeted sedation—so that any swings in blood pressure or other vital signs are kept in check.

This hands-on, early preparation not only tries to smooth out the rough spots during surgery but also reflects a genuine commitment to high-quality, tailored patient care (Cunningham et al., 2024).

8.5.3. Postoperative Care and Monitoring

Patients coming out of surgery need close attention—especially when MAC is involved. Right after the procedure, things can get a bit tricky; providers check heart rate, blood pressure, breathing, and a few other vital cues to spot any issues before they turn serious. Generally speaking, catching these signs early means a faster, smoother fix. Since anesthesia can alter normal body reactions, the team follows well-tested routines to lower any risks. It's a bit like juggling: all that careful watching mixes with the demands of performing anesthesia, balancing pain management with steady recovery (Navarro et al., 2021). Communication isn't just a buzzword out here. When the surgical crew and recovery staff chat and coordinate—even if it means a few handoffs here and there—the whole process flows better from the OR to areas where patients need even tighter monitoring. Newer drugs (think Desflurane) remind us how key it is to note not only how much of a drug is given but also how long it lasts; studies show this careful tracking can boost safety and even make surgeries run more efficiently. In many cases, what happens post-surgery becomes just another part of anesthesia management—keeping problems at bay while nudging recovery along (Karim et al., 2016). Then there's the whole human side of it. Postoperative care isn't just about the numbers; it involves looking after how patients feel physically, emotionally, and even mentally. Sometimes, if pain isn't dialed in carefully, it amps up stress and slows things a scenario no one wants. So, each patient and every procedure might need its mix of pain relief, with the team altering approaches as needed. A little extra reassurance, especially when someone's anxious or a bit off after surgery, can make a difference. To summarize, putting all these pieces together underlines a broad, team-driven approach that lifts patient outcomes and satisfaction in surgical settings (Navarro et al., 2021) (Figure 8.16).

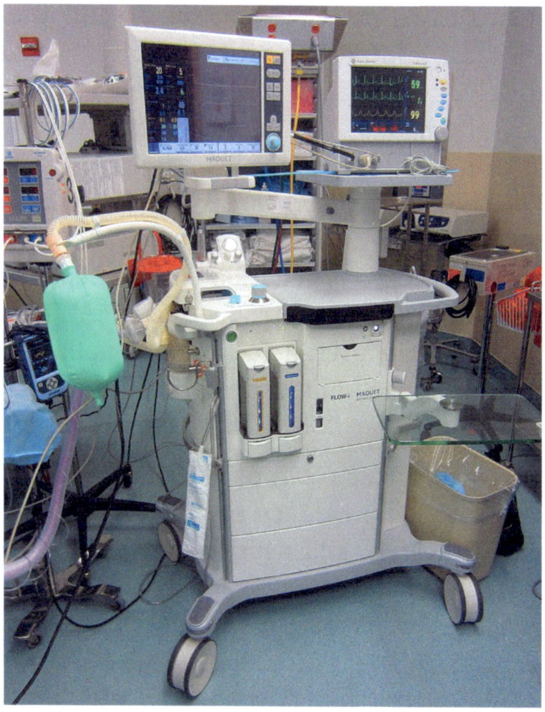

Figure 8.16. Post-anesthesia monitoring.

Source: By DiverDave - Own work, CC BY-SA 3.0, https://commons.wikimedia.org/w/index.php?curid=19899416.

Test Your Knowledge

1. What are the responsibilities of anesthesiologists and nurse anesthetists?
2. Why are preoperative assessments important?

SUMMARY

MAC is being used in many different medical settings these days, in large part due to the fact that it helps keep patients safe and procedures running smoothly. It's all about using a mix of sedatives and painkillers—administered by trained individuals—to make procedures less stressful than they might otherwise be. You might find MAC in settings like endoscopy suites or even for MRI procedures, where patient cooperation is a significant consideration. Through continuous observation and titration of sedation in real time, this practice helps to maintain patients in a stable condition as they get the care they need (Shah et al., 2024). In short, a balance between patient comfort and favorable outcomes provides evidence for the delivery of MAC as a routine component of anesthesia care.

Comparative studies, for the most part, point out that the integration of MAC and local infiltration anesthesia can be a game-changer. Evidence supports that when these techniques are combined, patients experience less pain during and after procedures. In a recent study, patients who received both local infiltration and MAC not only had lower pain scores but also shorter operative times and fewer early postoperative complications than patients who received local anesthesia alone; these findings, while not always dramatic, are encouraging (Fang et al., 2024). It seems that MAC can be mixed in to enhance both procedural efficiency and patient satisfaction, a quite significant added bonus as healthcare systems evolve toward better care. Overall, the literature on MAC is clear in that it can enhance outcomes in a very wide variety of settings. Being careful with the balance of depth of sedation with patient safety is still most important—especially where anxiety or discomfort might intrude. Using MAC has the potential to streamline the whole process and is in line with the overall goal of personalized patient care. With healthcare continuing to evolve, the adoption of such innovative practices as MAC seems to be an imperative for the enhancement of safety, comfort, and overall success of procedures (Fang et al., 2024; Shah et al., 2024).

When you move into MAC and sedation grounds, you'll discover that there's not entirely technique, it's a balance art. MAC is at its best when patients need to stay awake; that mix of pain medication and sedatives gives them a little wakefulness, which is absolutely essential in procedures such as spinal cord stimulation (SCS). Even a survey has shown that some 77% of physicians prefer deep sedation for the placements of SCS, an unmistakable vote in favor of the theory that patient involvement can be of value. This technique, blending patient wakefulness and adequate pain relief, is one instance of how anesthesia can be useful and secure. In keeping with the additional impact of MAC on other groups, there is additional complexity, especially concerning postoperative recovery. Advanced age, as various studies show, is known to enhance the risk for postoperative cognitive dysfunction (POCD) overall.

Further research even cites anesthesia with an increased permeability of the blood–brain barrier, potentially enhancing the manifestation of cognitive deterioration. In an intriguing study, elderly mice showed a pronounced elevation of matrix metalloproteinase-9 (MMP-9) levels after anesthesia—a finding for which the authors express concern over possible neurotoxic side effects. Such a discovery highlights the need to tailor sedation plans so that older individuals not only endure surgery but bounce back well in the long run. And then there is the so-called reality of real-world practice versus official safety guidelines. It appears what doctors actually do in the real world varies with set guidelines sometimes. Consider for example that around 45% of practitioners said they used GA to undergo certain SCS implants, even though complications are rare. This kind of disparity—albeit seemingly subtle—suggests that we still have some work to do in aligning "real life" practice with best practice guidelines. Overall, the observations lend themselves to an on-going debate regarding how MAC and sedation continue to evolve within the context of contemporary healthcare, reminding us that on-going research and debate are essential to helping ensure that patient care continues to be innovative and safe.

KEY TERMS FROM THIS CHAPTER

- Anesthetic care
- Hemodynamic stability
- Moderate sedation
- Opioid-free anesthesia
- Patient consent
- Sacral neuromodulation
- Sedation
- Task-management
- Deep sedation
- Minimal sedation
- Monitored Anesthesia Care
- Orthopedic interventions
- Respiratory function
- Safety standards
- Surgical practices

CRITICAL THINKING QUESTIONS

1. **Monitored anesthesia care (MAC) primarily involves:**
   a. General anesthesia with mechanical ventilation
   b. Regional anesthesia with sedation
   c. Sedation, analgesia, and patient monitoring
   d. Complete loss of consciousness
2. **In MAC, the level of sedation commonly aimed for is:**
   a. Minimal sedation
   b. Moderate sedation (conscious sedation)
   c. Deep sedation
   d. General anesthesia
3. **Which of the following is an indication for MAC?**
   a. Procedures requiring minimal invasiveness
   b. Patients unable to tolerate general anesthesia
   c. Surgeries where rapid recovery is needed
   d. All of the above
4. **Which of the following drugs is commonly used during MAC for sedation?**
   a. Propofol
   b. Midazolam
   c. Fentanyl
   d. All of the above
5. **Essential monitoring during MAC includes:**
   a. Electrocardiogram (ECG)
   b. Pulse oximetry
   c. Capnography
   d. All of the above

Short Answer Questions

1. What is monitored anesthesia care (MAC)?
2. Why is sedation important in medical procedures?
3. List the types of sedation.
4. Describe the benefits of monitored anesthesia care.
5. What is the role of anesthesia providers?

Answers to Critical Thinking Questions

1. (c); 2. (b); 3. (d); 4. (d); 5. (d)

REFERENCES

1. Apfelbaum, J. L., Hagberg, C. A., Connis, R. T., Abdelmalak, B., Agarkar, M., Dutton, R. P., Fiadjoe, J. E., et al. (2021). 2022 American Society of Anesthesiologists practice guidelines for management of the difficult airway. *Anesthesiology, 136*, 31–81. https://doi.org/10.1097/aln.0000000000004002.
2. Ayoub, C., Chalhoub, V., El-Achkar, A., Abou Heidar, N. F., Tamim, H., Maroun-Aouad, M., & El Hajj, A. (2023). Sedation as an alternative anesthetic technique for frail patients in transurethral resection of the prostate. *Therapeutic Advances in Urology, 15*. https://www.semanticscholar.org/paper/1891e3f0861fd6002615dad5182b2ad43a50002b (accessed on 20 May 2025).
3. Azghadi, A., Sharpe, M., Mikofalvy, K., El-Abtah, M., Sunshine, K. S., Shah, V., Maravillas, M. A., et al. (2025). Role of modified enhanced recovery after surgery (mERAS) in awake craniotomy performed under monitored anesthesia care (MAC); a single center retrospective study. *BMC Anesthesiology, 25*. https://www.semanticscholar.org/paper/0460bd3901944a72a9ed72289e11532694eb9605 (accessed on 20 May 2025).
4. Berger, M., Schenning, K. J., Br, C. H., Deiner, S., Whittington, R. A., & Eckenhoff, R. G. (2018). Best practices for postoperative brain health. *Anesthesia & Analgesia, 127*, 1406–1413. https://doi.org/10.1213/ane.0000000000003841.
5. Calkins, H., Hindricks, G., Cappato, R., Kim, Y. H., Saad, E., Aguinaga, L., Akar, J. G., et al. (2017). 2017 HRS/EHRA/ECAS/APHRS/SOLAECE expert consensus statement on catheter and surgical ablation of atrial fibrillation: Executive summary. *Journal of Arrhythmia, 33*, 369–409. https://doi.org/10.1016/j.joa.2017.08.001.
6. Cannesson, M. (2018). From invention to innovation: Bringing perioperative physiological closed-loop systems to the bedside. *Anesthesia & Analgesia*. https://www.semanticscholar.org/paper/7e623829afef6d64161f52f63da76a8dcc6f8085 (accessed on 20 May 2025).
7. Cappellari, M., & Toni, D. (2020). Response by Cappellari and Toni to letter regarding article, "General anesthesia versus conscious sedation and local anesthesia during thrombectomy for acute ischemic stroke." *Stroke*. https://www.semanticscholar.org/paper/a8a2338f05fd5d5b9549eb7e20366d003db2c5ee (accessed on 20 May 2025).
8. Caron, M., Parrot, A., Elabbadi, A., Dupeyrat, S., Turpin, M., Baury, T., Rozencwajg, S., et al. (2021). Pain and dyspnea control during awake fiberoptic bronchoscopy in critically ill patients: Safety and efficacy of remifentanil target-controlled infusion. *Annals of Intensive Care, 11*. https://www.semanticscholar.org/paper/d9cd98ffba26d940c5c3966d74156d1a6265db55 (accessed on 20 May 2025).
9. Chaniotakis, I., Spyrliadis, A., Katsimpoulas, M., & Kostomitsopoulos, N. (2018). The mouse and the rat in surgical research. The anesthetic approach. *Journal of the Hellenic Veterinary Medical Society, 67*(3), 147–162. https://doi.org/10.12681/jhvms.15633.
10. Cho, J. S., Ham, W. S., Lee, B., Kim, H. I., & Park, J. H. (2025). Comparison of remimazolam-based monitored anesthesia care and inhalation-based general anesthesia in transurethral resection of bladder tumor: A randomized-controlled trial. *Cancers, 17*. https://www.semanticscholar.org/paper/187c3e77dd578cdc01b2643a52712a11f2893523 (accessed on 20 May 2025).
11. Claassen, J. A. H. R., Thijssen, D. H. J., Panerai, R. B., & Faraci, F. M. (2021). Regulation of cerebral blood flow in humans: Physiology and clinical implications of autoregulation.

Physiological Reviews, 101, 1487–1559. https://doi.org/10.1152/physrev.00022.2020.

12. Cunningham, J. J., Braun, A. S., Hussey, P., Momaya, A., & Kukreja, P. (2024). Regional anesthesia for arthroscopic knee repair in a patient with hypertrophic obstructive cardiomyopathy (HOCM) under monitored anesthesia care with dexmedetomidine infusion. *Cureus, 16*. https://www.semanticscholar.org/paper/a9924fc86ac0f42af9ab5e7bdf38492a294bcef9 (accessed on 20 May 2025).
13. Das, S., & Ghosh, S. (2015). Monitored anesthesia care: An overview. *Journal of Anesthesiology, Clinical Pharmacology, 31*, 27–29. https://www.semanticscholar.org/paper/b546e9ab1e7a18339cc6f7d05c466590cd57ad0b (accessed on 20 May 2025).
14. Fang, L., Shen, J., Zhang, H., Zhang, L., Zheng, X., Zhao, H., & Zhang, J. (2024). A retrospective study of the safety and efficacy of peritoneal dialysis catheter placement under combined local infiltration anesthesia and monitored anesthesia care. *BMC Anesthesiology, 24*. https://www.semanticscholar.org/paper/8dffd6a996028266fab7cbaa091a25339bf9fd10 (accessed on 20 May 2025).
15. Gaya da Costa, M., Kalmar, A. F., & Struys, M. (2021). Inhaled anesthetics: Environmental role, occupational risk, and clinical use. *Journal of Clinical Medicine, 10*, 1306. https://doi.org/10.3390/jcm10061306.
16. Goldman, H. B., Lloyd, J. C., Noblett, K., Carey, M., Castaño Botero, J. C., Gajewski, J. B., Lehur, P. A., et al. (2018). International Continence Society best practice statement for use of sacral neuromodulation. *Neurourology and Urodynamics, 37*, 1823–1848. https://doi.org/10.1002/nau.23515.
17. Grey, P. M. (2014). *An Evaluation of Sedation Level Using BI spectral Index (Bis) And Correlated Adverse Events in Patients Undergoing Colonoscopies* (NC DOCKS at Western Carolina University). https://core.ac.uk/download/345080085.pdf (accessed on 20 May 2025).
18. Hasoon, J., Urits, I., Viswanath, O., Varrassi, G., Simopoulos, T., Kohan, L., Gutierrez, G., et al. (2021). Percutaneous spinal cord stimulation lead placement under deep sedation and general anesthesia. *Pain and Therapy, 10*, 1719–1730. https://doi.org/10.1007/s40122-021-00332-2.
19. Huang, L., Tian, W., Chen, X., Xu, H., Dai, W., Zhang, Y., Wu, X., et al. (2022). Peripheral neutrophils-derived matrix metallopeptidase-9 induces postoperative cognitive dysfunction in aged mice. *Frontiers in Aging Neuroscience, 14*. https://doi.org/10.3389/fnagi.2022.683295.
20. Hung, K., Chen, J. Y., Hsing, C., Chu, C., Lin, Y. T., Pang, Y., Teng, I. C., et al. (2023). Conscious sedation/monitored anesthesia care versus general anesthesia in patients undergoing transcatheter aortic valve replacement: A meta-analysis. *Frontiers in Cardiovascular Medicine, 9*. https://www.semanticscholar.org/paper/7e9277eb5ca12e60455420d0111c411bece3dd22 (accessed on 20 May 2025).
21. Karim, H. M. R., Sailo, L., Sangma, S. J. N., Syiemiong, et al. (2016). Pharmacoeconomics of desflurane based minimal flow anesthesia for different durations of surgery. https://core.ac.uk/download/543134029.pdf (accessed on 20 May 2025).
22. Kim, J. H., Nam, J. S., Seo, W. W., Joung, K. W., Chin, J., Kim, W. J., Choi, D., et al. (2024). Effects of remimazolam versus dexmedetomidine on recovery after transcatheter aortic valve replacement under monitored anesthesia care: A propensity score-matched, non-inferiority study. *Korean Journal of Anesthesiology, 77*, 537–545. https://www.semanticscholar.org/paper/4aa01ffdfdaaf7b4f3b0d5e3d379c0767f46f21c (accessed on 20 May 2025).

23. Klein, A. A., Meek, T., Allcock, E. A., Cook, T., Mincher, N., Morris, C., Nimmo, A. F., et al. (2021). Recommendations for standards of monitoring during anesthesia and recovery 2021. *Anesthesia, 76*, 1212–1223. https://doi.org/10.1111/anae.15501.

24. Majewski, L., & Tselonis, P. K. (2017). Task-management training for recognition, prioritization and decision-making for the SRNA. *College of Science and Health Theses and Dissertations, 213*. https://via.library.depaul.edu/csh_etd/213 (accessed on 20 May 2025).

25. Mazanikov, M. (2013). Patient-controlled sedation for endoscopic retrograde cholangiopancreatography. https://core.ac.uk/download/14927898.pdf (accessed on 20 May 2025).

26. Mehta, S. P., Bhananker, S. M., Posner, K. L., & Domino, K. B. (2013). Operating room fires. *Anesthesiology, 118*, 1133–1139. https://doi.org/10.1097/aln.0b013e31828afa7b.

27. Miyasaka, K., Shelley, K. H., Takahashi, S., Kubota, H., Ito, K., Yoshiya, I., Yamanishi, A., et al. (2021). Tribute to Dr. Takuo Aoyagi, inventor of pulse oximetry. *Journal of Anesthesia, 35*, 671–709. https://doi.org/10.1007/s00540-021-02967-z.

28. Navarro, K. L., Huss, M., Smith, J. C., Sharp, P., Marx, J. O., & Pacharinsak, C. (2021). Mouse anesthesia: The art and science. *ILAR Journal, 62*(1-2), 238–273. https://doi.org/10.1093/ilar/ilab016.

29. Poziombke, J. L. (2014). An evaluation of sedation level using bispectral index (BIS) and correlated adverse events in patients undergoing colonoscopies. *NC DOCKS at Western Carolina University*. https://core.ac.uk/download/345080087.pdf (accessed on 20 May 2025).

30. Shah, D., Sen, J., & Bawiskar, D. (2024). Non-operating room anesthesia (NORA): A comprehensive review of monitored anesthesia care. *Cureus, 16*. https://www.semanticscholar.org/paper/b78d10d1fef6bcd9342d0a357f8442c15b6ad954 (accessed on 20 May 2025).

31. Singla, A., & Singla, S. K. (2024). Evaluation of surgical conditions during elective endoscopic sinus surgery with total intravenous anesthesia and monitored anesthesia care. *An International Journal Clinical Rhinology*. https://www.semanticscholar.org/paper/a01afd13dbf8759c2dbb821ebccb6094c7580ecd (accessed on 20 May 2025).

32. Soffin, E. M., Wetmore, D. S., Beckman, J. D., Sheha, E., Vaishnav, A. S., Albert, T. J., Gang, C. H., et al. (2019). Opioid-free anesthesia within an enhanced recovery after surgery pathway for minimally invasive lumbar spine surgery: A retrospective matched cohort study. *Neurosurgical FOCUS, 46*, E8. https://doi.org/10.3171/2019.1.focus18645.

33. Ulusan Sayali, F. O., Kovac, A., Becker, M., Bhavsar, D., Nickerson, D., Golson, K., & Nazir, N. (2024). Satisfaction of patient, burn nurse/tech and anesthesia provider for monitored anesthesia care burn dressing change. *Journal of Burn Care & Research, 45*, 210. https://www.semanticscholar.org/paper/550c22d9d8f3a1b75cb0cc6fd2f8ff07716d7a63 (accessed on 20 May 2025).

34. Ulusan Sayali, F., Bhavsar, D., Nickerson, D., Slater, J., Golson, K., Nazir, N., & Kovac, A. (2025). Evaluating medication number and effect administered during monitored anesthesia care for burn dressing change. *Journal of Burn Care & Research: Official Publication of the American Burn Association, 46*, S346–S347. https://www.semanticscholar.org/paper/28cef71a601476a542696d6e67d67d71ec0cc15e (accessed on 20 May 2025).

35. Weerink, M. A. S., Struys, M., Hannivoort, L. N., Barends, C., Absalom, A., & Colin, P. (2017). Clinical pharmacokinetics and pharmacodynamics of dexmedetomidine. *Clinical Pharmacokinetics, 56*, 893–913. https://doi.org/10.1007/s40262-017-0507-7.

36. Wehrmann, T., Riphaus, A., Eckardt, A. J., Klare, P., Kopp, I., von Delius, S., Rosien, U., et al. (2023). Updated S3 guideline "Sedation for gastrointestinal endoscopy" of the German Society of Gastroenterology, Digestive and Metabolic Diseases (DGVS)–June 2023–AWMF-Register-No. 021/014. *Festschrift für Gastroenterology, 61*, e654–e705. https://doi.org/10.1055/a-2165-6388.

37. Welter, L. V., & Fonseca, L. F. (2016). Patient recovery assessment in post-operative recovery room in absence of anesthetic. *Journal of Nursing Ufpe Online, 10*, 2091–2099. https://www.semanticscholar.org/paper/30782eaa101aa56a1b37d477a7d715299c24557d (accessed on 20 May 2025).

38. Zhan, L., Zhang, Y., & Wang, J. X. (2021). Combined fascia iliaca compartment block and monitored anesthesia care for geriatric patients with hip fracture: Two case reports. *World Journal of Clinical Cases, 9*, 8268–8273. https://www.semanticscholar.org/paper/d45596534cc116dea7cc6c2f95f4f3de0ebc322c (accessed on 20 May 2025).

PEDIATRIC ANESTHESIA

9

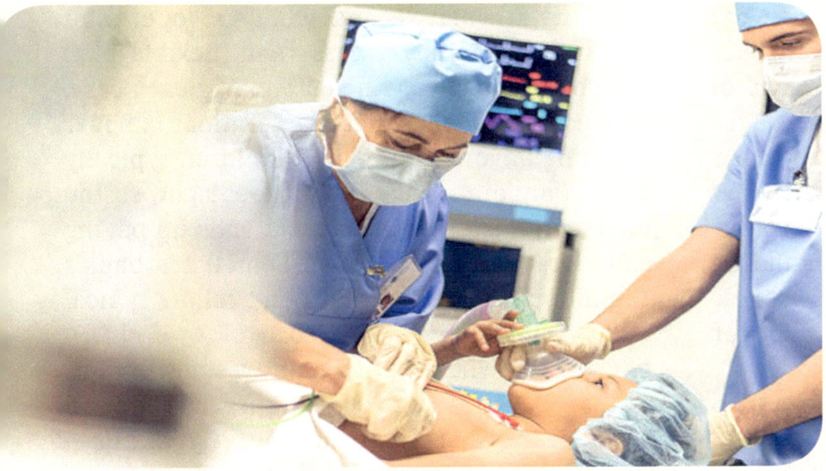

LEARNING OBJECTIVES

After studying this chapter, you will be able to:

1. Describe the physiological differences in children.
2. Explain the types of anesthesia used in pediatrics.
3. Perform necessary preoperative assessment for children.
4. Understand the intraoperative management.
5. Describe the postoperative care.

Introduction

Dealing with children who need anesthesia is sensitive work. Their brains and bodies develop in ways to make them different from adults—different anatomy, faster or slower metabolism, and even different social signals mean that a single approach just won't fit. Skilled management of anesthetic drugs is simply not possible without effective relief of pain, reduction of fear, and upkeep of recovery in a smooth manner. Doctors as a whole must remain current about new concepts and changing standards because a small mistake can have huge consequences. Pediatric anesthesiologists, for instance, must master a range of skills and to learn how to overcome the unique challenges of working with tiny patients, creating a patient setting that is both safe and comfortable in a natural, often not-so-perfect way. Some groups highlight that strong standards in pediatric anesthesia are crucial. The case is the action of the European Society for Paediatric Anesthesiology's Pain Committee, which advocates for a staged approach to perioperative pain management (Adamek et al., 2018). The approach suggests multi-layered methods that respond to each case of surgery as well as resource variability. Overall, obeying these standards manifests commitment to more secure outcomes—helping to speed recoveries and maintain health. Relying on evidence-based care allows anesthesiologists to trace the convoluted path of pediatrics so that their work continues to be viable and loyal to current methodologies. Pediatric anesthesia is not strictly operating room procedure; it even applies to careers like dentist anesthesiologists. Recent studies indicate that these specialists give a reasonable amount of secure anesthesia to children in office settings (Gabriel et al., 2017). Their successful, at times unexpected methods in meeting the needs of young patients offer a variety of possibilities for care. This specialization not only makes it easier for children to have their dentistry done safely, but it shows how the profession constantly evolves. Discovery of these varied approaches could be critical to enhanced overall care, guiding what new research must address, and altering education for future anesthesia providers (Figure 9.1).

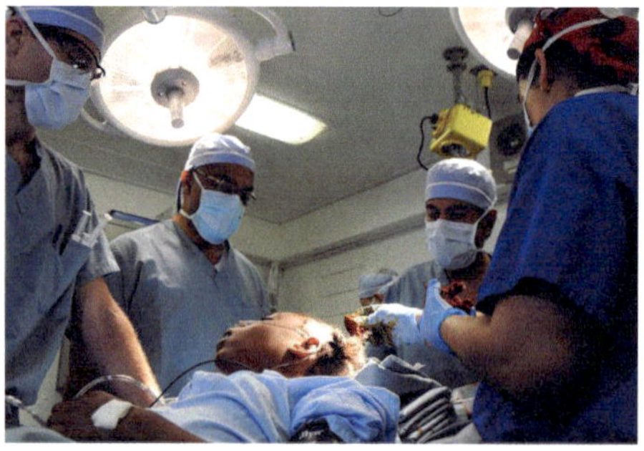

Figure 9.1. Pediatric anesthesia.

Source: By United States Navy - http://weblogs.baltimoresun.com/health/gupta%20haiti.jpg, Public Domain, https://commons.wikimedia.org/w/index.php?curid=16960834.

Definition of Pediatric Anesthesia

Pediatric anesthesia is not just baby versions of adult care—children require a completely different sense of how little bodies work. Kids, whether they're fragile newborns or on the brink of adolescence, all possess their own combination of physical and emotional traits that affect the administration of anesthesia. It's not only about being technically competent but also about knowing how a child's body grows, how there is difference in body composition, metabolic rate, and how they respond to medications. Because these patients are children, they risk losing too little or too much of the treatment due to the varying anatomy and chemistry of kids, so everyone works very closely with each other to create plans considering the age of the child, health status, and what the operation demands. Generally, a less rigid, flexible plan can come a long way in customizing each case. Staying awake for pediatric operations is never anything anyone can ignore. Children typically can't complain if they do not feel right, so the team administering anesthesia ends up paying extra close attention to them. Sometimes, babies exhibit complications that don't follow typical adult trajectories, which can slow d down figuring out where things went wrong (Ferriero et al., 2019). Even for most surgeries—when risks in general are comparatively minor—the likelihood of complications depends on a child's age and the type of procedure. With criteria and best practice continually evolving, practitioners have to have one foot forward gazing toward new technology and improved techniques. Simulation training and other hands-on classes are increasingly seen as the important tools to allow anesthesiologists to cope with these special challenges. And let's not forget the emotional side of anesthesia. Most kids are quite nervous or even outright scared to have a surgery, and that level of stress can actually change how their bodies react to anesthesia (Rosen et al., 2018). Pediatric anesthesiologists try not only to manage the physical but to soothe fears—whether in the guise of soft, childlike explanation, games, distractions, or plain old reassuring words. When both bodily and emotional needs are taken care of, the entire surgical process tends to proceed more smoothly, reducing anxieties for everyone involved. Lastly, improving our knowledge of pediatric anesthesia does not only lead to better clinical outcomes; it creates a kinder atmosphere that reassures families and makes children feel ever so slightly better at these challenging times.

Importance in Pediatric Surgery

Pediatric anesthesia in surgery isn't always about checking boxes on an inventory list—it's about getting the little ones through okay without taking either short-term or long-term risks too high. The age and development of a child can change their reaction to drugs, so physicians typically adjust their strategy to accommodate those special needs. For example, in general studies, non-invasive technology like near-infrared spectroscopy (NIRS) monitoring maintains the level of oxygen in the brain constant throughout a procedure. Keeping the brain in healthy function is directly related to the quality of neurological recovery afterwards. But it is peculiar that in applications other than for the heart, NIRS is not given any consideration; sometimes this lack leads to suboptimal regulation of blood flow to the brain, revealing a clear necessity for higher utilization of such sophisticated techniques in everyday practice (Weber et al., 2019).

Children and their families usually dive into surgery with a big dose of nerves and skepticism. And it is also the case that pre-op nervousness isn't always a child's problem—it's also a ripples-over-into-caregivers situation, complicating and making more challenging the induction process. Even theories exist that some measure of playfulness being involved, like a Cl Doctor popping in, can lift parents' moods, even while it may not completely alleviate the child's nervousness. Not surprisingly, this form of emotional support appears to make the entire process less clinical and more humane, validating the premise that attending to these emotions is equally critical to any technical step in surgery (Arriaga et al., 2016).

Aside from monitoring and providing emotional support, choosing the right medications for pediatric anesthesia matters. Kids process drugs differently from adults because of their dissimilar body chemistry; therefore, drug dosage is normally adjusted based on age and weight to avoid complications while providing effective pain relief. Restriction of how much of such anesthetic drugs a kid receives is also supported, since large quantities have long-term effects on their growing nervous system. In the overwhelming majority of cases, this fine balancing act has stimulated additional investigation of new drugs and approaches—a reminder that the interplay of wise monitoring, caring feeling, and customized treatment holds the secret to meeting the physical and psychologic needs of young patients on the operating table (Figure 9.2).

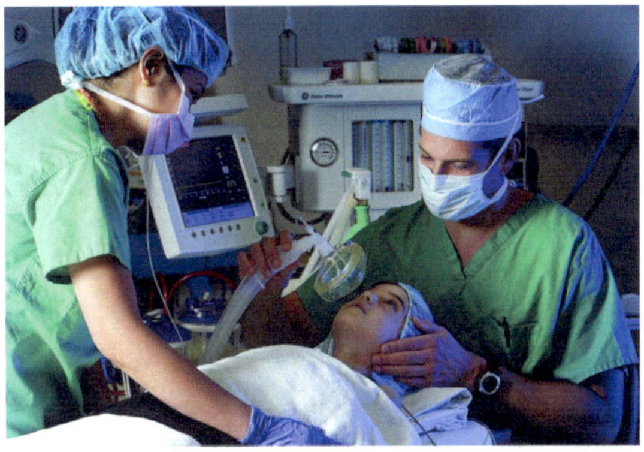

Figure 9.2. Importance of anesthesia in pediatric surgery.

Source: https://wpcdn.us-midwest-1.vip.tn-cloud.net/www.healthandlifemags.com/content/uploads/data-import/3e7e34de/042112SC5ii_133-1024x683.jpg.

9.1. Physiological Differences in Children

Learning Outcome

1. Understand the anatomical differences in kids versus adults.
2. Get the drug dosing right in kids.
3. Get the right anesthetic dosage for pediatric patients.

Children's bodies grow up differently than adults, and that's something to keep in mind when it comes to anesthesia. For example, a kid's breathing and heart systems aren't fully developed yet—this means how drugs work can vary quite a bit. In most cases, children show a faster metabolism and need more oxygen, so even small doses of anesthesia have to be picked carefully. Their makeup is also unique, with generally more water and less fat in their bodies; this shift affects how medicine spreads and leaves the body. All these points, when taken together, point to the need for anesthesia plans that fit each child's unique physiology—ensuring safety and effectiveness in the OR. Pain management in children isn't a straightforward matter either. According to the ESPA Pain Management Ladder, matching pain relief to the level of surgical stress and the natural differences in pain responses is key. Kids don't merely grow desensitized to repeated discomfort—they often report more distress even when they've been through similar experiences before. So, it's not all about the drugs; it's also about blending in psychological approaches, like using cognitive-behavioral therapy alongside proper prep, to calm nerves and help them cope better. Generally speaking, this mixed approach, which taps into the little nuances of childhood physiology, plays an important role in making the surgical process less overwhelming for young patients (Adamek et al., 2018). Handling procedural pain in children requires recognizing not just the physical differences but also the emotional ups and ds they experience. Take young patients in oncology, for instance—they often face a string of painful treatments that can add to their distress and overall sense of well-being. Approaches such as using local anesthesia and conscious sedation are tailored to meet the unique pain thresholds found in many of these cases. Beyond that, modern pediatric anesthesia protocols now stress careful pain evaluations and the use of several pain relief methods simultaneously—what some might call multimodal analgesia—to address a child's specific needs. As research keeps pushing forward, the focus on evidence-based, individualized pain management strategies remains crucial to safeguard both the physical and emotional health of children throughout their treatment journey (Liossi et al., 1999).

9.1.1. Differences in Anatomy and Physiology

Anatomical differences in kids versus adults play a huge role in pediatric anesthesia. Kids' airway structures differ quite a bit – think about it, in infants and toddlers the larynx sits higher in the neck, so the gap between the larynx and the tongue's base is shorter, which can trip up intubation. Their trachea is also slimmer and a bit more flexible, so handling the airway and keeping a good ventilation flow becomes more of a challenge. It's crucial for anesthesiologists to get these unique features because they bump up the risk of airway blockages, meaning that specialized techniques and equipment are usually necessary, as noted in the pediatric anesthesia literature (Kaye et al., 2020). But it doesn't stop with anatomy. The physiological side of things adds another layer of complexity when giving anesthesia to little ones. Kids tend to have their set of metabolic speeds, blood flow patterns, and breathing rhythms that differ from adults. Generally speaking, infants run a higher basal metabolic rate, so they need more oxygen and have a lower tolerance for pauses in breathing – even a short spell of apnea can turn into a serious issue, requiring quick moves to avoid complications. Plus, with kidneys and livers that aren't fully mature, drug behavior in the body ends up being a bit unpredictable, which calls for extra caution when adjusting dosages and timing to prevent side effects. These unique bodily responses underline why standard anesthesia protocols just don't fit when it comes to pediatric patients (Engelhardt et al., 2019). Overall, these anatomical and physiological quirks seriously affect clinical practice, especially in the realm of airway management. Airway troubles are far more common in pediatric anesthesia, so it doesn't work to simply adapt adult methods on a smaller scale. The lack of well-defined, kid-specific guidelines makes handling airway emergencies even tougher and ramps up the risks for young patients. Since most current algorithms lean on adult models, it's clear that approaches need to be tailored to fit the developmental and anatomical factors of children. In most cases, creating detailed, kid-focused frameworks is essential for guiding anesthesiologists through safe airway management and proper anesthesia administration (Engelhardt et al., 2019) (Figure 9.3).

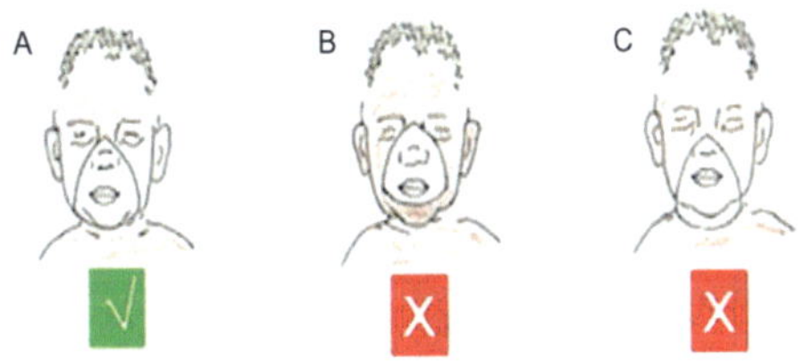

Figure 9.3. Anatomy of adults versus pediatric airway.

Source: Ibarra-Sarlat, M., Terrones-Vargas, E., Romero-Espinoza, L., Castañeda-Muciño, G., Herrera-Landero, A., & Núñez-Enríquez, J. C. (2018). Endotracheal Intubation in Children: Practice Recommendations, Insights, and Future Directions. InTech. doi: 10.5772/intechopen.70356.

9.1.2. Impact on Drug Metabolism

Getting drug dosing right in kids is no easy task. A mix of factors—enzyme quirks, organ maturity, and natural body differences—can change how a drug behaves. Take anesthetics, for instance. The way metabolic pathways slowly come online has a big say in how these agents work; in kids, propofol's journey through the body reveals just how varied things can be. Recent studies generally suggest that allometric scaling works pretty well for predicting its movement among different groups, but in the first year of life, those models need some serious altering because developmental changes run wild. So, clinicians, by and large, must stay on their toes to adjust dosing safely during procedures. Sometimes, though, the picture grows even more complicated. Certain treatments, like extracorporeal membrane oxygenation (ECMO), wind up shifting a child's physiology in unexpected ways, thereby upsetting the usual drug models. Kids on ECMO often show exposure changes that may weaken a drug's desired effect while upping the risk for side effects—an interplay that, in most cases, is drug-specific and still not fully figured out. In effect, this means that tailoring dosing strategies especially for these vulnerable patients isn't just a nice idea—it's an absolute must. New monitoring techniques also bring a breath of fresh air to this tricky scenario. Honest truth: traditional anesthetic depth monitors might not measure up correctly for children, yet emerging tech seems to offer a better glimpse into how anesthetics trigger pharmacodynamic responses. This extra clarity can help fine-tune dosing in ways that were hard to imagine before, particularly when data on pediatric anesthetic responses to agents like propofol is rather scarce. Overall, mixing a good grasp of drug metabolism nuances with these technological advances might just be the key to improving safety and outcomes in pediatric anesthesia.

9.1.3. Considerations for Anesthetic Dosage

Getting the right anesthetic dosage for pediatric patients is a real juggling act. Kids aren't just mini adults—their metabolic rates, body makeup, and organ maturity all vary, so a dose that works for grown-ups often just doesn't fit. Because children tend to process medications faster, using standard adult doses usually misses the mark. Sometimes, if the dosage isn't tuned to their needs, complications like emergence agitation can crop up. Research generally shows that when anesthetic techniques are adapted for each child, adverse effects drop and outcomes improve. In bridging textbook guidelines and everyday practice, healthcare teams can end up crafting personalized plans that make a difference (Cockrell et al., 2020). Monitoring anesthetic levels during procedures is just as crucial. A child's age, weight, and any pre-existing conditions all factor into finding that perfect dose—it isn't a one-size-fits-all deal. Paying close attention to these details helps reduce risks while ensuring the medicine does exactly what it's supposed to. Modern monitoring tech allows practitioners to catch changes in real time sometimes, and adjust doses on the fly, keeping things safe yet effective. Even emerging evidence suggests that a custom approach not only boosts patient safety but also cuts recovery times and minimizes post-surgery hiccups. By focusing on these tailored strategies, doctors can improve care and reduce on distressing side effects, leaving everyone more satisfied overall (Piccini et al., 2024). Meanwhile, fresh research into drug development and delivery methods adds new twists to the story of pediatric anesthetic dosing. Newer agents and refined techniques now let clinicians alter how deep and long anesthesia runs, offering sharper control than ever before. Understanding how these drugs move and work inside the body is key—because even a slight miscalculation might result in unwanted issues like heightened anxiety during recovery. In most cases, evidence-based guidelines paired with ongoing studies underscore the need to keep practices updated. That's why regularly refreshing pediatric anesthesia protocols with the latest scientific insights is so important for safeguarding these vulnerable patients (Cockrell et al., 2020).

Test Your Knowledge

1. What are the anatomical differences between adults and children?
2. How to get the right anesthetic dosage for pediatric patients?

9.2. Types of Anesthesia Used in Pediatrics

Learning Outcome

1. Describe the general anesthesia and regional anesthesia
2. Understand the sedation techniques

Anesthesia for kids can be truly tricky—children simply don't react the same way as adults. Generally speaking, many operations lean on general anesthesia (GA) to knock a patient into a deep sleep where pain and awareness are pretty much muted. Still, dosing calls for a tailored touch since youngsters break down medications in their unpredictable way. Just consider that in some cases—for example, kids with achondroplasia needing a dynamic MRI—doctors must assess the cervical spine with great care to avoid complications (Masarwy et al., 2025). Clearly, picking the right anesthesia isn't just another step; it's essential for keeping safety high and treatment effective. RA has been gaining ground in pediatric care too, mainly because it limits the overall exposure to drugs while still keeping pain in check. Techniques like nerve blocks and epidurals now crop up to target very specific areas, often reducing the necessity for all-out GA with all its possible drawbacks. For instance, a lumbar plexus block can be especially useful for children undergoing lower extremity surgery, making the discomfort more manageable and helping speed up recovery. This method fits snugly with the current trend toward multimodal pain relief—in line with enhanced recovery after surgery (ERAS) protocols that aim to reduce on opioids. Meanwhile, ongoing improvements in ultrasound technology only boost the safety and effectiveness of these regional techniques. Sedation, on the other hand, plays its crucial role, particularly for non-invasive procedures where a full anesthetic might be overkill. Some new agents like remimazolam have caught attention because they're fast acting and wear off quickly usually causing minimal respiratory depression (Bai et al., 2024). This quick turnaround is a big plus for young patients, many of whom become quite anxious or upset during procedures. Even so, the use of remimazolam in children still sparks debate; there isn't a clear consensus yet on its safety and benefits. More research and clinical studies are definitely needed to iron out proper guidelines and keep pace with the ever-evolving field of pediatric anesthesia, ensuring that kids receive the best possible care (Figure 9.4).

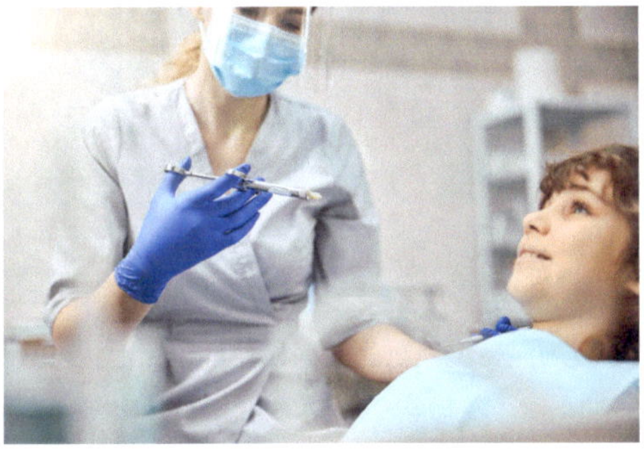

Figure 9.4. Anesthesia for kids.

Source: https://srikrishnahospitals.co.in/wp-content/uploads/sites/22/2024/08/Pediatric-Anesthesia.png.

9.2.1. General Anesthesia (GA)

Kids in dentistry often bring a mix of challenges. Treating little ones, especially those who don't easily cooperate or who present special healthcare needs (SHCN), can stir up extra complications. GA steps in as a key helper here—it's not just about putting a patient to sleep but about letting dentists carry out thorough dental rehab in ways that keep everyone safe and things under control. It's clear that when behavior issues pop up during treatments, GA isn't only a tool for numbing pain; it also helps overcome the emotional hurdles that can trip up the process, especially with kids whose age or behavior makes treatment trickier. If you take a closer look at the profiles of patients receiving GA, you start noticing some interesting differences between generally healthy kids and those with SHCN. Research generally shows that the latter tend to be older and often face more complex treatments, like extractions, which in turn lead to longer hospital stays and a need for more preoperative consultations (Al-Khotani A et al., 2025). These facts raise questions about tailoring dental care so that each unique patient's needs are met. As dental teams try out different approaches and alter their methods, the patterns in these studies keep nudging them toward creating more individual care plans that work well regardless of a child's overall health. Then there's the whole logistics side of GA in pediatric dentistry. When you dig into the details, factors like how long the anesthesia lasts and a patient's overall health play a big role. Many kids treated with GA fit into the American Society of Anesthesiologists physical status groups, with most falling under ASA I – which means they have little to no systemic disease (Dinc et al., 2024). This emphasizes the need for careful pre-op evaluations to catch any potential risks. Also, knowing that the average GA length often hinges on the dental procedure's complexity can help clinics run a bit more smoothly. To summarize, these insights not only shape best practices in pediatric anesthesia but also steer us toward better health outcomes for young patients (Figure 9.5).

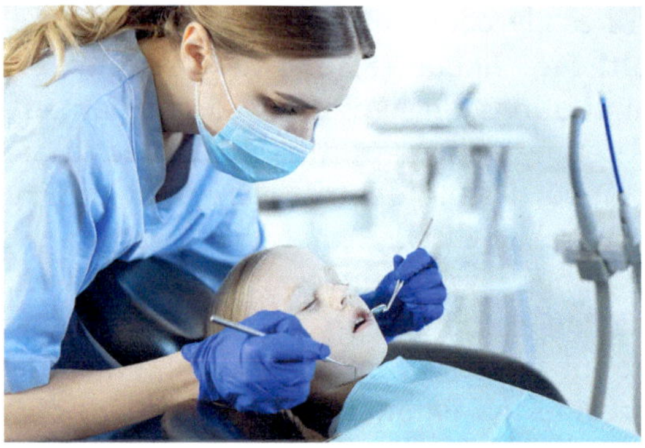

Figure 9.5. General anesthesia for children during dental procedures.

Source: https://www.drmichaels.com/wp-content/uploads/2022/02/images_blog_2018_general-anesthesia-for-kids.webp.

9.2.2. Regional Anesthesia (RA)

RA in kids uses a mix of methods to ease pain while keeping overall side effects low. Kids tend to feel pain differently and react in their ways—so altering these techniques is pretty important. For instance, nerve blocks can reduce on the pain kids experience after surgeries like hernia repairs or orthopedic fixes. Generally speaking, research shows that when experienced providers do these blocks, they usually boost pain relief and help kids bounce back faster, often shortening hospital stays. Outpatient procedures have also benefited; many children now face less anxiety and enjoy smoother recoveries, which boosts satisfaction for both them and their caregivers. Looking at anesthesia providers, it's hard not to notice the special role played by dentist anesthesiologists in pediatric care. Recent studies reveal that these specialists often handle GA for young children, especially during dental rehabilitation for early childhood caries. This practice, which is quite different from the typically adult-focused, often shorter duration procedures in hospitals, stands out as unique. To put it in perspective, when comparing 7133 office-based anesthetic encounters done by dentist anesthesiologists with 106,420 predominantly operating room anesthetics, the numbers underscore their knack for managing more complex pediatric cases. Overall, these findings point to the critical part these specialized providers play in improving surgical outcomes and streamlining pediatric anesthesia care (Saxen et al., 2017). Even though advancements in RA have been well documented, making these techniques accessible in low- and middle-income countries (LMIC) remains a challenge. There are noticeable barriers in these regions that create a significant gap in pediatric surgical care. Quite a few kids in LMIC suffer from conditions that RA could handle effectively, yet the services are still very limited. Practical initiatives aimed at boosting surgical care in these areas often require genuine, context-specific collaborations between institutions. While the awareness of disparities in pediatric surgical care has grown, ramping up the use of RA services in such settings could improve outcomes for some of our most vulnerable populations (Fezeu et al., 2018) (Figure 9.6).

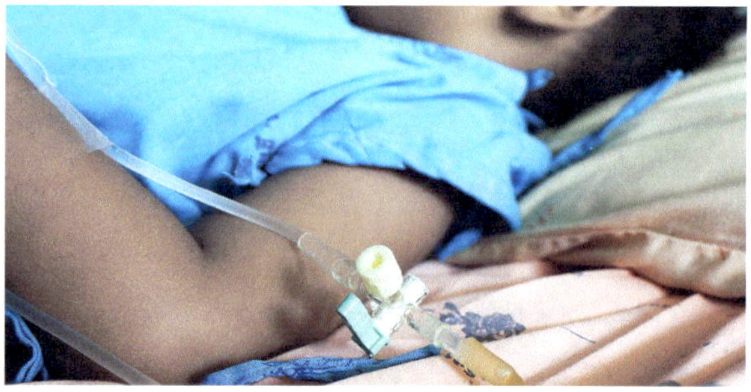

Figure 9.6. Pediatric regional anesthesia (RA).

Source: https://www.upstate.edu/anesthesiology/images/headers/header-pediatric-regional-anesthesiology.jpg.

9.2.3. Sedation Techniques

Handling anesthesia for kids can be a real puzzle. Doctors need to juggle different sedation methods to keep young patients both safe and comfortable. Lately, many have turned to RA—a method that zeroes in on pain and lowers whole-body complications. With ultrasound guidance in play, specialists can deliver more accurate nerve blocks that respect the small anatomical details unique to children. This trick lessens the heavy reliance on systemic opioids and even lowers the risk of breathing issues and other mishaps. Studies, in most cases, show that RA can smooth out recovery and improve surgical outcomes, making it a handy part of the pediatric anesthesia toolkit (Reysner et al., 2025). Trying out new twists, some clinicians are also exploring pediatric hypnosis as an alternative way to ease anxiety and pain during procedures. There's evidence suggesting that mixing in hypnosis—think guided imagery and simple relaxation techniques—can enhance a child's overall experience before and during an intervention. This method cuts back on the need for powerful drugs, reducing side effects and even lessening environmental impact, which fits a more sustainable care model. As more practitioners notice that a calm mind can change a body's response, hypnosis is slowly becoming a promising partner to traditional sedation methods (Lauder et al., 2024). Rolling out these varied sedation techniques underscores the need for specialized training and hands-on expertise among healthcare teams. Kids aren't just little adults—their physical makeup and emotional responses are uniquely different. For example, the choice between a regional block or adding hypnosis depends on factors like the child's developmental stage, past medical history, and the specific demands of the procedure. In most cases, staying updated through ongoing education and fresh research is key to fine-tuning these methods and exploring newer alternatives for improved outcomes. To summarize, the evolution of sedation practices isn't only about managing pain and easing anxiety; it's also about keeping patient safety and overall comfort at the heart of every intervention (Lauder et al., 2024; Reysner et al., 2025) (Figure 9.7).

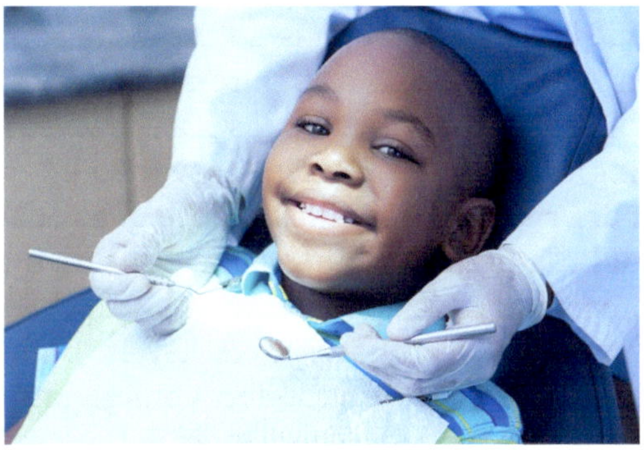

Figure 9.7. Sedation techniques for children.

Source: https://www.titan-dental.ca/wp-content/uploads/2022/05/types-of-sedation-techniques-for-children.jpg.

Test Your Knowledge

1. What is general anesthesia?
2. What do you mean by sedation techniques?

9.3. Preoperative Assessment

Learning Outcome

1. Understand the importance of medical history.
2. Discuss physical examination protocols.
3. Understand the psychological considerations for pediatric patients.

A solid preoperative check is essential when kids are headed for anesthesia. It's not just a checklist—it's about spotting anything that might tip the balance on safety or how smoothly the anesthesia and surgery come out. Kids have unique bodies and feelings, so the usual routine often needs a custom twist. Pre-surgery anxiety hits many of these little ones hard, sometimes setting them up for longer recoveries or extra pain afterward. Sometimes, a dose of a sedative and a little understanding can cut through that tension; it all adds up to a smoother experience. Getting these aspects right is key in building a safe, supportive space for young patients (Stant et al., 2025). Then there's the fasting issue, which plays a big role too. Longer fasting times not only stress out kids but also weigh on their families, occasionally even leading to complications once the surgery's over. The American Society of Anesthesiologists now suggests that kids can have clear liquids right up to about two hours before the operation. This change is meant to shrink those hunger gaps and help get better cooperation on surgery day. Sadly, many surgical centers haven't fully caught on to these updated guidelines, which means pre-surgery care can be a bit all over the place. Some systematic steps—like quick educational sessions for the nurses—might go a long way toward making sure families feel looked after and in the know (Mickolyzck et al., 2023). In the end, the preoperative review isn't just about flagging risks; it also builds a bridge for real conversation between medical teams and families. It digs into not only a child's medical history and physical state but also gets a sense of their everyday life. When anesthesiologists and surgical teams take the time to see what makes each child unique, they can whip up care plans that truly match the situation. Family insights, along with personal experiences, add an extra layer that builds trust across the board. These collaborative efforts often lead to smoother outcomes and leave everyone feeling more confident about the process. Ultimately, a well-thought-out preoperative assessment goes beyond just the clinical facts—it helps foster an environment of care and understanding for both kids and their families (Mickolyzck et al., 2023; Stant et al., 2025) (Figure 9.8).

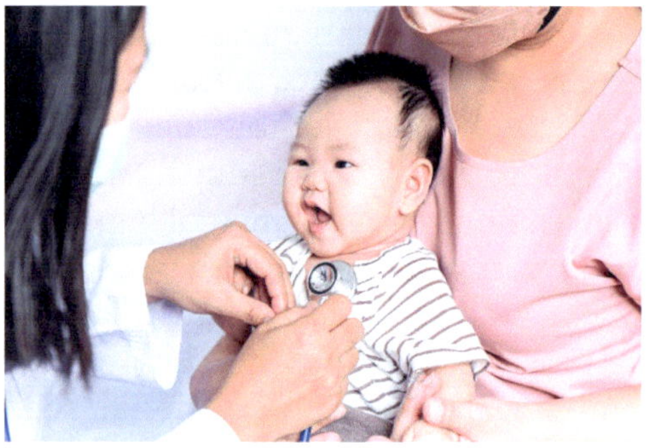

Figure 9.8. Pediatric preoperative assessment.

Source: https://montrealchildrenshospital.ca/wp-content/uploads/2013/03/AdobeStock_519816440-scaled.jpeg.

9.3.1. Importance of Medical History

Knowing a child's past health details plays a key role when planning anesthesia for young patients. It isn't merely a file of records – it tells us about prior conditions, surgeries, and any unusual responses to anesthesia. Kids often react differently than adults, and certain anesthetic agents may not be handled as well by them. Having this background helps spot things like asthma, allergies or even developmental hurdles that might call for a special approach. In most cases, a careful look at the history lets anesthesiologists lower risks and fine-tune care for both safety and effectiveness. In pediatric surgery the emotional state of both the young patient and the caregiver matters a lot. Knowing a childs' history—yes, all the details from past procedures—helps address worries that might pop up during pre-op chats. Sometimes, snippets from earlier surgeries guide doctors in tackling preoperative jitters, which can be common among kids and their families. For example, one study on Clown Doctors found that caregiver anxiety is linked to the child's overall health and past surgical experiences (Arriaga et al., 2016). This kind of background not only builds rapport, but it also fosters an environment where both sides feel understood and supported. Sharing a complete history among healthcare providers genuinely boosts teamwork. When surgeons, anesthesiologists and other team members are on the same page about a child's health background, even the trickier cases with coexisting issues tend to be handled better. This kind of collaboration is often highlighted by initiatives like those mentioned in the University of Iowa Department of Anesthesia newsletter, where better info sharing paves the way for improved outcomes. Ultimately, having a detailed record does more than inform decisions—it helps weave a holistic approach to pediatric anesthesia that prioritizes both safety and overall care.

9.3.2. Physical Examination Protocols

Pediatric anesthesia is tricky—it pushes us to rethink how we carry out exams designed just for kids. Every child's development shifts how we evaluate them, so doing a proper preop check isn't optional if we want things to be both safe and effective. Instead of following a fixed formula, the process dives into a child's medical history—spotting preexisting conditions and flagging potential anesthesia issues along the way. A hands-on physical exam, which often uncovers unique anatomical quirks or subtle physiological differences among young patients, plays a big role here. In taking note of these details, clinicians build up a real, in-depth picture of what each patient needs, allowing them to tailor anesthesia management to fit the individual health profile. This careful, family-focused approach ultimately helps forge a solid bond with both the child and the parent, highlighting its importance, especially in pediatric anesthesia (Sbaraglia et al., 2024). E-learning has been shaking up the way we train for these kinds of pediatric physical exams. Recent training modules, for instance, show genuine promise in boosting both theoretical know-how and hands-on skills—especially when examining tricky cases like Juvenile Idiopathic Arthritis (JIA). With structured online content, trainees get to practice key maneuvers and even interact with the material so that the learning sticks better. Data generally suggest that when practitioners measure things like maximal incisal openings and facial symmetry, they often perform better in real clinical settings. In most cases, this kind of formalized digital education underlines why having ongoing, standardized protocols isn't just a bonus but a necessity for honing pediatric examination skills (Pan et al., 2024). At the end of the day, mixing established exam methods with fresh educational ideas is shifting the care landscape in pediatric anesthesia. Using solid physical exam routines arms clinicians with the practical sense to make informed choices that boost both patient safety and overall anesthesia results. Plus, a commitment to continual learning and a methodical approach to assessments doesn't just standardize practice—it builds confidence among healthcare providers trying to deal with the unique twists of pediatric cases. When young patients come in with their very physiological challenges, sticking to these structured checks becomes even more crucial. In short, fusing detailed physical assessments with innovative training has set the stage for a real paradigm shift, one that aims for optimal anesthesia practices and better health outcomes for our most vulnerable patients (Sbaraglia et al., 2024) (Figure 9.9).

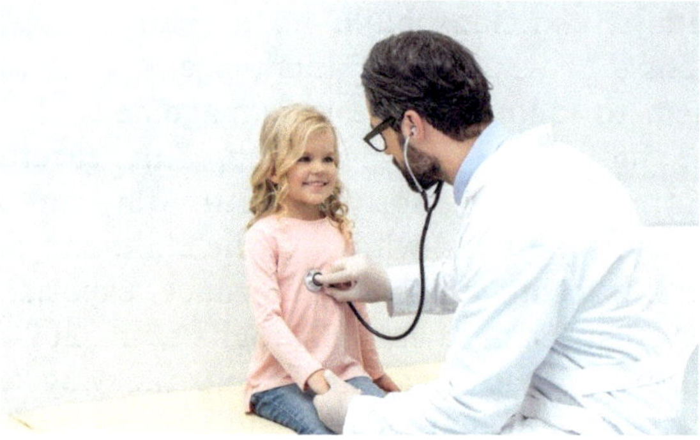

Figure 9.9. Physical examination.

Source: https://lagunabeachuc.com/wp-content/uploads/2024/04/child-physical-exam-.jpeg.

9.3.3. Psychological Considerations for Pediatric Patients

Many things affect how kids feel when they go under anesthesia. Kids get pretty anxious – it's a mix of being in a strange place, not having their parents nearby, and just being scared of getting hurt. Before any procedure, talking things through in a way they understand can help ease those worries. For instance, if you explain what's going on in simple, kid-friendly language, it kind of makes the whole experience less mysterious and even gives them a sense of control. Parents, of course, add a lot of comfort by being there. When they're involved, it tends to make the whole atmosphere a bit more relaxed, even though that underlying anxiety can still mess with not just how a kid feels, but also how well the anesthesia works overall. Deciding whether or not to sedate a child isn't only about the technical side of things – there's a whole other layer of emotional and ethical factors to consider. Take one situation: a parent, maybe due to previous experiences in a different system, asks for an unsedated esophagogastroduodenoscopy (EGD). This choice immediately stirs up some tricky ethical debates about what's best for the kid. Typically, sedation is the way to go, with the anesthesia, GI, and OR teams all saying it's key for the child's comfort and safety. Generally speaking, balancing what parents want with sound medical ethics isn't simple, yet it's vital for keeping the child emotionally safe. Such a balance not only leads to informed decisions but also builds trust and teamwork between the parent and the provider, as noted in (Calciano et al., 2024). Beyond managing anxiety, it's also important to consider how the body and mind work together when figuring out oxygen levels for kids under GA. There's still plenty of debate about what the best oxygen saturation levels should be because, well, kids aren't just tiny adults. Their stage of development means they react differently to anesthesia, which complicates how interventions should be handled. Any plan for managing oxygen has to think about both the physical mechanics and the emotional side of things – if oxygen levels stray too far from optimal, it might not only ramp up preoperative anxiety but also cause some post-surgery issues. In most cases, a rounded approach that mixes evidence about physical outcomes with the psychological impacts seems to be the best way forward, as elaborated in (Cho, 2023).

Test Your Knowledge

1. Why is history taking important in pediatrics?
2. What are the psychological considerations for pediatric patients?

9.4. Intraoperative Management

Learning Outcome

1. Learn about monitoring techniques.
2. Understand the anesthetic agents and their effects.
3. Describe the role of the anesthesiologist.

Managing anesthesia for kids during surgery isn't a one-size-fits-all deal—it calls for a careful, almost artisanal approach that fits each child's unique body needs. Age, weight, and any existing health issues all mix into the decision on which anesthetic techniques to use and how to keep a steady watch on the patient. You end up constantly checking vital signs like heart rate, blood pressure, and oxygen levels because there's barely any room for error with pediatric patients. Getting the anesthesia depth just right is crucial, not only to keep the child unaware during the operation but also to manage their pain properly. And when the surgery gets trickier—as with cases dealing with congenital heart defects—the process ramps up with a need for more advanced monitoring and quick, on-the-fly decisions to keep everything, like blood flow, running smoothly (Saracoglu and Salman, 2025). Picking the right anesthesia method is a big part of the job too; it's about more than just comfort—it actually helps steer the overall surgical outcome. Increasingly, doctors are turning to a mix of regional with GA, a trend that's hard to ignore nowadays. For example, using local anesthetics during procedures like circumcision has shown, in most cases, to lessen pain and improve the experience for the patient (Haqi et al., 2025). Surgeons and anesthesiologists typically team up closely, double-checking their plans to reduce on physiological stress. This kind of cooperation is built on a clear sense of what each technique brings to the table, its ups and downs, and making sure that pain management not only works well but also fits with the broader goals of caring for these young patients. Talking things over openly is another key ingredient. Whether it's a quick chat among the team or a more detailed conversation with the child's guardians, clear communication goes a long way. When families understand the planned techniques and what to expect after surgery, it builds trust and eases their worries—even if just a bit. And when the whole crew keeps the lines open, potential problems can be spotted and handled pretty fast. Overall, effective intraoperative management depends on a solid grasp of pediatric physiology, a team that jells together, and communication channels that aren't too fussy but work well to keep safety and comfort front and center (Haqi et al., 2025; Saracoglu and Salman, 2025) (Figure 9.10).

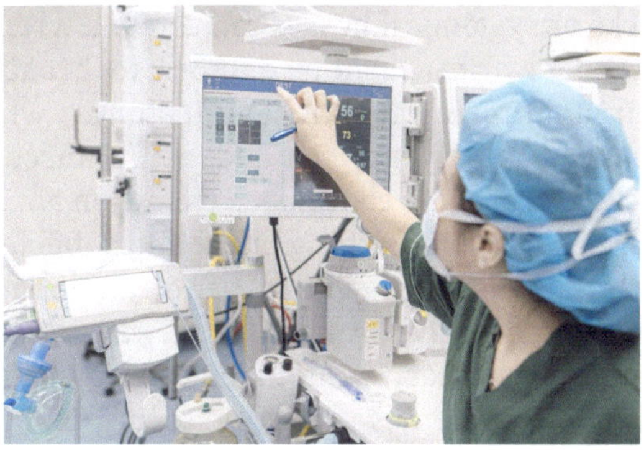

Figure 9.10. Intraoperative Management.

Source: https://xenonhealth.com/wp-content/uploads/2021/05/intraoperativehypertension.jpeg.

9.4.1. Monitoring Techniques

Kids aren't just miniature adults – their bodies work differently, which makes keeping an eye on them during anesthesia super important. Their development isn't a straight line, so doctors rely on advanced monitoring systems that dish out real-time info on things like heart rate, blood pressure and oxygen levels; even a slight wobble might signal trouble. Capnography, for example, checks carbon dioxide levels, which matters for little ones who can be extra prone to breathing hiccups. All these bits of data let anesthesiologists decide on the fly and keep things on track during surgery. Recent research has shown that monitoring methods need a personal touch when it comes to kids. Studies like APRICOT and NECTARINE—yes, real European comparisons—reveal wide gaps in how different clinics handle pediatric cases. In many cases, particularly with low-weight or very young infants, even small errors in keeping tabs on vital signs can have big consequences. Generally speaking, blending a mix of invasive and non-invasive techniques helps form a robust system, and these findings shed light on creating faster, more effective response plans for kids undergoing anesthesia (Castellheim et al., 2025). Tough pediatric airways add another layer of complexity. Conditions such as congenital quirks or systemic illnesses can throw a wrench into the works, pushing doctors to broaden their monitoring toolkit. For instance, when advanced airway devices and neuromuscular blockers are in use, continuous checks on airway openness and breathing mechanics become essential—missing even a beat can lead to dire outcomes like hypoxia or airway trauma. A multidisciplinary, sometimes even a slightly messy, approach to tracking these changes can make a difference in keeping these young patients safe during and after their procedures (Michał Łepik et al., 2024).

9.4.2. Anesthetic Agents and Their Effects

Pediatric anesthesia isn't just about putting kids to sleep—it's about considering what these drugs might quietly do to a child's developing brain. One study with around 200 children found an interesting pattern: when doctors use volatile agents or mix several anesthetics together, there's a notable IQ dip—about 9.1 points in cases where multiple agents are used. Propofol, on the other hand, seems to be a bit gentler, showing only around a 3.2 point drop, which in most cases suggests it could be a safer option. All this makes it clear that choosing the right drug matters, and clinicians need to keep an eye on potential long-term effects that might sneak in later (Dandemmanavar et al., 2025). Beyond just choosing the anesthetics, the way we monitor kids during these procedures has seen some big changes recently. Intraoperative electroencephalography (EEG) now gives us a live peek into a child's brain response, so dosing can be adjusted on the fly—even if sometimes the details get a bit tangled. This kind of real-time brain feedback is especially handy for children who don't follow the typical developmental script or when the surgery brings extra challenges; it helps avoid overly deep sedation that can happen with older dosing methods. In a sense, EEG-guided management is like adding a safety net—one that reduces risks in ways that traditional methods just can't match, making it part and parcel of modern pediatric anesthesia (Bong et al., 2024). The impact of these anesthetic choices stretches way beyond the operating room, affecting long-term cognitive outcomes in ways that aren't always immediately obvious. Post-procedure assessments show mixed results, hinting that not only does longer exposure tend to correlate with lower IQ scores, but each drug comes with its set of risks. Generally speaking, this complexity calls for more research and for clinicians to revisit and fine-tune their protocols over time. It's a puzzle where strategies like parental education, probing safer drug alternatives, and blending in neurophysiological monitoring all seem to play key roles in aiming for the best possible outcomes for these young patients (Bong et al., 2024; Dandemmanavar et al., 2025).

9.4.3. Role of the Anesthesiologist

Giving anesthesia to kids isn't just about dropping a drug. It starts with a thorough check-up—digging into the child's history, spotting any red flags, and planning out the approach since little ones react in their quirky ways. Generally speaking, a full pre-surgery review often means chatting with parents and caregivers to clear up what's coming, ease any worries, and build that all-important trust; after all, calming a child's nerves can shape both the emotional experience and how smoothly everything goes (Davenport et al., 2020). Sometimes, the process feels more like a conversation than a checklist, with each detail weaving into the next. Inside the operating room, things don't simply fall into a neat routine. The anesthesiologist keeps a close eye on vital signs, administers fluids, and stays ready for any hiccups that show up unexpectedly. Kids can throw curveballs—rapid shifts in their condition demand that the doc be nimble and ready to switch gears in real-time. A moment of calm decisiveness can change the outcome when, say, a sudden spike in stress throws the situation off balance (Polites and Azarow, 2020). In this fast-paced setting, ensuring the drugs work right means less discomfort and fewer issues after surgery. Finishing the surgery isn't the end of the story; recovery kicks off another crucial phase where the anesthesiologist still plays a big part. Kids might experience everything from mild discomfort to bouts of nausea or unexpected breathing challenges if things haven't gone exactly as planned. Here, doctors stick around to manage pain, watch for issues like airway blockages, and even explain what to expect as recovery unfolds. They spend time educating parents on aftercare and what warning signs to look out for (Davenport et al., 2020; Polites and Azarow, 2020). To summarize, the approach hangs on a blend of technical know-how and simple, honest communication—both key for keeping things as safe and smooth as possible (Figure 9.11).

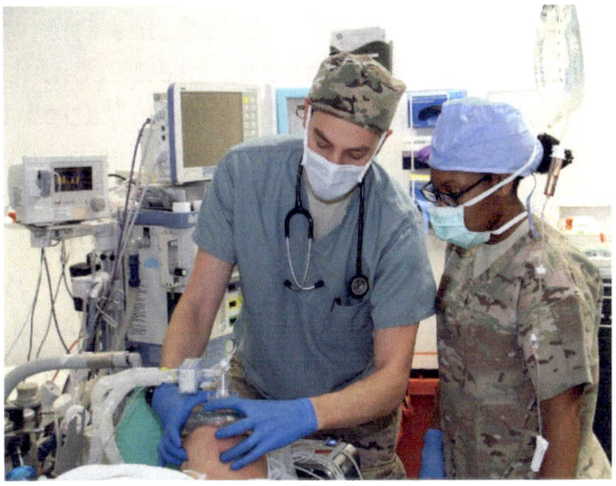

Figure 9.11. Anesthesiologist.

Source: https://upload.wikimedia.org/wikipedia/commons/7/74/Physician_anesthesiologist.jpg.

Test Your Knowledge

1. Describe the anesthetic agents and their effects.
2. What is the role of the anesthesiologist?

9.5. Postoperative Care

Learning Outcome

1. Understand the recovery room protocols.
2. Describe the pain management strategies.
3. Understand the potential complications and their management.

Postoperative care for kids is vital—it's not just about cleaning up after a procedure but also about easing the unwanted side effects of anesthesia. Kids can wake up pretty confused; this kind of pediatric emergence agitation not only drops satisfaction ratings but also hikes up care costs and can lead to more complications. We still aren't 100% sure why it happens, though research points to a mix of factors, so even small changes in how anesthesia is given might help. A systematic review even pointed out that what we know from evidence doesn't always match what happens in real life, which kind of throws the spotlight on the need for clear best-practice guidelines. The way these guidelines were developed and later double-checked by experts shows that a bit of thoughtful altering in pediatric anesthesia can boost outcomes and lower post-op issues (Cockrell et al., 2020). Pain management also plays a huge role in recovery, especially for young patients undergoing surgeries below the belly button. GA used to be the default, but since it isn't great at keeping pain at bay for long periods, folks have started looking at other methods. For example, mixing in caudal blocks with GA has shown to work better for controlling pain and reducing on opioid use after surgery. This method even helps stabilize heart rates during recovery—a bonus when you consider all the ups and downs that can happen. Using models like the Johns Hopkins Evidence-Based Practice approach, looking back at old case data offers some solid insights for setting up pain management protocols that fit how kids respond (Allen et al., 2023). When it comes to making sure kids recover well overall, you can't just focus on pain. Broad, all-around postoperative care also means offering a bit of psychological support and keeping a close watch for any anesthesia side effects. Take the FLACC (Face, Legs, Activity, Cry, and Consolability) scoring system, for instance; it lets healthcare providers get a read on pain levels in kids who can't exactly explain how they feel—helping to catch issues before they get worse. And when parents or caregivers get involved in creating a supportive recovery setting, it makes a difference for everyone involved. In short, mixing expert-approved guidelines, smart pain control, and a dose of emotional support seems to be the key to making the whole post-op experience a whole lot smoother for pediatric patients (Cockrell et al., 2020) (Figure 9.12).

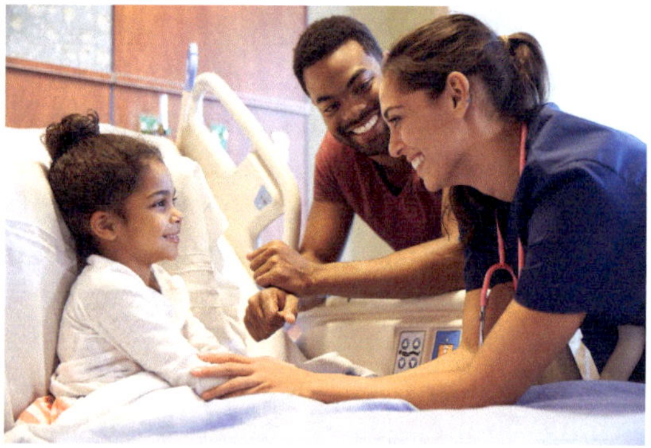

Figure 9.12. Postoperative care for kids.

Source: https://www.newarkadvocate.com/gcdn/presto/2021/10/15/PNEW/66047610-9b7b-458e-bda7-f8e401c09fed-Active_Fit_Surgery.jpg.

9.5.1. Recovery Room Protocols

Pediatric anesthesia cares deeply about how kids bounce back after surgery. Kids can react in many ways—physically and emotionally—so, right after the operation, it's crucial to watch things like heart rate, blood pressure, and oxygen levels closely to catch problems like breathing hiccups or unstable circulation early. The recovery room isn't just a sterile space, either; it's a place that should feel a bit comforting—having a favorite toy, a familiar blanket, or something of that sort can ease a child's anxiety. In many cases, tailoring care to match what each child seems to need makes a difference in how quickly they recover. How you sedate the patient plays a big role, too. Recent work suggests that mixing an initial, slightly dissociative dose of ketamine with the usual propofol can actually speed things up in the recovery phase (Ahmed et al., 2016). One study, for instance, tossed around two methods: one relying only on propofol and the other using both ketamine and propofol. Generally speaking, the kids in the mixed group recovered faster even though their procedures lasted a bit longer. This seems to be because adding ketamine lets doctors use less propofol overall, which means less lingering sedation after surgery and a quicker return to stability.

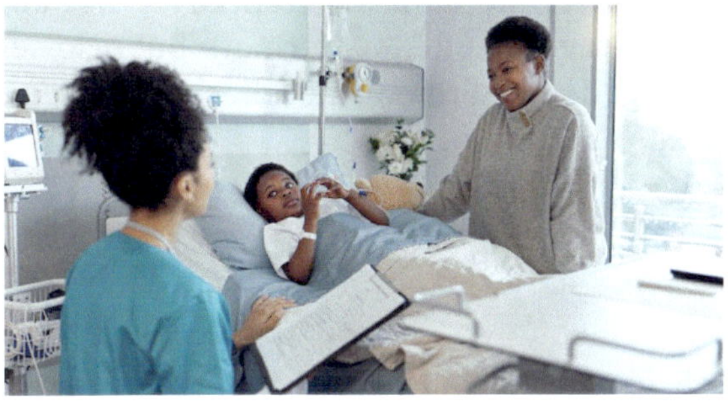

Figure 9.13. Recovery room protocols.

Source: https://img.freepik.com/premium-photo/mother-nurse-black-kid-patient-hospital-recovery-surgery-congenital-heart-disease-checkup-sick-cardiology-medical-worker-with-african-mom-child-postoperative-care_590464-456414.jpg.

Getting everyone to work together—the surgeons, anesthesia providers, and nurses—is another piece of the puzzle in these routines. Clear, on-the-fly communication means that post-op checks happen without delay and any issues are caught quickly. In many cases, recovery protocols in the post-anesthesia care unit (PACU) include steps like using the Aldrete scoring system, which looks at how alert a kid is, how active they are, and whether their circulation is steady. When every team member is in the loop and follows a shared set of guidelines, it creates a kind of well-rounded, patient-focused approach that helps kids get back on track after their procedures (Figure 9.13).

9.5.2. Pain Management Strategies

Kids' pain management needs special care because their bodies and minds don't just work like adults.' Using RA methods—like epidural analgesia—has started to catch the eye of many experts. In fact, some studies show that placing a thoracic epidural, even for children with mild spina bifida undergoing big surgeries, can be pretty safe. One study even found that those kids ended up needing far fewer opioids while keeping pain levels stable (Cain et al., 2018). All of this seems to help make the overall surgical experience far more kind and effective for the kids. There's also a big push to mix in psychological approaches along with drugs. Many kids facing painful procedures related to serious illnesses often seem more upset at the idea of pain than the pain itself (Liossi et al., 1999). Techniques like cognitive-behavioral therapy and simple preparation steps are proving useful in calming nerves. I mean, by helping kids see and think about pain in a different light—and even by using distraction methods such as virtual reality or interactive play—doctors are noticing improvements in how well kids handle both the discomfort and the fear. In most cases, these added layers help ease both body and mind during those tricky pre- and post-surgery moments. On top of that, blending drug-based with non-drug methods is key to covering all the bases. Generally speaking, customizing pain relief to each child's quirks can make a huge difference. For example, aside from using local anesthetics and sedation, it's vital that healthcare providers know just how to assess pain levels with scales that take into account what makes pediatric patients unique. Open, sometimes imperfect, communication among medical teams, the patients, and their families also plays a big part - even if the wording isn't always spot-on. To summarize, this well-rounded approach—which ties together care for both the body and the mind— shows a solid commitment to patient-centered pediatric anesthesia care.

9.5.3. Potential Complications and Their Management

Pediatric anesthesia isn't just about putting a kid to sleep—it's a tricky adventure where things might go sideways if not kept in check. Kids have their style; their bodies and innate quirks, like congenital issues and systemic quirks, demand a special approach when handling their airways. It's not hard to see how something as seemingly simple as a poor mask fit might turn into a failed intubation or leave them short on oxygen. A careful, hands-on check before surgery, along with a real sense of what risks might pop up, usually goes a long way in dodging these pitfalls. A diverse crew—pediatric anesthesiologists, ENT specialists, and a few other pros—often comes together to use smart airway devices, constant monitoring, and, yes, plenty of thoughtful aftercare to keep everything on track. Meanwhile, a shift toward regional techniques, like thoracic epidural analgesia (TEA), has been catching on as another way to sidestep complications. In most cases, doctors have found that such methods reduce the reliance on heavy opioids while keeping post-surgery pain under better control. Take, for example, those kids with low-level spina bifida facing major lower urinary tract reconstruction; using a thoracic epidural not only didn't spark any major neurological mishaps but also slashed the need for opioids noticeably. This goes to show that when it comes to pain relief for young ones, tailoring the approach can help avoid the downsides of systemic drugs on developing brains—and often gets them back on their feet a bit faster. Then there's the whole issue of keeping a close watch after the procedure. Kids tend to be more unpredictable, and even small swings in their vital signs or side effects from anesthesia can matter a great deal. Regular checks of breathing, pain levels, and overall response in a controlled setting become a key step in nipping problems like aspiration or airway injuries in the bud. In many instances, when something unexpected does crop up, a quick, combined effort from both the anesthesia and surgery teams makes all the difference. This kind of thorough, sometimes even spur-of-the-moment monitoring not only helps in the immediate aftermath but also sets the stage for healthier, smoother recoveries of the line (Figure 9.14).

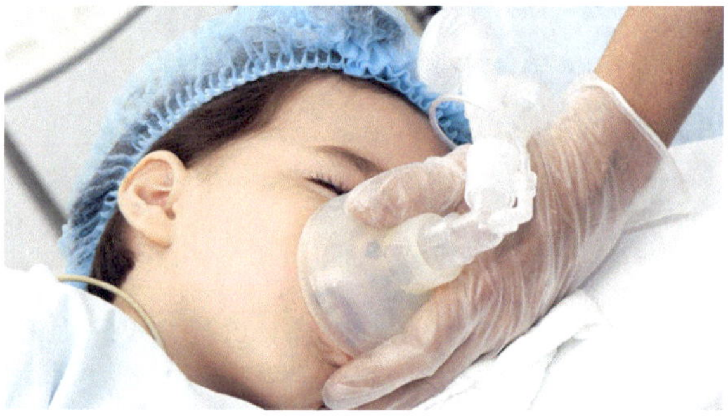

Figure 9.14. Avoiding anesthesia complications for kids.

Source: https://nortonchildrens.com/wp-content/uploads/anesthesia-1.jpg.

Test Your Knowledge

1. What are the pain management strategies?
2. Describe the potential complications and their management.

SUMMARY

Innovations in pediatric anesthesia keep advancing as we keep learning more about what children need both physically and psychologically. Research shows that severe accidents within procedures such as bone marrow aspirates or lumbar punctures happen but rarely, with serious complications reaching around 1.7%. Of course, at times in situations like premature birth and last-minute emergencies danger increases the possibility of respiratory complications (Dagher et al., 2024). This requires stringent pre-surgery testing to determine who might be at greater risk, and subsequently individualized anesthesia schedules to keep risks low.

Reducing preoperative anxiety is also an important consideration; it can decide how cooperative a child will be during procedures, and even affect the way they feel afterwards. Surveys reveal that, overall, there is significant heterogeneity in how physicians and nurses manage anxious children—newer practitioners or long-time practitioners sharing guidelines online. Ironically, working professionals online might not be exposed to as much specialized training, but still employ similar strategies used by experienced practitioners (Sablewski et al., 2024). And this leads us to the implication of taking on some principles in general so that everyone involved will have a good plan in place for managing anxiety, which should then make the whole thing easier for the child. In summary, pediatric anesthesia is a fine balance of safety, effectiveness, and even well-being. The data, it seems, highlights pre-surgical meticulous risk evaluations, though also indicates that being more unified in the treatment of anxiety is actually very important in general. For most, as this form of procedure increases, further research is essential in being able to bring forth best practices that ensure both physical health and comfort for young patients. Synthesizing these observations, the healthcare community is able to slowly close gaps in present practices—working to improve not only surgical outcomes but overall experience for our tiny tots.

Pediatric anesthesia is never the same from one moment to the next—new studies and day-to-day clinical events keep the pot boiling. Take, for instance, the handling of children's wrist fractures; this situation shows how messy and variable anesthetic practice in children can be. Treatments differ extensively by country, and that very often speaks to the need for guidelines that take into account fracture type as well as available medical resources. Sometimes, issues like not having enough anesthesia or missing out on cutting-edge equipment can knock patient outcomes off balance. In most cases, ironing out these inconsistencies is pretty vital if we're to set up reliable best practices in pediatric fracture care and, as a result, boost the overall quality of care in pediatric anesthesia (Labianca et al., 2024). In recent times, there's been a noticeable surge in educational activities among pediatric practitioners.

The Academy of Pediatric Physical Therapy, for example, has been driving efforts to remodel what they call the Essential Core Competencies, especially now that the field is speeding ahead with new advancements. Blending modern terminology with practice, skills-based strategies has helped to ensure practitioners are equipped to manage the unique difficulties of anesthetizing children. Clearly, such reforms in the way we teach not only enhance career growth but also advance daily clinical practices that directly impact pediatric anesthesia care (Schreiber et al., 2024). Emerging research and the publication of real-world, evidence-based guidelines continue to be a key area in shaping the future of pediatric anesthesia. RCTs, especially, are vital—they help build a growing body of knowledge about the special needs of children who undergo surgery. By keeping research quality high, healthcare teams are able to make decisions that lead to better patient outcomes and improved safety measures. In conclusion, the implementation of a broad range of research evidence into everyday practice is crucial to advancing the subspecialty of pediatric anesthesia and to delivering a higher standard of care to our youngest patients (Labianca et al., 2024).

KEY TERMS FROM THIS CHAPTER

- Breathing rhythms
- Educational programs
- Evidence-based practices
- Metabolism
- Nervous system
- Pediatric care
- Smart monitoring
- Cognitive-behavioral therapy
- Emotional support
- Extracorporeal membrane oxygenation
- Near-infrared spectroscopy
- Pediatric anesthesia
- Personalized medication

CRITICAL THINKING QUESTIONS

1. **Why is sevoflurane preferred for induction in pediatric patients?**
   a. Minimal airway irritation
   b. Strong analgesic properties
   c. Long duration of action
   d. Low cost
2. **In pediatric patients, the narrowest part of the airway is:**
   a. Vocal cords
   b. Cricoid cartilage
   c. Epiglottis
   d. Trachea
3. **The most common premedication used for pediatric anesthesia is:**
   a. Diazepam
   b. Midazolam
   c. Ketamine
   d. Propofol
4. **The preferred induction method in pediatric patients is:**
   a. Intravenous induction with propofol
   b. Inhalational induction with sevoflurane
   c. Intramuscular ketamine
   d. Oral midazolam followed by IV induction
5. **Which breathing circuit is most commonly used for pediatric patients?**
   a. Mapleson A
   b. Mapleson D
   c. Bain circuit
   d. Jackson-Rees modification of Mapleson F

Short Answer Questions

1. Define pediatric anesthesia.
2. What are the physiological differences in children?
3. List the types of anesthesia used in pediatrics.
4. What is the preoperative assessment?
5. What is intra-operative management?

Answers to Critical Thinking Questions

1. (a); 2. (b); 3. (b); 4. (b); 5. (d)

REFERENCES

1. Adamek, A., Akin, A., Al-Zaben, K., Alm, C., Amminnikutty, M., Amoli, M. M., Anderson, B. J., et al. (2018). Postoperative pain management in children: Guidance from the pain committee of the European Society for Pediatric Anesthesiology (ESPA Pain Management Ladder Initiative). https://core.ac.uk/download/157582937.pdf (accessed on 20 May 2025).
2. Aebi, C., Shah, A. G., Anderson, B., Arlt, M., Barr, D., Barthelemy, R., Beiderlinden, M., et al. (2017). Medication complications in extracorporeal membrane oxygenation. https://core.ac.uk/download/129191716.pdf (accessed on 20 May 2025).
3. Ahmed, S. S., Nitu, M., Hicks, S., Hedlund, L., Slaven, J. E., & Rigby, M. R. (2016). Propofol-based procedural sedation with or without low-dose ketamine in children. *Journal of Pediatric Intensive Care, 5*(1), 1–6. https://doi.org/10.1055/s-0035-1568152.
4. Al-Khotani, A., Ajabnoor, H., Koshak, R., Alshehri, S. A., & Meisha, D. E. (2025). Clinical profiles and treatment outcomes of dental rehabilitation in patients treated under general anesthesia: A comparison between healthy and special healthcare needs children. *Frontiers in Pediatrics.* https://www.semanticscholar.org/paper/c3dc60f990ead3bf6dc5514c38563ac9c848368f (accessed on 20 May 2025).
5. Allen, R. (2023). *Guidelines for Performing Caudal Blocks in Pediatric Sub-Umbilical Surgeries* (Doctoral dissertation, Otterbein University). Doctor of Nursing Practice Scholarly Projects, 131. https://digitalcommons.otterbein.edu/stu_doc/131 (accessed on 20 May 2025).
6. Arriaga, P., & Pacheco, C. (2016). Effects of cl doctors on child and caregiver anxiety at the entrance to the surgery care unit and separation from caregivers. https://core.ac.uk/download/46603912.pdf (accessed on 20 May 2025).
7. Bai, C., Xu, M., Guo, Y., Jin, Y., & Zhao, X. (2024). Clinical application and research progress of remimazolam for pediatric patients. *Drug Design, Development and Therapy, 18*, 1221–1229. https://www.semanticscholar.org/paper/6c25776d47520145a6000e6dbfdd931e557f7562 (accessed on 20 May 2025).
8. Bong, C. L., & Yuan, I. (2024). The utility of electroencephalography in guiding general anesthesia in children. *Anesthesia and Analgesia.* https://www.semanticscholar.org/paper/071984586bbd330f0044725277873c1b45aea111 (accessed on 20 May 2025).
9. Cain, M. P., Green, M. C., Horn, N. D., Misseri, C., et al. (2018). Epidural analgesia decreases narcotic requirements in low level spina bifida patients undergoing urologic laparotomy for neurogenic bladder and bowel. https://core.ac.uk/download/160755276.pdf (accessed on 20 May 2025).
10. Calciano, C. S., et al. (2025). Ethical considerations of unsedated esophagogastroduodenoscopy in pediatric patients. *Narrative Inquiry in Bioethics, 15*(1), 69–77. https://dx.doi.org/10.1353/nib.2025.a957206.
11. Cappellini, I., Bavestrello Piccini, G., Campagnola, L., Bochicchio, C., Carente, R., Lai, F., Magazzini, S., & Consales, G. (2024). Procedural sedation in emergency department: A narrative review. *Emergency Care and Medicine, 1*(2), 103–136. https://doi.org/10.3390/ecm1020014.
12. Castellheim, A., Habre, W., & Hansen, T. G. (2025). Clinical practice and outcomes in European pediatric cardiac anesthesia: A secondary analysis of the APRICOT and NECTARINE studies. *Acta Anesthesiologic Scandinavica, 69.* https://www.semanticscholar.org/paper/84202c5207e6fb9ee47bd84038cd1cb9fedc816b (accessed on 20 May 2025).

13. Cho, S. A. (2023). What is your optimal target of oxygen during general anesthesia in pediatric patients? *Anesthesia and Pain Medicine, 19*, S5–S11. https://www.semanticscholar.org/paper/cf3a5af768162518f625b1958098aea62d67cff4 (accessed on 20 May 2025).

14. Cockrell, M. (2020). *Pediatric Emergence Agitation: Best Practice Guideline for Certified Registered Nurse Anesthetists* (Doctoral project No. 147). The University of Southern Mississippi. https://aquila.usm.edu/dnp_capstone/147 (accessed on 20 May 2025).

15. Dagher, K., Benvenuti, C., Virag, K., & Habre, W. (2024). The incidence of postoperative complications following lumbar and bone marrow punctures in pediatric anesthesia: Insights from APRICOT. *Journal of Pediatric Hematology/Oncology, 46*, 165–171. https://www.semanticscholar.org/paper/a190bf0bf9253dfd6387187af799ca3b7d0a711c (accessed on 20 May 2025).

16. Dandemmanavar, V., KN, V., R, V., Bandyopadhyay, S., Gakhar, H., & Dey, A. (2025). The impact of anesthetic agents on neurocognitive outcomes in pediatric patients. *Journal of Neonatal Surgery, 14*(10S), 153–161. https://www.jneonatalsurg.com/index.php/jns/article/view/2774 (accessed on 20 May 2025).

17. Davenport, M., Pakarinen, M. P., Tam, P. K. H., Laje, P., & Holcomb, G. (2020). From the editors: The COVID-19 crisis and its implications for pediatric surgeons. *Journal of Pediatric Surgery, 55*, 785–788. https://doi.org/10.1016/j.jpedsurg.2020.04.009.

18. Department of Anesthesia. (2010). *University of Lowa.* https://core.ac.uk/download/18608345.pdf (accessed on 20 May 2025).

19. Engelhardt, T., Fiadjoe, J., Weiss, M., Baker, P., Bew, S., Echeverry Marín, P., & von Ungern-Sternberg, B. V. (2019). A framework for the management of the pediatric airway. *Pediatric Anesthesia, 29*, 985–992. https://www.semanticscholar.org/paper/4f8016ad9faa1775dea6de7d9043ae72b764a4bf (accessed on 20 May 2025).

20. Ferriero, D. M., Fullerton, H. J., Bernard, T. J., Billinghurst, L., Daniels, S. R., DeBaun, M. R., deVeber, G., et al. (2019). Management of stroke in neonates and children: A scientific statement from the American Heart Association/American Stroke Association. *Stroke, 50*. https://doi.org/10.1161/str.0000000000000183.

21. Fezeu, F., Ramesh, A., Melmer, P. D., Moosa, S., Larson, P. S., & Henderson, F., Jr. (2018). Challenges and solutions for functional neurosurgery in developing countries. *Cureus, 10*(9), e3314. https://doi.org/10.7759/cureus.3314.

22. Haqi, A., Ridwansyah, R., Kurniawan, C., Hidayat, R. N., & Soenendar, R. A. (2025). Comparative analysis of anesthesia techniques and circumcision methods on pain outcomes in pediatric mass circumcision: An observational study. *Open Access Indonesian Journal of Medical Reviews.* https://www.semanticscholar.org/paper/6f7542d3a7384f8c83917ee2ae40d0f063806df6 (accessed on 20 May 2025).

23. Kaye, A., Jeha, G., Renschler, J. S., Fuller, M. C., Pham, A. D., & Cornett, E. (2020). Anesthetic agents in pediatric patients: A comprehensive review of pharmacological considerations in clinical practice. *Medical Research Archives, 8.* https://www.semanticscholar.org/paper/3711182274f8f2b8cef4a278dac4a1d74fe24528 (accessed on 20 May 2025).

24. Labianca, L., Calderaro, C., & Maffulli, N. (2024). Pediatric wrist fractures: Variations in management across countries. *British Medical Bulletin.* https://www.semanticscholar.org/paper/f609d8ee434d7fb077fe2ae0cbb748fd97dd858a (accessed on 20 May 2025).

25. Lauder, G. R., & Kuttner, L. (2024). Innovative change not as yet fully integrated in pediatric anesthesia. *Pediatric Anesthesia, 34*, 697–700. https://www.semanticscholar.org/paper/ff3e4edc0f0b0fac1cff7b90256e5646e469b4e0 (accessed on 20 May 2025).

26. Łepik, M., Uszok, Z., Rosiak, K., Płeska, K., Reguła, K., Waloch, K., Wojtania, J., Piaszczyński, S., Czajka, A., & Szymański, B. (2024). Difficult pediatric airway in anesthesia practice and future sport performance. *Quality in Sport, 18*, 50920. https://doi.org/10.12775/QS.2024.18.50920.

27. Liossi, C. (1999). Management of pediatric procedure-related cancer pain.

28. Masarwy, A., Watterson, C., Tuchman, A., & Danielpour, M. (2025). Flexion–extension cervical MRI imaging in pediatric patients with achondroplasia unsupervised by neurosurgery or radiology, is it safe? *Child's Nervous System, 41*. https://www.semanticscholar.org/paper/23d25aafa061beccd6ca4bee61dc90cefc8924e7 (accessed on 20 May 2025).

29. Mickolyzck, B. (2023). *Pediatric Preoperative Fasting Guidelines Update and Education: A Quality Improvement Project* [Unpublished DNP project]. Sacred Heart University.

30. Muslu Dinc, B., & Arun, F. (2024). The effect of patient-specific variables on the need for dental treatment under general anesthesia in children: A retrospective study. *Necmettin Erbakan Üniversitesi Diş Hekimliği Dergisi (NEU Dent J)*. https://www.semanticscholar.org/paper/c4ed3910b8e0b4a392d56bee96c3833d73e481e3 (accessed on 20 May 2025).

31. Pan, N., Sadun, R., Lerman, M., Resnick, C. M., Bost, J. E., Stoustrup, P., Twilt, M., et al. (2024). A randomized controlled educational study to evaluate an e-learning module to teach the physical examination of the temporomandibular joint in juvenile idiopathic arthritis. *Pediatric Rheumatology, 22*. https://www.semanticscholar.org/paper/77fe7176856ead814232c9bd9cb92e3220195ec6 (accessed on 20 May 2025).

32. Polites, S. F., & Azarow, K. S. (2020). Perspectives on pediatric appendicitis and appendectomy during the Severe Acute Respiratory Syndrome Coronavirus 2 pandemic. *Journal of Laparoendoscopic & Advanced Surgical Techniques, 30*, 356–357. https://doi.org/10.1089/lap.2020.0197.

33. Reysner, T., Wieczorowska-Tobis, K., Mularski, A., Kowalski, G., Daroszewski, P., & Reysner, M. (2025). Revolutionizing pediatric surgery: The transformative role of regional anesthesia—A narrative review. *Surgeries*. https://www.semanticscholar.org/paper/2fa00e236a8dba236b479af4d537099f1a2b6c40 (accessed on 20 May 2025).

34. Rigby-Jones, A. E., & Sneyd, J. R. (2011). Propofol and children—what we know and what we do not know. https://core.ac.uk/download/29817530.pdf.

35. Rosen, R., Vandenplas, Y., Singendonk, M., Cabana, M. D., DiLorenzo, C., Gottrand, F., Gupta, S. K., et al. (2018). Pediatric gastroesophageal reflux clinical practice guidelines. *Journal of Pediatric Gastroenterology and Nutrition, 66*, 516–554. https://doi.org/10.1097/mpg.0000000000001889.

36. Sablewski, A., Eimer, C., Nemeth, M., & Miller, C. (2024). Preoperative anxiety management practices in pediatric anesthesia: Comparative analysis of an online survey presented to experts and social media users. *JMIR Pediatrics and Parenting, 8*. https://www.semanticscholar.org/paper/e7d143392a73360b3708ed7c1f3f0cfb6aaf1b13 (accessed on 20 May 2025).

37. Saracoglu, G., & Salman, N. (2025). Anesthetic management in pediatric cardiac surgery. *Surgery on Children, 2*, 66–71. https://doi.org/10.51271/SOC-0038.

38. Saxen, M. A., Urman, R. D., Yepes, J. F., Gabriel, R. A., & Jones, J. E. (2017). Comparison of anesthesia for dental/oral surgery by office-based dentist anesthesiologists versus operating room-based physician anesthesiologists. *Anesthesia Progress, 64*(4), 212–220. https://doi.org/10.2344/anpr-65-01-04.

39. Sbaraglia, F., Cuomo, C., Della Sala, F., Festa, R., Garra, R., Maiellare, F., Micci, D. M., et al. (2024). State of the art in pediatric anesthesia: A narrative review about the use of preoperative time. *Journal of Personalized Medicine, 14*. https://www.semanticscholar.org/paper/21c8aef10cdc8fa528e4e0ec84632cd976870d9d (accessed on 20 May 2025).

40. Schreiber, J., Rapport, M., Anderson, D., Lundeen, H., Moore, J., & Furze, J. (2024). Revision of the essential core competencies: Domains of competence and associated competencies for pediatric physical therapy professional education. *Pediatric Physical Therapy*. https://www.semanticscholar.org/paper/4d37b5c0434a6ba225a40df98488719c2c92b698 (accessed on 20 May 2025).

41. Stant, W. R. (2025). *Development of Evidence-Based Clinical Practice Guidelines for Pediatric Preoperative Anxiety*. https://core.ac.uk/download/616421797.pdf.

42. Weber, F., & Scoones, G. P. (2019). A practical approach to cerebral near-infrared spectroscopy (NIRS) directed hemodynamic management in noncardiac pediatric anesthesia. *Pediatric Anesthesia, 29*, 993–1001. https://doi.org/10.1111/pan.13726.

OBSTETRIC ANESTHESIA

10

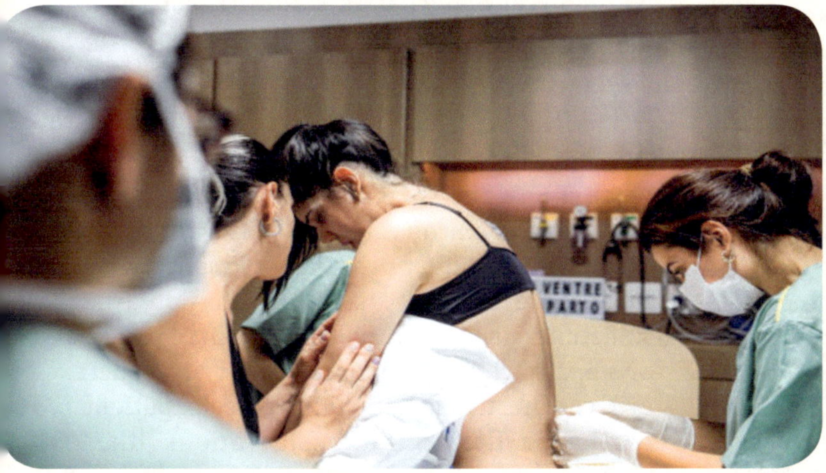

LEARNING OBJECTIVES

After studying this chapter, you will be able to:

1. Describe the types of obstetric anesthesia.
2. Indicate obstetric anesthesia use.
3. Understand the benefits of obstetric anesthesia.
4. Describe the risks and complications of obstetric anesthesia.

Introduction

Obstetric anesthesia is the key to keeping mothers healthy and comfortable throughout labor, even as their bodies undergo some pretty drastic changes. Knowing different ways to keep pain off—from epidurals to spinal blocks— makes a difference to mom and baby. Sometimes, complications such as post dural puncture headaches (PDPH) occur and remind us that having a deep practical knowledge matters. Too many cases of PDPH mean that clearly there is a genuine necessity to devise clever means of preventing and rectifying these issues, most often involving ongoing learning and education tailored to childbirth situations. In the end, obstetric anesthesia is not so much a matter of technical skill—it's also an integral part of maternal health and can really improve the whole birthing process. With advancements in obstetric anesthesia, it is met with a mix of concerns from ensuring that patients are secure to possessing the right people who can perform the job, especially when finances are limited. Training non-physician anesthetists is recently a contentious topic because it seems like the perfect way of addressing gaps when there aren't enough specialist doctors present. Médecins Sans Frontières has tried this, for example, in Haiti; there, they trained nurse anesthetists in an extremely interactive way, which managed to provide emergency anesthesia to patients when they needed it most. Some studies even indicate that, with adequate training, these non-physician providers can provide anesthesia safely—perhaps a giant step towards more even health care. Global health programs are shifting too, and the potential of mixing types of anesthesia providers could be just what's needed to increase good outcomes for mothers in resource-limited areas (Rosseel et al., 2009).

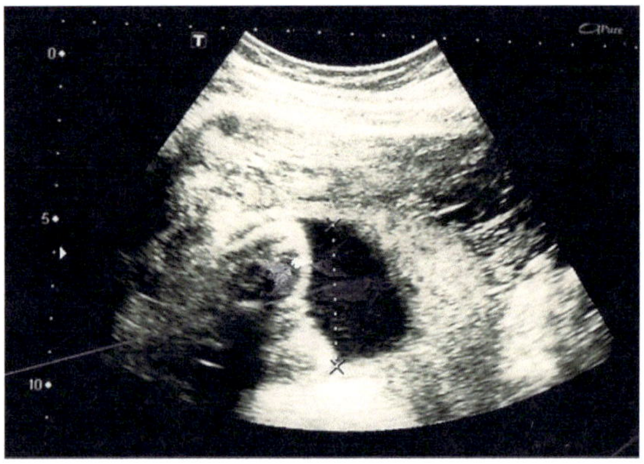

Figure 10.1. Obstetric anesthesia.

Source: By Dahab AA, Aburass R, Shawkat W, Babgi R, Essa O, Mujallid RH - https://www.ncbi.nlm.nih.gov/pmc/articles/PMC3216095/figure/F3/, CC BY 2.5, https://commons.wikimedia.org/w/index.php?curid=36870447.

The issues of PDPH also support that ongoing research and innovative thinking are essential to maximize obstetric anesthesia. Statistics show dural punctures occur roughly 0.5% to 2.5% of the time while performing epidurals, and such hiccups can be painful for patients' egos. These problems usually make new mothers struggle with daily activities and slow down recovery by more than usual. While most women do end up defeating a PDPH on their, quick relief is nonetheless uber important. Various treatments—e.g., epidural blood patches and others—are continually under consideration as practitioners work toward identifying the best, evidence-based practices for alleviating these agonizing incidents. A multidisciplinary strategy that combines education, in-practice training, and cutting-edge research remains vital to the progress of obstetric anesthesia and general maternal outcomes (Holzer et al., 2009) (Figure 10.1).

Definition of Obstetric Anesthesia

Obstetric anesthesia is required—especially when a new life is coming. In essence, it's not only about pain numbing but also addressing the body and mind needs of a pregnant patient. Doctors are known to mix and match approaches, sometimes using neuraxial methods like epidurals or spinals, while in other scenarios using general or local anesthesia depending on each patient's particular demands. Considerations like a mother's overall health, the baby's status, and specifics of delivery or surgery—like life-and-death scenarios with C-sections where timely effective relief is critical—come into play in making this decision. In most cases, it's not so much to reduce pain but to improve overall outcomes for both mother and child at one of the most critical junctures in life. In the past few years, the obstetric anesthetic scene has altered dramatically. Advances have taken safety levels just that bit higher, and issues of low blood pressure due to spinal anesthesia (SA) have led many to explore further on how to better manage maternal circulation. Broadly speaking, methods like fluid loading and optimal use of vasopressors come in to counteract hypotension, especially in cesarean section. All in all, the incorporation of up-to-date, evidence-based guidelines into practice keeps the team on track—even though, occasionally, there are minor differences in how protocols are implemented—and keeps everyone running together in harmony (Mladenovic et al., 2024). It is not just about physical management, though; the patient's mental health is a concern big time.

The anesthetizing choice can make a difference for years in a woman's birthing experience, sometimes gliding over anxiety and uncertainty that most commonly accompany labor. There is frequent repetition in research in which proper pain control is not only demonstrated to improve the short-term experience but may also reduce on instances of postpartum depression. If you look at it, obstetric anesthesia is not only a technical procedure—it's a holistic practice that honors comfort, sound clinical outcomes, and a better psychological experience for mothers at delivery (Engbers, 2018) (Figure 10.2).

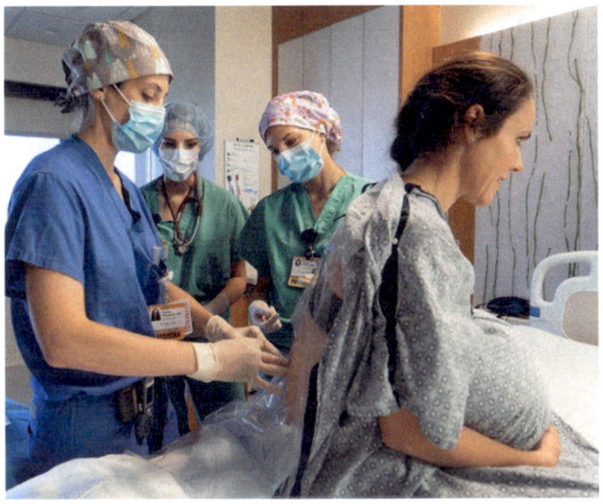

Figure 10.2. Definition of Obstetric Anesthesia.

Source: https://cdn.atriumhealth.org/-/media/wakeforest/school/images/page-content/education-and-training/residencies-and-fellowships/anesthesiology-residency/anes-res-curr-obstetric-anes-2.jpg?h=646&w=800&rev=bb7f85fe3be34686a8fb139f2b0e4690&hash=F3AADFADB2C2ADF98E0BA7582FA45282.

Importance in Maternal and Fetal Health

Good obstetric anesthesia is important in ensuring mother and baby are safe during labor and childbirth. It is not just about getting the lady through the pain—stress reduction for the baby is also important. Any procedure should be accompanied by a sound plan that duly takes into consideration a woman's past medical history and complications prior. Too often, bringing together a diverse group of experts is the core, especially in rural areas where subspecialized services are lacking. The CDC's LOCATe tool, for instance, typically concludes that both mother and baby outcomes tend to be contingent on the amount of care available. Including risk-savvy anesthesia practices, as supported by organizations like the American College of Obstetricians and Gynecologists, can enhance overall wellness. Maternal health is far from straightforward. The issues pile up in the blink of an eye, so close attention and timely intervention are often supported by excellent obstetric anesthesia. Research tells us that many obstetric patients ultimately need intensive care—a testament to just how complex things have become. In the overwhelming majority of cases, the use of a special critical care approach with high-risk patients has produced better outcomes (see Dudas, 2014). Refining anesthetic techniques, as well as co-management between a variety of different healthcare providers, is necessary to an answering the evolving needs of maternal health. At other times, the manner in which these practices converge might have a measure of an ad hoc quality to it, but they aim to ensure that care is both timely and targeted. In another sense, good care isn't necessarily about the technicalities—it is also about guaranteeing that everybody involved is properly trained. In actuality, ongoing learning and even a small amount of hands-on experience are necessary because no two labor and delivery situations are ever the same. Training staff in the recognition of complications like hypertension or heavy bleeding can be a matter of life and death. On occasion, using obstetric triggers in nursing assessments (emphasizes the need for teamwork. Eventually, these ongoing education efforts help healthcare teams better care for patients while strengthening the system overall. Embracing an attitude of ongoing learning and the occasional minor mishaps along the way can eventually lead to safer birthing experiences for all parties concerned (Dudas, 2014).

10.1. Types of Obstetric Anesthesia

Learning Outcome

1. Define the epidural anesthesia.
2. Describe the spinal anesthesia.
3. Understand the general anesthesia.

Pain management for childbirth has come a long way. Doctors now stress the importance of using methods that are both safe and get the job done. Neuraxial techniques like epidurals and spinal blocks—methods that let the mother stay engaged with the process—have become go-to options. Take the combined spinal-epidural (CSE) block, for instance; it kicks in quickly and generally needs less local anesthetic, which many find appealing. Studies, in most cases, show that this method offers faster relief and often ups the odds of a spontaneous vaginal birth, improving the overall labor experience and boosting maternal satisfaction. Choosing the right method depends on the unique situation of each patient's labor, so individual care is key (Reale et al., 2021). Another layer to obstetric anesthesia involves handling patients who face extra challenges, such as those with von Willebrand disease (vWD). This bleeding disorder, which complicates the usual decision process, forces practitioners to weigh their options carefully. One paper, for instance, found that neuraxial methods were given safely to most pregnant patients with vWD—provided that thorough, and sometimes, repetitive preoperative assessments and team consultations were in play. The specific approach was tailored based on vWD type, severity, and the patient's overall status. Often, treatment plans mixed in desmopressin or factor concentrates to help the blood clot better, thereby offering effective pain control while curbing the possible risks of bleeding issues (Reale et al., 2021). Not all cases suit neuraxial techniques. Sometimes, general anesthesia (GA) is the fallback, especially during emergency cesarean deliveries or when a quick onset of anesthesia is critical and neuraxial methods just won't do. Sure, GA carries its set of risks—challenges with managing the airway and potential impacts on the baby—but advancements in drugs have, generally speaking, improved its safety profile quite a bit. In planned cases, a careful pre-anesthetic check and close monitoring are essential to keep things as safe as possible. Knowing the ins and outs of these different techniques helps healthcare providers choose the best option that puts both maternal and neonatal safety first (Angélica de et al., 2018) (Figure 10.3).

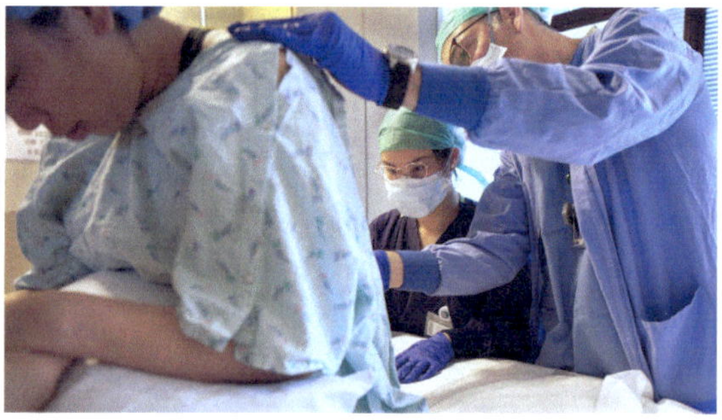

Figure 10.3. Types of Obstetric Anesthesia.

Source: https://anesthesiology.uw.edu/wp-content/uploads/2023/03/OB-Montlake-10-scaled.jpg.

10.1.1. Epidural Anesthesia

Regional anesthesia (RA)—epidurals especially—has become a cornerstone in obstetric care today. It works by blocking pain signals in targeted spots so that labor feels less overwhelming. In many cases, this means mothers can remain alert and truly involved in their birthing experience while enjoying solid pain relief. Sometimes doctors even opt for a continuous infusion to tailor the relief to each woman's needs, which may foster a closer, positive connection between mother and baby. Clinical studies usually back up this approach, showing that epidurals handle pain effectively while keeping both mom and baby safe, a reason they're widely recommended. Preeclampsia, for instance, throws an extra wrench into things when using epidurals. This high blood pressure disorder complicates labor and delivery so that careful, individualized anesthetic plans become essential to keep blood flow stable. CRNAs (certified registered nurse anesthetists) play a key role here, employing advanced techniques that help lower the risks tied to RA. Research often points out the ups and downs of various methods, comparing epidural approaches against spinal ones. Overall, the evidence suggests that epidurals not only offer solid pain alleviation but also allow for necessary interventions in high-risk situations, thereby guarding maternal safety and comfort during and after labor (Potter et al., 2008).

Another consideration is the mother's position during the second stage of labor, especially when an epidural is in use—this can affect outcomes for both her and the baby. The common practice of directed pushing while lying on the back has come under some debate, with some studies hinting that it might contribute to less-than-ideal results. Instead, letting women trust their natural, sometimes involuntary, pushing cues can enhance the experience. Evidence seems to underscore that personalized care approaches, tuned to the body's natural rhythms, are key. When combined with effective pain relief from an epidural, such strategies can ease complications and create a more supportive setting for childbirth (American College of Obstetricians and Gynecologists et al., 2007) (Figure 10.4).

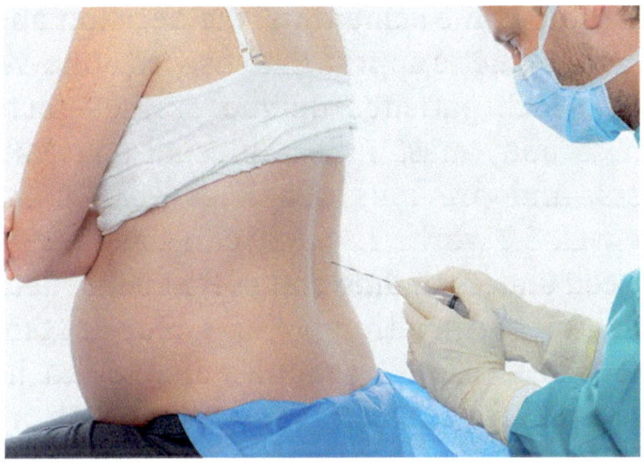

Figure 10.4. Epidural anaesthesia.

Source: https://cdn.cdnparenting.com/articles/2018/07/220165417-H.webp.

10.1.2. Spinal Anesthesia (SA)

SA has become a go-to technique in obstetric care, especially when things move fast—like during an emergency cesarean. When a delivery demands immediate action and the usual labor epidural just isn't doing enough, doctors often lean toward this method because it gives a deep, reliable pain block. The safety of both mother and baby hangs on choosing the right anesthetic, and surveys reveal that, in category-one cesarean sections, anesthesiologists frequently pick SA over topping up an epidural (Desai et al., 2019). This trend kind of nudges us to update protocols and adjust established guidelines more naturally. Using SA in maternity care comes with its advantages and its challenges, all mixed together in a rather complex picture. Generally speaking, studies show that this technique lowers maternal morbidity—mainly by keeping the widespread effects of GA at bay. It kicks in quickly, which is a big deal when every second counts. Clinicians keep a careful eye on the sensory block, and if it doesn't quite hit the mark, they might try a CSE technique that marries immediately rapid relief with some added flexibility. This blended approach seems to boost the overall safety and effectiveness of cesarean deliveries, even if it sometimes requires on-the-spot adjustments (Tawfik et al., 2016). At the same time, the decision about which anesthetic approach to use isn't one-size-fits-all. Each patient's unique profile—factors such as body mass index, unusual anatomical twists, and previous surgeries—can change how well SA works. In many clinical settings, a nuanced understanding of these personal details is key to getting things right. For instance, some places use ultrasound guidance to help place epidural catheters, and while that often improves success, the results can vary among patients. Ultimately, blending clinical insight with the latest technology and working together as a team remains essential. As the field steadily evolves, ongoing research and a willingness to adapt are vital for keeping maternal care at top-notch levels (Desai et al., 2019) (Figure 10.5).

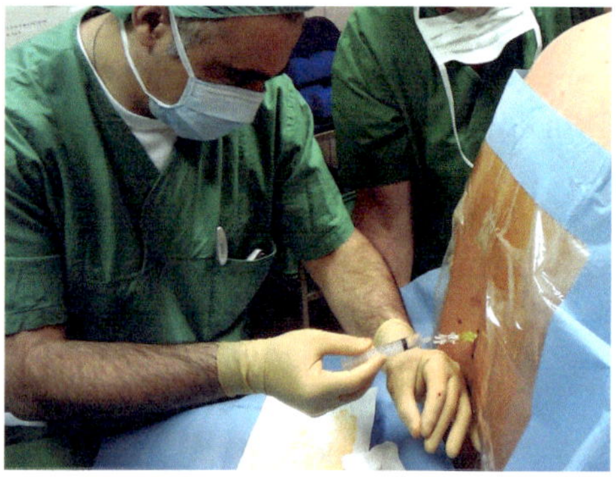

Figure 10.5. Spinal anesthesia in labor and childbirth.

Source: By User: MrArifnajafov - Own work - Privatarchiv Foto von MrArifnajafovYükl⊠y⊠nin öz işi, CC BY 3.0, https://commons.wikimedia.org/w/index.php?curid=15113448.

10.1.3. General Anesthesia (GA)

Obstetric anesthesia can be pretty tricky. Doctors need to know a range of techniques because sometimes the usual regional methods just don't work out. For most deliveries, labor analgesia is the first choice, yet emergencies—say, when urgent surgery is needed or maternal health issues rule out regional methods—force a switch to GA. This method kicks in fast and takes control of the mom's airway right away, making it an indispensable option when every second counts. A clinician's skill with these techniques matters, impacting both maternal and fetal outcomes; hence, thorough training is a must, especially in those high-pressure moments. At the same time, using GA in obstetric settings brings up extra safety concerns for both mother and baby. Pregnancy comes with changes—like increased airway swelling and altered drug metabolism—that make dosing anesthetics more complicated, and the risks of aspiration or respiratory issues can get higher. Anesthesiologists have to balance giving enough medication while not jeopardizing the baby's well-being. Generally speaking, this balancing act stresses how important it is to choose the right technique in every situation. When a labor epidural fails to do its job, managing anesthesia becomes even more of a challenge. In these cases, an obstetrician might find that simply converting the epidural into a solid anesthetic for a cesarean just doesn't cut it. Survey data often shows that practitioners weigh the effectiveness of the initial epidural along with the mother's condition before deciding what to do next. If even a top-up can't provide a reliable sensory block, many clinicians lean toward SA—or, in more dire circumstances, GA. All of these varied approaches underscore a pressing need for well-established guidelines to help steer decision-making in such complex scenarios, ensuring optimal care during obstetric procedures (Figure 10.6).

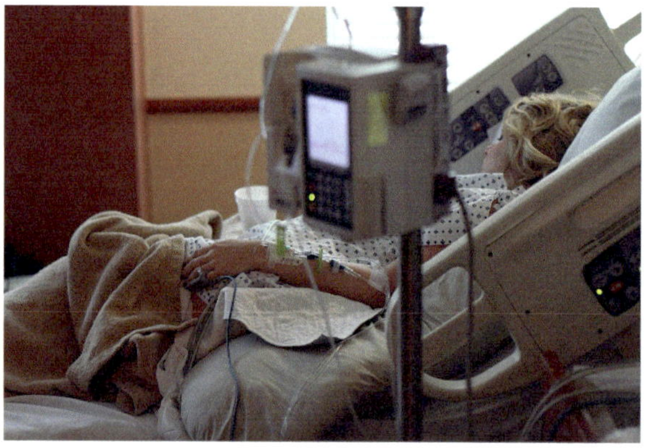

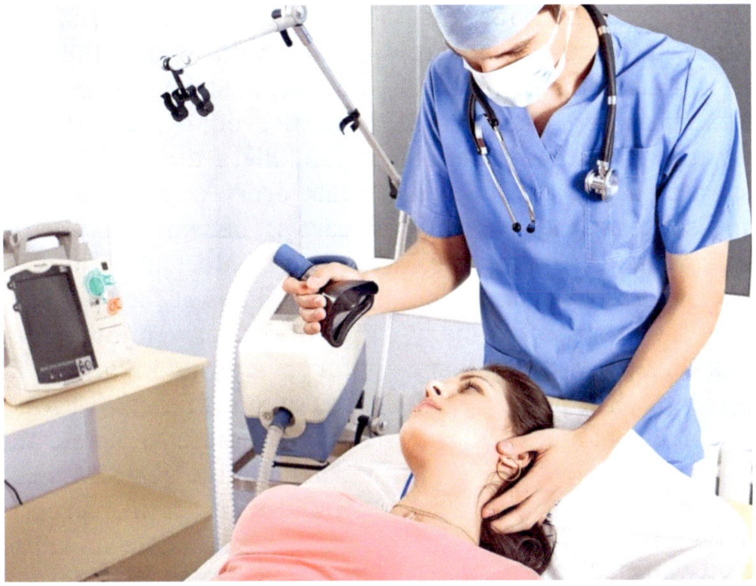

Figure 10.6. General anesthesia (GA) used during labor.

Source: By Pixabay - user:Parentingupstream - https://pixabay.com/en/hospital-labor-delivery-mom-840135/, CC0, https://commons.wikimedia.org/w/index.php?curid=76037830.

Test Your Knowledge

1. What is epidural anesthesia?
2. What is general anesthesia?

10.2. Indications for Use

Learning Outcome

1. Understand pain management during labor.
2. Understand the surgical interventions.
3. Describe the special considerations for high-risk pregnancies.

GA in C-sections isn't just a routine choice—it often reveals deep differences in patient care that many might not immediately notice. Often, a laboring patient ends up getting GA, typically when conditions like maternal or fetal distress demand quick action. A retrospective look into these practices showed, in most cases, that Black and Hispanic patients experience higher rates of GA compared to non-Hispanic White patients. Yet, when a patient already has neuraxial labor analgesia in place, the decision seems to level out, with the use of both general and neuraxial methods not differing much across racial lines (Thomas et al., 2024). This detail, though subtle, underscores how a better grasp of such indicators plays a key role in making care more equitable and in shaping anesthetic methods for diverse populations. Maternal health, especially during infectious outbreaks like COVID-19, throws another layer of complexity into the mix. Pregnant women—uniquely vulnerable to viral complications—end up needing specialized and timely care, which brings home the idea that every situation can be a bit different. Severe respiratory issues mean that both the mother and the baby must be watched very closely, and healthcare teams often adjust anesthetic choices on the fly to meet these pressing needs. Given all the physiological changes that pregnancy brings about, it's crucial for providers to alter their strategies accordingly. For example, handling COVID-19 in expectant patients has led many hospitals to bring together multi-disciplinary teams, aiming to balance the risks posed by the virus with the intricate needs of maternal care (Liang et al., 2020).

In most cases, this just reinforces how careful we all need to be when facing new health challenges in obstetric anesthesia. At the same time, the choice of anesthetic method reaches far beyond a single patient case—it reflects broader, systemic trends within maternal healthcare. Knowing when to use GA can tip the scales in high-risk or emergency deliveries, where every minute counts. For anesthetists and other care providers, being clued in about a patient's demographics and medical history becomes indispensable, even if sometimes the details might seem repetitive. Meanwhile, as guidelines shift—especially with new data from infectious outbreaks—ongoing education and constant adaptation prove necessary. These evolving practices not only boost the safety and effectiveness of anesthesia interventions but also help push the overall system toward fairer healthcare for all (Liang et al., 2020; Thomas et al., 2024).

10.2.1. Pain Management During Labor

Childbirth is a turning point—a moment when easing pain can change the whole experience for a mom and her baby. Over time, the ways to manage pain during labor have shifted a lot, largely thanks to improvements in obstetric anesthesia. Nowadays, techniques like spinal and epidural anesthesia are common; they deliver solid pain relief while still letting women move around more than the older, full-body painkillers did. There's a growing awareness that every woman's body reacts in its way, so care is becoming more personalized to help boost comfort and safety. When caregivers lean on methods backed by real evidence, it tends to create a warmer, more supportive atmosphere for everyone involved. Certified registered nurse anesthetists (CRNAs) have stepped into an even more vital role these days, especially when things get complicated in the delivery room. In cases like preeclampsia—where the risks with anesthesia shoot up—the seasoned skills of CRNAs come into play. Recent writings generally point out that truly grasping how preeclampsia works can help in picking the right pain relief plan. Research indicates that using regional methods tends to help stabilize patient conditions more effectively.

Teaming up with the rest of the obstetric crew, CRNAs help shape a care strategy that considers each patient's unique needs, thereby boosting both safety and overall satisfaction during labor and delivery. Today's approach also puts a strong emphasis on letting women make informed choices about their pain management. Some care models, like letting the laboring process follow natural bodily cues (often referred to as "laboring down"), highlight how tailored care can reduce on the stress linked to rigid pushing techniques. There's even some evidence that sticking with prolonged Valsalva maneuvers might lead to unwanted outcomes, nudging clinicians toward more supportive, patient-centered methods. By questioning the old idea of universal instructions during the pushing stage, many practitioners are now leaning toward strategies that honor a woman's signals and preferences. This gradual shift doesn't only improve outcomes; it builds a more compassionate healthcare vibe that looks after both physical ease and emotional well-being—even if a few commas end up being a bit misplaced along the way (Figure 10.7).

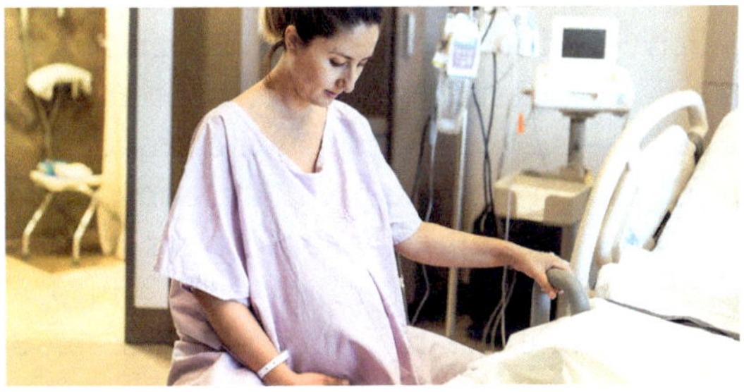

Figure 10.7. Managing pain during labor.

Source: https://www.lancastergeneralhealth.org/-/media/images/lancaster%20general/images/healthhub/motherhood/lgh_healthhub_motherhood_template_1200x600_pain_during_labor.ashx?mw=1200&mh=600.

10.2.2. Surgical Interventions (e.g., Cesarean Sections)

Obstetric surgeries, especially cesarean sections, come with their set of challenges. Cesarean deliveries sometimes happen because the health of the mother or baby forces a quicker decision, even when surgery itself isn't risk-free. The choice of anesthesia—whether it's a neuraxial method or GA—plays a huge role in shaping outcomes for both parties. Generally speaking, GA is saved for those moments when other techniques just don't fit the bill. Research shows that roughly 20% of cesarean procedures end up using GA (Padalko et al., 2025). This option, effective as it can be, carries risks like potential awareness during surgery and a spike in stress responses, meaning that every decision about it must be made with great care. New multimodal anesthesia methods are kind of reshuffling how these surgeries are done. Recent studies suggest that mixing in adjuvants—say, clonidine and IV acetaminophen—can noticeably improve the recovery process for moms and boost newborn health outcomes. This method helps steady things like blood pressure and heart function and attenuates the typical neuroendocrine stress response that surgery often brings along (Padalko et al., 2025). In most cases, such findings nudge us toward refining our anesthetic practices so that both maternal and neonatal well-being remain front and center. It's a trend that urges continuous, careful rethinking of how anesthesia is administered during obstetric procedures.

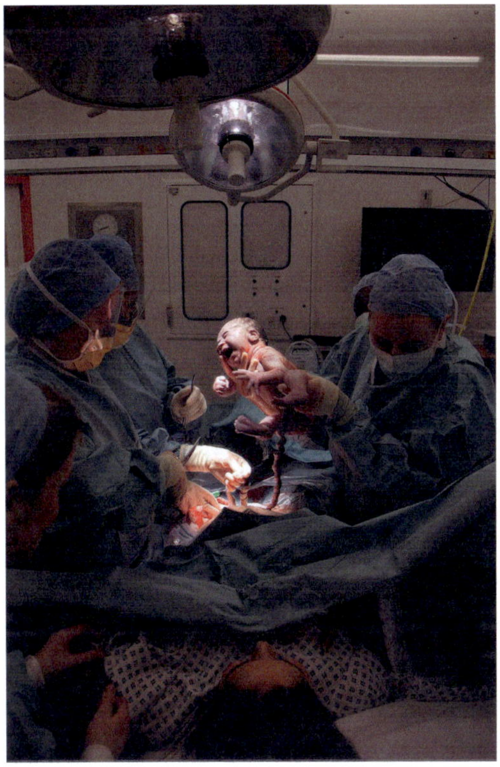

Figure 10.8. Caesarian section.

Source: By Salim Fadhley - Edit by Diliff This image can be cited as: Fadhley, Salim (2014). "Caesarean section photography." Wikiversity Journal of Medicine 1 (2). DOI:10.15347/wjm/2014.006. ISSN 20018762. - This file was derived from: Cesarian the moment of birth.jpg, FAL, https://commons.wikimedia.org/w/index.php?curid=4280288.

When patients have unique conditions, like Noonan syndrome, things get even trickier. Such individuals often come with extra challenges—

ranging from heart irregularities to clotting issues—that complicate the usual anesthetic plans. In these instances, a tailored approach—which factors in everything from anticoagulant status to breathing function—is pretty much essential. Experts generally agree that the best outcomes rely on a tight-knit multidisciplinary team coordinating throughout the surgery, leaving no stone unturned when it comes to managing risks. This situation underscores the need to adapt anesthetic strategies to each patient's unique profile while staying true to the core principles of obstetric anesthesia (Figure 10.8).

10.2.3. Special Considerations for High-Risk Pregnancies

Managing high-risk pregnancies can be tricky—it calls for a mix of experts, especially when anesthesia is involved. It's not just a checklist; a mother's health and the baby's well-being can both be affected by the choices made. In most cases, anesthesiologists need to grasp how drugs might impact both sides, and keeping an eye on the baby's heartbeat is key. A sudden dip or erratic pulse might simply hint at distress from the anesthesia or even just how the mom is positioned. Some case studies have pointed out that not watching the blood flow between the uterus and placenta closely may lead to complications during surgery. All of this, taken together, ends up shaping the decisions and protocols for high-risk pregnancies—aiming to get the best outcomes for both mother and child (Schwarzkopf et al., 2013). When surgery comes into the picture for these delicate situations, teamwork takes center stage. Obstetricians, anesthesiologists, and the surgical crew have to be in sync, passing vital info around rapidly—even if it means a few pauses here and there. For instance, if a pregnant woman with traumatic injuries needs an operation immediately, the anesthesiologist might have to switch tactics based on what they see about the baby's condition at that very moment. I've seen cases where sudden surprises during surgery led to an emergency C-section right then, showing just how crucial constant, sometimes even impulsive, communication is. This kind of close coordination ensures that interventions aren't just quick—they also respect the unique, ever-changing nature of the pregnant body. In most cases, understanding these nuances builds an environment that puts safety first and drives better results overall (Kuckowski et al., 2007). Then there's the whole matter of picking the right medications. Generally speaking, a pregnant body handles drugs a bit differently because of natural changes in metabolism and excretion. Anesthetics and pain relievers must be chosen with care so they don't negatively affect the baby's development while still managing the mother's pain.

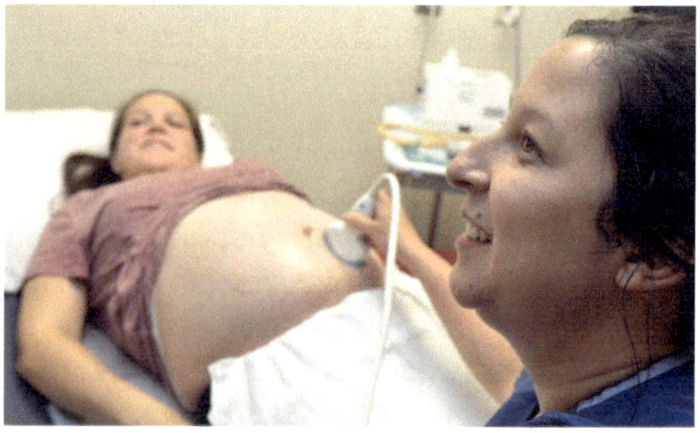

Figure 10.9. High-risk pregnancy.

Source: By Jacob Sippel - https://health.mil/News/Gallery/Photos/2017/04/27/During-Pregnancy, CC BY-SA 4.0, https://commons.wikimedia.org/w/index.php?curid=74814735.

It's a delicate balance, which is why clear, practical guidelines for dosages and drug choices become essential—especially in high-pressure emergency situations. Regular, sometimes even sporadic, checks on how both mom and baby respond to these substances help catch any issues early on. By setting up robust protocols and making sure everyone on the team is on the same page, the risks tied to anesthesia in high-risk pregnancies can be kept to a minimum, paving the way for a safer experience for both mother and child (Schwarzkopf et al., 2013) (Figure 10.9).

Test Your Knowledge

1. How do you manage pain during labor?
2. What are the special considerations for high-risk pregnancies?

10.3. Benefits of Obstetric Anesthesia

Learning Outcome

1. Enhance maternal comfort.
2. Improve fetal outcomes.
3. Reduce the stress and anxiety during labor.

Obstetric anesthesia isn't just about taking the edge off labor pain; it shapes the whole birth experience for both mom and baby. In high-pressure moments—say, during a cesarean—it can turn an otherwise daunting process into an opportunity for early connection. Research generally suggests that many providers, even in the face of clinical hurdles, now favor immediate skin-to-skin contact after a C-section, a practice that's seen as vital for bonding and jump-starting breastfeeding. Of course, real-world obstacles can sometimes block this positive step from becoming routine, which is why a smart, well-planned anesthetic approach is so crucial. In short, when pain is managed well, mothers can share those precious early bonding moments that set the stage for both immediate comfort and long-term health benefits (Balatero et al., 2018). Obstetric anesthesia also becomes a key player when complications crop up during labor. For instance, issues like fetal distress or an unusually long labor might force an urgent move toward surgical solutions, such as a cesarean section—a situation that can naturally spike anxiety. Yet a good anesthetic technique not only eases discomfort but also offers a sense of control. The ability to rapidly deploy regional blocks—like epidurals or spinal injections—lets healthcare teams jump in quickly when unexpected challenges arise. This quick response doesn't just ease maternal worry; it also empowers teams to steer the situation toward safer outcomes, even when things seem a bit unpredictable (Keith-Brown et al., 2017). There are longer-lasting benefits, too, that touch on mental health and recovery. Painful, traumatic childbirth experiences can sometimes leave a lasting mark, even contributing to issues like PTSD or postpartum depression. By easing pain and softening the rough edges of labor, obstetric anesthesia can help lessen these negative effects, making the transition to motherhood a bit smoother. Additionally, mothers who feel supported during birth are often more inclined to engage in nurturing, responsive care afterward—a positive cycle that boosts both their mental well-being and the baby's development. In this way, well-administered obstetric anesthesia not only brings immediate comfort but also lays d the foundation for a healthier postnatal recovery (Balatero et al., 2018).

10.3.1. Enhanced Maternal Comfort

Childbirth is a life-changing moment, yet it usually comes with a bundle of physical strain and emotional ups and downs. In most cases, easing the pain during labor isn't just about feeling better in the moment—it helps reduce on the stress that comes with intense uterine contractions and cervical dilation. Many turn to methods like epidurals or a CSE, which are often seen as the top choice because they focus on the pain with fewer side effects; this, in turn, creates a calmer space for both mom and baby. Mixing modern pain relief approaches into labor care is essential for boosting comfort and overall satisfaction—a point supported by current clinical research (Ismail et al., 2025). Besides using medications, non-drug methods also play a big role in lifting maternal comfort. Techniques such as guided imagery, simple relaxation exercises, and consistent support during labor often help women feel more in control of the birthing process. There's plenty of evidence suggesting that when moms are more engaged and actively supported, their pain tends to ease up, which might even reduce anxiety and let labor roll along more smoothly. For example, the assistance of a doula is increasingly seen as a worthwhile addition to childbirth education and standard obstetric care. In many cases, blending drug and non-drug strategies works out as a winning formula for enhancing comfort and, ultimately, leads to better outcomes for newborns (Munro et al., 2020). In settings where resources are scarce, making sure mothers are comfortable demands creative, tailored strategies. When advanced medical infrastructure isn't available, prioritizing safe anesthesia and effective pain relief becomes even more critical. Training local healthcare providers through dedicated educational programs can make a noticeable difference—these efforts often boost the use of targeted pain control methods, which directly benefits expectant moms. Establishing clear protocols for both regional and GA helps ensure that, even in tough conditions, maternal comfort isn't overlooked. Ultimately, addressing the gaps in access to obstetric anesthesia is key to fostering a general culture of maternal well-being, leading to healthier outcomes for both mothers and their babies (Ismail et al., 2025) (Figure 10.10).

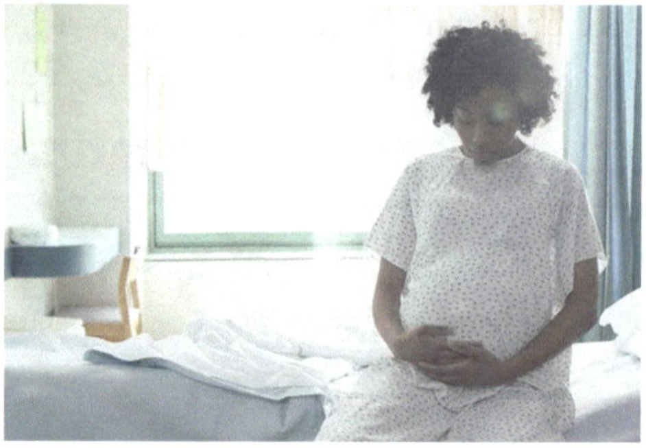

Figure 10.10. Comfort and pain relief during labor.

Source: https://images.ctfassets.net/2ql69mthp94m/7nUMWtE67QQLj8HiNAm2Y3/8b266d0b5c0303b5e0babbf03d625202/Comfort-measures-during-labor.jpeg?fm=webp&q=70.

10.3.2. Improved Fetal Outcomes

Obstetric anesthesia is a cornerstone in keeping things safe for both mother and baby during labor. Managing pain well not only brings comfort to the mother but also lowers stress that might otherwise unsettle the baby's delicate balance. Doctors often turn to regional techniques like epidurals or spinal blocks—methods that help ease pain while keeping uteroplacental blood flow steady. Unchecked pain can trigger a spike in catecholamines, which, in most cases, messes with fetal oxygen levels. It pays off to look after each woman's unique physical and emotional needs, creating an environment that supports both her well-being and that of the baby. Looking at the second stage of labor, evidence these days suggests that sticking with old methods like directed pushing might not always be the best bet—sometimes it can lead to lower oxygen for the fetus and even minor injuries for the mother. Instead, techniques such as "laboring down," which lets moms follow their natural urge to bear down, may help reduce stress on the baby and improve oxygen delivery during contractions. Generally speaking, when healthcare providers mix in the latest scientific findings with a bit of common sense in positioning and pushing, the outcomes tend to improve. Such tailored approaches not only empower mothers but also smooth the way for the physiological processes that are so crucial for neonatal health. Finally, having quality resources and solid training in medical facilities makes a difference. In areas where staffing is light and essential equipment—like oxygen, blood products, and safe anesthesia practices—is in short supply, risks can quickly ramp up. For example, a shortage of these vital tools often jeopardizes the safety of both mother and baby during complications. Addressing these systemic issues, as some studies have pointed out, is key to lowering maternal and perinatal mortality rates. When healthcare systems focus on improving resources and training, they build a foundation that lessens risks and ultimately leads to much better outcomes for diverse populations (American College of Obstetricians and Gynecologists et al., 2007; Manasyan et al., 2013).

10.3.3. Reduction of Stress and Anxiety During Labor

Childbirth isn't just about the physical process—mental comfort plays a huge role for caregivers. Anxiety during labor can touch both the mom and baby in ways that clearly call for some thoughtful help. Lowering tension seems to not only brighten the experience for the birthing person but also helps labor move along more naturally. For example, having a trusted face nearby when the neuraxial pain relief is set up has been seen to lessen those uneasy feelings. More and more, caregivers are noticing that a little extra emotional backup can create a calmer, more reassuring atmosphere for delivery (Burns et al., 2018). Beyond having someone supportive by your side, non-drug ways of coping with labor pain and worry are getting a lot of attention. Techniques like massage, a bit of acupressure, and reflex touches have been talked about nowadays because they seem capable of easing discomfort without extra medication. Research generally shows that these caring, alternative therapies lower pain levels at different parts of labor, which in turn helps smooth out emotional ups and downs. When such approaches mix with standard medical treatments, care teams end up offering a wider toolkit for pain management. This rounded strategy not only gives women a sense of power during labor but also meets their emotional needs, reducing overall stress and anxiety (Yenter et al., 2024). Healthcare is always on the move, and blending different care strategies remains key to better outcomes during labor. Seeing how reducing stress can help labor progress guides obstetric anesthesiologists to fine-tune treatments that care for both body and mind. Evidence like having a supportive visitor around during neuraxial placement reminds everyone that a good labor environment should combine solid clinical skills with genuine kindness. That kind of holistic care boosts a woman's sense of independence and comfort, making childbirth a more positive experience. Ongoing efforts to mix both drug-based and alternative methods show a real commitment to perfecting obstetric care, ensuring that stress and anxiety are managed well throughout the process (Burns et al., 2018; Yenter et al., 2024) (Figure 10.11).

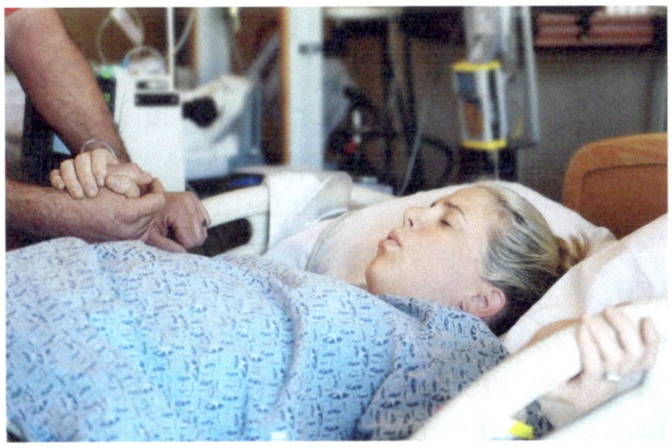

Figure 10.11. Reduction of stress and anxiety during labor.

Source: https://www.parents.com/thmb/E1LikLqnxm6gRLm0qb82l3aC4MU=/1500x0/filters:no_upscale():max_bytes(150000):strip_icc()/woman-in-labor-in-hospital_0-07a86fb1da7a4158a2690f23482fc1af.jpg.

Test Your Knowledge

1. What is maternal comfort?
2. How to reduce stress and anxiety during labor?

10.4. Risks and Complications

Learning Outcome

1. Understand the potential side effects for the mother.
2. Describe the risks to the fetus.
3. Describe the long-term implications of anesthesia use.

Obstetric anesthesia carries plenty of hidden hazards that can unexpectedly affect both mothers and their babies. Pain management for pregnant patients dealing with opioid-use disorder is especially tricky and often throws up challenges that don't always fit the textbook. During labor, while effective pain relief is needed, it comes with its set of issues—like the risks of developing tolerance, going through withdrawal, or even slipping back into substance use. A group of experts—SOAP, SMFM, and ASRA among them—has put together a consensus filled with evidence-backed recommendations for better pain management. Generally speaking, their guidance pushes for a case-by-case approach that puts the well-being of both mom and baby first, all while keeping an eye on the complications linked to OUD during the peripartum phase (Lim et al., 2024). Anesthesiologists, on the other hand, often face emergencies that seem to appear out of nowhere—whether it's during pregnancy, labor, or even the postpartum period. Emergencies like severe bleeding before or after birth, or high blood pressure episodes seen in conditions such as pre-eclampsia and eclampsia, have long been major contributors to risks for both mother and child, globally speaking. It gets even more complicated when patients come in with other health issues that only add to the mix. One case series, for instance, showcased various anesthetic techniques used during high-risk C-sections, underlining just how critical swift, coordinated intervention can be. In many cases, that rapid response makes all the difference for both maternal and neonatal outcomes (Bhowmik et al., 2024). There's also the risk of adverse reactions to anesthesia drugs and techniques, a factor that can spiral into serious complications. Whether using GA or regional methods, each approach carries dangers like respiratory depression, unstable heart function, or delayed recovery in the mother—which can, in turn, have a ripple effect on the newborn.

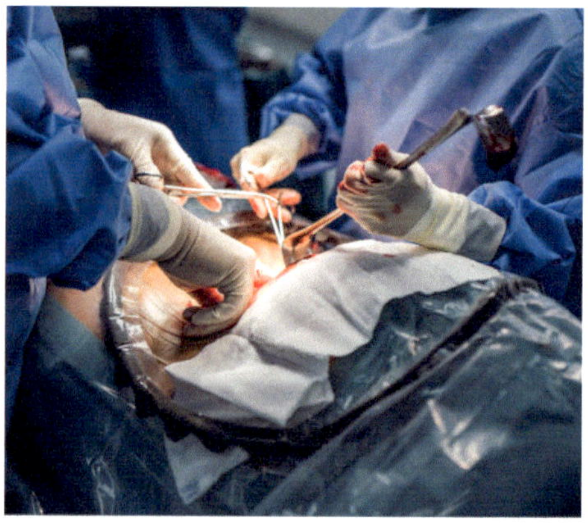

Figure 10.12. C-Section Injuries: risks and complications.

Source: https://www.birthinjuryguide.org/wp-content/uploads/2020/12/csection-500x430.jpg.

Because these issues crop up fairly often, clinicians usually take a proactive stance, carefully assessing each patient's risks before administering any anesthesia. Given that pregnancy brings about a host of physiological changes that might alter drug metabolism and blood flow, anesthesiologists need to be extra vigilant. By sticking with rigorous monitoring protocols and performing thorough preoperative checks, healthcare teams can reduce the odds of complications and steer obstetric anesthesia toward much safer practices (Figure 10.12).

10.4.1. Potential Side Effects for the Mother

During a cesarean, keeping the mom comfortable is crucial. Sometimes, though, the very measures that ease pain end up bringing unwelcome baggage – for example, episodes of nausea or vomiting that can disrupt the whole procedure and force the team to take extra steps. It's pretty common for these side effects to pop up, and while preventative anti-nausea medications generally help, they can themselves cause added complications, especially when using a mix of spinal and epidural (CSE) anesthesia. In the end, making sure both mom and baby are safe is what matters – which is why anesthesiologists and obstetricians have to juggle these issues while managing recovery and patient expectations (Levin et al., 2025). Another twist is that some anesthetic agents can cross the placenta, subtly affecting the mom's health. In emergency situations, GA is often deployed and gets extra scrutiny because fast-acting drugs like thiopental and succinylcholine work almost instantly. They kick in quickly to sedate, but then risks like prolonged recovery, respiratory depression, and even postpartum problems may follow; interestingly, even small delays between anesthesia induction and delivery seem to pile on additional risks such as uterine atony and neonatal depression (Pintarič, 2019). So, closely watching the mom's status throughout the process becomes a must to curb these risks and deliver top-notch care. Lastly, easing labor pain with opioids can sometimes be a bit messy. When drugs like fentanyl are administered—whether through an epidural or IV—they can occasionally lead to breathing issues for both the mother and the newborn, often requiring quick fixes right after delivery. Plus, any lingering effects might interfere with those crucial early bonding moments between a new mom and her infant. On the flip side, alternatives such as remifentanil clear from the body rather rapidly, which usually lowers the risk for the baby; still, individual responses can vary and complicate the overall outcome. To summarize, getting a nuanced grip on how these choices affect maternal and neonatal well-being is key to fine-tuning clinical practices in obstetric settings (Pintarič, 2019) (Figure 10.13).

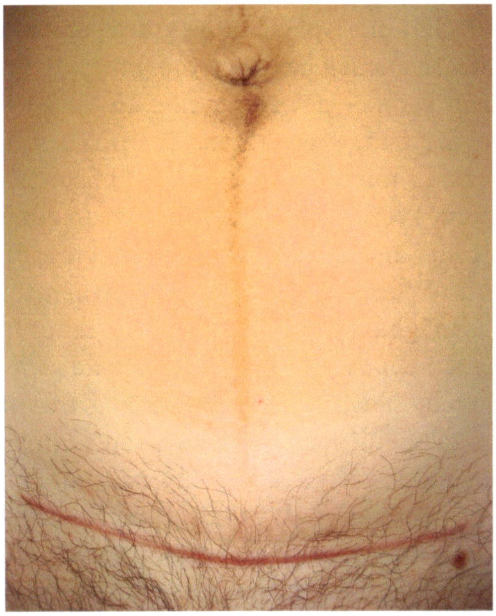

Figure 10.13. C-Section delivery side effects.

Source: By Azoreg - Own work, CC BY-SA 3.0, https://commons.wikimedia.org/w/index.php?curid=5188946.

10.4.2. Risks to the Fetus

Obstetric anesthesia is tricky and demands we understand how a fetus might be affected. When anesthesia is used, even minor shifts in a mother's physiological state or the way medications work can stress the fetus unexpectedly. For example, positioning during surgery might block the blood flow between the uterus and placenta, which in turn can lead to hypoxia. One case involved an expectant mom who, after suffering trauma, needed surgery; despite diligent pre-op monitoring, her baby showed signs of distress and ultimately required an emergency cesarean section.

This incident, among others, clearly shows why a well-coordinated team is so important for both the mother's and the baby's safety (Schwarzkopf et al., 2013). Preeclampsia brings its set of challenges with high blood pressure and extra complications that make anesthesia management more demanding. Regional techniques like spinal or epidural anesthesia have to be chosen based on the patient's ability to keep stable—not something to take lightly when the baby's well-being is on the line. In most cases, nurse anesthetists and obstetricians join forces to strike a balance between effective pain relief and ensuring safety. A review of the literature generally suggests that, when things are managed carefully, RA eases labor pain without negatively affecting outcomes for the mother or newborn. Understanding the nitty-gritty of conditions such as preeclampsia is pretty essential for achieving safe labor and delivery (Potter et al., 2008). Other conditions, like maternal obesity, diabetes, and even some heart issues, add extra layers of risk during obstetric anesthesia. Providers need to be on their toes—sometimes monitoring vital signs closely or switching up anesthetic techniques—to help keep the baby well-oxygenated and avoid complications. It's all about teamwork; nurses, anesthesiologists, and obstetricians must come together (even if their roles occasionally blur) to craft a plan that puts both maternal health and fetal safety first. By tackling these varied challenges in a flexible, evidence-driven way, teams can lift the quality of care for pregnant patients and better safeguard fetal outcomes.

10.4.3. Long-Term Implications of Anesthesia Use

Obstetric anesthesia brings along some lasting worries that we shouldn't ignore. There's always that chance—even if it's small—that a patient might, by accident, become aware during GA, and that unexpected moment can shake someone's mental balance. Some studies say roughly one in every 670 cesarean sections ends up in this situation, mostly because the dosage isn't always adjusted perfectly for all those pregnancy-related changes. Things like anxiety, unsettling nightmares, or even full-blown post-traumatic stress have been noted, which kind of underlines why managing these risks is key. With alternatives such as neuraxial analgesia catching on more these days, it's important to remind healthcare folks about the need for spot-on dosing and steady monitoring (Corner et al., 2024). There's also another angle to consider: postoperative complications, notably acute kidney injury (AKI). Research has linked AKI that happens after surgery with higher long-term mortality rates, a fact that adds another level of care needed for obstetric patients whose bodies are constantly shifting. In these cases, careful and ongoing observation becomes crucial. Lately, new machine learning methods have started showing promise in predicting which patients might run into issues after surgery—apparently even outperforming traditional statistical models in accuracy. These advancements, in most cases, allow clinicians to craft more precise, tailored interventions meant to boost survival rates and speed up recovery (Choi et al., 2024). Lastly, as obstetric anesthesia continues to evolve, a mixed approach involving various specialists is becoming all the more important. When anesthesiologists, obstetricians, and nurses work together—sometimes in unexpected ways—the best practices can naturally develop, shaping clinical guidelines and the way patients are educated. Regular training sessions and updates on the latest findings about anesthesia complications help build a kind of safety-first culture in healthcare facilities. Keeping a constant, if sometimes imperfect, check on potential issues like AKI or even those rare moments of unintended awareness can lower the risk of long-term harm. In general, deepening our understanding of these challenges while putting patient education and safety front and center leads to more informed decisions about using anesthesia in obstetric care (Choi et al., 2024; Corner et al., 2024) (Figure 10.14).

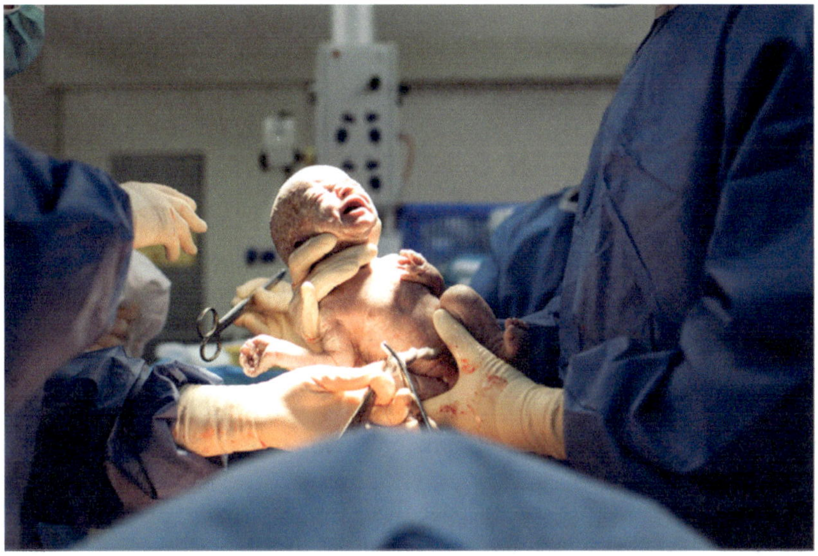

Figure 10.14. Obstetric Anesthesia Patient Safety: Practices to Ensure Adequate Venous Access and Safe Drug Administration During Transfer to the Operating Room for Emergency Cesarean Delivery.

Source: https://www.apsf.org/wp-content/uploads/newsletters/2015/Oct/image/Depositphotos_4526179_l-2015.png.

Test Your Knowledge

1. Describe the potential side effects for the mother
2. What is a risk for the fetus?

SUMMARY

Obstetric anesthesia has come a long way in recent years—it's not simply about reducing labor pain but also seems to be linked to mothers' mental states afterward. There is more buzz regarding whether the painkillers used during labor might also affect the risk of or even the extent of postpartum depression and anxiety. While effective pain relief is, for the most part, the main goal, there remains a lot of scope for exploration into whether and how such methods might combine with long-term mental health. What we do know at present could be the starting point for further research, allowing us to refine pain relief more effectively and improve mother's well-being after birth (Munro et al., 2020).

In the meantime, as neuraxial anesthesia becomes increasingly common, attention's needed on the other side. Consider the post-dural puncture headache (PDPH) as an example—it's a fairly significant problem that can de-escalate the quality of care in obstetric procedures. Certain recent efforts at quality improvement, such as the testing of neostigmine and atropine as potential PDPH treatments, remind us all that practice at the bedside is ever-changing and being current is imperative. Evidence-based practices that build provider competence might well be the solution to more clinical ease in such complications, with better outcomes in the delivery room (Morato et al., 2024). Briefly, the synergy of pain relief, maternal mood disturbances, and complications that may arise from obstetric anesthesia bears testament to how multidisciplinary this field can be. Further research, in the meantime, is necessary to cover the gaps and gain a more complete understanding of how anesthetic choice affects body and mind. Joint effort between mental health professionals, obstetricians, and anesthetists can open the door to overall care that values the well-being of mothers and infants. Finally, the evolution of obstetric anesthesia is not solely a matter of first-rate pain relief—it's also one of enhancing overall maternal health on those trying postpartum days (Morato et al., 2024; Munro et al., 2020).

New developments in obstetric anesthesia reveal that providing maternal care just so is not just a check-off box – it matters in everyday situations where education rates are rising. Take the MacArthur Foundations' efforts in Mexico, where promoting professional midwifery is seen as an actual game changer. They're not just focused on increasing midwifery training but trying to spark increased demand for skilled care. A simple baseline measurement – really more of a "where are we now?" snapshot – helps track whether or not these changes are making a difference (Keith-Brown et al., 2017). Really, a well-trained staff with real know-how can actually make a difference in maternal health outcomes in substantial ways. Across the United States, discussions of pain relief during labor have turned toward nitrous oxide—an approach that's been declining in practice since the 1880s.

Some reports mention that many providers are not that well acquainted with it, which only adds to the challenge of putting it into practice. A new quality improvement project aimed to tackle that directly by instituting educational modules for anesthesia providers, detailing the use of nitrous oxide in labor in simple language. The result was beneficial: people not only learned more, but they were also more inclined to try nitrous oxide as a part of their toolkit. It seems that when education stimulates curiosity, it has the ability to increase the mechanisms through which we get laboring women to feel ease during labor (Alfonso et al., 2023). Education and accessibility of a range of anesthesia options are certainly interconnected when talking about obstetric services.

The Mexican midwifery movement's success stories and the nitrous oxide education in the United States indicate that the solution is more confident caregivers. When practitioners get a good sense of what it is like to work with many techniques—and in the process hone their skills—communities are left with more resilient systems for dealing with labor pain and maternal care in general. This kind of change not only guarantees that laboring women are provided with the customized care they need but also nudges the whole system towards safer, more comfortable practices in general (Alfonso et al., 2023; Keith-Brown et al., 2017).

KEY TERMS FROM THIS CHAPTER

- Airway swelling
- Body mass index
- Combined spinal-epidural
- Emergency cesarean
- Fetal distress
- Labor analgesia
- Maternal health
- Post dural puncture headaches
- Bleeding
- Childbirth
- Drug metabolism
- Excretion
- Hypertension
- Maternal care
- Obstetric anesthesia
- Preeclampsia

CRITICAL THINKING QUESTIONS

1. **The primary goal of obstetric anesthesia is to:**
   a. Provide pain relief during labor
   b. Maintain maternal and fetal safety
   c. Facilitate cesarean delivery if required
   d. All of the above
2. **The most commonly used regional anesthesia for labor pain management is:**
   a. Spinal anesthesia
   b. Epidural anesthesia
   c. General anesthesia
   d. Local infiltration
3. **Which of the following local anesthetics is commonly used in epidural anesthesia for obstetrics?**
   a. Lidocaine
   b. Bupivacaine
   c. Procaine
   d. Articaine
4. **Absolute contraindications to epidural anesthesia in obstetrics include:**
   a. Patient refusal
   b. Coagulopathy
   c. Severe hypovolemia
   d. All of the above
5. **Which regional anesthetic technique is most commonly used for cesarean delivery?**
   a. Epidural anesthesia
   b. Spinal anesthesia
   c. Combined spinal-epidural (CSE) anesthesia
   d. General anesthesia

Short Answer Questions

1. Define the obstetric anesthesia.
2. Why is obstetric anesthesia important in maternal and fetal health?
3. List the types of obstetric anesthesia.
4. What are the benefits of obstetric anesthesia?
5. What are the risks and complications of obstetric anesthesia?

Answers to Critical Thinking Questions

1. (d); 2. (b); 3. (b); 4. (d); 5. (b)

REFERENCES

1. American College of Obstetricians and Gynecologists, Roberts, J., Hanson, L., Lothian, J., Ponkey, S. E., Rothman, B. K., Simkin, P., et al. (2007). *Best Practices in Second Stage Labor Care: Maternal Bearing Down and Positioning.* https://core.ac.uk/download/213087164.pdf (accessed on 20 May 2025).
2. Balatero, J. S. (2018). Obstetric nurses' perceived barriers to immediate skin to skin contact after cesarean birth. https://core.ac.uk/download/159401074.pdf (accessed on 20 May 2025).
3. Bhowmik, J. D., & Kumar, D. (2024). Anesthetic challenges and management of obstetric emergencies in a secondary care hospital in a remote mining area: A case series. *Cureus, 16.* https://www.semanticscholar.org/paper/e0232cdc481568e53480831a622a6c30c1485928 (accessed on 20 May 2025).
4. Braga, A. de F. de A., Carvalho, V. H., Braga, F. S. da S., & Pereira, R. I. C. (2018). Bloqueio combinado raquiperidural para-analgesia de parto: Estudo comparativo com bloqueio peridural contínuo. *Brazilian Journal of Anesthesiology, 69*, 7–12. https://doi.org/10.1016/j.bjan.2018.08.002.
5. Burns, M. A., Inchiosa Jr, M. A., Kubal, K. P., Kumaraswami, et al. (2018). Anesthesiologists' preferences regarding visitor presence during placement of neuraxial labor analgesia. https://core.ac.uk/download/217336177.pdf (accessed on 20 May 2025).
6. Choi, B. Y., Choi, W., Min, J., Chung, B. H., Koh, E. S., Hong, S., Ban, T. H., et al. (2024). Predicting long-term mortality of patients with postoperative acute kidney injury following noncardiac general anesthesia surgery using machine learning. *Kidney Research and Clinical Practice.* https://www.semanticscholar.org/paper/315eb58635c5e297dcc549f516ca9f128f501261 (accessed on 20 May 2025).
7. Corner, H., Barley, M., & Metodiev, Y. (2024). The use of processed electroencephalography (pEEG) in obstetric anesthesia: A narrative review. *Obstetric Anesthesia Digest.* https://www.semanticscholar.org/paper/de51b1c63f4607d3d4691e64c371e733b1b37eb3 (accessed on 20 May 2025).
8. Desai, N., Gardner, A. J., & Carvalho, B. (2019). Labor epidural analgesia to cesarean section anesthetic conversion failure: A national survey. *Anesthesiology Research and Practice, 2019*, 1–7. https://doi.org/10.1155/2019/6381792.
9. Dudas, L. (2014). Creating a comanaged obstetric/intensive care unit. *Journal of Obstetric, Gynecologic, & Neonatal Nursing, 43.* https://www.semanticscholar.org/paper/5a4770e65f78854dad0dc74249a63990f4de31cf (accessed on 20 May 2025).
10. Engbers, F. (2018). Is unconsciousness simply the reverse of consciousness? *Anesthesia, 73.* https://www.semanticscholar.org/paper/d16dc5f7251ca654f1b15950cce494932daf4e9c (accessed on 20 May 2025).
11. Garcia, E. N., Alfonso, F., & Orta, E. (2023). The return of nitrous oxide uses in the United States: An educational module. *Nicole Wertheim College of Nursing Student Projects, 234.* https://digitalcommons.fiu.edu/cnhs-studentprojects/234 (accessed on 20 May 2025).
12. George, R. (2017). Obstetrics and gynecology in low-resource settings: A practical guide. *Anesthesia & Analgesia.* https://www.semanticscholar.org/paper/63da218074a32a708a30acafb3507dba8f5f2f68 (accessed on 20 May 2025).

13. Holman, C., Glover, A., Fertaly, K., & Nelson, M. (2023). Operationalizing risk-appropriate perinatal care in a rural US state: Directions for policy and practice. *BMC Health Services Research, 23.* https://www.semanticscholar.org/paper/43bd0aebbf00a7f395190d4aa5d8272370bfcf48 (accessed on 20 May 2025).

14. Holzer, T. (2009). Treatment of post dural puncture headaches in the obstetric population. https://core.ac.uk/download/567882515.pdf (accessed on 20 May 2025).

15. Ismail, M. F., & Ismail, N. (2025). Labor analgesia and its impact on maternal and neonatal outcomes: Balancing benefits, risks, and unresolved questions. *Asian Journal of Medicine and Health.* https://www.semanticscholar.org/paper/5a79e42b4f73a5fc9883cbbad8a112eb60c2007f (accessed on 20 May 2025).

16. Keith-Br, K., & Atkin, L. C. (2017). MacArthur Foundation's initiative to promote midwifery in Mexico, complete baseline report. https://core.ac.uk/download/89473016.pdf (accessed on 20 May 2025).

17. Kuckowski, K., & Van Zundert, A. (2007). Anesthesia for pregnant women with valvular heart disease: The state-of-the-art (Review). https://core.ac.uk/download/55881363.pdf (accessed on 20 May 2025).

18. Levin, D., Levin, S., & Cohen, S. (2025). Effectiveness of P6 stimulation and transdermal scopolamine patch for the reduction of nausea and vomiting during caesarean section under combined spinal–epidural anesthesia: A randomized clinical trial. *Journal of Clinical Medicine, 14.* https://www.semanticscholar.org/paper/808456e51e56c22df469698022018e3f1140aa14 (accessed on 20 May 2025).

19. Liang, H., & Acharya, G. (2020). Novel corona virus disease (COVID-19) in pregnancy: What clinical recommendations to follow? *Acta Obstetrician et Gynecological Scandinavica, 99,* 439–442. https://doi.org/10.1111/aogs.13836.

20. Lim, G., Carvalho, B., George, R. B., Bateman, B. T., Brummett, C. M., Ip, V. H., Landau, R., et al. (2024). Consensus statement on pain management for pregnant patients with opioid-use disorder from the Society for Obstetric Anesthesia and Perinatology, Society for Maternal-Fetal Medicine, and American Society of Regional Anesthesia and Pain Medicine. *Anesthesia and Analgesia.* https://www.semanticscholar.org/paper/a23c137048c1e622f1ef18114781fdc3391aca5a (accessed on 20 May 2025).

21. Lozada, M. J., Babazade, R., & Vadhera, R. B. (2018). Obstetric analgesia and anesthesia. In J. P. Phelan, L. D. Pacheco, M. R. Foley, G. R. Saade, G. A. Dildy, & M. A. Belfort (Eds.), *Critical Care Obstetrics* (ch. 19). https://doi.org/10.1002/9781119129400.ch19.

22. Manasyan, A., Saleem, S., Koso-Thomas, M., Althabe, F., Pasha, O., Chomba, E., Goudar, S. S., Patel, A., Esamai, F., Garces, A., Kodkany, B., Belizán, J., McClure, E. M., Derman, R. J., Hibberd, P., Liechty, E. A., Hambidge, K. M., Carlo, W. A., Buekens, P., Moore, J., & EmONC Trial Group. (2013). Assessment of obstetric and neonatal health services in developing country health facilities. *American Journal of Perinatology, 30*(9), 787–794. https://doi.org/10.1055/s-0032-1333409.

23. Meskine, A., Elwartiti, L., Moujahid, A., Elghadbane, H. A., & Drissi, M. (2025). Anesthetic management of a cesarean section in a patient with Noonan syndrome: A multidisciplinary approach. *International Journal of Advanced Research, 13*(1), 1271–1274. https://www.journalijar.com (accessed on 20 May 2025).

24. Mladenovic, D., Kostic, S., Ivanović, K., Jovanovic, I., Petronijevic, M., Petronijevic, M., & Vrzić Petronijević, S. (2024). Depressive symptoms during pregnancy and the postpartum period: A tertiary hospital experience. *Medicina, 60*. https://www.semanticscholar.org/paper/e35f194e7701e7071b83be7e0890c70f6627baba (accessed on 20 May 2025).

25. Mohamed Tawfik, M. M., Atallah, M. M., Elkharboutly, W. S., Allakkany, N. S., & Abdelkhalek, M. (2016). Does preprocedural ultrasound increase the first-pass success rate of epidural catheterization before cesarean delivery? A randomized controlled trial. *Anesthesia & Analgesia, 124*, 851–856. https://doi.org/10.1213/ane.0000000000001325.

26. Morato, A., Vera, C. D., & Gattorno, J. C. (2024). Elevating the standard of post-dural puncture headache treatment: An educational module. *Nicole Wertheim College of Nursing Student Projects*, 299. https://digitalcommons.fiu.edu/cnhs-studentprojects/299 (accessed on 20 May 2025).

27. Munro, A., MacCormick, H., Sabharwal, A., & George, R. B. (2020). Pharmacologic labor analgesia and its relationship to postpartum psychiatric disorders: A scoping review. *Canadian Journal of Anesthesia, 67*(5), 588–604. https://doi.org/10.1007/s12630-020-01587-7.

28. Padalko, A. A., & Dziuba, H. A. (2025). Justification and implementation of the multimodal general anesthesia model for elective cesarean section into clinical practice. *Zaporozhye Medical Journal, 27*(1), 56–64. https://zmj.zsmu.edu.ua/article/view/317596 (accessed on 20 May 2025).

29. Pintarič, T. (2019). ESRA19-0628 maternal anesthesia/analgesia and fetal/neonatal drug uptake. *Regional Anesthesia & Pain Medicine, 44*, A10–A11. https://www.semanticscholar.org/paper/1cbfa7f248547b1d581f6b9f175eddd1a41488f3 (accessed on 20 May 2025).

30. Potter, L. M. (2008). Spinal versus epidural anesthesia for the management of patients with preeclampsia undergoing elective or urgent cesarean section. https://core.ac.uk/download/567882393.pdf (accessed on 20 May 2025).

31. Reale, S. C., Farber, M. K., Lumbreras-Márquez, M. I., Connors, J. M., & Carabuena, J. M. (2021). Anesthetic management of Von Willebrand disease in pregnancy: A retrospective analysis of a large case series. *Anesthesia & Analgesia*. https://doi.org/10.1213/ane.0000000000005502.

32. Rosseel, P., Trelles, M., Guilavogui, S., Ford, N., & Chu, K. (2010). Ten years of experience training non-physician anesthesia providers in Haiti. *World Journal of Surgery, 34*(3), 453–458. https://doi.org/10.1007/s00268-009-0192-2.

33. Schwarzkopf, R., Gross, S. C., Coopersmith, A., & Gidumal, R. (2013). Ankle fracture surgery on a pregnant patient complicated by intraoperative emergency caesarian section. *Case Reports in Orthopedics, 2013*, 962794. https://doi.org/10.1155/2013/962794.

34. Thomas, C. L., Lange, E. M. S., Banayan, J. M., Zhu, Y., Liao, C., Peralta, F., Grobman, W. A., et al. (2024). Racial and ethnic disparities in receipt of general anesthesia for cesarean delivery. *JAMA Network Open, 7*, e2350825. https://doi.org/10.1001/jamanetworkopen.2023.50825.

35. Yenter, E. (2024). Efficacy of complimentary manual therapies for labor pain management. *Physician Assistant Scholarly Project Papers, 212*. https://commons.und.edu/pas-grad-papers/212 (accessed on 20 May 2025).

GERIATRIC ANESTHESIA

11

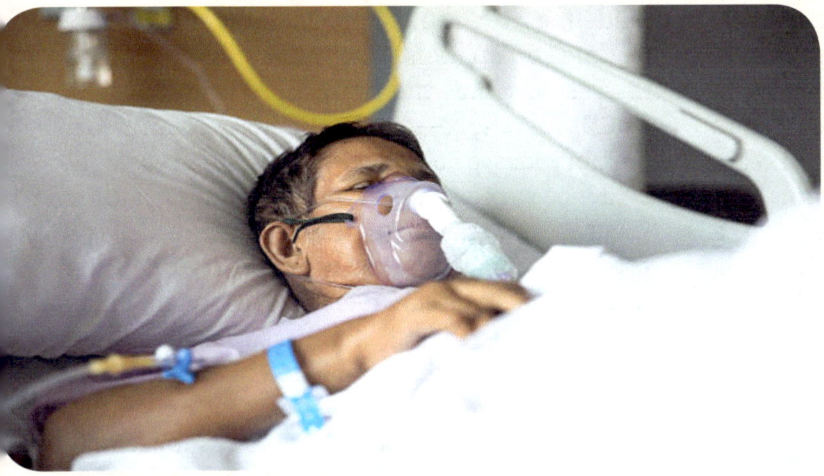

LEARNING OBJECTIVES

After studying this chapter, you will be able to:

1. Describe the physiological changes in the elderly.
2. Learn about common anesthetic agents used in geriatric patients.
3. Perform the preoperative assessment in geriatric patients.
4. Understand the intraoperative management considerations.
5. Discuss about postoperative care and complications of geriatric anesthesia.

Introduction

With our population growing older, medicine—especially the handling of anesthesia—creates a whole host of problems. The body does not work quite so well anymore; organs don't function as well and drugs respond differently. This brings about a kind of rethinking of the standard anesthesia regimens. Older patients have more baggage in the form of multiple medical conditions and an arsenal of medications that complicate things. All of which implies that anesthesia must be customized to each patient, not only to reduce risk but also to maximize surgical result. And then there is the brain part. Every now and then, we will find that after surgery, older patients receive a kind of mental clouding—often called postoperative cognitive dysfunction, or POCD. Evidently, the anxiety of surgery and the anaesthesia itself can actually trigger a small amount of brain inflammation, which in most cases will make these mental hiccup moments. Overall, physicians need to be a bit more cautious by performing strict check-ups beforehand and keeping an eye out for mental alertness afterward. It also raises the possibility that examination of treatments intended to calm this inflammation can be very worthwhile in the balancing of brain health with anesthetic practice in these patients. Second, screening for overall physical health—typically by means of body composition analysis—gives crucial information about a patient's overall health and nutritional status. Procedures such as dual-energy X-ray absorptiometry (DXA) and bioelectrical impedance analysis (BIA) are good at signaling shortfalls that would most probably disrupt recovery. With such advice under one's belt, anesthetic treatment and post-op protocols can be adapted on the fly. Overall, because the issues of aging add more dimensions of risk to safe anesthesia, it would be wise to use a team approach that gathers information from both body scans and psychological tests. Finally, a more integrated method may result in safer, more person-centered care (Figure 11.1).

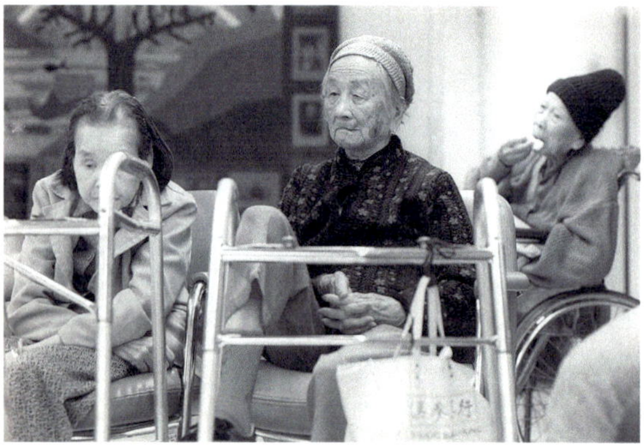

Figure 11.1. Geriatric anesthesia.

Source: By Nancy Wong - Own work, CC BY-SA 4.0, https://commons.wikimedia.org/w/index.php?curid=81990672.

Definition of Geriatric Anesthesia

Aging and anesthesia have become quite a partnership, and this union has spawned a specialty in geriatric anesthesia. Old patients come with their own set of idiosyncrasies—organs slow down, and drugs respond differently—which raises the risk for complications in the operating room. Doctors, especially anesthesiologists, now have to give special attention to each patient, balancing meticulously the special way an old body metabolizes drugs. It's an intimate knowledge of how those bodies metabolize drugs that is the key to designing a suitable plan of safety, and thus being able to obtain the optimal amount of pain relief, sedation, and level of anesthesia is the most important thing. In most cases, this isn't really about adhering to standard guidelines; it's about tuning care to the internal rhythms of a patient. There's actually a genuine interest in what the brain does after surgery. POCD, for short—can show up as confusion, memory loss, or outright agitation. Increasingly, evidence suggests that some brain inflammation (neuroinflammation) is a major cause, which has prompted many to call for pre-surgical brain testing. The tests can detect those who might be more prone to mental slumps. Unraveling these signs to inflammation could lead to better ways of avoiding or even preventing those cognitive dips. However, as every patient's response may vary, further research and more consistent practices are a requirement (Safavynia et al., 2019). Another key ingredient in making surgery safe for elderly patients is teamwork. It's not something a person does all by themselves—there are surgeons, anesthesiologists, geriatricians, and nurses who all have a hand in grasping the complexity of the care. Protocols typically refer to early identification of at-risk patients and close monitoring during and post-surgery to intercept problems such as delirium. Open, occasionally spontaneous, communication between the team facilitates leaping on complications ahead of time. And frequent training for all involved creates a culture in which the special requirements of the elderly are not just noted but welcomed. All this collaboration can actually reduce lower errors and improve patient safety, strengthening the justification for geriatric anaesthesia to be part of modern surgical practice (Aldecoa et al., 2017) (Figure 11.2).

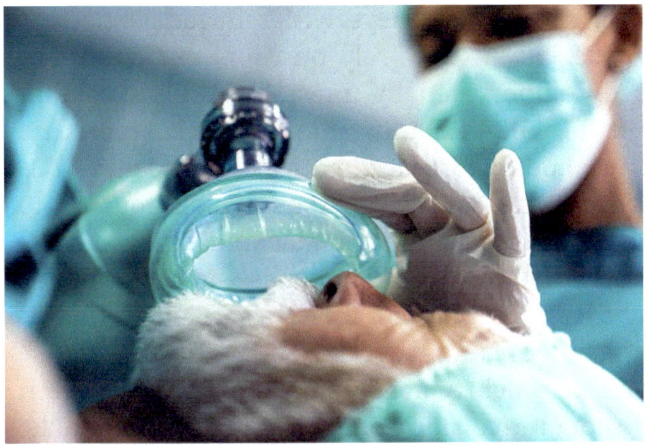

Figure 11.2. Definition of Geriatric Anesthesia.

Source: https://sagahq.org/wp-content/uploads/2023/07/procedure-of-anesthesia-for-surgery-to-treatment-p-2022-07-28-23-55-39-utc.jpg.

Importance of Anesthesia in the Elderly

Older patients undergoing anesthesia need to take a close examination of how the body's machinery is rewired by aging—this is not merely a matter of drugs interacting with receptors, but of appreciating that as humans age, their system for metabolizing these drugs alters in ways both surprising and subtle. Seniors often carry with them a combination of other medical conditions, such as heart issues or lapses in memory, which raise the stakes on any surgical intervention. For the most part, doctors need to select their medications, dosages, and monitoring devices with caution to suit each patient's true needs. Processed EEG monitoring, which peeks into brain activity, can typically catch adverse reactions before they're a problem; however, because patient reactions are so varied, even with EEG, finding a one-size-fits-all solution remains difficult (Drover et al., 2018). It's also necessary to consider how the use of anesthetics aligns with the mental recovery after surgery. Recent research, like the study on Dexmedetomidine (DEX), collectively shows that lower infusion rates go hand in hand with better short-term cognitive performance – measured on tests like the Mini-Mental State Examination (MMSE). This is not simply a function of the body acclimating to the anesthesia; it's also about having a solid mind afterwards. Even minor modifications in anesthetic administration can help minimize the risk of confusion and delirium postoperation and support a good quality of life (Dhiraj et al., 2024). Individualized anesthetic protocols are more than an adjunct recommendation—now it is essential for effective and safe surgery in elderly patients. One must gain an overall sense of a patient's prior state of health, medicines currently being taken, and potential drug confusion prior to choosing a method, since aging can affect the way drugs are processed, and increase the older population's susceptibility to desired as well as undesired side effects. This necessitates a bit of coordination: anesthesiologists, surgeons, and geriatricians must often coordinate together in a loose but significant fashion to find the best way. Ongoing studies, with their highs and lows, are what continually shape such approaches, thus placing patient safety at the very heart of all surgical results.

11.1. Physiological Changes in the Elderly

Learning Outcome

1. Understand the cardiovascular system adaptations.
2. Describe the respiratory system considerations.
3. Understand the neurological changes affecting anesthesia.

Aging creates changes that affect surgery in unexpected ways. The kidneys and liver, for example, no longer work as they once did, so medications remain in the system longer than expected. The liver—its enzyme function normally lower—can interfere with how drugs are metabolized, and that can mean anesthetics can stay around, elevating the risk of complications during surgery. Kidneys, with reduced glomerular filtration rate, also can permit drugs to build up, especially if they rely on renal excretion. For most cases, dosing needs to be adjusted and closely supervised by anesthesiologists so that any deleterious effects can be avoided (Bhadani et al., 2024). Fluid balance and temperature also don't always obey the rules in the elderly. As the bodies lose acclimatization to continuous thermoregulation, getting too cold under anesthetic becomes a critical issue, which goes on to complicate recovery as well. Physicians have to resort to trusting warming machines and carefully planned fluid management—frequently resorting to blending techniques at times—to hold control. Body composition alterations (e.g., losing muscle and gaining additional fat) also lead to liquids and drugs spreading unpredictably, altering the dosing and the impact of drugs (Lapid et al., 2024). And then there is the problem of cognitive impairment, which typically adds confusion where it is needed least regarding anesthesia management. Preoperative slownesses in the brain can make it hard to identify new proof of delirium post-surgery, a condition that can easily be missed. Pain, certain medications, and even hospital stressors can contribute to further disturbing a patient's brain. It is vital to identify these alterations in advance, since unnoticed delirium can result in patients remaining in the hospital longer and performing worse in the long term. Typically, an elderly anesthetic plan will be one that decreases sedatives and tries other, non-pharmacologic approaches to help decrease postoperative cognitive glitches. All of which is why team-based, multidisciplinary care is so vital when managing these patients (Bhadani et al., 2024) (Figure 11.3).

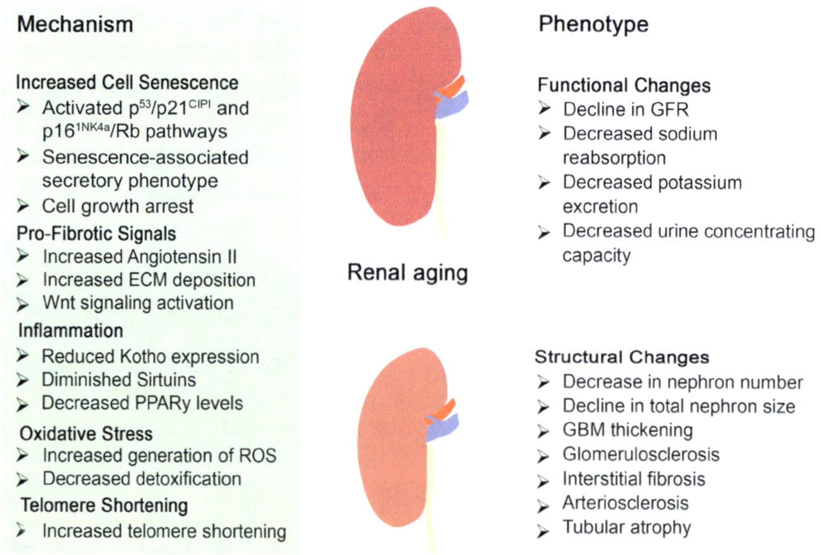

Figure 11.3. Factors that increase and decrease age-related changes in the kidney.

Source: Liu F, Chen J, Li Z, Meng X. Recent Advances in Epigenetics of Age-Related Kidney Diseases. *Genes*. 2022; 13(5):796. https://doi.org/10.3390/genes13050796.

11.1.1. Cardiovascular System Adaptations

Aging brings about many bodily shifts—especially in how the heart works—that change the game for anesthesia in older patients. As people grow older, their hearts tend to get a thicker muscle and become less flexible. This isn't just a cosmetic change; it often means that the heart can't pump as robustly, so there's a higher chance of low blood pressure and poor blood flow during surgery. At the same time, blood vessels lose some of their bounce, which can push systolic pressure up, adding another layer of challenge when managing anesthesia. Generally speaking, it's essential that anesthesiologists grasp these changes, because a one-size-fits-all approach just won't cut it when precise control over fluids and circulation is so crucial. Beyond these structural alters, the way older bodies handle medications also shifts noticeably. In most cases, elderly patients don't metabolize drugs the same way younger bodies do—often due to a slowdown in liver and kidney function—so what might be a routine dose for one person can be a lot more potent for another.

This means that standard anesthetic agents might have unexpectedly strong effects or linger longer, for reasons that sometimes even catch clinicians by surprise. It's a delicate dance: doctors need to adjust dosages carefully and stay alert to any side effects that creep in from drugs building up in the system. Research too has a say in this whole matter. Many studies, for instance (Almutairi et al., 2022), have highlighted that a thorough preoperative checkup is indispensable to understand each patient's cardiovascular risks. There's a growing consensus that a tailored anesthesia plan—one that accounts for individual heart health—can help reduce post-surgery problems like delirium or lingering cognitive hiccups. With more older adults heading into surgery these days (Kanaparthy et al., 2025), it makes sense to lean on this specialized knowledge about how the heart ages. To summarize, a customized approach that takes into account the natural, and sometimes unpredictable, changes in cardiovascular function is key to keeping elderly patients safe and improving their outcomes.

11.1.2. Respiratory System Considerations

Breathing becomes a major concern when dealing with older patients during anesthesia. With age, lungs get stiffer and the chest wall loses some of its springiness, meaning there's less room left over in the lungs. In many cases, this drop in lung capacity increases the risk of low oxygen levels or too much carbon dioxide when under anesthesia—a real worry for those giving the anesthesia. That's why it all starts with a good look at one's breathing before surgery, using tests to check ventilation and oxygen levels. Knowing these limits helps in picking the right anesthetic method and extra therapies, which in turn tailors the approach for each elderly patient and tries to keep risks low. Many seniors also bring along other breathing troubles like COPD, interstitial lung disease, or even sleep apnea. These extra conditions just add to the mix and make managing anesthesia trickier. They sometimes force providers to use more advanced airway techniques and mess with the normal dosing of anesthetic drugs. Anesthesia teams must stay extra alert after surgery too, since older patients can easily develop pneumonia or have portions of their lungs collapse. This makes thorough pre-surgery evaluations and careful post-op monitoring key—there's a real need to keep an eye on how the lungs are behaving. The issues with breathing in older folks don't stop at the surgery door either. Studies—including those looking at centenarians having surgery—often point out that breathing mishaps can mean longer hospital stays and higher costs (Krishna et al., 2020). After procedures, there's still the puzzle of adjusting for changes in the pulmonary mechanics and how efficiently they exchange gas. Simple tactics, like using incentive spirometry or getting moving a bit sooner, can nicely boost lung function post-surgery and help speed up recovery. Generally speaking, understanding these age-related breathing challenges is crucial for anesthesiologists, so they can navigate through these complexities with a strategy that keeps patient safety first (Figure 11.4).

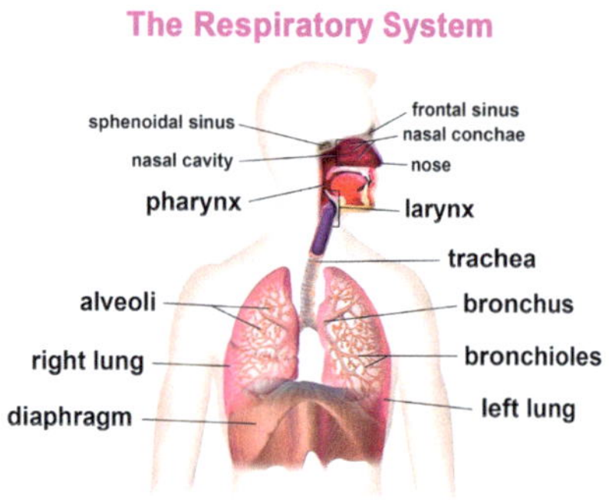

Figure 11.4. Respiratory system.

Source: https://i.ytimg.com/vi/ZB7uA5o0mS4/maxresdefault.jpg.

11.1.3. Neurological Changes Affecting Anesthesia

Aging and anesthesia don't mix in a straightforward way. As people grow older, their brains change—not in one neat overhaul, but through subtle shifts in how neurons connect and how neurotransmitters work. These quiet adjustments can alter how someone responds to anesthetic drugs, sometimes making them more vulnerable to issues like cloudy thinking after surgery. In most cases, recent studies point out that elderly patients behave differently when it comes to medication effects, partly because their bodies handle drug processing in a changed manner. This irregularity in reaction often bumps up the risk of complications and makes it clear that anesthesia plans need to take these neurological alters into account, making the case for personalized care. A big worry for older adults centers on POCD, where the mind simply doesn't bounce back as expected after an operation. Research shows that the specific anesthetic used can deeply influence these outcomes; for example, one study comparing sevoflurane with desflurane found that both temporarily lower MMSE scores, though sevoflurane seems to hit a bit harder. Many clinicians now lean on techniques like processed electroencephalography (EEG) to better gauge anesthesia depth, which generally helps reduce on the chance of cognitive hiccups (Meineke et al., 2014). On top of that, medications like benzodiazepines might actually add fuel to the fire of cognitive decline, since age-induced changes in brain receptor sensitivity can lead to prolonged sedation and slower recoveries. Some are even exploring unconventional alternatives—think lavender oil aromatherapy—as a softer option to calm nerves before surgery, potentially reducing the reliance on traditional anxiolytic drugs and offering safer overall care for these patients (Gonzalez et al., 2022).

Test Your Knowledge

1. What are the cardiovascular system adaptations?
2. Describe the neurological changes affecting anesthesia.

11.2. Common Anesthetic Agents Used in Geriatric Patients

Learning Outcome

1. Describe the inhalational anesthetics and intravenous anesthetics.
2. Understand the regional anesthesia techniques.

Choosing the right anesthetic for older patients isn't a straightforward task. As people get older, everything from heart function and lung capacity to kidney work and metabolism starts to change in ways that matter when it comes to how drugs act in the body. Drugs like midazolam and DEX are popular choices because they typically have a safer profile, but extra caution is needed. For example, midazolam works well for sedation, yet if someone's liver isn't cutting it, the drug can linger—which may lead to extended effects and even breathing issues. That's why careful dose alters and constant monitoring during surgery become a must (Paschoal et al., 2025). There are also alternatives like clonidine and DEX that have made their mark in the anesthetic scene for older folks. These medications not only help ease anxiety but also tend to keep blood pressure steady—a real bonus for patients juggling several health issues. Instead of a one-size-fits-all approach, doctors often consider the full picture: a patient's complete medical history, their current medications, and any underlying conditions.

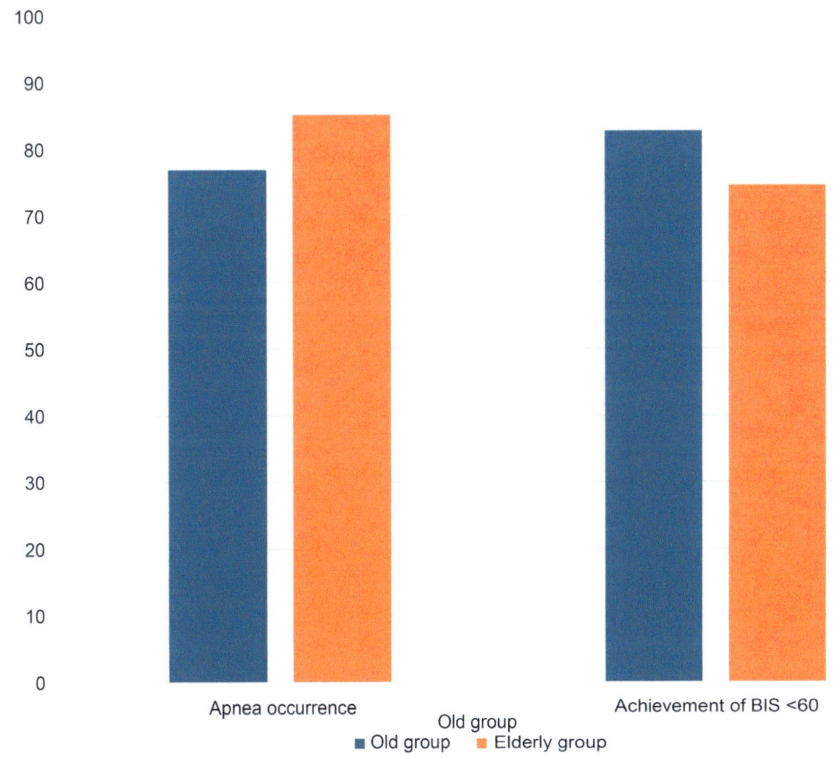

Figure 11.5. Clinical pharmacology of anesthetic agents in elderly.

Source: Chae MS, Lee N, Koh HJ. Age-Related Response to Remimazolam among Older Patients Undergoing Orthopedic Surgery: A Single-Center Prospective Observational Study. *Medicina*. 2024; 60(10):1616. https://doi.org/10.3390/medicina60101616.

This broader look naturally boosts patient safety and helps tailor the anesthetic to what the individual needs (Shaji et al., 2024). In the end, finding the perfect anesthetic for this demographic is a bit of a juggling act. It isn't only about getting the desired effect; minimizing risk plays a huge role too. Studies generally show that differences in drug metabolism—for instance, variations in plasma protein levels—can lead to unpredictable responses in older patients. With that in mind, a solid grasp of how these medications work is essential. Continuous learning, periodic dose adjustments, and a commitment to evidence-based protocols all help ensure that elderly patients enjoy safer and smoother surgical outcomes (Paschoal et al., 2025; Shaji et al., 2024) (Figure 11.5).

11.2.1. Inhalational Anesthetics

Surgery today often relies on the quick action and simplicity of inhalational anesthetics. They're popular because they kick in fast and are easy to use. Still, things aren't so straightforward when it comes to older patients – their bodies handle these substances in a way that's quite distinct from younger ones. With aging, the way these drugs interact with the body shifts, changing not only how deep the anesthesia goes but also how long it takes for someone to bounce back. Studies generally show that older adults sometimes react more intensely, and that can bring about unwanted side effects like delirium and other cognitive hiccups. Getting the right type and dose becomes important to keep things safe and effective during operations. There's also the matter of how these anesthetics link to problems with thinking after surgery, known as postoperative cognitive dysfunction (POCD). Research suggests that exposure to these agents might spark off a kind of brain inflammation—something that's even more pronounced in folks who already have some memory or thinking challenges. This inflammation seems to be influenced both by the stress of surgery and the drugs themselves, which makes managing elderly patients even trickier. In most cases, doctors need to check a patient's mental starting point carefully and choose their anesthesia plan with extra caution. Plus, emerging strategies to ward off brain inflammation could soon pave the way for more personalized anesthetic plans that focus on protecting cognitive health (Seyed et al., 2019). Another key issue is watching over neuromuscular blockers when inhalational anesthetics are in play with older patients. It's important to monitor muscle function objectively, since that helps stop any lingering drug effects that could lead to breathing problems or other complications. A recent consensus from a panel of clinician scientists pointed out that using quantitative methods — like tracking the train-of-four ratio — is crucial for confirming that muscle function is truly bouncing back (Naguib et al., 2017). Neglecting this kind of monitoring could result in prolonged respiratory distress and further postoperative challenges. Simply put, pairing inhalational anesthetics with rigorous neuromuscular monitoring is essential to merging effective anesthesia with patient safety, especially in our elderly population (Figure 11.6).

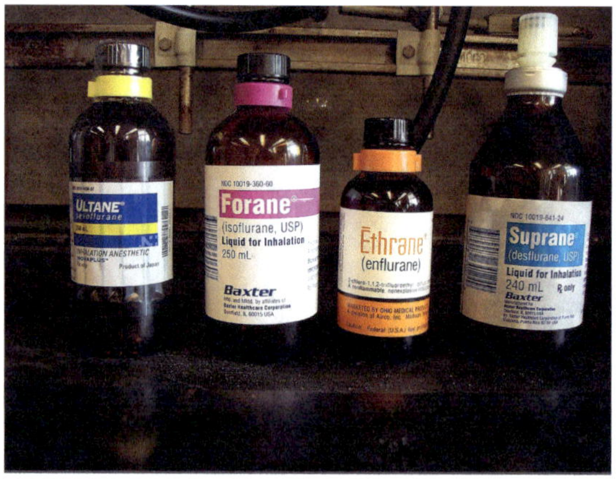

Figure 11.6. Inhaled anesthetics.

Source: By Diesel-50 (talk) - Own work (Original text: I created this work entirely by myself.), Public Domain, https://commons.wikimedia.org/w/index.php?curid=65246942.

11.2.2. Intravenous Anesthetics

Intravenous anesthetics are playing an ever-larger role in treating older patients, largely because as folks age, their bodies handle medications in peculiar ways. Aging brings changes—liver and kidney functions shift, which then messes with how drugs are metabolized and flushed out. For this reason, doctors need to pick anesthetic agents with extra care so they don't leave patients sedated for too long or trigger lingering cognitive fog. Lately, there's been a push to use drugs that help patients snap back to clear thinking more quickly. Take, for example, colorectal surgeries where propofol was compared to sevoflurane; the evidence hinted that those on propofol bounced back cognitively faster (Dushin et al., 2025). Dosing and delivering IV anesthetics require some extra thought when dealing with the elderly, since the usual amounts might not fit every individual—health conditions and body differences come into play. A recent study even dug into the effects of ciprofol versus propofol during hip replacements and found that patients on propofol woke up and had their breathing tubes removed sooner than those on ciprofol. This difference underlines that it's not just the choice of drug, but also how it's administered, that matters a lot (Yang et al., 2024). At the same time, accumulating research on IV anesthetics in older populations calls for constant checks on patient outcomes and complication rates. Since seniors are often more sensitive to medications, careful dosing and close monitoring before, during, and after surgery are key. The common occurrence of cognitive issues after surgery demands that we use evidence-based approaches to keep these risks in check. Anesthetic methods that encourage rapid recovery—like the ones involving propofol—seem to help reduce both the length and intensity of cognitive hiccups after surgery, ultimately boosting care quality for the elderly (Dushin et al., 2025). As the field of geriatric anesthesia keeps evolving, ongoing research will be crucial in fine-tuning these practices to ensure the best results for these vulnerable patients (Figure 11.7).

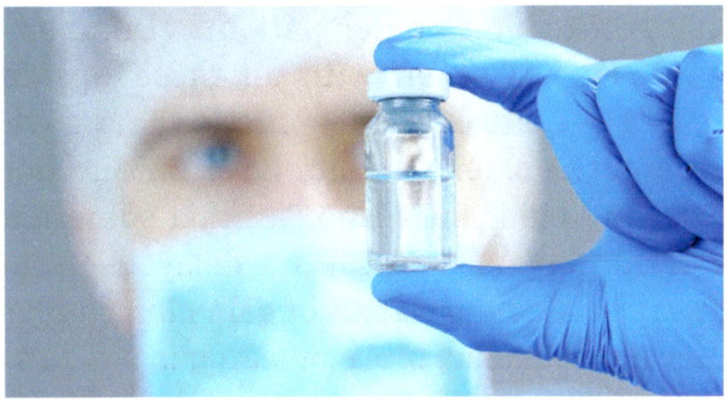

Figure 11.7. Intravenous anesthetics.

Source: https://chblob.icloudhospital.com/images/1-649fce17-abf9-4e5d-b157-eac949eefa62.jpg.

11.2.3. Regional Anesthesia Techniques

Elderly patients facing surgery have plenty of hurdles to overcome. Regional anesthesia (RA), for example, keeps popping up in studies as a promising tool—especially when it comes to hip fractures. Some reports even hint that using techniques like nerve blocks can cut back on heart and breathing mishaps that usually show up with general anesthesia (GA). In many recent comparisons, better safety numbers and fewer after-surgery issues seem to stress how smart it is to pick the right anesthesia for older folks, which can boost recovery and even keep the mind clearer in many cases (Li et al., 2025). When it comes to calming pain before surgery, peripheral nerve blocks (PNBs) have stepped into the spotlight for patients with hip fractures. This approach can sometimes lower reliance on heavy-duty painkillers—yes, even opioids—and tackle the rising worries over opioid side effects. Reports on methods like the femoral nerve block or the fascia iliaca compartment block have backed them up; studies show these methods not only offer lasting relief but also encourage patients to get moving sooner after their operation. To summarize, these nerve blocks play a key role in easing pain early on, which many feel can help dodge the kind of post-surgery confusion that often troubles older patients (Dönmez et al., 2024). Still, even with all these upsides, bringing RA into everyday practice isn't a walk in the park. Older patients have unique body quirks and medicine responses that sometimes mean surgery might even be delayed—issues that can muddy the waters of pain management. Generally speaking, more research is needed to pinpoint exactly how different nerve block styles stack up. Ongoing studies, with all their nuanced findings, should help fine-tune treatment plans that work better for these patients—boosting both surgery outcomes and overall safety. In the end, weaving RA into standard care for older individuals seems like a smart move to raise the bar for quality treatment (Figure 11.8).

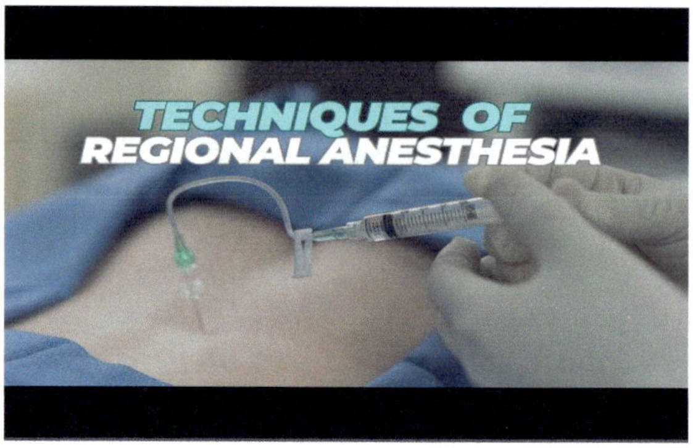

Figure 11.8. Techniques of regional anesthesia.

Source: https://i.ytimg.com/vi/uH52H7GSrLE/sddefault.jpg.

Test Your Knowledge

1. What are the intravenous anesthetics?
2. Describe the regional anesthesia techniques.

11.3. Preoperative Assessment in Geriatric Patients

Learning Outcome

1. Review the comprehensive medical history.
2. Evaluate the functional status.
3. Describe the risk assessment tools.

Managing anesthesia in older patients starts with a solid preoperative check. It's not only about pinning down existing health problems, but also about getting a real sense of how healthy someone is overall. Research generally shows that digging deep—spotting hints of frailty or long-term conditions—makes a big difference, since these issues can unexpectedly complicate any surgery. Age changes how drugs behave in the body, so there's no one-size-fits-all plan here. When these details are caught early on, it becomes possible to craft a more individualized anesthetic strategy, one that matches the patient's unique medical history and the specific surgical demands, ultimately leading to a safer experience (Souza et al., 2024). The process usually isn't a solo act either; it's very much a team effort. Often, anesthesiologists, surgeons, nurses, and even geriatric experts all share their perspectives to form a more complete picture of the patient's health. Working together like this, clinicians can bring in ERAS protocols, a set of practices that many studies note helps boost recovery—especially in cases like hip fractures. These protocols lean on things like premedication, solid nutritional support, and effective pain control, each playing its part in reducing the risks after surgery. To summarize, such comprehensive preoperative reviews help fine-tune anesthetic approaches, tailoring them to each individual and generally smoothing out the recovery process (Uppalapati et al., 2024). Finally, it helps to remember that looking after a patient's mind is just as key as checking their body. Many older patients face anxiety or depression, which can add another layer of challenge to both surgery and healing. By catching these psychological factors early, healthcare teams can roll out supportive measures—sometimes a bit of counseling or a clear explanation goes a long way in easing worries. This kind of approach, which blends the physical with the emotional, not only gives patients a greater sense of control but also tends to encourage sticking to the recovery plan. In most cases, accounting for both mental and physical well-being helps build a more effective anesthetic strategy that's just right for elderly patients (Souza et al., 2024).

11.3.1. Comprehensive Medical History Review

Assessing a patient's medical background is key to managing anesthesia—especially when it comes to older folks. As people age, they tend to pick up a mix of health issues that can sometimes make surgery trickier than expected. Knowing all the ins and outs of someone's past illnesses lets anesthesiologists gauge risks and craft a plan that feels tailor-made. This point becomes extra important with frailty, which is simply when someone's natural reserves are lower, sometimes leading to hiccups after an operation. In most cases, using straightforward tools like the Memorial Sloan Kettering Frailty Index (MSK-FI) gives a richer picture of vulnerability than merely checking age or relying on scores like ASA-PS. It all just goes to show that digging deep into a patient's history isn't a mere formality—it's a real safeguard for better surgical outcomes. Anesthetic effects truly can vary, largely due to the unique twists hidden in a senior's health story. It's not only about the numbers; everyday factors like functional ability, social support, and even nutrition plays huge roles in how the body handles anesthetics—and then how recovery pans out. Looking over a patient's full background gives clinicians a multi-layered view, sometimes flagging risks that might otherwise slip by unnoticed. Take cognitive impairments, for example, which aren't uncommon among older adults; they might well nudge the team to alter both the anesthesia method and subsequent care.

Generally speaking, this broader, sometimes slightly messy perspective enables healthcare providers to catch potential pitfalls early on, painting a picture of not just physical but also mental health that ultimately helps in shaping a more individualized anesthetic plan. Finally, folding a complete medical history into pre-surgery checks has sparked some neat advancements in managing postoperative pain. Recent research has even started leaning away from the classic, one-size-fits-all opioid approach, since older patients often react differently.

For example, methadone has shown promise in easing pain after procedures, sidestepping several of the issues that traditional opioids tend to bring along—something particularly important given seniors' heightened sensitivity to side effects. In most cases, this lively discussion about fresh pain management techniques underscores just how pivotal a thorough history review is. By blending insights from various medical specialties and not shying away from even the small details, care teams can better navigate the quirks of geriatric anesthesia. All of this, in the end, aims to foster smoother recoveries and greater satisfaction for patients, even if the process sometimes feels a bit imperfect (Figure 11.9).

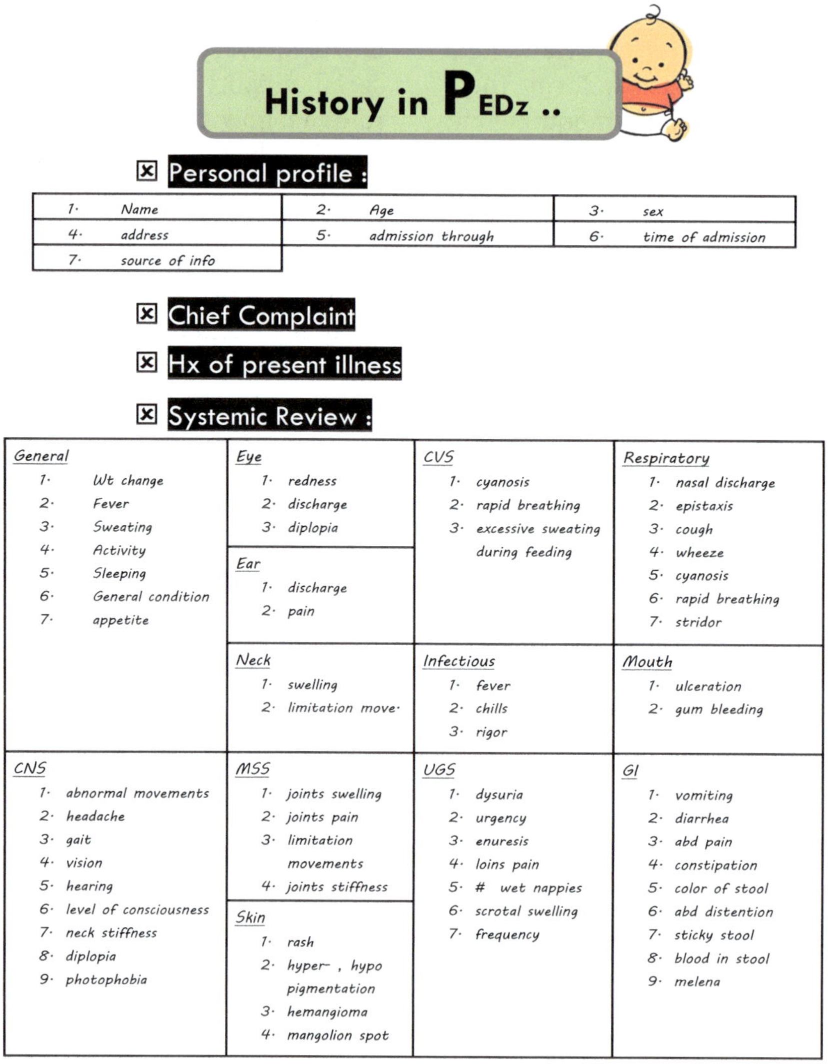

Figure 11.9. Medical history review.

Source: https://en.wikipedia.org/wiki/File:Hx_in_PEDz.pdf.

11.3.2. Evaluation of Functional Status

Evaluating how older patients function is key in managing anesthesia for seniors—it affects surgical outcomes and the recovery process. With many elderly individuals facing a host of health issues like frailty and other medical challenges, knowing their usual level of function becomes pretty important. In busy hospitals, targeted programs such as occupational therapy have shown they can help preserve mobility during a patient's stay. For instance, a study at an Acute Geriatric Unit revealed that older individuals who took part in an Occupational Therapy program generally left with better mobility scores at discharge (Sidoli et al., 2024). This kind of result hints at how closely a patient's functional assessment ties into the bigger picture of anesthetic care, stressing the need for broad evaluations. There's also more to functional status than just keeping up mobility. It plays a role in managing pain and guiding rehabilitation for older folks. One retrospective study looking at caudal epidural steroid injections in patients aged 65 and up showed notable improvements in both pain perception and how well patients recovered functionally. By using common pain scales and disability measures, the study pretty much made it clear that effective pain management can boost overall function (Ali et al., 2023). Keeping function intact doesn't only speed up postoperative recovery—it also helps maintain independence, which is crucial for many older adults. Making sure that functional evaluations become part of the anesthetic care plan is pretty critical if we want the best surgical outcomes. A well-rounded assessment should cover things like mobility, pain levels, and the capacity to handle daily tasks. Such evaluations can help guide plans both before and after surgery, ensuring care is tailored to each person's unique situation. In geriatric anesthesia, noticing issues that might hold back recovery—like cognitive decline or other preexisting conditions—allows a more proactive approach to tackle these risks. To summarize, putting a spotlight on functional status not only refines anesthetic management for older patients but also supports a more holistic approach to care, ultimately making surgical success and patient satisfaction that much more achievable.

11.3.3. Risk Assessment Tools

Treating older patients under anesthesia isn't as cut-and-dry as it might seem. Seniors often come with a host of different health issues, and the usual checklists—think of the old ECOG Performance Status—might not pick up on the small yet important changes that happen with age. Research, generally speaking, shows that these traditional tools can miss key details when it comes to predicting recovery after surgery. That's where newer approaches come in. Geriatric assessment tools, especially those that fall under what some call comprehensive geriatric assessment (CGA), take a broader look. They check out things like frailty, cognitive sharpness, and nutrition; all these bits play a big role in not just handling immediate anesthesia risks but also figuring out how patients will do in the long run. One interesting study even pointed out that these CGA methods do a pretty solid job of flagging patients who might be in trouble for complications like confusion or long hospital stays. It kind of makes sense—if you know ahead of time who's more likely to have a rough ride, anesthesiologists can alter their approach for each individual. By throwing CGA scores into the pre-op mix, doctors get a peek at details that typical metrics might skip over. In most cases, folks flagged as frail by these assessments end up showing a higher probability of complications.

To summarize, it suggests that making these assessments a regular part of the process could change how we manage care for elderly patients. Another angle to consider is how these assessments can help tailor both pre- and post-surgery care. Once you figure out exactly what risks are kicking around, you can set up specific strategies—say, better nutritional plans or dedicated physical rehab sessions—to help out before and after the operation. Research has shed some light on how using CGA helps guide whether a surgical plan should lean more toward aggressive, curative measures or if a palliative approach might be better. Essentially, having a clearer picture of a patient's strengths and vulnerabilities means that surgical teams are more prepared for the unique challenges that come with aging. This not only lowers the chances for a drop in overall function but also, in a real way, improves the quality of life once the surgery is over. In short, switching up the standard preoperative routine to include these tools isn't just a minor alter—it's a game changer for safer, more patient-focused care (Figure 11.10).

☒ **Past Medical Hx**

1. Previous admission	2. Previous surgeries	3. Hx of blood transfusion
4. Hx of allergy	5. Accidents , injuries	6. Previous investigations

☒ **Perinatal Hx**

a. Prenatal :

1. Mother's age	2. Maternal fever or rash	3. Maternal diabetes	4. Drugs taking
5. Exposure to radiation	6. Antenatal care	7. Prolonged rupture of membrane > 18-24 h	8. Duration of pregnancy

b. Natal :

1. Delivery mode	2. Crying	3. Birth wt

c. Post-natal :

1. Neonatal admissions	2. Neonatal jaundice

☒ **Nutrition Hx**

1. Breast feeding (frequency, duration)	2. Bottle feeding (frequency, amount, reason for bottle)	3. Wt gain
4. Weaning	5. Table food (type, amount)	

☒ **Developmental Hx**

1. Gross motor	2. Fine motor	3. Language
4. Social	5. School performance	

☒ **Vaccination Hx**

1. Type of vaccine	2. Age of vaccine
3. According JNP, UNRWA	4. complication

☒ **Family Hx**

1. Mother's age	2. Father's age	3. Consanguinity
4. # children and similar conditions	5. Genetic diseases	6. Early deaths

☒ **Social Hx**

1. House (rooms, ventilation)	2. Occupation of father	3. Income
4. Insurance	5. Animals	6. Smoking

☒ **Psychiatric Hx**

1. anxiety	2. emotional problem	3. temper	4. school refusal
5. mental problem	6. behavioral problem	7. mood disorders	

Figure 11.10. Treating older patients under anesthesia.

Source: https://en.wikipedia.org/w/index.php?title=File:Hx_in_PEDz.pdf&page=2.

Test Your Knowledge

1. Evaluate how older patients function in the management of anesthesia for seniors.
2. What are the tools of risk assessment?

11.4. Intraoperative Management Considerations

Learning Outcome

1. Understand the monitoring techniques for elderly patients.
2. Understand the dosage adjustments for anesthetic agents.
3. Discuss on management of comorbidities in older adults.

Managing surgery for older adults isn't a straightforward task. Often, you deal with bodies that don't have the same backup as they used to—so hidden medical issues and shifting physiology become part of the equation. In most cases, that means clinicians have to pick anesthetic drugs carefully, avoiding sudden blood pressure swings or unexpected mental fog. Keeping a non-stop watch on the heart—catching any arrhythmia or a shift in blood pressure—can be a lifesaver, literally. At the same time, mixing pain relief methods often eases discomfort after the operation while reducing on heavy narcotic use, which in turn reduces breathing issues. All told, crafting an anesthetic plan that's personalized pays off by speeding recovery and generally shortening hospital stays. Deciding between SA and GA tends to stir up plenty of questions among professionals working with the elderly. Recent research generally hints that SA might offer a couple of clear upsides, like getting pain relief set up faster immediately after surgery and even reducing blood loss during the procedure—a real bonus for this age group. Yet, one can't ignore that picking the right patients is crucial, especially for those with heart problems that can get aggravated (Buren et al., 2025). And when it comes to GA, it requires careful planning to manage the airway, since things can sometimes get tricky. It's almost a given that the right medication and precise dosages are critical, because older bodies often react differently to drugs, meaning adjustments are sometimes needed to sidestep unwanted side effects. In short, a tailored approach goes a long way in keeping things safe and, frankly, making patients more satisfied with their care. Managing what goes on during surgery extends far beyond just giving the patient anesthesia. There's an entire team involved—anesthesiologists, surgeons, nurses—all needing to chat and coordinate in real-time to keep up with the ever-changing conditions in the OR. The particular vulnerabilities of older patients demand a proactive, hands-on method to keep vital signs steady throughout the procedure. Generally speaking, following tried-and-true guidelines—like those from the American College of Cardiology and the American Heart Association—helps teams work through risk assessments and make better anesthetic choices, especially for patients with cardiovascular issues (Okolo et al., 2025). This kind of teamwork not only helps prevent surprises during surgery but also contributes to smoother, quicker recoveries and, ultimately, higher overall quality of care (Figure 11.11).

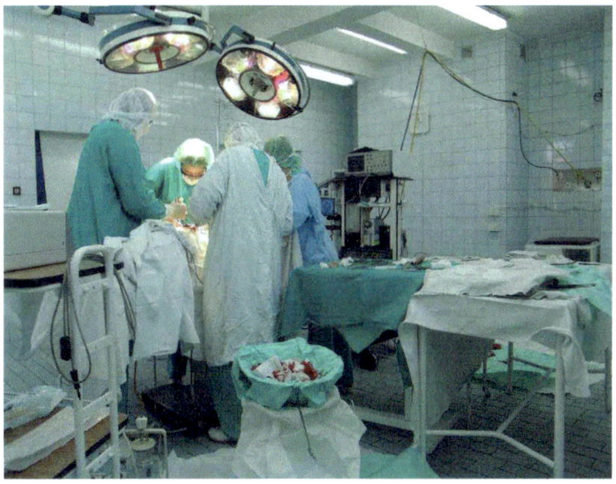

Figure 11.11. Intraoperative management.

Source: By Piotr Bodzek, MD - Uploaded from http://www.ginbytom.slam.katowice.pl/25.html with author permission., CC BY-SA 3.0, https://commons.wikimedia.org/w/index.php?curid=372117.

11.4.1. Monitoring Techniques for Elderly Patients

Managing older patients during anesthesia isn't a walk in the park. Aging tends to bring about a decline in how well organs work, so doctors have to be extra cautious—keeping a constant eye on things like heart rate, blood pressure, and breathing. In many cases, this close watch helps catch sudden blood flow changes due to other health problems, and tools such as capnography and pulse oximetry play their part by flagging early signs of breathing trouble. It's a sort of round-the-clock vigilance that not only upholds patient safety but also lowers the chances of post-surgery hiccups like delirium or cognitive issues (Souza et al., 2024). ERAS protocols have turned the traditional approach on its head, especially when it comes to caring for elderly patients. These guidelines push for a team-based style—starting with thorough checks before surgery, then carefully tailoring anesthetic plans, and finally, keeping tabs throughout the recovery process. Doctors regularly assess vital signs in real-time and monitor fluid balance to keep things in check, given the usual age-related changes. Since every patient brings a mix of conditions like frailty and other illnesses, the approach has to be adjusted to match their very specific needs—a strategy that, in most cases, helps smooth out recovery and reduce complications (Uppalapati et al., 2024). After surgery, managing pain becomes just as critical. Older adults often respond differently to pain relievers such as opioids—so clinicians stay alert for side effects like sluggish breathing or moments of confusion. They check pain levels consistently, even when it feels redundant to look again, and they keep an eye out for signs of delirium or other post-surgery issues. Patient feedback sometimes gets sprinkled into these assessments, allowing providers to alter pain management on the fly. Ultimately, success isn't found solely in the choice of anesthetic agents but in a relentless, watchful presence throughout the entire surgical journey, reinforcing a broad, careful approach to geriatric anesthesia (Souza et al., 2024) (Figure 11.12).

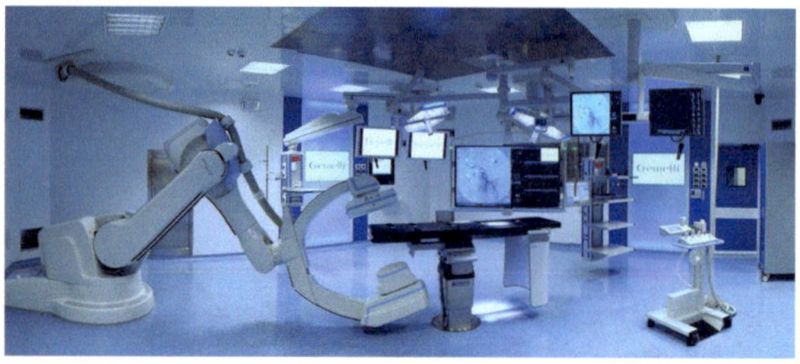

Figure 11.12. Anesthesia monitoring in geriatric surgeries.

Source: By Pfree2014 - Own work, CC0, https://commons.wikimedia.org/w/index.php?curid=36622337.

11.4.2. Dosage Adjustments for Anesthetic Agents

Geriatric anesthesia demands extra care when it comes to altering drug doses. Older patients often come loaded with various health issues and their bodies tend to handle medications in unexpected ways. Checking kidney function, liver work, and overall physical resilience is important—even though it might seem obvious. For example, drugs like benzodiazepines and opioids can sometimes linger too long in the system, leading to extended sedation or even breathing trouble, which might worsen other conditions. Adjusting the dosage according to each patient's unique traits helps to lower unwanted side effects while still controlling pain. Clinicians, in most cases, are advised to lean on research-backed guidelines that reflect the distinct drug-processing characteristics of the elderly, aiming for safer surgical outcomes. The choice of anesthetic agent also plays a big role in how well someone bounces back after surgery. Think about propofol and DEX: these agents are popular—largely thanks to their favorable properties—but in older patients, the amount needed for the same sedative effect is generally much lower than that used in younger folks.

There's always the concern that, if not adjusted properly, these medications could contribute to postoperative confusion or memory issues. New drugs and enhanced monitoring techniques have started to make a difference, offering more personalized care at the bedside. It turns out that combining solid pharmacological science with a natural, individual approach to patient care is becoming more and more essential as practices evolve. Using a preoperative delirium risk tool may be a game-changer when nailing down the right doses of commonly used anesthetic agents. Ongoing studies show that, by spotting who's more at risk, clinicians can fine-tune their anesthetic plans; this helps reduce the chances for complications such as POCD and postoperative delirium (POD). Adjusting the amounts of drugs like midazolam, DEX, ketamine, and fentanyl-based on these risk checks can lead to smoother recoveries and fewer mishaps. To summarize, paying attention to these assessments before surgery not only cuts down potential risks but also brings clinical practice more in line with the latest evidence-based standards (Cappellini et al., 2024; Detwiler et al., 2023).

11.4.3. Management of Comorbidities

Elderly patients face more health challenges than ever, which makes giving anesthesia especially tricky. Many seniors deal with heart issues, breathing problems, and even metabolic disorders – a mix that calls for a deep look at their overall health rather than just one aspect. In most cases, planning anesthesia must factor in an increased risk of problems after surgery. A thorough preoperative check-up remains a key step, letting anesthesiologists tailor plans to fit each patient's unique needs. When doctors consider everything—from daily functionality to social circumstances—they're better able to foresee bumps in the road, leading to smoother outcomes both immediately and in the long run (Uppalapati et al., 2024). Using enhanced recovery practices is now seen as essential to handle these intertwined conditions, especially when surgery comes into play. Many rely on the ERAS approach—Enhanced Recovery After Surgery—which generally reduces the body's stress and helps patients recover faster using methods proven by research. This strategy takes care of everything from ensuring proper nutrition to mixing different pain management techniques aimed at older adults.

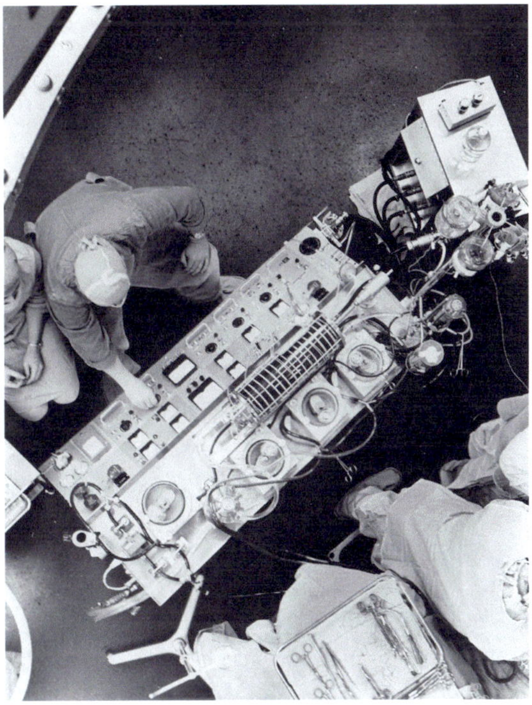

Figure 11.13. Managing multiple comorbidities.

Source: By The U.S. Food and Drug Administration - Hospital Operating Room (FDA 042), Public Domain, https://commons.wikimedia.org/w/index.php?curid=33628031.

Even though the specifics of every anesthetic method aren't laid out here, weaving in these protocols often means shorter hospital stays and fewer post-surgery complications. By putting the body's basic needs first, clinicians can help pave the way to both better immediate recoveries and improved long-term health for seniors facing complex issues (Uppalapati et al., 2024). Among the many anesthesia methods available, PNBs have emerged as a promising alternative for those with multiple health problems. For example, the method known as Single-Insertion Multiple Nerve Block Anesthesia (SIMBA) has shown encouraging results in treating femur fractures. This technique not only tends to keep swings in blood pressure and other hemodynamic markers in check, but it also delivers good pain relief after surgery—a crucial benefit since these patients are generally at higher risk. Some studies even indicate that SIMBA works well for patients with heart complications, highlighting its value for more vulnerable cases. Mixing such forward-thinking approaches into a comprehensive preoperative plan can go a long way in managing comorbidities, ultimately leading to better surgical outcomes (Figure 11.13).

Test Your Knowledge

1. What are monitoring techniques for elderly patients?
2. Describe the management of comorbidities in older adults.

11.5. Postoperative Care and Complications

Learning Outcome

1. Describe the common postoperative complications in the elderly.
2. Understand the pain management strategies for elderly patients.
3. Understand the importance of early mobilization.

Older patients need close watch after surgery—it's not just routine care but a tailored approach that accounts for their often fragile state. Many older folks come with their challenges like weaker organs and a higher chance of complications, so keeping an eye on things like breathing becomes extra important. Sometimes, if breathing gets tough, options like a tracheostomy might pop up; knowing this ahead of time can help the team set up the operating room better, which may influence how things turn out. Observations suggest that being ready sooner rather than later can stave off a host of issues while smoothing out recovery, especially when it comes to anesthesia for these patients (Farrell et al., 1959). Multiple health issues, such as high blood pressure, diabetes, or heart troubles, add another layer of difficulty to the post-surgery phase. These extra burdens not only amp up the risk of surgical mishaps but can also muddle pain management and other care aspects. In most cases, steady monitoring and early action reduce on complications quite a bit. Getting a thorough check before surgery lets the healthcare team guess what hurdles might pop up later on. This comprehensive way of handling care helps craft specific anesthesia and surgical plans that consider the quirks of aging biology, leading to better overall outcomes for this vulnerable group (Amornyotin et al., 2021). Anesthesia-related problems after an operation can interfere with recovery in older patients, so staying alert and flexible is key. Issues like delirium or lingering sedation appear more frequently in this crowd, so adjustments in how anesthesia is managed become necessary. Regularly checking on a patient's alertness and mental state helps reduce these risks. It also pays off to set up a supportive setting where patients and their families can have candid chats—this kind of communication makes the recovery process feel a bit more natural and less forced. Sharing what to expect after surgery lets everyone get involved, boosting both emotional and physical healing. Such a hands-on approach not only improves immediate recovery but also supports long-term health and independence (Amornyotin et al., 2021; Farrell et al., 1959) (Figure 11.14).

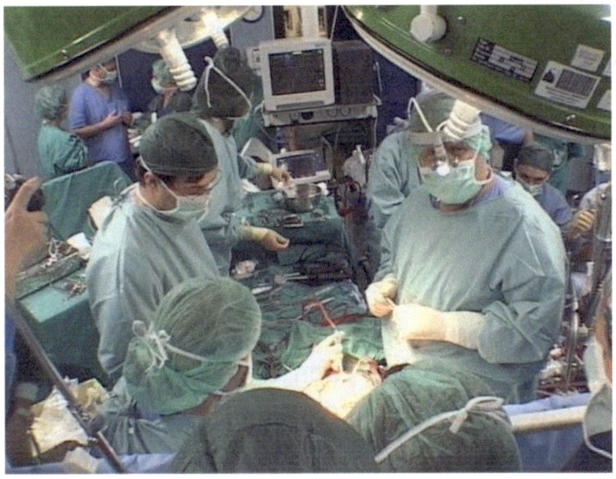

Figure 11.14. Post-operative care for elderly patients.

Source: By Frp17580 – Own work, Public Domain, https://commons.wikimedia.org/w/index.php?curid=5244864.

11.5.1. Common Postoperative Complications in the Elderly

Managing postsurgical issues in older patients is one of those hurdles that keeps healthcare providers on their toes. Complications can vary wildly – sometimes they're just minor bumps in the road, and other times they hit hard, even threatening lives. Heart problems, for instance, like irregular heartbeats or even heart attacks, pop up quite frequently. Often, the root of this vulnerability is the patient's pre-existing conditions, mixed up with naturally lower bodily reserves. It's a clear sign that getting a thorough check-up before surgery is a must – not just a look at physical health but also a peek into mental and nutritional well-being since all these factors combine to influence recovery. In most cases, using detailed assessment tools helps anticipate the issues and plan out the right interventions (Miao et al., 2023). Then there's POD – a complication that seems to hit older adults more often. It comes on suddenly, with confusing spells and shifts in one's state of awareness, which can slow d how quickly someone bounces back. Research generally points to age, certain medications, and even changes in the environment as triggers for this condition. It's especially worrisome because delirium can drag out hospital stays and raise medical costs. Some strategies, like enhanced recovery protocols that mix in pre-surgery planning with a range of interventions, appear to lower its chances. There's even some discussion about how different anesthetic techniques might alter the risk, hinting at more layers to unravel (Yoshimura et al., 2022).

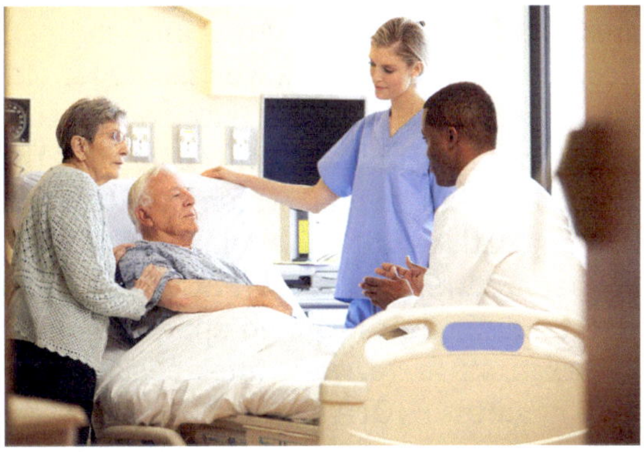

Figure 11.15. Common postoperative complications in the elderly.

Source: https://madeforthismoment.asahq.org/wp-content/uploads/2017/10/iStock-465446791.jpg.

When surgeries are in the mix, existing illnesses often add extra complications – things like infections or delays in healing can snowball quickly. Seniors frequently come in with a tangle of past medical issues that throw off the usual recovery path. That's why keeping a sharp eye on signs of infection after surgery becomes so critical. Factors such as a weakened immune response and slower wound repair push us toward getting a more collaborative approach on board – involving surgeons, anesthetists, and even specialists in geriatric care. Risk-assessment tools that factor in nutrition and frailty can sometimes offer valuable clues, helping doctors put together tailored care plans for each patient (Miao et al., 2023). To summarize, these wide-ranging strategies should, ideally, lower the risks and boost recovery outcomes (Figure 11.15).

11.5.2. Pain Management Strategies

Pain management for elderly patients facing surgery is a big deal in anesthesia. Good pain control lifts a patient's comfort and often speeds up recovery—helping them head home quicker. Studies now show RA works wonders, especially when treating hip fracture cases. RA has been known to reduce on those nasty postoperative issues like cognitive hiccups and delirium, which, let's face it, are extra worrisome for older adults. In short, RA offers better pain relief after surgery, trimming the need for opioids and their bothersome side effects, which boosts overall safety and satisfaction (Li et al., 2025). Doctors have been rethinking pain strategies as our understanding grows. Opioid-sparing methods have taken off in geriatric anesthesia. Opioid-Free Anesthesia (OFA) pops up as a strong choice for easing pain without triggering the messy neuroinflammatory side effects tied to opioids. Research, in most cases, suggests that teaming OFA with techniques like the iliofascial nerve block noticeably improves recovery and lowers the risk of perioperative neurocognitive dysfunction (PND) in older patients. By cutting back on opioid use, OFA tackles that immediate pain and even seems to support long-term brain health—a double win for modern anesthesia tailored to seniors (Zhi et al., 2025). Effective pain care goes beyond just easing the immediate hurt—it plays a key role in long-term quality of life too. Keeping pain levels under control helps boost mobility and can let older adults bounce back to their regular routines more swiftly. Some patients even find themselves rediscovering their pre-surgery strength sooner than expected. When anesthesia protocols put advanced pain management first, it's not only about keeping a patient comfortable; it's an investment in overall geriatric healthcare, potentially cutting future costs from longer hospital stays and rehab needs. This blend of strategies, woven into everyday practice, speaks to a broader, more holistic approach to improving surgical results and overall well-being.

11.5.3. Importance of Early Mobilization

After surgery, older patients face some tricky hurdles that demand a care plan focused on getting them back to their everyday selves. Early movement is the real game-changer here—research generally shows that getting seniors up and moving soon can boost recovery. Getting them to take even a few steps right away seems to lower the chances of problems like blood clots in the legs or lungs, issues that crop up more easily when mobility drops off. It even helps spark better heart function and muscle strength so they can regain the independence they once had. In several multidisciplinary studies, experts have pointed to the value of mixing rehabilitation efforts with early ambulation as a way to fight off the deconditioning that often follows surgery in older adults (Saur et al., 2022). When it comes to starting movement, timing and technique are crucial. In the realm of geriatric anesthesia, clinicians generally need to be extra sensitive to how older bodies react post-surgery. A guided walk, combined with supportive measures tailored to each patient's needs, can make a world of difference. Research tends to show that when seniors are helped to start moving shortly after their procedures, the risk for further complications drops noticeably. Plus, teams made up of nurses, physical therapists, and geriatricians all contribute not only physical support but also that much-needed emotional backup – which is particularly important for this vulnerable group (Olotu et al., 2019). Integrating early mobilization into the overall care plan isn't just about fixing up the body; it touches on mental well-being too. Jumping into physical activity can ease feelings of anxiety and even depression that sometimes settle in after surgery. Often, when older patients join these mobility programs, they end up feeling a newfound sense of control and empowerment. Not to mention, early movement tends to shorten hospital stays and even reduce on healthcare costs—a side benefit that shouldn't be overlooked. To summarize, making early mobilization a standard part of surgical care for elders is essential; it helps address both the physical and psychological sides of recovery (Nicole et al., 2022) (Figure 11.16).

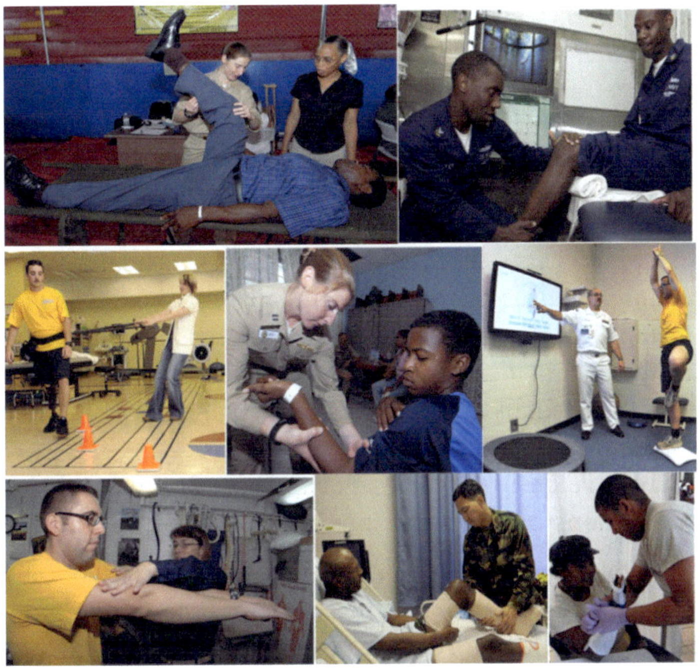

Figure 11.16. Importance of early mobilization.

Source: Composite image. Photos by the U.S. Navy and U.S. Air Force, including works by Mass Communication Specialists Anastasia Puscian, Joshua Karsten, and others. Public domain. Wikimedia Commons, https://commons.wikimedia.org/w/index.php?curid=14511419.

Test Your Knowledge

1. What are the common postoperative complications in the elderly?
2. Describe the pain management strategies for elderly patients.

SUMMARY

Geriatric anaesthesia is changing because our aging patients bring their own set of issues—and to be honest, the rate of change astounds many. Older and older patients are being operated on, so it's reasonably clear that practice anaesthesia needs a tailor-made twist. It's not a question of replacing drugs; it's about understanding what growing older does for us in terms of what it throws at us, like not just more disease but changes in brain function. Overall, research (Larsson et al., 2018) suggests that POCD is a valid concern, so pre-surgical assessment needs to take into account not just medical history but also mental state and ordinary health. Sarcopenia, that loss of muscle and strength, is another thorn in the side when scheduling surgery on older patients. Aging, the majority of the time, leads to a considerable decline in muscle strength, and correcting these changes early in life can improve rehabilitation and general welfare.

At the cellular level, the processes behind muscle loss indicate why early rehabilitation of the body and specific muscle treatment are necessary—a fact even recorded in some research studies (Larsson et al., 2018). Proactively preserved strength and mobility have the potential to reduce on falls, injury, and other hospital visits, lessening the strain on our healthcare system. In conclusion, geriatric anesthesia certainly requires a broad, occasionally untidy approach that balances essential surgical needs with the vulnerable zones of aging. Professionals in the field must develop and fine-tune evidence-based strategies that range from pre-surgical assessments to aftercare following the procedure, considering all those small things that count. With continued attempts to prevent POCD in the first place and confront muscle loss directly (Kotekar et al., 2018), there is every likelihood for further upbeat outcomes in elderly surgeries. For the vast majority, a balanced, customized plan not only creates safer operations but also enhances the quality of life for our elderly population.

Geriatric medicine is evolving, and care that's tailored specifically to older people is beginning to deliver some tangible benefits. Consider the Acute Geriatric Community Hospital (AGCH) for example—mixes specialist care with more generic in its approach. This arrangement, as a rule, centers on the extremely particular requirements of older patients. They even developed 13 different rules for admitting just this population. These guidelines assist in selecting the appropriate candidates for admission and, in most instances, establish a better cohesive approach to care—even if the complexity of caring for older adults can be quite daunting. It all seems to be making a huge amount of difference these days as our healthcare systems increasingly, if not completely, rethink how they handle all of it, now that care is shifting from the big institutions into community settings (Kroeze et al., 2024).

Looking at the training the next generation of geriatric experts receives, there's a vast range. Analysis of Polish undergraduate courses in this area shows that while everything starts from a shared national standard, the actual curriculum swings pretty wildly from one institution to another. This kind of inconsistency, in most cases, makes it tough for students to prepare for the changing demographics we're all expecting soon. It would not be out of place to merge such programs and give them a new spin so that teaching catches up with the times. This transition should, in theory, place graduates in a position to learn the skills needed to navigate the messy side of geriatric care. As populations shift and new problems emerge, ensuring that what is taught in the classroom—always imperfectly at times—is up to date with these trends matters more and more (Kupis et al., 2024). All of it—better education and novel care—suggests a genuine need for reform in how we handle geriatric anesthesia. If you think about it, an integration of AGCH's admission practices with improved educational standards can help to some extent to counter the special challenges brought by older patients to the operating room. Geriatric anesthesia training not only enables physicians and nurses to appreciate the frequently subtle effects of aging, but also enhances patient safety and outcomes. Together, the cooperation between schools and hospitals opens the door to serious innovation in care for the elderly, reminding us that both curricula and daily practice need to change if we are ever to keep up with an aging population.

KEY TERMS FROM THIS CHAPTER

- Bioelectrical impedance analysis
- Body composition
- Cardiovascular system
- Cognitive hiccups
- Delirium
- Dexmedetomidine
- Dual-energy X-ray absorptiometry
- Electroencephalography
- Geriatric anesthesia
- Glomerular filtration rate
- Inhalational anesthetics
- Intravenous anesthetics

CRITICAL THINKING QUESTIONS

1. **In elderly patients, the reduction in cardiac output is primarily due to:**
   a. Decreased heart rate
   b. Decreased stroke volume
   c. Increased systemic vascular resistance
   d. Myocardial stiffening
2. **In geriatric patients, the volume of distribution (Vd) for lipid-soluble drugs is:**
   a. Decreased due to reduced fat stores
   b. Increased due to higher body fat percentage
   c. Unchanged due to homeostasis
   d. Variable based on hydration status
3. **What is the most common preoperative risk factor in elderly patients?**
   a. Cardiac disease
   b. Renal impairment
   c. Cognitive dysfunction
   d. Respiratory disease
4. **Elderly patients are more sensitive to anesthetic agents due to:**
   a. Increased hepatic metabolism
   b. Increased renal clearance
   c. Decreased central nervous system (CNS) reserve
   d. Increased protein binding
5. **Which of the following is a risk factor for postoperative delirium in elderly patients?**
   a. Preexisting dementia
   b. Prolonged surgery duration
   c. Use of benzodiazepines
   d. All of the above

Short Answer Questions

1. Define the geriatric anesthesia.
2. Why is anesthesia important in the elderly?
3. What are physiological changes in the elderly?
4. Describe the common anesthetic agents used in geriatric patients.
5. What is the preoperative assessment in geriatric patients?

Answers to Critical Thinking Questions

1. (d); 2. (b); 3. (a); 4. (c); 5. (d)

REFERENCES

1. Aldecoa, C., Bettelli, G., Bilotta, F., Sanders, R. D., Audisio, R. A., Borozdina, A., Cherubini, A., et al. (2017). European Society of Anesthesiology evidence-based and consensus-based guideline on postoperative delirium. *European Journal of Anesthesiology, 34*, 192–214. https://doi.org/10.1097/eja.0000000000000594.
2. Almutairi, A. M. A., Alshammari, M. T. S., Al Shammari, F. A. F., Alanazi, A. S. A., Alanazi, H. M. M., Alanazi, A. O. K., Alshammari, J. H., Almutairi, M. B. S., Alanazi, B. S. A., Alharbi, M. K. M., Almutiri, O. M., Alshammari, A. H., Alshammari, A. M. K., Alanazi, H. S. H., Alanazi, M. S. F., & Alanazi, A. T. Z. (2022). Effect of general anesthesia on postoperative cognitive function in elderly patients. *Journal of Population Therapeutics and Clinical Pharmacology, 29*(04), 3653–3665. https://doi.org/10.53555/jptcp.v29i04.5961.
3. Amornyotin, S. (2021). Anesthetic consideration for geriatric patients. In *Update in Geriatrics*. IntechOpen. http://dx.doi.org/10.5772/intechopen.97003.
4. Bhadani, J. S., Kumar, A., Shyam, A., & Mukhopadhaya, J. (2024). A multidisciplinary approach to managing delirium in elderly orthopedic patients: Integrating best practices for optimal outcomes. *Journal of Orthopedic Case Reports, 14*, 1–3. https://www.semanticscholar.org/paper/0789fab62697891d7fa128a70e17a6d362c01d16 (accessed on 20 May 2025).
5. Buren, M. A., & Cil, H. (2025). Anesthetic considerations and management of spine surgery performed under neuraxial anesthesia. *Current Anesthesiology Reports*. https://www.semanticscholar.org/paper/9c1dc96e9b4c0dc4d11b815711b41d0fdca374b8 (accessed on 20 May 2025).
6. Cappellini, I., Bavestrello Piccini, G., Campagnola, L., Bochicchio, C., Carente, R., Lai, F., Magazzini, S., & Consales, G. (2024). Procedural sedation in emergency department: A narrative review. *Emergency Care and Medicine, 1*(2), 103–136. https://doi.org/10.3390/ecm1020014.
7. Detwiler, C. (2023). *Delirium Risk Assessment and The Effect on Administration of Four Adjuvant Anesthetics* (Doctoral dissertation, University of North Carolina at Chapel Hill). https://core.ac.uk/download/596785693.pdf (accessed on 20 May 2025).
8. Dhiraj, S., Kumari, P., & Kumari, R. (2024). Assessing the effect of dexmedetomidine dosages on short-term cognitive function in geriatric patients undergoing head and neck cancer surgery: A cross-sectional study. *Student's Journal of Health Research Africa, 5*(3), 7. https://doi.org/10.51168/sjhrafrica.v5i3.1104.
9. Dönmez, B., Vanhonacker, D., Lammens, R., & Bhutia, J. (2024). Role of peripheral nerve blocks in the preoperative pain management of hip fractures in the elderly: A narrative review. *Acta Anesthesiologic Belgica*. https://www.semanticscholar.org/paper/122947fc0d40eea0536ca8adcd076eeaa1856eef (accessed on 20 May 2025).
10. Donoghue, T. J. (2021). Using the Memorial Sloan Kettering Frailty Index to identify patients at high risk for postoperative intensive care unit admission, specialized advanced care unit admission, and 30-day readmission. https://core.ac.uk/download/390087913.pdf (accessed on 20 May 2025).
11. Drover, C. M., Drover, D. R., Vaughn, D. A., MacIver, M. B., Cohen, M. S., et al. (2018). Do complexity measures of frontal EEG distinguish loss of consciousness in geriatric patients under anesthesia? https://core.ac.uk/download/323076544.pdf.

12. Dushin, I. N., Tetenich, A. A., Kazantceva, M. O., Kotov, A. A., Emelkina, A. V., Haustov, R. I., Savina, E. N., et al. (2025). Experience of using composite Z-score to assess delayed cognitive recovery in elderly patients who underwent surgery for colorectal cancer under intravenous or inhalation anesthesia: A prospective observational pilot study. *Messenger of Anesthesiology and Resuscitation, 22*(1), 16–23. https://doi.org/10.24884/2078-5658-2025-22-1-16-23.
13. Farrell, J. J., Meyer, W. H., & Starzl, T. E. (1959). Prophylactic tracheostomy in aged and poor risk general surgical patients. https://core.ac.uk/download/12203425.pdf (accessed on 20 May 2025).
14. Gonzalez, M. A., Campbell, Y. D., & Rodriguez-Diaz, A. (2022). Lavender aromatherapy compared to midazolam for quality improvement of preoperative anxiety in elderly surgical patients: An educational module. *Nicole Wertheim College of Nursing Student Projects, 107*. https://digitalcommons.fiu.edu/cnhs-studentprojects/107 (accessed on 20 May 2025).
15. Güler, A., Şenol, Y. C., Akpinar, A. E., Çiftçi, H. E., Yiğit, M., Öz, Z. G., Orhun, E., et al. (2023). Effectiveness of ultrasonography-guided caudal epidural steroid injection in improving pain and functional status of geriatric patients with spinal pain. *Turkish Journal of Geriatrics, 26*(3), 258–266. https://doi.org/10.29400/tjgeri.2023.352.
16. Kanaparthy, A., Kanaparthy, R., Pillai, A., Sandhu, et al. (2025). Geriatric endodontic. https://core.ac.uk/download/pdf/267953527.pdf (accessed on 20 May 2025).
17. Kotekar, N., Shenkar, A., & Nagaraj, R. (2018). Postoperative cognitive dysfunction–current preventive strategies. *Clinical Interventions in Aging, 13*, 2267–2273. https://doi.org/10.2147/cia.s133896.
18. Krishna, B., & Pathak, N. (2020). Perioperative management of geriatric patients for orthopedic surgeries. https://core.ac.uk/download/539905066.pdf (accessed on 20 May 2025).
19. Kroeze, E., de Groot, A. J., Smorenburg, S. M., Mac Neil Vroomen, J. L., Van Vught, A., & Buurman, B. M. (2024). A case vignette study to refine the target group of an intermediate care model: The Acute Geriatric Community Hospital. *European Geriatric Medicine, 15*, 977–989. https://www.semanticscholar.org/paper/bec9ac206d021a1a3af81bf6b1380d64b06c8808 (accessed on 20 May 2025).
20. Kupis, R., Perera, I., Targowski, T., Gąsowski, J., & Piotrowicz, K. (2024). Is geriatric medicine teaching homogeneous? The analysis of geriatric medicine courses at Polish undergraduate medical programmers. *European Geriatric Medicine, 15*, 1523–1532. https://www.semanticscholar.org/paper/c70f8f8b10a316de16828d41f4b5d642e5c1198f (accessed on 20 May 2025).
21. Lapid, M. I., Petrides, G., Hermida, A. P., & Forester, B. P. (2024). S2: Neuromodulation in geriatric psychiatry: Innovations and insights in ECT, TMS, tDCS, and cannabinoid therapies. *International Psychogeriatrics, 36*(9). https://www.semanticscholar.org/paper/1b6d154d1e0065731888183d67d5f08b0a687202 (accessed on 20 May 2025).
22. Larsson, L., Degens, H., Li, M., Salviati, L., Lee, Y. I., Thompson, W. J., Kirkland, J. L., et al. (2018). Sarcopenia: Aging-related loss of muscle mass and function. *Physiological Reviews, 99*, 427–511. https://doi.org/10.1152/physrev.00061.2017.
23. Li, P., Li, X., Peng, G., Deng, J., & Li, Q. (2025). Comparative analysis of general and regional anesthesia applications in geriatric hip fracture surgery. *Medicine, 104*. https://www.

semanticscholar.org/paper/6fe2d192a24a28037376e2aa5daaab3b9c2da42d (accessed on 20 May 2025).

24. Marra, M., Sammarco, R., De Lorenzo, A., Iellamo, F., Siervo, M., Pietrobelli, A., Donini, L. M., et al. (2019). Assessment of body composition in health and disease using bioelectrical impedance analysis (BIA) and dual energy X-ray absorptiometry (DXA): A critical overview. *Contrast Media & Molecular Imaging, 2019*, 1–9. https://doi.org/10.1155/2019/3548284.

25. Miao, X., Ding, L. Y., Hu, J., Zhu, H., Zhao, K., Lu, J., Jiang, X., et al. (2023). A web-based calculator combining Geriatric Nutritional Risk Index (GNRI) and Tilburg Frailty Indicator (TFI) predicts postoperative complications among young elderly patients with gastric cancer. *Geriatrics & Gerontology International, 23*, 205–212. https://www.semanticscholar.org/paper/b31dfc9be69e14e39fd37603240fed0d2ef5f470 (accessed on 20 May 2025).

26. Mohamed Naguib, S. J., Kopman, A. F., Hunter, J. M., Fülesdi, B., Arkes, H. R., Elstein, A. S., et al. (2017). Consensus statement on perioperative use of neuromuscular monitoring. *Anesthesia & Analgesia, 127*(1), 71–80. https://doi.org/10.1213/ane.0000000000002670.

27. Okolo, D., Ugorji, W. S., Gopep, N. S., Oragui, C. C., Ubajaka, C. C., & Okobi, O. (2025). Perioperative management of anesthesia in patients with cardiovascular disease: A review of current guidelines in the United States. *Cureus, 17*. https://www.semanticscholar.org/paper/2f0f2adefd28628e444237315d80eed35c0fe377 (accessed on 20 May 2025).

28. Olotu, C., Weimann, A., Bahrs, C., Schwenk, W., Scherer, M., & Kiefmann, R. (2019). The perioperative care of older patients. *Deutsches Ärzteblatt International, 116*(5), 63–69. https://doi.org/10.3238/arztebl.2019.0063.

29. Paschoal, J., Santos, I., Malaquias, D., Freitas, K., Leão, M., Silva, A., Silva, K., Mazurek, M., Menezes, M., Fernandes, R., Oliveira, M., Silva, L., Araújo, A., Pereira, T., Rita, L., Paula, K., Silva, L., Preto, G., Montes, A., & Bezerra, T. (2025). Comparative analysis of the best drug of choice for sedation in a surgical procedure in elderly patients: Pros and side effects of sedatives. *Journal of Anesthesia, 10*, 1–14. https://doi.org/10.52338/joa.2025.4595.

30. Pschirrer, H., & Tocco, C. (2024). Methadone. https://core.ac.uk/download/621638201.docx (accessed on 20 May 2025).

31. Safavynia, S. A., & Goldstein, P. A. (2019). The role of neuroinflammation in postoperative cognitive dysfunction: Moving from hypothesis to treatment. *Frontiers in Psychiatry, 9*. https://doi.org/10.3389/fpsyt.2018.00752.

32. Saur, N. M., Davis, B. R., Montroni, I., Shahrokni, A., Rostoft, S., Russell, M. M., Mohile, S. G., et al. (2022). The American Society of Colon and Rectal Surgeons clinical practice guidelines for the perioperative evaluation and management of frailty among older adults undergoing colorectal surgery. *Diseases of the Colon & Rectum, 65*(4), 473–488. https://doi.org/10.1097/dcr.0000000000002410.

33. Seddighi, R., & Doherty, T. J. (2012). Anesthesia of the geriatric equine. *Veterinary Medicine (Auckland, N.Z.), 3*, 53–64. https://doi.org/10.2147/VMRR.S34162.

34. Shaji, A., & Herakal, G. I. (2024). Evaluating the effects of anesthetic agents on geriatrics to enhance perioperative care practices: A narrative review. *International Journal of Scientific and Research Publications, 14*(01). http://dx.doi.org/10.29322/IJSRP.14.01.2023.p14533.

35. Souza, L. M., Silva, N. M., Rocha, D. G. V. B., Lima, L. P. A. S., Barros, A. B. N., Zanetti, I. G., Almeida,

L. A., et al. (2024). Management of anesthesia in elderly patients, special considerations and challenges. *International Seven Journal of Health Research*. https://www.semanticscholar.org/paper/fd45a44a2dd63f829f7c9920bf7ef48a2f257bca (accessed on 20 May 2025).

36. Tang, X. J., Lee, J. S. X., Chan, E. H. L., De Mel, S., Chee, Y. L., Chng, W. J., Lim, N. A., Chan, J. Y., Lim, S. T., Choong, S. H. C., Ooi, M. G. M., & Poon, M. L. (2024). Outcomes of elderly patients with DLBCL and utility of geriatric assessment tools to predict chemotoxicity. *Blood, 144*(Supplement 1), 3660. https://doi.org/10.1182/blood-2024-208906.
37. Theodorakis, N., Nikolaou, M., Hitas, C., Anagnostou, D., Kreouzi, M., Kalantzi, S., Spyridaki, A., et al. (2024). Comprehensive peri-operative risk assessment and management of geriatric patients. *Diagnostics, 14*. https://www.semanticscholar.org/paper/fb2f4ddd694f721c2776a79d09d2447198be9bd3 (accessed on 20 May 2025).
38. Tong, Z., Wei, S., Kuang, J., Zhou, S., Yu, D., Gao, T., Lei, L., et al. (2025). Effects of opioid-free anesthesia combined with iliofascial nerve block on perioperative neurocognitive deficits in elderly patients undergoing hip fracture surgery: Study protocol for a prospective, multicenter, parallel-group, randomized controlled trial. *Trials, 26*. https://www.semanticscholar.org/paper/25e5a6ef10935b606508ffc9ee4ce985daf6bea7 (accessed on 20 May 2025).
39. Uppalapati, T., & Thornton, I. (2024). Anesthesia management of hip fracture surgery in geriatric patients: A review. *Cureus, 16*. https://www.semanticscholar.org/paper/be01f630fff71e505df7695c09fddaeeabdaed22 (accessed on 20 May 2025).
40. Yang, D., Zhou, J., Sun, L., Li, M., & Zhang, J. (2024). Comparison of postoperative awakening between ciprofol and propofol in elderly patients undergoing hip replacement surgery: A single-blind, randomized, controlled trial. *Minerva Anesthesiologic*. https://www.semanticscholar.org/paper/5ba7ca704ff9e87254e0731a20454090e0fc5481 (accessed on 20 May 2025).
41. Yoshimura, M., Shiramoto, H., Koga, M., Yoshimatsu, A., & Morimoto, Y. (2022). Comparing the effects of peripheral nerve block and general anesthesia with general anesthesia alone on postoperative delirium and complications in elderly patients: A retrospective cohort study using a nationwide database. *Regional Anesthesia & Pain Medicine, 47*, 521–526. https://www.semanticscholar.org/paper/3bcfceb23772bcdf90bd9b092cc824806282098a (accessed on 20 May 2025).

ANESTHESIA FOR PATIENTS WITH COMORBID CONDITIONS

12

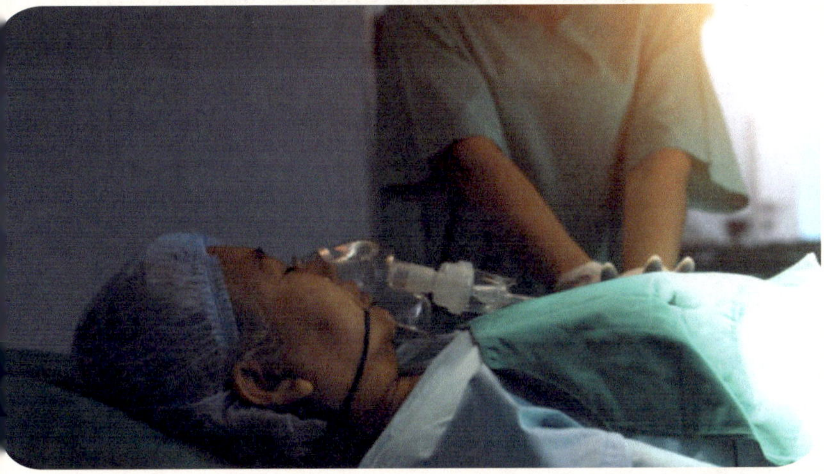

LEARNING OBJECTIVES

After studying this chapter, you will be able to:

1. Describe the common comorbid conditions.
2. Understand the preoperative assessment.
3. Describe the anesthetic considerations for specific conditions.
4. Describe the risks and complications of anesthesia.

Introduction

Modern medicine is not a solo air. Patient factors come into play in unexpected ways when it comes to surgery. Look at comorbidities, for instance—when an individual already has some health issues, the mode of action of anesthesia can be altogether different. Doctors are now, generally speaking, leaning towards care created around the patient, so they learn how anesthesia and pre-existing health challenges interact. It's not solely life-of-the-mind small talk either; miscalculating these specifics can extend recovery times or enhance complications risks, so anesthetic teams need to be awake on their feet because changing conditions alter drug requirements and safety overall—a need for double-checking and having backup plans that are appropriate for each patient's unique circumstance. Over 230 million procedures occur every year around the world, necessitating pain control in this setting to be thorough. An estimated 30% of people—yes, almost a third—struggle with chronic pain, so the individual and societal costs mount. That's why adding pain management to anesthesia isn't optional, especially for individuals who are managing other health conditions. Precision medicine has, by and large, revolutionized things, making possible the combination of drugs with therapies, lifestyle changes, and sometimes even invasive measures. These combinations of techniques work for better healing and less complication, and this indicates the critical role of anesthesiology in operating rooms of today (Aslanidis et al., 2023). Airway management is another issue that complicates matters, especially in difficult situations. For both emergency as well as elective operations, both maintaining the patient's airway open is significant, but it becomes even more significant when patients have other conditions as well. Every now and then, patients demonstrate uncommon anatomical characteristics or physiologic responses that baffle traditional approaches. An immediate effective solution in airway management can actually be the difference between life and death. Medical personnel need to be current on best practice, whether it is adapting to new, at times imperfect techniques. Ultimately, proper anesthesia is not as much a matter of obtaining drugs that are properly dosed as it is surviving challenges that come with other medical issues, and ongoing training and learning always prioritizing patient safety (Aslanidis et al., 2023) (Figure 12.1).

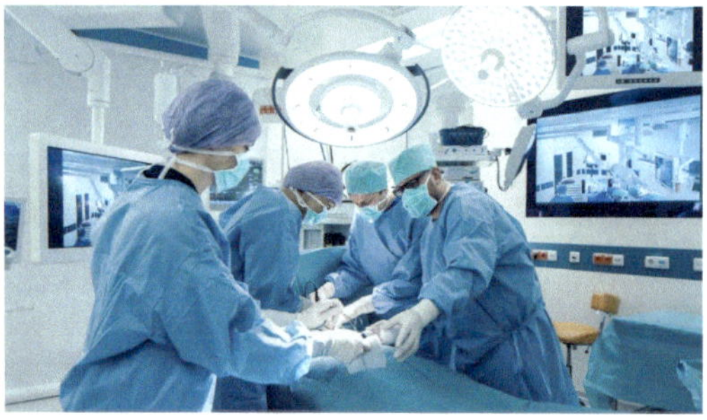

Figure 12.1. Anesthesia for Patients with Comorbid Conditions.

Source: https://i0.wp.com/anaesthesianews.wordpress.com/wp-content/uploads/2024/02/istock-864574770.jpg?fit=1200%2C675&ssl=1.

Definition of Anesthesia

Anesthesia is not just about putting someone under for surgery—it is an art of techniques and drugs that take a patient through a series of states, from relaxing into deep unawareness. It becomes increasingly complicated when there are medical issues building up; those with other conditions can behave in unpredictable ways compared to healthier individuals. Take, for example, patients with chronic pain in the muscles. They are more likely to have underlying mood pathology that, in a way, obscures the usual dynamics of pain control and overall care (Salazar et al., 2013). So, understanding what anesthesia guards against is not so much about prevention of pain—it's also about anticipating surprise complications when a patient's history is more involved. Beyond the general principle, there's that American Society of Anesthesiologists-Physical Status (ASA-PS) Classification that most utilize. Overall, it's a machine intended to quantify risk, scoring patients based on their general health. However, not every anesthetist uses it the same way, which can lead to varying estimates of risk—especially for high-stress cases of trauma when one doctor's evaluation of a patient's additional conditions might influence the choice (Naidu et al., 2018). A proper comprehension of the ASA-PS system in all its glory and failure enables medical teams to modify their strategy such that patients with more health issues are given the close, watchful monitoring that they need for surgery. In the end, the world of anesthesia is always evolving, and that takes greater, more flexible knowledge—especially for those dealing with multiple health issues. With new technologies available all the time, the more tailored approach to practice is not only helpful, but imperative. This type of care helps with better clinical outcomes and patient satisfaction. Add this to the repeated correlation between chronic pain and hidden mood disorders (Salazar et al., 2013), it only highlights how essential it is to study anesthesia in a more broad, general sense. Ultimately, constant investigation and keeping abreast of emerging wisdom are essential to helping anesthesiologists navigate this complicated landscape (Figure 12.2).

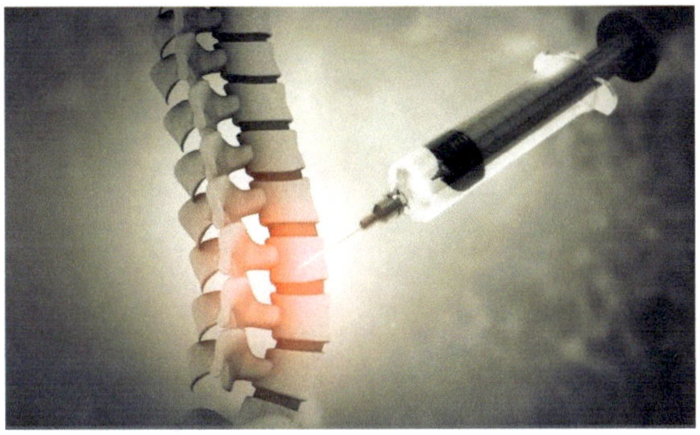

Figure 12.2. Anesthesia.

Source: https://www.relainstitute.com/wp-content/uploads/2022/12/Anesthesia_1-1.jpg.

12.1. Common Comorbid Conditions

Learning Outcome

1. Recognize how anesthesia interacts with cardiovascular issues.
2. Understand the respiratory disorders.
3. Describe the diabetes mellitus.

Managing anesthesia for patients with extra health issues can be tricky. Sometimes, hidden vulnerabilities become worse, raising the chance of complications both during and after surgery. For example, someone with heart problems like high blood pressure or heart failure might run into issues such as unpredictable rhythms or unstable blood flow under anesthesia. That's why a full pre-surgery check is pretty important—it lets the team adjust the anesthesia plan just right. Some research generally points out that ketamine-based mix-ups may lower complications inside the operating room and help with patient cooperation during less invasive procedures like radiofrequency ablation (Akhilesh et al., 2024). When there are several conditions in play, things can quickly get complicated—especially with older patients. Aging brings its changes, and when you add diabetes or COPD into the mix, the way anesthesia works in the body can get all tangled up. These patients sometimes react differently to medications, which makes it tougher to keep things balanced during surgery. In most cases, using a mix of pain-relief techniques (multimodal analgesia) helps control pain while reducing on opiates—a must for patients at risk of breathing issues (Heo et al., 2024). Understanding exactly how these extra conditions affect anesthesia choices is essential for patient safety and smoother surgical results. On top of that, these common health problems don't just affect what happens during surgery—they can influence recovery afterward too. For instance, people with a history of irregular heartbeats or atrial fibrillation might see their heart rate bouncing around during and after procedures, which can make getting better more challenging. Some studies suggest that a careful use of dexmedetomidine (DEX) might help stabilize the heart rate in such cases (Heo et al., 2024). Overall, anesthesiologists need to stay on their toes, ready to alter their approach based on each patient's mix of conditions. Dealing with these complexities not only ups immediate surgical safety but also sets the stage for better long-term recovery for patients facing multiple health challenges.

12.1.1. Cardiovascular Diseases

Recognizing how anesthesia interacts with cardiovascular issues is crucial—it can shape patient outcomes. Many surgical patients already have hidden heart conditions, so a thorough pre-surgery check is needed to uncover risks related to anesthesia. Often, patients with underlying heart problems become more vulnerable during the operation, especially in major non-cardiac surgeries. These vulnerabilities might show up as heart attacks, kidney injuries, or other serious events. In many cases, the bodily processes—like unstable blood flow and extra heart stress—play a big role in these complications, and addressing them helps lower the chance of adverse outcomes. This insight lets anesthesiologists design custom anesthesia plans that focus on steady blood flow and reduced risks for those carrying extra health burdens. Some recent research indicates that patients with added heart conditions are, in general, at a noticeably higher risk during surgery. The mix of surgical stress, anesthesia-driven blood pressure shifts, and the patient's preexisting issues creates a complex picture. Fluctuations in blood pressure during the operation—especially bouts of low blood pressure—are often tied to an uptick in heart injuries and kidney problems (Hallqvist et al., 2020). With surgery numbers on the rise, these findings kind of underline the need for targeted management strategies during anesthesia. For example, continuous hemodynamic monitoring right through the surgical process lets the team catch and respond to worrisome changes quickly, which in turn helps safeguard vital organs. These measures are key to boosting clinical outcomes and lowering both morbidity and mortality linked with non-cardiac surgeries in these vulnerable groups. Adding to these challenges, infectious diseases like COVID-19 have layered on extra complexity when managing patients with heart issues under anesthesia. Patients infected with SARS-CoV-2, particularly those already struggling with heart conditions, have an elevated risk of severe respiratory and cardiovascular problems. The virus acts by lowering angiotensin-converting enzyme 2 (ACE2), which can further worsen heart function (Alyari et al., 2020). This situation calls for a team-based approach that weaves together insights from both cardiology and infectious disease expertise. Anesthesia protocols, therefore, may need to be adjusted to ease stress responses and keep blood flow as stable as possible. As healthcare continues to evolve—especially amid ongoing global challenges—a well-rounded understanding of how cardiovascular issues and anesthesia interact remains vital to enhancing patient care and outcomes (Figure 12.3).

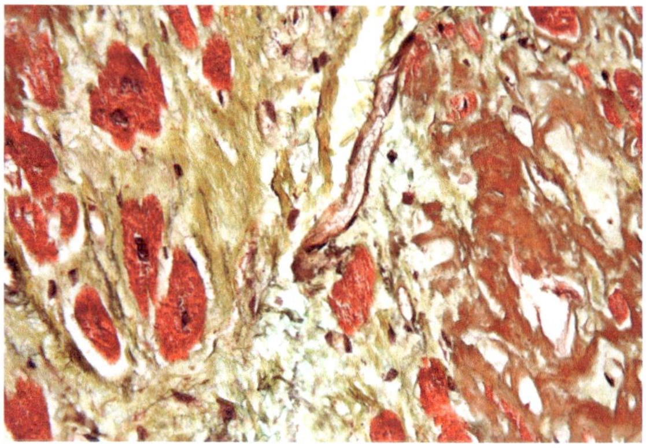

Figure 12.3. Cardiovascular diseases.

Source: By Nephron - Own work, CC BY-SA 3.0, https://commons.wikimedia.org/w/index.php?curid=8674830.

12.1.2. Respiratory Disorders

Surgery isn't just about the procedure – often, breathing issues shape how anesthesia is handled and affect recovery. Patients may come in with trouble breathing, like COPD, asthma, or even laryngomalacia, and these problems tend to mix with other issues such as obesity or chronic lung disease. In many cases, these overlapping concerns can bump up the risk of complications around the time of surgery. It's important, then, to look at how these respiratory complications jive with the effects of anesthesia; small adjustments in drug delivery, ventilation methods, and how the patient is monitored during the operation can make a big difference in keeping things safe and smooth. Take laryngomalacia, for example. This condition often grabs attention in young patients – though its influence can linger sometimes into later years. It's mainly about the collapse of the tissues above the voice box, and it often comes hand-in-hand with other airway issues like tracheomalacia or bronchomalacia. Research has hinted that when multiple airway problems crop up together, breathing difficulties can worsen, which in turn makes managing anesthesia trickier. In most cases, a solid checkup before surgery – including an endoscopic look and a review of the patient's history – proves vital to spot those at higher risk.

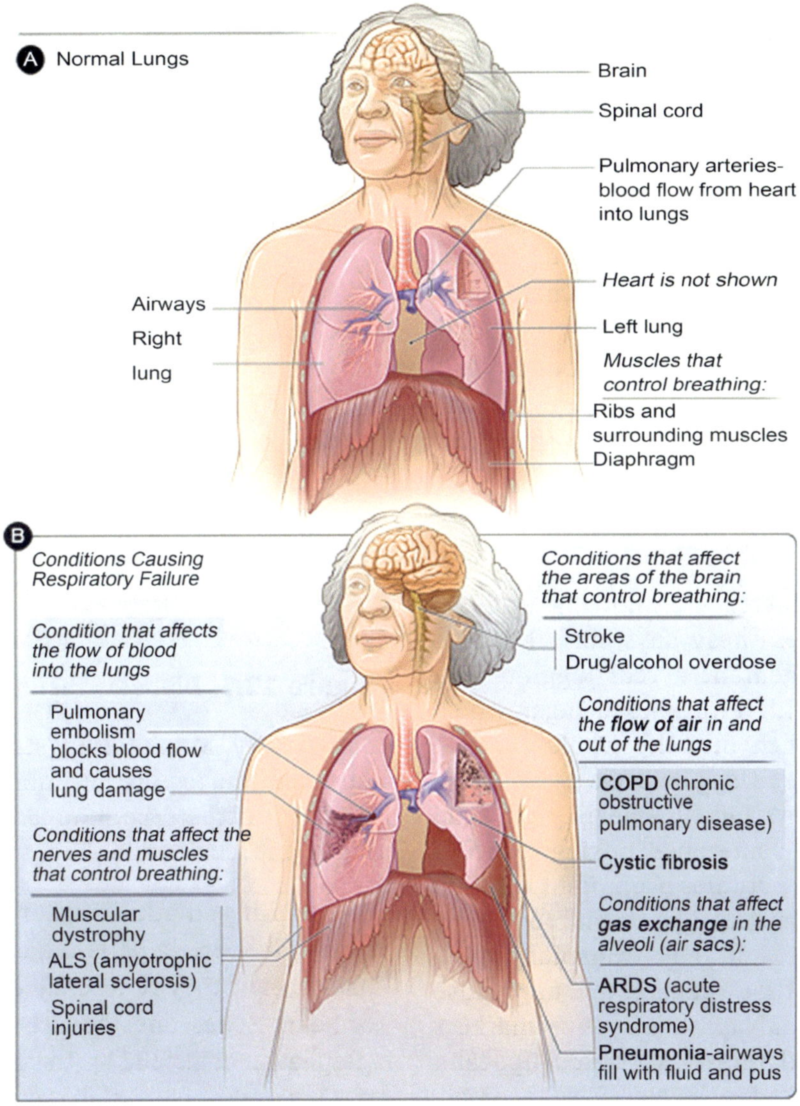

Figure 12.4. Respiratory disorders.

Source: By National Heart Lung and Blood Institute (NIH) - National Heart Lung and Blood Institute (NIH), Public Domain, https://commons.wikimedia.org/w/index.php?curid=29588225.

Figuring out the specific type of laryngomalacia, even if it means rethinking standard classifications, helps determine which airway tools and anesthetic plans will work best to reduce post-surgery issues (Kusak-Jarosz et al., 2017). Then there's the tricky side of anesthesia itself, which seems to play with both brain and breathing functions – a matter that gets even more delicate when older patients are involved. Studies generally show that even small alters in the depth of anesthesia can lead to a range of outcomes, from temporary memory slips to bouts of breathing trouble (Allard et al., 2014). For instance, comparing agents like desflurane and sevoflurane has revealed that each can cause a slight, short-lived drop in cognitive performance, though the effects aren't identical across the board. It underscores that a one-size-fits-all approach just doesn't cut it, especially for seniors already dealing with lung issues. Anesthesiologists, juggling these challenges, need to fine-tune their methods - balancing the right anesthesia depth while doing their best to keep a patient's breathing capabilities intact, even if that means sometimes reworking traditional protocols (Figure 12.4).

12.1.3. Diabetes Mellitus

Patients with diabetes are showing up with more health issues these days, and it makes anesthesia management a real juggling act. Diabetes brings with it high blood sugar, which can throw a wrench into the whole surgical process. When blood sugar levels spike, risks like poor blood flow and slow healing can crop up unexpectedly—sometimes making recovery a lot tougher. Some studies even point out that during critical moments, like when blood flow comes back after a kidney transplant, high sugar can worsen tissue damage and may cause kidney function to fall apart, as seen by markers like neutrophil gelatinase-associated lipocalin (NGAL) and creatinine levels (Parekh et al., 2011)., keeping blood sugar steady becomes key, and anesthesia teams play an increasingly crucial role in that balancing act. The drug side of things isn't any simpler either. Diabetes doesn't just disrupt body functions—it messes with how anesthetics and pain relievers work alongside diabetic meds. This mix sometimes forces doctors to take extra time to review everything before surgery. It demands a custom plan, since the way anesthetic agents jostle with glucose controls means insulin can behave in unpredictable ways. In practice, those handling anesthesia have to be extra watchful about when insulin is given—too little or too much can easily trigger dangerous blood sugar drops or spikes.

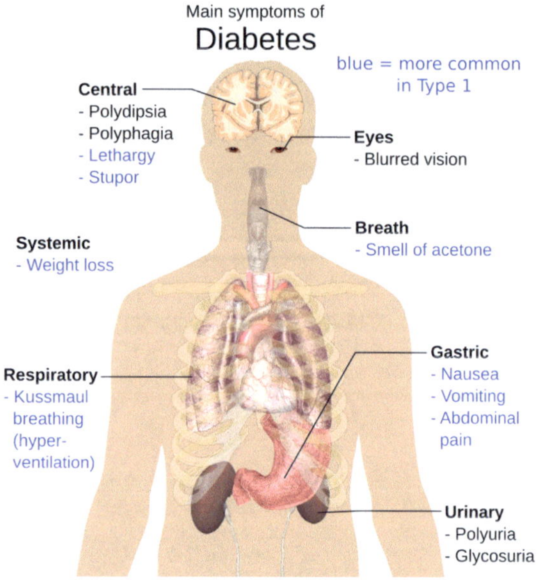

Figure 12.5. Diabetes mellitus.

Source: By Mikael Häggström - See above. All used images are in public domain., Public Domain, https://commons.wikimedia.org/w/index.php?curid=6055528.

And if you add in other details like which type of diabetes a patient has, how long they've had it, or if they're already dealing with nerve or heart issues, anesthesia can get even trickier (Raghavan et al., 2011). To summarize, knowing the ins and outs of diabetes is vital for patient safety. Even once the surgery wraps up, diabetes can keep causing headaches. Patients tend to wake up slower from anesthesia, and that delay might open the door to problems like infections—especially around the surgery site. In fact, if diabetes isn't well managed, the risk for infections goes up, potentially worsening other health problems. These challenges drive home the need for doctors from different specialties—endocrinologists, anesthesiologists, and others—to band together in planning out care. Tackling the many twists and turns of diabetes during anesthesia not only helps with the immediate win at surgery but also sets the stage for a better recovery down the road, boosting the overall quality of care for those with diabetes (Figure 12.5).

Test Your Knowledge

1. How anesthesia interacts with cardiovascular issues?
2. What are 3 major respiratory disorders?

12.2. Preoperative Assessment

Learning Outcome

1. Evaluate medical history.
2. Discuss on physical examination and diagnostic testing.

A preoperative evaluation is key for planning how anesthesia will be handled in patients juggling multiple health issues. Often, this starts with a casual but detailed run down of past illnesses, a physical check, and a few lab tests that fit each person's unique profile. When doctors sift through these details, they can generally sense which added medical problems might stir up complications during surgery. Take, for example, patients with obstructive sleep apnea (OSA)—a condition that, in many cases, flies under the radar but can cause breathing troubles during anesthesia (Gray-Cunningham et al., 2019). Using screening tools like the STOP-Bang Questionnaire helps catch these risks early, meaning that extra monitoring after surgery or alters to the anesthetic approach might be put in place just in time. Lately, efforts to speed up preoperative assessments have been making a difference not just to patient outcomes but also to how surgical schedules run. Some newer initiatives have reshaped how pre-op clinics operate—staffing them with dedicated nursing teams to trim waiting times and catch details that might otherwise lead to day-of-surgery cancellations. Change management techniques, in most cases, have led to fewer avoidable delays and a noticeable boost in patient satisfaction (Flint et al., 2016). This kind of strategy doesn't only smooth out the preoperative experience for individuals with extra health issues, but also gives anesthesia providers a bit more room to think through the risks and plan their approach. A deeper look before surgery also shines a light on the specific anesthesia challenges tied to different health conditions.

For instance, a patient with heart issues might need a distinct set of anesthetic drugs or monitoring than someone primarily dealing with lung troubles. This kind of personalized plan can help lower risks like erratic heart rhythms or low oxygen levels after surgery—issues often seen in patients with several overlapping conditions (Gray-Cunningham et al., 2019). Sometimes, when patients understand the particular risks they face, it builds a sort of teamwork feel between them and their healthcare crew, encouraging them to follow pre-surgery instructions more carefully. In essence, a thoughtful, individualized preoperative check-up doesn't only make anesthesia safer—it lays the groundwork for a smoother recovery afterwards (Figure 12.6).

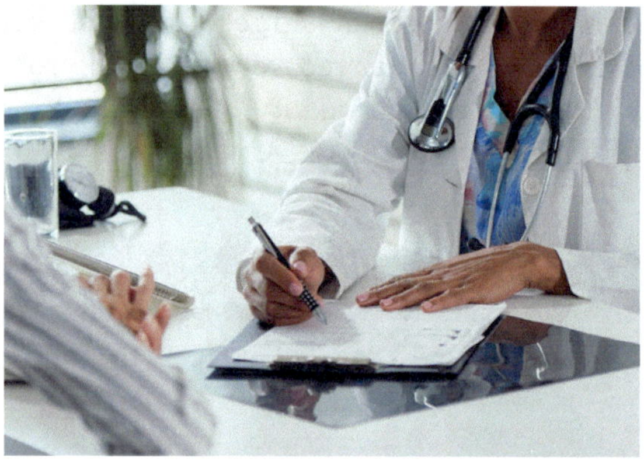

Figure 12.6. Preoperative Assessment.

Source: https://drpulerammego.co.za/storage/2022/08/secondary-service-image-2.jpg.

12.2.1. Medical History Evaluation

Taking a deep dive into a patient's health history is where you usually begin planning anesthesia—this step is especially important when multiple conditions are involved. You have to check out everything—from any chronic diseases and regular medications to past bumps with anesthesia. This kind of overall review not only hints at which anesthetic approach might work best, but it also plays a role in figuring out care before and after surgery. In many cases, patients dealing with OSA can be trickier because they tend to run into breathing problems while under anesthesia; nailing d an accurate OSA diagnosis and weighing its risks is key for safe anesthesia delivery and setting up the proper safety measures (Parafianowicz et al., 2024). Patients with heart conditions, like coronary artery disease, also require extra attention when planning their anesthetic care. Generally speaking, it's crucial to grasp their cardiovascular status—details like how well they function day-to-day and any recent heart-related events help shape the plan. Nurse anesthetists, in particular, need to be sharp at spotting even subtle hints of myocardial ischemia and be ready to jump into action if any trouble spots come up during surgery. This attention to detail can go a long way toward reducing the risk of complications, ensuring that even non-cardiac surgeries run more smoothly (Maund et al., 2003). Also, the way each comorbid condition might sway the choice of anesthesia shouldn't be overlooked. It's especially relevant for patients with breathing or metabolic issues, since these problems can sometimes complicate managing the airway or how drugs are broken d. People can react in unexpected ways to anesthetic agents, so a personalized approach—one that considers each patient's unique health background—is often the best bet. By carefully sifting through all these factors, anesthetists can craft a more predictable, and safer surgical journey. In most cases, this level of individualized care ends up boosting both the surgical outcomes and the overall satisfaction of the patient (Parafianowicz et al., 2024).

12.2.2. Physical Examination

Checking a patient's physical state is important when handling anesthesia, especially if other health problems are in play. A full evaluation not only reveals the overall condition but also hints at hidden risks. For example, taking a detailed history along with a hands-on physical check can bring to light heart or breathing troubles that might complicate an anesthetic course. The American Society of Anesthesiologists (ASA) system often leans on these findings to sort patients into various risk levels—a way of grouping that generally guides how anesthesia is adjusted for each individual. In most cases, this exam forms the bedrock of pre-surgery planning, influencing both the anesthesia approach and broader safety decisions. Sometimes, though, it isn't just about the physical exam; imaging like chest X-rays also plays a part. Recent studies, for instance, have shown that these pictures can uncover issues—such as blocked airways or lung problems—that might not show up otherwise. In one cohort study, checking radiographs in animals delivered some surprising evidence of respiratory lesions. This means it's not only the patient's clinical story or physical check that counts, but also what the radiographs reveal. By spotting potential complications sooner, anesthesiologists can often craft more refined strategies that help ease risks—especially for folks already dealing with extra health concerns. Another angle picking up steam is the use of biomarkers in these assessments. Generally speaking, evaluating levels of B-type natriuretic peptide (BNP) appears to go hand in hand with gauging pneumonia severity, offering another window into a patient's preoperative state. One study on pneumonia patients found that elevated BNP levels came along with higher odds of complications and even mortality. In this light, physical exam findings mixed with blood markers can provide a more complete picture of someone's condition. All told, these comprehensive checks—though sometimes a bit messy in their details—equip anesthesiologists to make better, more human-centered decisions that prioritize safety and aim for the best surgical outcomes (Figure 12.7).

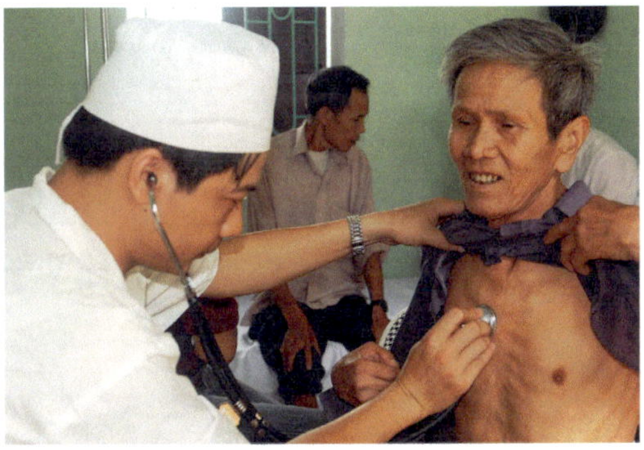

Figure 12.7. Physical exam before surgery.

Source: By JoAnn Moravac, U.S. Army - http://www.army.mil/; VIRIN: 44812-2009-07-15-170720, Public Domain, https://commons.wikimedia.org/w/index.php?curid=9735692.

12.2.3. Diagnostic Testing

Diagnostic testing plays a big part when patients come to surgery with multiple health issues. Getting a good read on someone's condition beforehand – through tests like blood work, imaging, or even heart assessments – helps shape how anesthesia is given. In many cases, routine check-ups reveal unexpected details about a patient's overall state, and with these insights, anesthesiologists can adjust their approach to lower risks and boost safety. This kind of personalized strategy tends not only to deal with the immediate surgery but also to account for any lingering health factors that could influence anesthesia outcomes. New developments in testing techniques have turned preoperative assessments into a more dynamic process. Sometimes, advancements in technology or updated testing methods let doctors pick up subtle issues that might otherwise be missed – consider how an echocardiogram might unexpectedly show left ventricular dysfunction in a patient with heart concerns. Clearly, when these findings pop up, they can lead to changes in the anesthesia plan, whether that means choosing a different drug or setting up additional monitoring. Redesigning screening clinics to better manage resources and patient flow has even helped reduce on last-minute cancellations while boosting overall satisfaction and safety (Flint et al., 2016). Even the broader treatment plan can shift when diagnostics uncover abnormalities. Data from tests – even studies in veterinary contexts, like those using an abdominal ultrasound – remind us that catching a problem early can change what happens next, even if those examples are just indirectly related to human medicine. Generally speaking, when routine AUS detects issues, the whole care pathway might change, enabling anesthesiologists to craft more tailored, patient-focused interventions that tackle individual challenges. In most cases, understanding these interdependencies helps improve both surgical outcomes and overall patient care (Blair et al., 2015) (Figure 12.8).

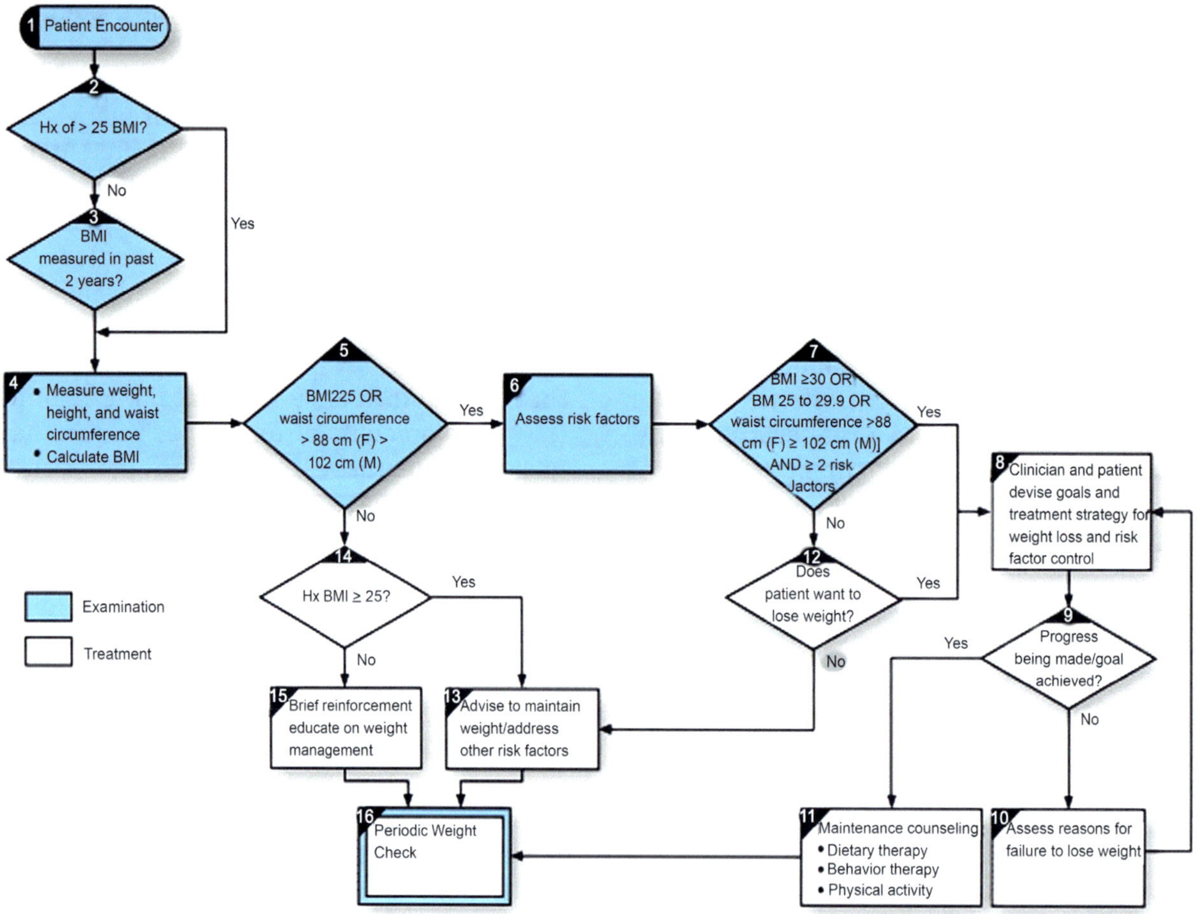

Figure 12.8. Diagnostic testing.

Source: By National Heart, Lung, and Blood Institute - Page at National Heart, Lung, and Blood Institute at the U.S. Department of Health & Human Services, Public Domain, https://commons.wikimedia.org/w/index.php?curid=11656201.

Test Your Knowledge

1. What is physical examination?
2. What is diagnostic testing?

12.3. Anesthetic Considerations for Specific Conditions

Learning Outcome

1. Understand the adjustments for cardiovascular patients.
2. Learn about strategies for managing respiratory issues.
3. Describe the protocols for diabetic patients.

Managing anesthesia in folks with extra health problems calls for extra care. Patients who have metabolic issues like isovaleric acidemia (IVA) tend to be more sensitive when the body is stressed by surgery. Often, this kind of sensitivity can lead to troubling events—for example, a bout of acute acidosis may occur if they have to endure prolonged fasting or an invasive procedure. Sometimes, when IVA pops up alongside mental health issues, things get even muddled because antipsychotic meds might mix badly with anesthetic drugs. This scenario usually forces clinicians to adjust their dosing, keep a sharper eye on the patient, and design a surgical plan that eases these risks. In most cases, having a team—anesthesiologists, surgeons, and primary care docs—work together is the best way to craft a plan that tackles all of these overlapping challenges (Chinen et al., 2022). Sleep apnea, specifically OSA, adds another twist to the whole picture. OSA not only makes it tougher to handle the airway but also cranks up a patient's sensitivity to sedatives, which can sometimes trigger severe respiratory depression during and shortly after surgery. Generally speaking, the whole anesthetic approach must take a longer view, starting with a thorough preoperative check to spot the risk factors connected to OSA. Things like smart patient positioning, steering clear of some sedatives, and keeping constant tabs on breathing function all play key parts in ensuring safety. When the anesthesia plan is customized based on these risk levels, it tends to boost both the safety and overall outcome for the patient (Parafianowicz et al., 2024). Overall, the unpredictable nature of managing anesthesia for patients with multiple health issues means that a one-size-fits-all method just won't do. When conditions like IVA join forces with psychiatric challenges, the usual anesthetic routines might not work as expected, so plans often need altering to suit each individual case. Similarly, encountering conditions like OSA signals that careful pre-op assessments and custom in-operation tactics are a must to create a safe and effective environment. All these complexities—sometimes even repeating similar care adjustments—underline the importance of ongoing learning and adapting in anesthetic practices, making sure providers are always ready for the evolving challenges in patient care (Chinen et al., 2022; Parafianowicz et al., 2024).

12.3.1. Adjustments for Cardiovascular Patients

For patients with heart issues, anesthesia management isn't just a set procedure—it's a careful balancing act. When risks like heart attacks and blood clots hang around, doctors lean on continuous monitoring so they can alter medications or fluid levels on the fly. That live look at heart stability lets them jump on any unexpected shifts in a patient's condition, and designing anesthesia plans around individual histories does make a difference (Pereira et al., 2024). Sometimes it's less about following a checklist and more about paying careful attention as things unfold. Teaming up across specialties has become a real game changer for those with complex heart problems facing surgery. Instead of working in isolation, anesthesiologists, cardiovascular specialists, and surgeons pool their expertise to mix general anesthesia (GA) practices with focused cardiac care. They keep preoperative heart medications going and choose techniques that dodge extra risks while also boosting communication among everyone involved, so key details rarely slip through the cracks (Zhao et al., 2024). In many cases, this mixed approach brings in fresh perspectives and smoother coordination. At the end of the day, making adjustments for heart patients isn't just an extra step—it's essential for better outcomes. Anesthesia strategies need to roll with our ever-growing understanding of heart risks and the benefits of personalized care. It's crucial to look at the full picture—a patient's entire medical history and current state, especially when severe cardiac issues are in play. By constantly learning on the job and pushing for innovative methods, healthcare teams can chip away at the barriers in anesthesia management. This effort not only fine-tunes care for each individual but also builds stronger, more adaptable protocols for those undergoing surgery with pre-existing heart conditions (Pereira et al., 2024) (Figure 12.9).

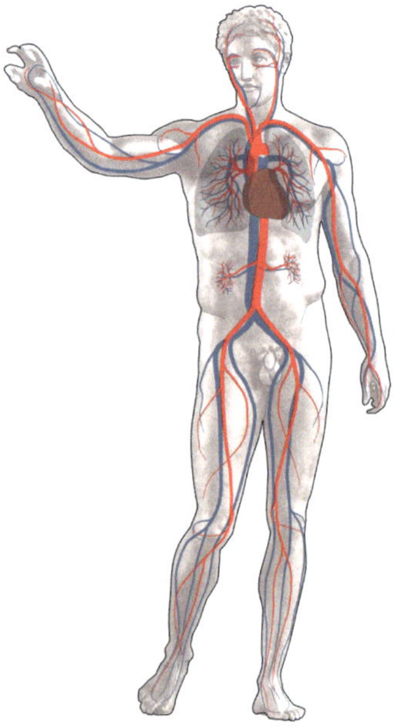

Figure 12.9. Caring for patients with cardiovascular disease.

Source: By User: Sansculotte - self-drawn, CC BY-SA 2.5, https://commons.wikimedia.org/w/index.php?curid=335448.

12.3.2. Strategies for Managing Respiratory Issues

Anesthesia and breathing problems are linked in ways that demand we get under the skin of pre-surgery checks and custom care. We kick off by spotting anyone who already has trouble breathing—think sleep apnea or asthma—and then weigh the risks to set up a plan that works for that person. It's not just about listing issues; it means looking at how sensitive someone might be to drugs and sorting out airway challenges, all while keeping in mind that guidelines matter when using drugs that might push lung issues over the edge. Each unique breathing profile gets its due attention throughout the process, with careful thought given to preventing mishaps by staying on top of the details.

A smart move during anesthesia is the use of top-notch monitors. Pulse oximetry and capnography, for example, offer live updates on oxygen levels and ventilation—crucial clues for spotting trouble early. In cases like OSA, the chances of airway blockages go up during sedation so that these monitors help catch issues just as they start, making way for quick fixes like positive pressure ventilation. In most cases, prepping the lungs ahead of time with bronchodilators pays off; every step in this process adds up to a safer overall experience, even if the approach can seem a bit all over the place sometimes. Talking things through with patients is another key piece. Laying out how their condition might mix with anesthesia not only builds trust but also gets them involved in their care. For instance, someone with asthma should, generally speaking, stick to their meds and keep an eye on known triggers—little reminders that can make a big difference. Chatting about any alters in the usual anesthesia game plan because of existing issues creates a sort of teamwork between the patient and care team. Even after the surgery, a bit of follow-up education goes a long way in catching any respiratory hiccups early. All this combined—a mix of tailored checks and clear, ongoing discussion—helps keep patients safe, a point underscored in recent reviews (Murray-Torres et al., 2021; Parafianowicz et al., 2024) (Figure 12.10).

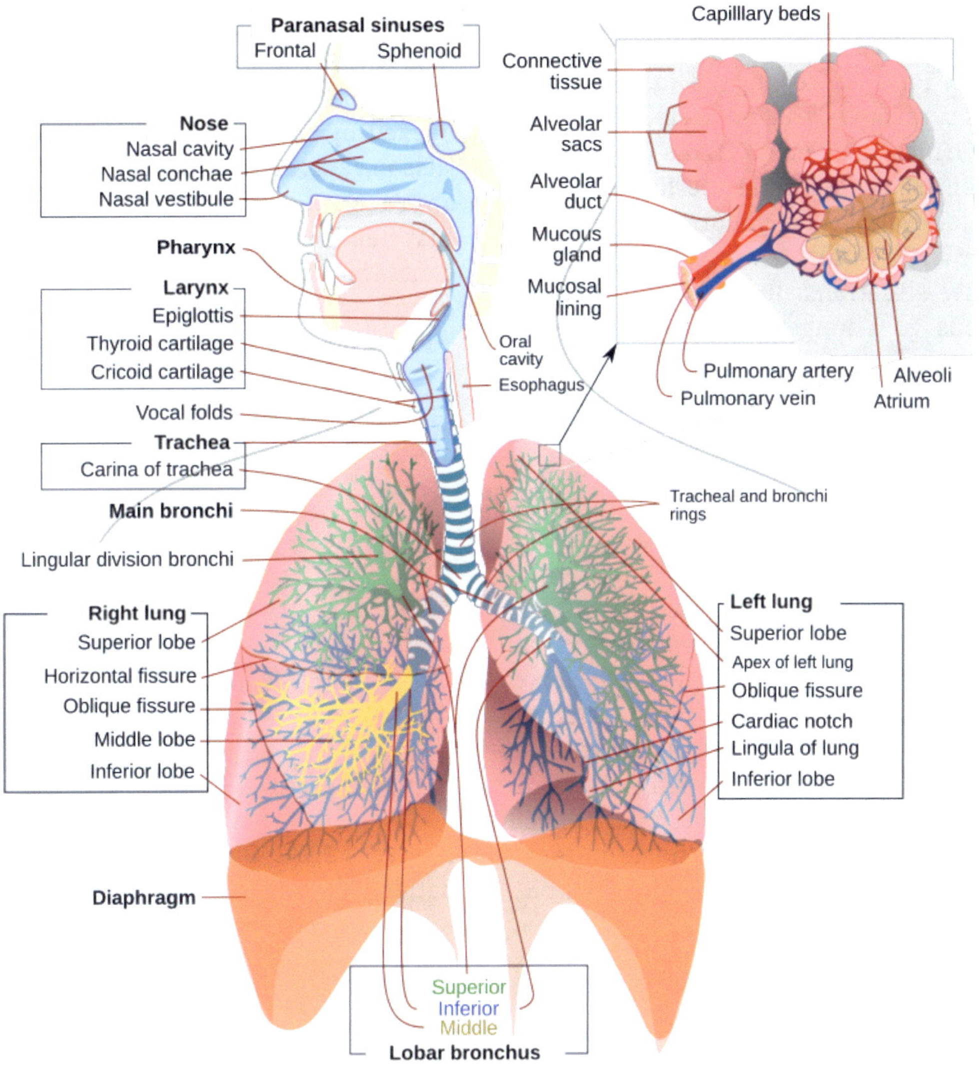

Figure 12.10. The respiratory system.

Source: By LadyofHats, Jmarchn - Own work using:Sobotta, Johannes (1982) Atlas der Anatomie des Menschen/ 2 Brust, Bauch, Becken, untere Extremitäten, Haut. (18th ed.), Munich: Urban & Schwarzenberg ISBN: 3-541-02828-9. OCLC: 260005032.Gray, Henry (1980) Gray's Anatomy (36th ed.), Edinburgh: Churchill Livingstone ISBN: 0-443-01505-8. OCLC: 7775214.Yokochi, Chihiro (1991) Atlas fotográfico de anatomía del cuerpo humano (3rd ed.), Mexico: Interamericana/McGraw-Hill ISBN: 968-25-1677-3. OCLC: 33318149.Also used several online diagrams like:[1][2], Public Domain, https://commons.wikimedia.org/w/index.php?curid=3945169.

12.3.3. Protocols for Diabetic Patients

Diabetic patients who need anesthesia call for a bit of extra attention—it's not just routine care. Detailed checks before any surgery are a must, with a strong focus on keeping blood sugar in a safe zone. Patients relying on insulin often have to get custom-tailored plans, meaning that as surgery nears, their medications might need readjustments. Take the fasting period before an operation, for example; it's important to monitor those sugar levels closely to dodge both too-high and too-low situations. In most cases, these careful steps go a long way toward reducing risks during anesthesia and help set the stage for a smoother recovery. During the operation, keeping glucose steady remains a top priority. Anesthesiologists, as you might expect, are on constant alert—sometimes using continuous monitors—to track any sudden changes. It's especially critical because blood sugar that wanders can trigger issues like infections, slow wound healing, or even a longer hospital stay. Generally speaking, sticking to these routines supports a patient's overall stability and jives with best practices in anesthesia care. In many instances, staying vigilant throughout the procedure can seriously affect both the immediate recovery and long-term outcomes. After surgery, things shift a bit but careful management is still key. Postoperative care means keeping an eye on how diabetes is managed since stress, diet changes, or fluctuations in activity might alter insulin needs. Hospitals usually set up protocols to regularly check and alter insulin plans according to the patient's current condition—which, admittedly, can change rapidly. Educating patients on how to check their glucose themselves and adjust medications naturally adds one more safety net. To summarize, these comprehensive guidelines, backed by solid evidence (Dowell et al., 2022, Nelson et al., 2019), highlight why a personalized approach matters so much. They remind us that handling the intricacies of diabetes in the context of anesthesia isn't one-size-fits-all—it's about easing recovery and paving the way for better overall health outcomes (Figure 12.11).

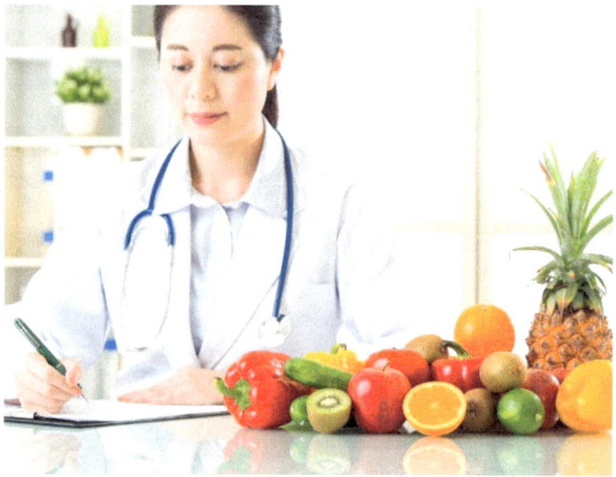

Figure 12.11. Dietary guidelines for diabetic patients.

Source: https://www.cdi.org.in/wp-content/uploads/2021/03/Dietary-guidelines-for-diabetic-Patients-1200x900.jpg.

Test Your Knowledge

1. What are the adjustments for cardiovascular patients?
2. What are the protocols for diabetic patients?

12.4. Risks and Complications

Learning Outcome

1. Describe the potential complications of anesthesia.
2. Manage increased risks in patients with comorbidities.
3. Understand the strategies to mitigate risks.

Patients who show up for anesthesia often come in with lingering health issues—take OSA for example, which pops up in adults more than you'd expect. Roughly speaking, about one in every four U.S. adults seems to have OSA, yet oddly enough, nearly 80–90% of those with moderate to severe cases go undiagnosed. This mismatch cranks up the risk during surgery, sometimes leading to problems like breathing troubles or even irregular heartbeats. The Society of Anesthesia and Sleep, for instance, advises a thorough pre-surgery check for OSA, and tools such as the STOP-Bang Questionnaire can sometimes spot high-risk patients before the operation begins (Gray-Cunningham et al., 2019). Then there's the twist with patients fighting end-stage renal disease (ESRD). These individuals tend to bear a heavier load of other health conditions, making them extra vulnerable when GA is in the mix. In many cases, alternatives like an ultrasound-guided transversus abdominis plane (TAP) block have started to win favor. This approach has proven useful for things like peritoneal dialysis catheter placement without the need to go under full GA—thereby reducing on systemic effects and reducing associated risks. Some research even shows that TAP blocks can be performed successfully in a fair number of ESRD cases, offering a more pinpointed anesthesia strategy that fits the unique health profile of these patients (Gršković et al., 2016). Mixing multiple health challenges with anesthesia management underlines the pressing need for a more individualized assessment. Surgical teams, overall, need to keep a close watch on the many factors that might shift a patient's risk profile in the perioperative period. As anesthetic practice keeps evolving—in ways that are sometimes unpredictable—there's an increasing push to tailor the approach to fit each patient's distinct challenges. This doesn't just mean choosing the right methods, but also setting up robust preoperative screening routines that catch issues early, ultimately paving the way for safer, more effective care for patients with complex medical histories (Gray-Cunningham et al., 2019; Gršković et al., 2016) (Figure 12.12).

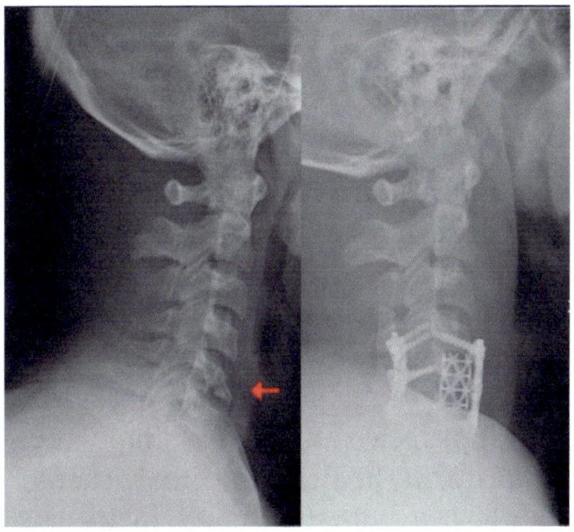

Figure 12.12. Spine surgery.

Source: By Moquito 17 at the English-language Wikipedia, CC BY-SA 3.0, https://commons.wikimedia.org/w/index.php?curid=7940879.

12.4.1. Potential Complications of Anesthesia

Anesthesia mixing with other health issues can stir up a host of problems that weigh d how patients recover. Older patients, for example, often suffer from bouts of post-op confusion that not only derail their recovery but also throw off their treatment routines, leading to a bump in overall risks—even mortality. One study looked at different ways to give anesthesia and found that seniors getting regional blocks had much less delirium (about 8.1% versus 20.6% with general anesthesia, P=0.012) during orthopedic surgeries. This finding hints that picking the right type of anesthesia is key, especially for those extra vulnerable patients (Delen et al., 2023). People with ongoing, chronic issues face their hurdles too. Take those with kidney troubles: they often battle fluid and electrolyte imbalances that raise the stakes during surgery. The stress from the operation, combined with the drugs used, can sometimes push them into sudden kidney failure, especially if heart problems are already on the table. Further, the blood flow changes that come with anesthesia might further upset kidney function—so keeping a close watch on fluids and electrolytes is crucial (Imtiaz et al., 2019). When patients juggle more than one condition, these concerns naturally grow in importance. Anesthesia care isn't just about the procedure itself; it's about matching the approach to the whole patient. Delirium and kidney issues aren't just random risks—they reflect a tangled interaction between how the body reacts and what the anesthesia does. Whether the team goes with a regional or general approach can deeply shape recovery and long-term health. In most cases, this means anesthesiologists need to be flexible, personalizing care and keeping an eye out for any bumps along the perioperative journey (Delen et al., 2023; Imtiaz et al., 2019).

12.4.2. Increased Risks in Patients with Comorbidities

Managing anesthesia for patients saddled with additional health issues can up the chances of things going awry during surgery. Patients with neurological conditions, for example, might not only face a decline in their cognitive abilities but also see a worsening in their symptoms post-anesthesia—something a fair bit of evidence hints at, particularly with conditions like epilepsy or dementia. Doctors, in most cases, have to essentially weigh the risks versus the perks, sometimes even exploring alternative methods to stick to the surgical objectives while keeping complications at bay. It's all about crafting that uniquely tailored plan that fits each patient's specific needs. Anesthetic risks, it turns out, can ripple out well beyond the operating room and have a lasting impact on overall health. Take individuals with cardiovascular issues: a bout of anesthesia might just trigger some unexpected heart instability during the procedure, which research generally suggests can lead to notable complications once surgery wraps up. This means thorough preoperative checks to pinpoint any cardiac vulnerabilities are a must; in many cases, these evaluations guide the anesthetic approach and help doctors steer clear of further problems. With solid, safety-first protocols in place, anesthesiologists can keep these risks in check, ensuring that even patients with layered health challenges get care that's both efficient and balanced. At the same time, the way other health conditions mix with anesthesia management calls for ongoing learning and adjustments in practice. A growing set of studies shows that anesthesia's physical effects on patients with multiple issues are only one part of the puzzle – there's also a broader impact on the whole healthcare delivery system. One systematic review, for instance, pointed out the need for inventive care models that address these specialized needs, a notion seemingly embraced by centers focusing on complex cases. Integrating such findings into everyday practice can help boost the overall safety and effectiveness of anesthetic protocols. Ultimately, considering both patient-specific factors and system-wide impacts might be our best bet at delivering truly equitable and comprehensive care.

12.4.3. Strategies to Mitigate Risks

Understanding a patient's medical past is key when planning anesthesia. A solid pre-surgery check-up helps sort out risks and, in most cases, uncovers hidden issues linked to other health problems. Sometimes, things like OSA show up unexpectedly—and this condition can change how an airway gets handled or how a person responds to sedative drugs. Parafianowicz et al. (2024) reminds us that nailing the diagnosis and designing a custom anesthesia plan usually goes a long way in keeping things safe. Matching the anesthetic approach to the patient's unique background not only smooths out the surgical process but also sets the stage for a better recovery. In essence, diving deep into the preoperative details makes sure that the methods used are in tune with each patient's physical limits, given their extra challenges. During the operation, the scene shifts and extra caution becomes a must—especially for folks with added health concerns. Anesthesiologists need to keep their eyes peeled, particularly for patients with known neurological issues or those at risk for some cognitive hiccups later on. GA can hit people differently if they've got preexisting brain or memory concerns, so it calls for a flexible strategy when dealing with sedative doses and ongoing checks. Research, as noted in (Jung Nho, 2023).), shows that these patients might face post-op cognitive slowdowns. It often means opting for lighter anesthesia or even swapping in alternative drugs to help safeguard brain function. This constant, watchful, and adaptive approach makes a difference in keeping complications at bay. After surgery, care doesn't take a back seat—it's every bit as critical, especially when other conditions are in the mix. The leap from the operating room to recovery shouldn't be rushed; it demands a plan tailored to each individuals specific needs. This stage can throw up its set of challenges, like managing pain, tracking breathing, and sometimes even seeing a flare-up of preexisting issues. For example, a patient with OSA might need extra help with their breathing, sometimes in the form of continuous positive airway pressure (CPAP) therapy when the situation calls for it. Plus, having the surgical team, the anesthesiologist, and recovery staff all in close, if not always perfectly smooth, communication amps up the overall care. As (Parafianowicz et al., 2024) points out, when everyone pulls together—even if things aren't always picture-perfect—the risks of post-op complications drop notably, paving the way for a safer, more effective recovery (Figure 12.13).

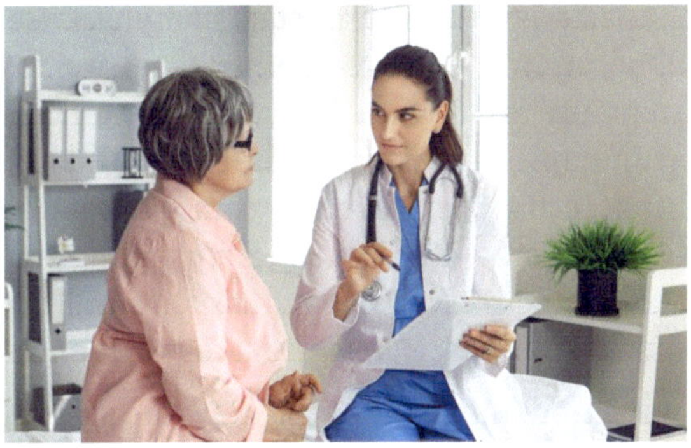

Figure 12.13. Strategies to Mitigate Risks.

Source: https://b764203.smushcdn.com/764203/wp-content/uploads/baxterassociatesllc-329663-doctor-patient-meeting-blogbanner-1-825x510.jpg?lossy=0&strip=1&webp=1.

Test Your Knowledge

1. What are the potential complications of anesthesia?
2. Describe the strategies to mitigate risks.

SUMMARY

It isn't always as simple as it may seem to deal with patients who have a multitude of health problems. Practitioners today have to get their minds around a mix of physical and psychological issues—you know, PTSD and liver disease—meaning old standbys for working with anesthesia might have to be re-thought hard. It appears that when psychiatric treatments are off the mark, it is even more crucial that professionals consider their decisions, especially in cases with co-morbidities like PTSD (Campbell et al., 2021). Putting body care together with psychiatric care can be the distinction between a rollercoaster and a cruise ride in surgery. Risk stratification can play an immense part in this too. Utilization of tried and true scoring systems like the Child-Turcotte-Pugh and Model for End-Stage Liver Disease helps to approximate surgical risk in patients with liver pathology (Kholili et al., 2016).

The greater amount of lost liver function, the more unpredictable the risks become, and thus anesthetic plans must be as unique as the patients themselves. This thorough, tailored evaluation not only dictates what anesthesia techniques to use—it also keeps the nurse care team on standby to handle any unexpected complications that might occur during the procedure. In the future, how anesthesia is delivered in such complex cases will rely on ongoing learning and interprofessional collaboration. The more familiar the providers are with how multiple health concerns interact, the better they are able to create thoughtful, effective plans. Evidence (Campbell et al., 2021) shows that an improved understanding of the manner in which conditions like PTSD influence the surgical portrait leads to improved outcomes for patients. It's most likely that building a culture of continuous learning-even with a few missteps along the way-will protect patients at risk from the problems of navigating multiple health issues simultaneously. Ultimately, expanding our knowledge is more about keeping pace with the latest evidence and less about being current with the latest studies.

It's not simple managing anesthesia for patients with other conditions. You must understand how the body works and how medications behave—especially when other challenges are added into the mix. Take psychiatric issues, for example; patients in that facility may need something different because they react more strongly to some medications and are prone to relapse in substance dependency. Studies even reveal that with the combination of personality disorders and other issues, risk of relapse is heightened (Gable et al., 2006). This most likely speaks volumes in terms of attention paid not only to patient safety but to also ensure improved surgery outcomes and fewer post-op hiccupps. Obstetric anesthesia—spinal anesthesia (SA), in particular—is something that can become extremely complicated. Maternal hypotension is a significant complication for both mother and baby.

There has been some recent evidence to suggest that norepinephrine is a better option than phenylephrine for the treatment of hypotension after a spinal anesthetic. Norepinephrine, with some beta-adrenergic activity, seems to maintain the cardiac output of the mother while not hindering uterine perfusion as much (Clarke et al., 2024). In most cases, this distinction becomes especially critical for patients with heart conditions who might react too strongly to more standard treatments. Getting these nuances right helps anesthesia providers decide on the best course of action, keeping both mother and baby safer during the procedure. Preoperative evaluations are, without a doubt, essential when you're dealing with extra health issues. It is worth having a team of several specialties examine the whole medical history—mental and cardiovascular illnesses as well—to pick up any red flags early. This kind of thorough check can guide the anesthesiology plan and post-anesthesia care. And, of course, routine refresher training in today's evidence-based practices, like norepinephrine for hypotension, is critical to better outcomes. Overall, bringing together the added conditions and control of the anesthetics calls for a careful, comprehensive approach. Even if things are not ideal, taking that extra minute to plan ahead can reward significant returns on planning as well as on-the-fly decision making.

KEY TERMS FROM THIS CHAPTER

Cardiovascular diseases
Diabetes
Heart failure
Laryngomalacia
Obstructive sleep apnea
Precision medicine
Radiofrequency ablation
Change management
Diagnostic testing
High blood pressure
Musculoskeletal pain
Physical examination
Preoperative evaluation
Respiratory disorders

CRITICAL THINKING QUESTIONS

1. **Which of the following is the primary goal of anesthesia management in a patient with ischemic heart disease?**
   a. Maintain high heart rate to improve cardiac output
   b. Avoid increases in myocardial oxygen demand
   c. Minimize preload and afterload
   d. Avoid the use of volatile anesthetics
2. **In patients with COPD, the most important anesthetic consideration is:**
   a. Avoiding nitrous oxide
   b. Preventing hyperventilation
   c. Ensuring low oxygen concentrations
   d. Maintaining adequate ventilation and avoiding air trapping
3. **In a diabetic patient undergoing surgery, intraoperative blood glucose levels should ideally be maintained within the range of:**
   a. 70-100 mg/dL
   b. 140-180 mg/dL
   c. 200-250 mg/dL
   d. 180-220 mg/dL
4. **In patients with chronic kidney disease, which of the following drugs requires dose adjustment?**
   a. Propofol
   b. Succinylcholine
   c. Rocuronium
   d. Morphine
5. **Which of the following anesthetic agents is most suitable for induction in a patient with asthma?**
   a. Thiopental
   b. Ketamine
   c. Propofol
   d. Etomidate

Short Answer Questions

1. Define the anesthesia
2. What is the most common comorbid condition?
3. What is preoperative assessment?
4. What are the anesthetic considerations for specific conditions?
5. Describe the risks and complications of anesthesia.

Answers to Critical Thinking Questions

1. (b); 2. (d); 3. (b); 4. (d); 5. (b)

REFERENCES

1. Alyari, M., Bakhtiarian, S., Gakharia, T., Nikandish, M., et al. (2020). The overview of the management of comorbid cardiovascular diseases and diabetes during COVID-19. https://core.ac.uk/download/493003542.pdf (accessed on 20 May 2025).
2. Annemans, L., De Regge, M., Duyck, P., Gemmel, P., et al. (2013). Physician-owned specialized facilities: Focused factories or destructive competition? A systematic review. https://core.ac.uk/download/55777137.pdf (accessed on 20 May 2025).
3. Aslanidis, T., Darcy, C., Alves Bersot, C. D., Barros, V. G., Carlos, D., Bersot, G., Dhir, M., et al. (2023). *Airway Management in Emergency Medicine*. IntechOpen eBooks. https://doi.org/10.5772/intechopen.110971.
4. Aydoğdu, Y. F., Örmeci, M., Özcan, A. H., Akdeniz, Y., Çalta, A. F., & Oğuz, S. (2024). The effect of comorbid conditions on postoperative morbidity in COVID-19 test positive patients undergoing emergency surgery. *Hippocrates Medical Journal*. https://www.semanticscholar.org/paper/8cb669082598503c091394fa65d93568bad55025 (accessed on 20 May 2025).
5. Bilgiç, E. B. (2025). Anesthetic risk analysis with routine preoperative thoracic radiography in dogs and cats. *Revista Científica de la Facultad de Ciencias Veterinarias*. https://www.semanticscholar.org/paper/d8c27eb9e43311303569a26a5b880505ed43cb3f (accessed on 20 May 2025).
6. Blair, W. H., Chen, R. X., Sturges, B. K., Taylor, A., et al. (2015). Effect of screening abdominal ultrasound examination on the decision to pursue advanced diagnostic tests and treatment in dogs with neurologic disease. https://core.ac.uk/download/323069729.pdf.
7. Campbell, Y., Gattorno, J., et al. (2021). A learning module in post-traumatic stress disorder (PTSD) and the use of 3,4-methylenedioxymethamphetamine (MDMA) assisted psychotherapies in patients who have PTSD and other alike disorders. https://core.ac.uk/download/484355156.pdf (accessed on 20 May 2025).
8. Chinen, Y., Goto, S., Goto, T., Kawano, K., et al. (2022). An unusual case of oral surgical management in a patient with isovaleric acidemia and schizophrenia: A case report. https://core.ac.uk/download/638964075.pdf (accessed on 20 May 2025).
9. Clarke, S., Miller, A., & Salgado, A. (2024). An educational module explaining the use of norepinephrine to treat post-spinal anesthesia-induced hypotension in parturient undergoing elective C-sections: A quality improvement project. *Nicole Wertheim College of Nursing Student Projects, 304*. https://digitalcommons.fiu.edu/cnhs-studentprojects/304 (accessed on 20 May 2025).
10. Delen, L., & Dişli, Z. (2023). A retrospective study of the effects of anesthesia methods on post-operative delirium in geriatric patients having orthopedic surgery: Anesthesia methods on post-operative delirium. *Journal of Surgery and Medicine, 7*, 324–328. https://doi.org/10.28982/josam.7710.
11. Dowell, D., Ragan, K., Jones, C. M., Baldwin, G., & Chou, R. (2022). CDC clinical practice guideline for prescribing opioids for pain—United States, 2022. *MMWR Recommendations and Reports, 71*(3), 1–95. https://doi.org/10.15585/mmwr.rr7103a1.

12. Flint, T. (2016). Gaining efficiency and reducing cost: The re-design of a preoperative screening clinic. http://deepblue.lib.umich.edu/bitstream/2027.42/137960/1/Flint2016.pdf (accessed on 20 May 2025).
13. Gable, G. K. (2006). Factors in relapse among physicians in recovery from substance dependence disorders. https://core.ac.uk/download/234120554.pdf (accessed on 20 May 2025).
14. Gray-Cunningham, C. (2019). The effect of obstructive sleep apnea screening on outcomes of adult surgical patients in a suburban hospital. https://core.ac.uk/download/270036191.pdf (accessed on 20 May 2025).
15. Gršković, A., Vujičić, B., Markić, D., Rahelić, D., Lasić, H., Božinović, I., Španjol, J., et al. (2016). Postavljanje katetera za peritonejsku dijalizu primjenom regionalne anestezije: Ultrazvučno vođeni TAP blok. https://core.ac.uk/download/481922457.pdf.
16. Gurrieri, C., Šprung, J., Weingarten, T. N., & Warner, M. E. (2017). Patients with glycogen storage diseases undergoing anesthesia: A case series. *BMC Anesthesiology, 17*, Article 42. https://doi.org/10.1186/s12871-017-0428-x.
17. Hallqvist, L. (2020). Perioperative risk factors and outcomes. https://core.ac.uk/download/361354309.pdf (accessed on 20 May 2025).
18. Handargal, N. H., & Usman, F. (2024). Prognostic value of B-type natriuretic peptide in hospitalized patients with pneumonia. *APIK Journal of Internal Medicine*. https://www.semanticscholar.org/paper/2fc9fe01b9f2b014f34df0e70a5ec3cfb06eb2eb (accessed on 20 May 2025).
19. Heo, M., Cho, M. J., Lee, S. I., & Kim, K. W. (2024). Dexmedetomidine as an effective alternative tool for heart rate control in atrial fibrillation during general anesthesia—A case report. *Saudi Journal of Anesthesia, 18*, 299–301. https://www.semanticscholar.org/paper/b2e00eb0121b5cb302fcccd331d17a320b7b7b32 (accessed on 20 May 2025).
20. Hoh, B. L., Ko, N., Amin-Hanjani, S., Chou, S., Cruz-Flores, S., Dangayach, N., Derdeyn, C. P., et al. (2023). 2023 guideline for the management of patients with aneurysmal subarachnoid hemorrhage: A guideline from the American Heart Association/American Stroke Association. *Stroke, 54*. https://doi.org/10.1161/str.0000000000000436.
21. Horsanali, B. Ö., Horsanali, M. O., & Tekgül, Z. T. (2017). Anesthesia for urological surgery. https://core.ac.uk/download/322429268.pdf (accessed on 20 May 2025).
22. Imtiaz, A., & Mahmood, R. (2019). Preoperative assessment in patients with kidney disease. *Annals of Abbasi Shaheed Hospital and Karachi Medical & Dental College*. https://www.semanticscholar.org/paper/e6ebfed577eb93a4909097f5f613442a7b3a216a (accessed on 20 May 2025).
23. Joshi, G. P., & Kehlet, H. (2019). Enhanced recovery pathways: Looking into the future. *Anesthesia & Analgesia, 128*(1), 5–7. https://doi.org/10.1213/ane.0000000000003746.
24. Jung Nho, M. (2023). General anesthesia, cognition, and neurological comorbidities. *Science Insights, 43*(4), 1097–1104. https://doi.org/10.15354/si.23.re815.
25. Kholili, U., & Syalini, D. A. (2016). Surgery in liver diseases: Perioperative evaluation & management. https://core.ac.uk/download/pdf/268594952.pdf (accessed on 20 May 2025).
26. Kusak, B., Cichocka-Jarosz, E., Jedynak-Wasowicz, U., & Lis, G. (2017). Types of laryngomalacia in children: Interrelationship between clinical course and comorbid conditions. *European*

Archives of Oto-Rhino-Laryngology, 274(3), 1577–1583. https://doi.org/10.1007/s00405-016-4334-5.

27. Maund, M. L. (2003). Coronary artery disease and noncardiac surgery: Considerations in anesthesia nursing. https://core.ac.uk/download/578218495.pdf (accessed on 20 May 2025).

28. Meineke, M., Applegate, R. L., 2nd, Rasmussen, T., Anderson, D., Azer, S., Mehdizadeh, A., Kim, A., & Allard, M. (2014). Cognitive dysfunction following desflurane versus sevoflurane general anesthesia in elderly patients: A randomized controlled trial. *Medical Gas Research, 4*(1), 6. https://doi.org/10.1186/2045-9912-4-6.

29. Murray-Torres, T. M., Naguib, A. N., Tobias, J. D., Winch, et al. (2021). Anesthesia for thoracic surgery in infants and children. https://core.ac.uk/download/480389082.pdf (accessed on 20 May 2025).

30. Naidu, S., & Singaram, S. (2018). Use of the American Society of Anesthesiologists Physical Status Classification in non-trauma surgical versus trauma patients: A survey of inter-observer consistency. https://core.ac.uk/download/478367779.pdf (accessed on 20 May 2025).

31. Nelson, G., Bakkum-Gamez, J. N., Kalogera, E., Glaser, G., Altman, A. D., Meyer, L. A., Taylor, J., et al. (2019). Guidelines for perioperative care in gynecologic/oncology: Enhanced Recovery After Surgery (ERAS) Society recommendations—2019 update. *International Journal of Gynecological Cancer, 29*(4), 651–668. https://doi.org/10.1136/ijgc-2019-000356.

32. Northrup, H., Aronow, M. E., Bebin, E. M., Bissler, J. J., Darling, T. N., de Vries, P. J., Frost, M., et al. (2021). Updated international tuberous sclerosis complex diagnostic criteria and surveillance and management recommendations. *Pediatric Neurology, 123*, 50–66. https://doi.org/10.1016/j.pediatrneurol.2021.07.011.

33. Pahade, A., Ashita, M., Joshi, V., Singh, V., & Chowdhury, I. (2024). Monitored anesthesia care for percutaneous radiofrequency ablation of oncological lesions: A retrospective analysis and literature review. *Anesthesia, Pain & Intensive Care*. https://www.semanticscholar.org/paper/ba85f110748e12a58298ec23ffc12a9024e92718 (accessed on 20 May 2025).

34. Parafianowicz, A., & Surma, A. (2024). Anesthetic management in obstructive sleep apnea: A narrative review. https://core.ac.uk/download/636385963.pdf (accessed on 20 May 2025).

35. Parekh, J., Niemann, C. U., Dang, K., & Hirose, R. (2011). Intraoperative hyperglycemia augments ischemia reperfusion injury in renal transplantation: A prospective study. *Journal of Transplantation, 2011*, Article 652458. https://doi.org/10.1155/2011/652458.

36. Patorno, E., Neuman, M. D., Schneeweiss, S., Mogun, H., & Bateman, B. T. (2014). Comparative safety of anesthetic type for hip fracture surgery in adults: Retrospective cohort study. *BMJ (Clinical Research Ed.), 348*, g4022. https://doi.org/10.1136/bmj.g4022.

37. Pereira, I. V., de Lima, C. V. R., Cavalcanti-da-Silva, M., de Souza, F. M., Gonzales, D. S., Ferreira, P. F. C. L., Borges, L. G. S., et al. (2024). Anesthesia and patients with cardiovascular diseases: Challenges and approaches. *Revita de Gestão Social e Ambiental*. https://www.semanticscholar.org/paper/9a63242855747a66cdd7160c285bb074954673c5 (accessed on 20 May 2025).

38. Raghavan, S. R. (2011). *Necrotizing Soft Tissue Infections Management: A Study About the Intervention with Long Incision Fasciotomies Over Other Types of Traditional Management*. https://core.ac.uk/download/288215683.pdf (accessed on 20 May 2025).

39. Salazar, A., Arnow, B., Baca, B., Ojeda, B., Gleicher, I., Failde, I., et al. (2013). Undiagnosed mood disorders and sleep disturbances in primary care patients with chronic musculoskeletal pain. https://core.ac.uk/download/161360209.pdf (accessed on 20 May 2025.

40. Zahoor, Q. A., Taj, A., & Khan, S. (2025). Safety and efficacy of isobaric ropivacaine for spinal anesthesia in cardiac patients undergoing lower limb surgeries: A prospective study. *International Journal of Advanced Research*, (Jan), 751–757.

41. Zhao, D., & Li, Y. (2024). A case of optimizing anesthetic management for an elderly patient with severe left ventricular dysfunction through a multi-disciplinary treatment approach. *International Journal of Anesthesia and Clinical Medicine.* https://www.semanticscholar.org/paper/5f8c9c21d572fadaab08d601730a0463843f6c18 (accessed on 20 May 2025).

INTRAOPERATIVE MONITORING AND CRISIS MANAGEMENT

13

LEARNING OBJECTIVES

After studying this chapter, you will be able to:

1. Describe the types of intraoperative monitoring.
2. Describe the technologies used in intraoperative monitoring.
3. Understand the role of anesthesiologists in monitoring.
4. Discuss common intraoperative crises and crisis management protocols.

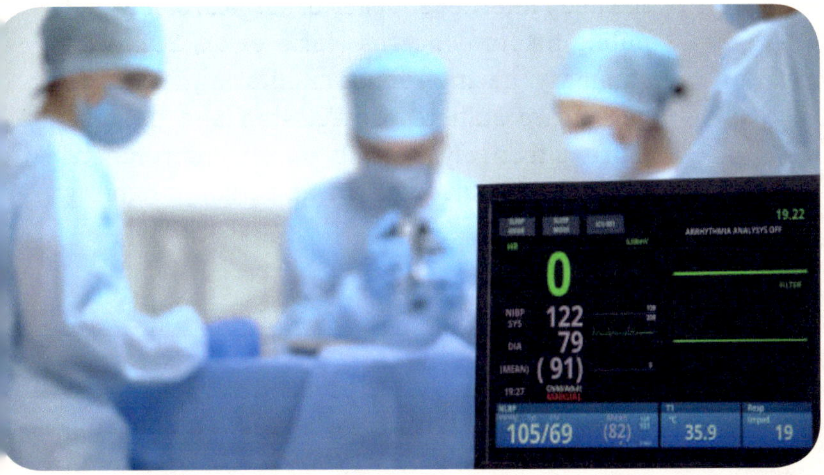

Introduction

Intraoperative monitoring and crisis management are now an absolute priority in the current healthcare environment. Fresh technology keeps redefining surgical procedures, yet there's always a genuine need to shield patients at every twist of an operation. Gathering information in real time with analysis in the fly enables groups to act quickly whenever unexpected complications emerge. This hands-on approach to surgery allows surgeons to make quicker decisions and address surprises—sometimes even before they fully emerge. With the added risks surgeries entail, particularly during global health crises, existing practices in monitoring come under scrutiny all the time to ensure that each patient receives proper treatment and that procedures go as smoothly as possible. Today's guidelines encourage taking another hard look at our reliable procedures when confronted by crises like global pandemics. In general, the idea is that a well-thought-out model for emergency management not only helps streamline an operation but also adds to better overall patient outcomes. For example, the 2023 Guideline for the Management of Patients With Aneurysmal Subarachnoid Hemorrhage emphatically puts patients first with recommendations that are in accord with current medical principles and the standards of today's tech (Hoh et al., 2023). It illustrates putting faith in actual evidence, meaning that monitoring in the operating room isn't a case of sitting back and waiting for things to happen—it's about developing a response that fits the specific circumstances of a given patient.

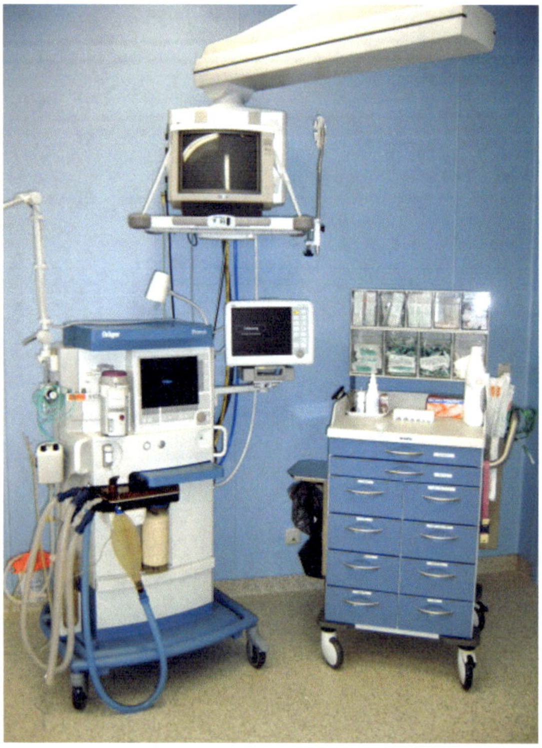

Figure 13.1. Equipment used for anaesthesia in the operating room.

Source: By No machine-readable author provided. Paunami assumed (based on copyright claims). - No machine-readable source provided. Own work assumed (based on copyright claims)., CC BY-SA 2.5, https://commons.wikimedia.org/w/index.php?curid=600832.

A good monitoring system not only protects physical health, but it also alleviates emotional and psychological weights brought about by surgery. While surprises are met by teams, there are more open lines of communications necessary. The feedback from continuous monitoring not just solves immediate problems, but it also directs the path to better plans for recovery of patients in the future. For the COVID-19 situation, for instance, heightened awareness of infection control became a core element in emergency management, highlighting the deep interdependency of surgical safety and public health concerns (Iorio et al., 2020). In summary, having robust monitoring facilitates healthcare staff to protect staff and patients more effectively, setting up an environment where good outcomes are an actual possibility (Figure 13.1).

Definition of Intraoperative Monitoring

Modern surgery is not as divergent from yesteryear's as it once was; patient monitoring now comes a long way with the advent of technology and enhanced management of safety. In most cases, intraoperative monitoring—, monitoring such parameters as heart rate, blood pressure, oxygenation, and even neuromuscular impulses—is paramount during conducting a procedure. The idea is simple: keep everything in harmony during surgery so that when something is amiss, the group can jump in at once. Of course, sudden changes can be troublesome, but watchfulness enables crises and simplifies the recovery process, ultimately creating a new path in surgical treatment. Reflect on how this monitoring increases an anesthesiologist's ability to react quickly. Monitoring vital signs in real time, healthcare workers rely on these readings to decide—often within fractions of a second—when to change anesthesia depth or adjust fluid infusion. More sophisticated machines, such as depth-of-anesthesia monitors and neuromuscular assessment equipment, give them a better understanding of the process even if the technique sometimes appears somewhat unwieldy. In general, this up-front checking reduces risks of anesthesia and surgery and is therefore an essential factor in avoiding adverse events and ensuring that patients are safe during the procedure. Standardized protocols also play a big part in keeping outcomes on track and care as effective as possible. Various guidelines suggest that reconciling monitoring rituals to the type of surgery and the patients specific needs can help teams with issues before they become uncontrollable. These setups tend to create a more relaxed, cooperative environment among surgical and anesthetic teams, which can lead to fewer infections and other delays—especially in high-risk groups. In most cases, a good and adaptive monitoring system not only ensures smoother postoperative recovery, but can also lower overall healthcare expenses. In conclusion, this dynamic system of monitoring patients illustrates how crucial it is in managing emergencies and delivering quality care in the OR (Figure 13.2).

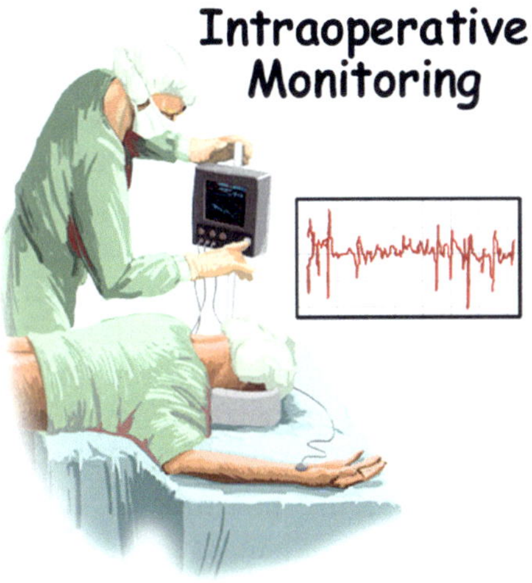

Figure 13.2. Intraoperative monitoring.

Source: https://eorthopod.com/sites/default/files/images/intraop_monitoring_intro01.jpg.

Importance of Crisis Management in Surgical Settings

Operating room crisis management is not an afterthought—it's the harsh reality when things start to go wrong. A piece of equipment breakdown, an unexpected shift in patient condition, or even a communication breakdown between team members can take things off the rails. Sometimes one simple detail can be a domino effect of issues that demand immediate, forceful intervention. Take cardiac implantable electronic devices (CIEDs), for instance: their presence can render otherwise simple surgery far more complex, especially if preoperative screening does not detect the risk of electromagnetic interference posing a threat to device function. By remaining alert to risk areas through continuous monitoring—and by encouraging less formal, ongoing communication between cardiology and surgical staff—health care organizations can deliver care that's safe as well as effective (Ariana et al., 2025). Monitoring doesn't cease once the surgery is initiated; it goes on right through pain management afterwards, particularly when opioids are employed. Surgeons, for the most part, must not only deal with the procedure but also keep their eyes on how pain is controlled post-surgery. An individualized approach—frequently one based on pharmacogenetics—is what can be applied to control pain more accurately while reducing the chance of dependence or abuse, especially in the midst of the ongoing opioid crisis. In a way, the barriers created by pain management emphasize the whole need for good, well-practiced crisis management procedures since any slip-up for a second can lead to major reversals. Hospitals that consistently employ good monitoring techniques and encourage feedback from a range of experts are likely to create a system which defends patient safety and overall surgical success (Rosendo et al., 2024). Briefly speaking, crisis management in surgery is hard to overestimate—it is closely related directly to patient safety and the procedure's success overall. The more sophisticated the surgical procedures become, the more urgently one needs to be flexible and think on their feet. Easy, clear communication with a set protocol that is well-established but sometimes adaptive guarantees that when something goes wrong, teams are able to immediately call upon the right ones. And by paying for ongoing training and real-world refresh for staff members, hospitals can create an environment that's both prepared and hardy. Implementing these ideas, as a general rule, leads to improved outcomes and helps build a patient-focused culture (Figure 13.3).

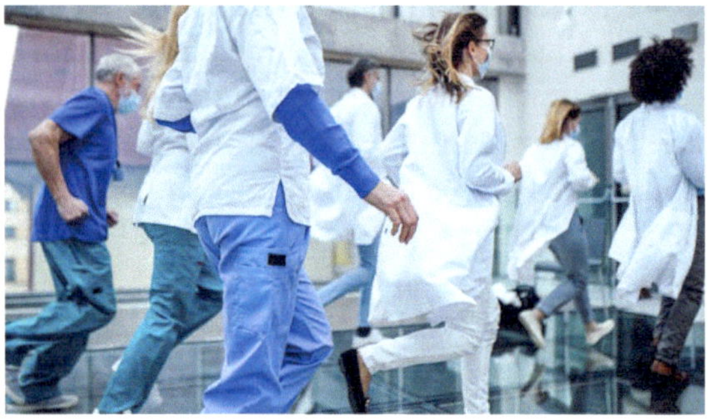

Figure 13.3. Crisis management in critical care and surgery.

Source: https://img.hpnonline.com/files/base/ebm/hpn/image/2023/04/16x9/AdobeStock_343585885.64343397abb70.png?auto=format,compress&fit=max&q=45&w=640&width=640.

13.1. Types of Intraoperative Monitoring

Learning Outcome

1. Perform physiological monitoring and neuromuscular monitoring during surgery.
2. Perform depth of anesthesia monitoring.

During surgery, keeping an eye on various factors is essential to protect the patient and steer the operation toward a good outcome. Hemodynamic monitoring, for example, offers an ongoing look at how the heart and blood vessels are holding up. You get nonstop blood pressure readings, pulse oximetry measurements, and checks on cardiac output that feedback crucial clues—clues which often help guide anesthetic choices and alert the team to issues like sudden low pressure or irregular heartbeats. Advanced tools like invasive arterial lines or central venous catheters, for instance, are used to snag real time, highly accurate data so that interventions can kick in without delay. Generally speaking, these methods also blend with newer guidelines promoting a more patient-focused approach during risky operations such as aneurysmal subarachnoid hemorrhage, which drives home the importance of comprehensive monitoring practices (Brian et al., 2023). Brain and nerve checks don't fall by the wayside either, especially when there's a potential threat to the head or spine. In these cases, methods like EEG and evoked potentials pop up to monitor neuronal function as things unfold in real time. EEG can, for example, pick up early hints of reduced blood flow or even over-sedation, providing a candid snapshot of how the brain's activity is flowing. At the same time, techniques that track somatosensory or motor signals deliver valuable bits of information about the spinal cord's integrity, enabling the surgical crew to react quickly when the numbers stray. This extra focus on neuromonitoring reinforces what many in modern anesthesiology have been saying—that keeping tabs on the brain and nerves is key to nipping potential complications in the bud (Michael Grant et al., 2021). Mixing multiple monitoring methods is shifting the way care is managed in the operating room. While traditional checks continue to have their merit, they often call for additional layers of assessment to get the full picture of a patient's state. Combining hemodynamic data with depth-of-anesthesia monitors, for instance, can offer a more rounded view; this lets the anesthesiologist tailor treatments on the fly. Such an approach is especially useful in complex surgeries where patient responses can be unpredictable. With emerging advances in fields like artificial intelligence (AI) and machine learning (MI), there's real potential for even smarter, real time analysis to assist in decision-making. In short, seamlessly integrating diverse monitoring tools ultimately hits at the core goal of surgical crisis management—cutting risks while boosting overall patient safety and operative success (Michael Grant et al., 2021).

13.1.1. Physiological Monitoring (e.g., Heart Rate, Blood Pressure)

During surgery, keeping track of a patient's body signals is a matter of urgency. Doctors need to watch heart rate and blood pressure because even small changes might hint at trouble—like low blood volume or an erratic heartbeat—that could require immediate steps. It's not just about numbers; when those figures stray from the usual, they serve as red flags that demand quick judgment. Sometimes, a sudden dip or spike is a sign that swift, informed action can make a difference to safety and outcomes. Looking at these vital signs goes beyond simply noting the numbers. In most cases, the same reading might mean something different from one patient to another. For example, a fluctuation in heart rate doesn't always trigger the same response—it could be influenced by things like previous health issues or current medications. Similarly, what counts as a "good" blood pressure can shift depending on the patient's age, overall heart health or even the type of operation underway. Generally speaking, doctors blend standard guidelines with personal insight to avoid misreading the situation, juggling both common rules and unique details that add layers of complexity. Recent technological advances have shifted the scene in monitoring during surgery. Modern devices—often boasting rapid, continuous readouts—can pick up fluctuations that older equipment might miss, making detection of adverse changes more timely. Yet, while these gadgets provide an impressive flow of data, they don't replace the seasoned judgment of a clinician; both elements need to be in play. As stated in current guidelines (Brian et al., 2023), mixing high-tech tools with real-world medical experience offers a more rounded and effective approach to patient care, ensuring that every crucial moment in the operating room is met with a balanced, informed response (Figure 13.4).

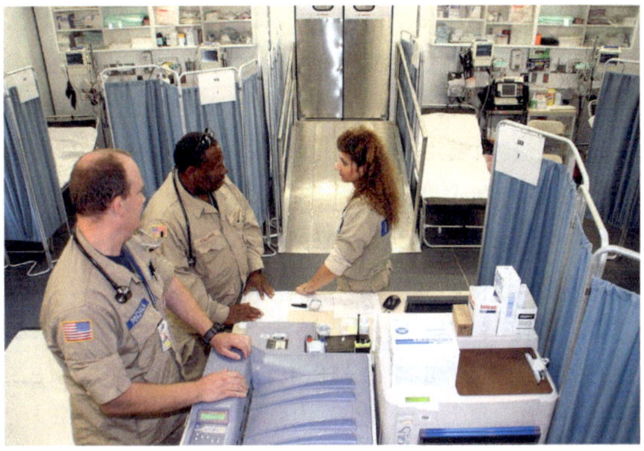

Figure 13.4. Arterial blood pressure monitoring during surgery.

Source: By Robert Kaufmann - This image is from the FEMA Photo Library (obsolete as of 2019). An archived copy may be found at the Wayback Machine (note: link may be permanently dead, as not all photos were backed up in this way).If the FEMA link is permanently dead, the photo can be found at NARA Access to Archival Databases (only works if photo was taken between 1989 and October 2004), or at City-data.com., Public Domain, https://commons.wikimedia.org/w/index.php?curid=8085463.

13.1.2. Neuromuscular Monitoring

Neuromuscular monitoring during surgery isn't just a procedural step—it keeps patients safe while fine-tuning anesthesia on the fly. By constantly checking how muscles react, clinicians can alter the dose and timing of drugs, which helps lower the chance of leftover paralysis when a patient wakes up. New research generally speaking pushes for measurable techniques over just going by what feels right; numbers often give a clearer picture than subjective impressions. Simple, effective protocols like these also seem to boost recovery after surgery and help dodge problems such as breathing difficulties, a point current guidelines often stress as central to accident prevention in the OR.

Newer monitoring gadgets are shaking up crisis management in the operating room. When devices stream continuous feedback on muscle function, anesthetists can quickly adjust treatments, reducing on risks that come when paralysis isn't fully reversed. This kind of real-time insight even makes team chats flow better—everyone gets a better read on the patient's current state. Integrating these monitors into broader decision-making systems, for instance, with tech like the Anesthesiology Control Tower (ACT), tends to elevate both surgical and anesthetic safety overall, ultimately steering care towards better patient outcomes (Gregory et al., 2018). Getting hands-on with neuromuscular monitoring and building awareness around it is just as crucial.

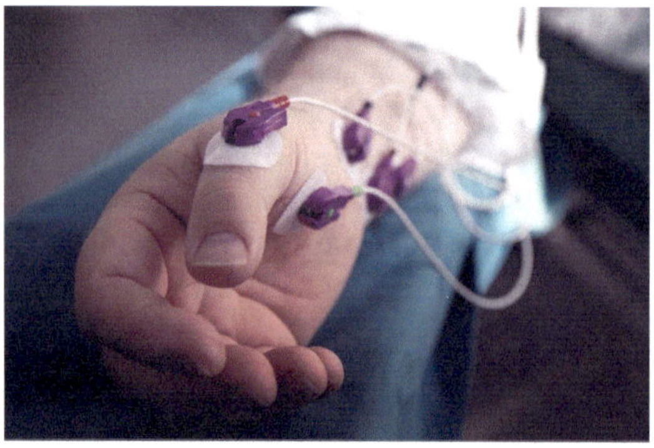

Figure 13.5. Neuromuscular monitoring.

Source: https://anaesthesianews.wordpress.com/wp-content/uploads/2022/01/41_cs_one-0533.jpg?w=1024&h=666&crop=1.

Lately, online courses and similar initiatives on perioperative pain control have popped up, reflecting a sincere push to bring fresh evidence into everyday practice. As providers get more used to these tools, they often show a boost in confidence when handling treatments—say, adjusting magnesium sulfate—possibly even shifting how postoperative pain is managed (Miller et al., 2023). In many cases, this kind of training nurtures a safety-first mindset that's essential in the high-pressure, fast-paced world of the operating room, where quick decisions and on-the-spot assessments can make a difference (Figure 13.5).

13.1.3. Depth of Anesthesia Monitoring

Surgical work isn't just about the skillful cut and stitch; it calls for keeping a close watch over anesthesia throughout the procedure. A solid monitoring routine not only helps keep patients safe but also shapes how the whole surgery turns out. One of the trickier parts is figuring out how deep the anesthetic goes—this helps reduce on the chances of the patient waking up or feeling pain. New tech keeps shaking things up with fresh insights into anesthetic depth. Take, for example, the recent push to use AI in the operating room; it can crunch live data in ways that seem to upend older methods of measuring depth and overall management (Jacob et al., 2024). All this change nudges care providers to keep learning and adjusting as methods evolve. It turns out that tracking anesthetic depth goes way beyond checking off a few basic numbers, and it often means tuning into the subtle differences that different clinical cases present. Think about obesity, which is becoming a more common challenge in the OR—when patients are heavier, it pushes for unique strategies to handle anesthesia safely. The extra risks linked with anesthetizing obese patients drive home why custom depth monitoring matters so much in these scenarios. Being thorough in checking and recording anesthetic depth can help ward off problems like airway issues or unstable blood pressure (Antonelli et al., 2016). In most cases, rolling out clear, evidence-based care pathways is key to upping the overall quality of care during surgery. When things go sideways mid-surgery, having a good read on anesthetic depth can be a lifesaver. Doctors need to be extra alert, spotting any odd changes that might hint at trouble—whether it's an upcoming crisis or just a sign the pain isn't well controlled. Quick, real-time checks become crucial here, and clever new tools like AI-driven analytics start to play a bigger role. Plus, it's generally important that anesthesia teams get enough practice both in reading these monitors and in acting when red flags appear, even if sometimes the instructions seem a bit all over the place. In the end, blending a strong monitoring setup with the know-how for rapid intervention keeps patient safety front and center; that's why pushing ahead with better anesthetic depth checks remains a cornerstone of today's anesthesiology (Jacob et al., 2024) (Figure 13.6).

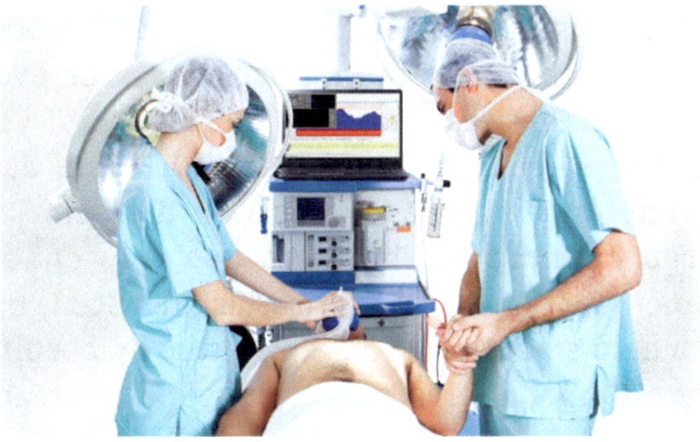

Figure 13.6. Anesthesia depth monitoring.

Source: https://neurosoft.com/files/catalog/catalog/1926/en/NINDEX_big.png.

Test Your Knowledge

1. How to do physiological monitoring of a patient during surgery?
2. How to monitor depth of anesthesia?

13.2. Technologies Used in Intraoperative Monitoring

Learning Outcome

1. Explain the electrocardiography (ECG).
2. Describe the pulse oximetry.
3. Understand the capnography.

Enhancing patient safety during surgery has meant turning to high-tech monitors that keep an eye on vital signs around the clock. Hospitals now use devices that track these signals continuously, so doctors can quickly act if something unexpected happens. Some monitors—like the Surgical Pleth Index and the Nociception Level— stand out for how they help steer pain management in the OR. They give live updates on how patients respond to pain, which in most cases allows clinicians to fine-tune opioid doses and sometimes speed up recovery. Early trials seem promising, yet researchers are still testing out newer systems like IoC2, especially among high-risk groups (Li et al., 2025). This way of adjusting pain treatment based on a person's signals shows just how tech can change how care is given. In another important area, watching over heart performance has become key during complex operations, especially for patients with significant cardiac risks. Tools like the pulmonary artery catheter—and even non-invasive bioimpedance devices—offer a real-time look at heart function and fluid balance. They churn out constant information on things like cardiac output and the resistance in blood vessels, which lets the team alter treatments almost on the fly. For example, in coronary artery bypass grafting, this kind of monitoring has been linked to fewer complications during and after the procedure. By keeping a steady watch, anesthesiologists and surgeons can better maintain the patient's balance and reduce severe problems such as arrhythmias or even shock (Coêlho de Sá et al., 2024). When you put these technologies together, it hints at a broader move toward precision medicine in surgery. Improved monitors not only enable immediate responses to crises as they occur but also help smooth out long-term care by keeping everything under steady control. The steady flow of data from these systems lets medical teams make quick, informed choices even when things get hectic. By investing in these cutting-edge tools, hospitals are boosting their crisis management skills and overall patient safety. This focus on advanced intraoperative checks—albeit with a few natural quirks here and there—reflects a solid commitment to turning operating rooms into safer and more adaptable environments, which ultimately leads to better patient outcomes in an increasingly complex medical world.

13.2.1. Electrocardiography (ECG)

Keeping an eye on the heart during surgery is critical, and one tool that makes a difference is electrocardiography—ECG, for short. This method gives live updates on the heart's electrical patterns, letting doctors spot arrhythmias, ischemia, and other irregularities pretty early on.

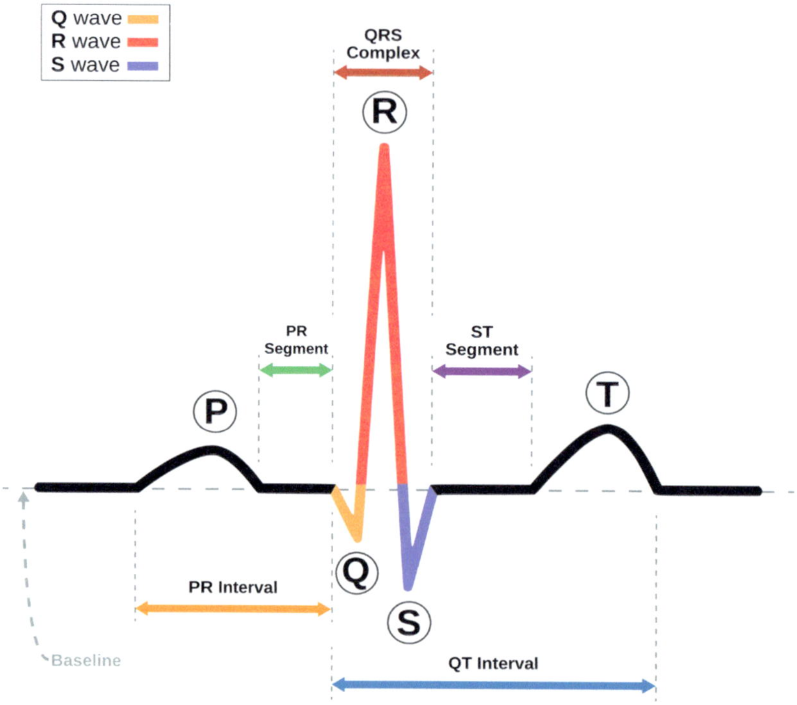

Figure 13.7. Electrocardiogram.

Source: By Created by Agateller (Anthony Atkielski), converted to svg by atom. - SinusRhythmLabels.png, Public Domain, https://commons.wikimedia.org/w/index.php?curid=1560893.

It's especially important for patients with a history of heart issues or in moments when the surgery itself becomes a stress fest—for example, when they work on a pheochromocytoma tumor, which can cause sudden shifts in blood pressure due to a burst of catecholamines (Irwanda et al., 2025). In most cases, continuous heart monitoring means the team can jump in quickly to ease any impending crisis, eventually boosting the overall outcome of the operation. ECG isn't just combined as a backup plan; it plays a key role in managing potential emergencies.

Variations in a patient's heart rate or rhythm during surgery can be dramatic, which forces the surgeons and anesthesiologists to sync up fast. By highlighting any fluctuating beats or odd signals, the ECG helps flag early signs of trouble. Take, for instance, those complicated cases or even robotic-assisted procedures where keeping a constant dialogue is crucial (Mahendran et al., 2024). With the help of these readings, healthcare pros are able to maintain situational awareness—and adjust medications or surgical techniques at a moment's notice—to steer clear of dangerous complications. There's also a big educational side to this whole ECG setup that often gets overlooked. As surgical techniques change and evolve, doctors need to be sharp not only in their hands-on skills but also in reading and making sense of what the ECG is telling them. This need gets even more pressing in robotic-assisted surgeries, where the clutter from multiple monitors and environmental distractions can throw off one's focus (Mahendran et al., 2024). Training programs that cover both the technical nitty-gritty and the softer, interpretive skills are essential for building a dependable surgical team. In most cases, well-rounded training like this ensures that when things go sideways, everyone is ready to react quickly and protect both the patient and the integrity of the procedure (Figure 13.7).

13.2.2. Pulse Oximetry

Surgical monitoring has taken a wild turn over the years. New tricks now let doctors check vital signs almost instantly, and pulse oximetry is a prime example of that change. It's a non-invasive tool that continually displays a patient's oxygen levels—a real lifesaver when catching early signs of low oxygen. The old methods can be so slow that they miss urgent moments, which is why, with its clear reliability and ease, pulse oximetry has become a staple in the operating room to flag respiratory issues as they start to develop (Shiraboina et al., 2025). When an unexpected crisis hits mid-surgery, accurate monitoring more than ever. Pulse oximetry not only provides a constant check but also steers decisions when things go off track—say, during sudden blood loss or respiratory distress. In most cases, quickly spotting a drop in oxygen saturation can be the fine line between preserving stability and hitting a critical failure. This rapid readout lets doctors adjust anesthetics or add supplemental oxygen on the fly. To summarize, mixing this modern technique with traditional practices seems like a smart, dual-approach to keeping patients safe (Alfaifi, 2024). Beyond the operating room, pulse oximetry proves its worth in other clinical spots too. For example, it's effectively used in NICUs to watch over preterm newborns, showing just how versatile it is. Some studies suggest that even though these advanced tools might not always yield dramatically better clinical outcomes than the old methods, they do round out a more complete monitoring strategy (Alfaifi, 2024). As surgical standards keep on shifting, blending in pulse oximetry within everyday protocols appears essential for truly safeguarding patient care, even if it means a little extra oversight in moments of crisis.

13.2.3. Capnography

Operating room monitoring has come a long way and, in many cases, patient safety has taken a real leap—especially when sedation and anesthesia are part of the deal. Capnography now stands out as one of those clever, ongoing checks that keeps a constant eye on exhaled CO_2 levels. It doesn't just tell doctors that ventilation is working; it also gives early hints of possible breathing issues like shallow breaths or even airway blockages. Generally speaking, when clinicians keep an eye on the capnogram waveform, they grab almost real-time insights into patient's respiratory status—letting them jump in quickly when needed. Newer guidelines have even bumped capnography up as a key monitoring method during sedation, a nod to how it boosts awareness and helps with crisis management in busy ORs (Sneyd, 2022). Its knack for visually laying out respiratory trends helps practitioners decide on patient care, particularly in high-pressure situations. Capnography's impact reaches far beyond just the routine checks. When it's woven into procedural sedation, it tends to substantially lower the number of airway mishaps. Studies, for the most part, show that using capnography keeps cases of hypoxia and airway mismanagement noticeably down. By offering a clear, almost intuitive picture of a patient's breathing patterns, it turns into an accessible, go-to tool for clinicians—improving situational awareness and helping them respond more effectively in a crisis. Plus, advances in capnographic technology, like newer sampling methods that work to reduce interference from ambient air, have overall upped the accuracy of measurements. This, in turn, often leads to better outcomes for patients—a fact that is especially important in outpatient settings where procedures demand fast and safe recoveries, further underlining how central capnography has become in modern anesthetic practice (Law et al., 2021). Of course, it's not all smooth sailing. While capnography clearly offers benefits, its rollout hasn't been uniform; different medical specialties have embraced it at their pace. Anesthetists generally champion its use, but some groups—dental professionals, for example—seem slower to make it a regular part of their routine. This difference points to a need for broader training and awareness campaigns to build a consistent standard of care across all fields using sedation. As healthcare keeps evolving, shifting more emphasis onto capnography might just lead to better safety protocols and more effective in-OR crisis management. If we can overcome the initial resistance, capnography could very well turn into the universal standard that ensures every healthcare provider is prepared to handle respiratory complications quickly and efficiently (Sneyd, 2022) (Figure 13.8).

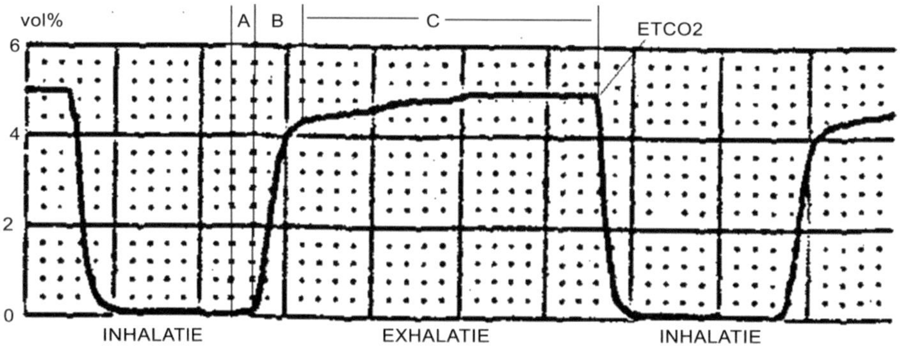

Figure 13.8. Capnography: assessing ventilation during anesthesia.

Source: By Rschiedon at Dutch Wikipedia, CC BY-SA 3.0, https://commons.wikimedia.org/w/index.php?curid=3260266.

Test Your Knowledge

1. What is called electrocardiography?
2. What is the capnography used for?

13.3. Role of Anesthesiologists in Monitoring

Learning Outcome

1. Understand the responsibilities during surgery.
2. Understand the communication with the surgical team.
3. Discuss decision-making in response to monitoring data.

Surgical operations are tricky, and keeping a close watch isn't just a nice-to-have—it's a must, especially while the surgery is happening. Anesthesiologists jump right into that mix, using modern gadgets and their judgment to keep everything steady. They check things like heart rate, blood pressure, oxygen levels—, all those vital details—and alter anesthesia on the fly when something unexpected arises. This nonstop monitoring often stops little issues before they snowball into bigger problems, helping patients do better during and after surgery. Their knack for regional anesthesia (RA), for instance, not only eases pain but also cuts down the need for opioids—which is important given the risks that come with long-term opioid use. In short, having these specialists and the surgeons working side-by-side ups the safety game in the operating room. Integrated monitoring systems have turned anesthesiology on its head, making it easier to jump into action when things look iffy. Modern tools now do more than just log vital signs—they pick up on odd little shifts before they escalate. Take blood glucose and body temperature, for example; these are kept under close watch, especially in patients burdened with other health issues. Then there's that decision support system, like the ACT, which offers real-time analytics and suggestions based on fresh patient data, allowing anesthesiologists to act fast. In most cases, this rapid-response setup helps tackle issues like postoperative breathing troubles and low blood pressure during surgery (Gregory et al., 2018). The role of an anesthesiologist goes well beyond the moment the surgery starts or ends.

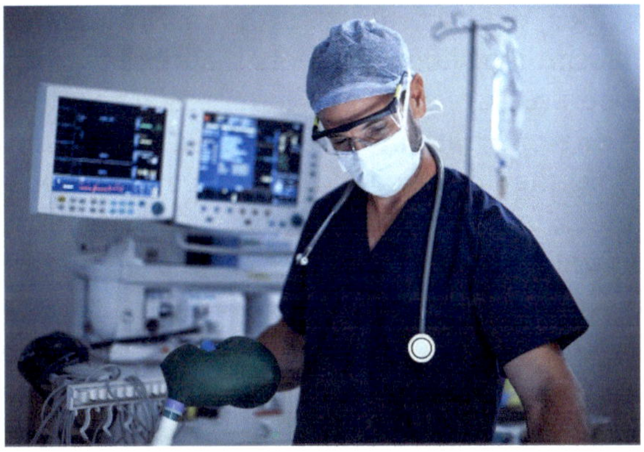

Figure 13.9. Anesthesia and the vital role of an anesthesiologist.

Source: https://www.summithealth.com/sites/default/files/2022-04/Anesthesiology_iStock-592648028.jpg.

They're involved from the get-go—handling preoperative evaluations, crafting custom anesthesia plans that consider each patient's quirks and risks, and even checking in after everything's done. With recovery paths that focus on getting patients back on track faster, these experts team up with surgeons to fine-tune care plans that reduce on extra treatments once patients leave the hospital, and they make sure pain relief is balanced enough to prevent any heavy reliance on opioids (Schwenk et al., 2018). To summarize, anesthesiologists aren't just there for the moment of crisis; their careful oversight before, during, and after the operation cements their place as a key part of modern surgical care—even if sometimes things get a bit messy (Figure 13.9).

13.3.1. Responsibilities During Surgery

In surgery, every detail matters for how well a patient does, so having a solid plan isn't just a luxury—it's essential. The team has to keep an eye on things nonstop, checking vital signs with many tech that spits out real-time info on the patient's state. Things get even trickier when dealing with conditions like pheochromocytomas, tumors that tend to throw blood pressure off balance. Generally speaking, getting the patient as optimized as possible before the operation is highly recommended—studies, for example, show that using adenosine to handle hypertensive crises during surgery can help. When every person on the team gets what their role is, it smooths out communication and helps keep any major mishaps from happening (Alonso et al., 2021). Pressure injuries and other problems also remind us that the surgical team's duties aren't simple. For those lengthy procedures—think spinal or orthopedic stuff—the need to assess and adjust on the fly becomes a constant challenge. Some interviews with the surgical staff even hint that current pressure relief systems don't always monitor enough, which sometimes ramps up the risk of pressure injuries. If the team can nail d design requirements for new tech that gives live feedback, managing patient comfort and lowering complications might just become a bit easier. This kind of proactive thinking not only helps right away but also seems to improve long-term outcomes and overall satisfaction with the surgical experience (Boszczyk et al., 2020). Sometimes, crises pop up out of nowhere in the OR, meaning that the whole crew has to be well-versed in teaming up to handle emergencies. Sudden changes in the plan are almost par for the course, and team members must identify and tackle any issues quickly so that the patient stays as stable as possible—even when complications emerge. Building an atmosphere of mutual respect and keeping communication open sets the stage for patient safety, even if things don't always go by the book. The interventions can vary a lot, depending on factors like patient comorbidities or surprises during the procedure, which stresses the need for adaptability and speedy decision-making. To summarize, this broad, flexible approach to managing responsibilities in the OR ends up boosting both safety and overall effectiveness (Alonso et al., 2021; Boszczyk et al., 2020) (Figure 13.10).

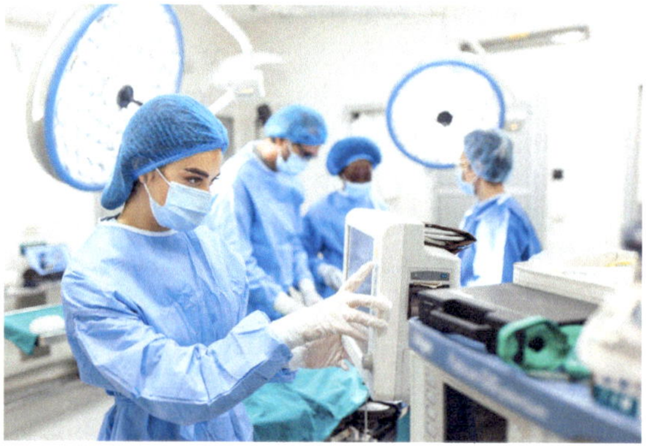

Figure 13.10. Responsibilities of anesthesiologist during surgery.

Source: https://static.joblist.com/static/job-descriptions/anesthesiologist.jpg.

13.3.2. Communication with the Surgical Team

Clear, straightforward talk among the surgical team is essential—it keeps patients safe and helps deliver better results during operations.

Sometimes, when messages aren't relayed properly or everyone isn't on the same page, mistakes happen that risk patient well-being and slow down the whole process. Simple tools like checklists or set protocols, for example, unite everyone around a common method of sharing details, dropping the chance for mix-ups. In many cases, a well-planned handoff system, as seen in some quality improvement projects, boosts the flow of key information, helping the team work together more naturally (Sosnick et al., 2024). When things go awry mid-surgery, quick and accurate communication can truly make a difference. In those hectic moments, passing on the right info at the right time might just change a patient's outcome.

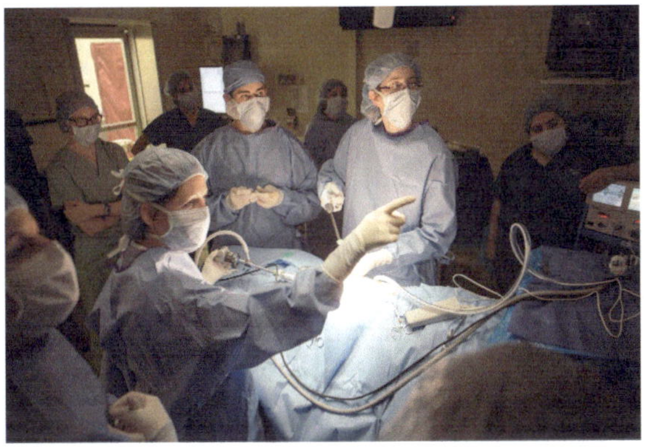

Figure 13.11. The importance of communicating in surgery.

Source: https://vetmed.tamu.edu/images/news/b17i5401[1].jpg.

Training staff members in simple, structured ways of talking not only builds a sense of accountability, but also gives them the confidence to speak up when something seems off. Regular check-ups on skills and ongoing learning sessions help each person fine-tune their dialogue, so that every single voice is heard and critical details aren't lost in the scramble (Franson et al., 2020). Good communication in the operating room also helps create a vibe of mutual trust and respect. When team members freely swap ideas, they're better ready to handle the unexpected—even under high pressure where split-second decisions matter. Some studies generally show that a strong communication base lifts morale and makes the work feel less stressful. Plus, smoother information sharing doesn't just improve patient care—it can also lower avoidable costs from errors, lending a boost to the financial health of healthcare providers (Sosnick et al., 2024) (Figure 13.11).

13.3.3. Decision-Making in Response to Monitoring Data

Rapid, in-the-moment choices drive good crisis management in healthcare. When surgery kicks off, a huge flood of data comes in at breakneck speed—vital signs, blood loss readings, neurological cues—and you suddenly need a solid, down-to-earth system to make sense of it all. Decision-makers can't simply react. They have to piece together raw numbers into something that suggests what to do next. Take interactive dashboards, for example; these tools mash up different data streams, letting doctors and nurses view the whole picture quickly—and sometimes even spot when things start to go sideways. Predictive analytics, in most cases, adds another layer by hinting at potential complications before they fully develop, which, in turn, helps in juggling resources more wisely and improving patient safety during crucial interventions (Ike et al., 2024). In essence, when crises erupt, this blend of speed and smart tech proves essential. Inside an operating room, monitoring isn't a neat, orderly checklist; it's a wild mix of metrics that demand constant scrutiny. The real challenge is turning all that complex info into clear, actionable steps. As machine learning techniques keep maturing—models like Auto Regressive Integrated Moving Average (ARIMA) come to mind—they open doors for a more forward-looking approach to what might happen next. This kind of predictive insight lets surgical teams act preemptively, tackling issues before they balloon into full-blown problems. Plus, when team members chat in plain language about these insights, everyone gets on the same page regarding the patient's current status and the next steps to take (Fatma et al., 2024). It's a reminder that even high-tech tools need to be communicated in regular, everyday terms, sometimes with a bit of repetition to drive the point home. Operating environments during surgery are messy and unpredictable, and those in charge must stay flexible and well-informed. Real-time monitoring—especially when boosted by modern analytics—can reveal small details that might just change the whole plan mid-surgery. In practice, combining straightforward dashboards with automated data alerts doesn't just crunch numbers; it reshapes how crises are managed. As surgical teams face unexpected hiccups, the pace at which they can refigure things and take action often makes the difference between a smooth fix and a major setback. In most cases, fostering an atmosphere of continuous adjustment and even a touch of trial-and-error goes a long way. Ultimately, by smartly embracing these advanced systems, healthcare workers tap into the living pulse of intraoperative data—helping them navigate tough moments in a way that keeps patient care firmly in focus (Ike et al., 2024).

Test Your Knowledge

1. Describe the responsibilities during surgery.
2. What is the decision-making process based on data?

13.4. Common Intraoperative Crises

Learning Outcome

1. Understand the anaphylactic reactions.
2. Describe the cause of cardiac arrest during surgery.
3. Understand the cause of hemorrhage during surgery.

Surgical procedures don't always stick to the plan—sometimes, unexpected crises hit, throwing everyone in the OR for a loop. Sudden drops in blood pressure, breathing struggles or major blood loss can all pop up without warning, and nothing prepares the team until it happens. In pediatric neurosurgery, for instance, kids' unique bodies tend to add extra complications to these unpredictable moments. New intraoperative neuromonitoring tools now catch things like cerebral ischemia sooner, which generally ups patient safety. These devices send out real-time signals about the patient's status, so anesthesiologists and surgeons can jump in quickly, cutting the crisis short (Domi et al., 2025). Handling these in-surgery surprises means you have to have a broad view of what might go wrong and use solid monitoring that works in real time. For example, using intraoperative parathyroid hormone (IOPTH) checks during endocrine surgeries shows the need for immediate feedback, helping guide split-second decisions. With conditions such as hyperparathyroidism on the rise, it's becoming even more critical to stick to regular IOPTH checks. Relying on these hormonal cues lets the surgical team adjust their techniques almost instantly, which, in most cases, leads to better results during parathyroidectomies. This merging of advanced monitoring with real-time decision-making underscores why regular training and flexibility are so important in today's surgical practice (Domi et al., 2025).

As surgical methods keep evolving, so too must the way teams deal with common crises in the OR. Enhanced recovery after surgery (ERAS) protocols have emerged— a way to work smart both before and during an operation with an eye on avoiding problems altogether. These methods don't just tackle issues as they arise; they form part of a broader plan aimed at smoother overall recovery. It appears that mixing cutting-edge technology with a hands-on approach to crisis management truly equips teams for the unpredictable nature of modern surgery. In the end, blending solid monitoring insights with a responsive plan is key to keeping patient care on track during even the most challenging cases (Domi et al., 2025) (Figure 13.12).

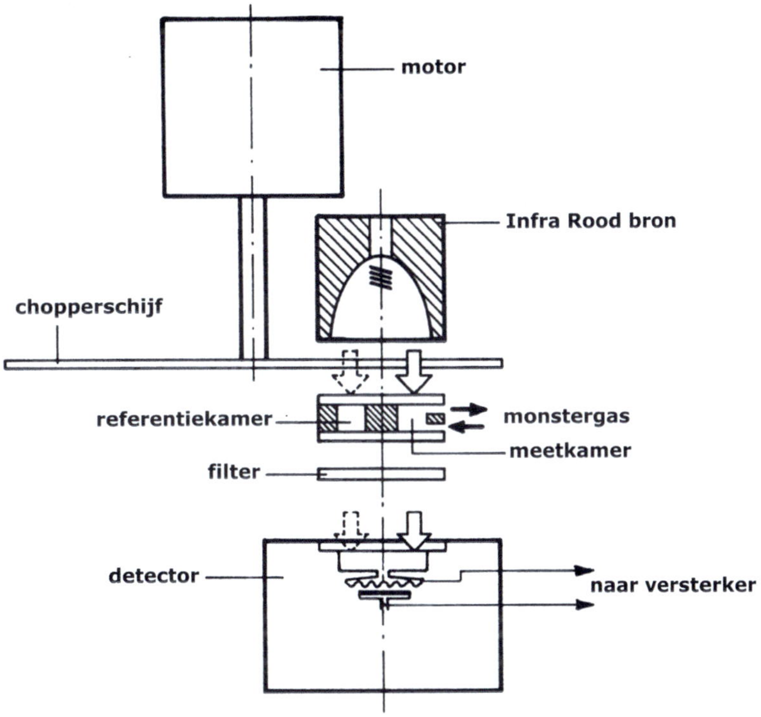

Figure 13.12. Schematic overview of a capnograph.

Source: By Rschiedon at Dutch Wikipedia, CC BY-SA 3.0, https://commons.wikimedia.org/w/index.php?curid=3260261.

13.4.1. Anaphylactic Reactions

Quick detection of severe allergic reactions during surgery is essential for patient safety. In the operating room, anaphylaxis—a sudden, serious allergic response—can occur without warning and create life-threatening challenges. One case, for example, involved a patient who suffered a grade III reaction almost immediately after receiving atracurium during a living donor nephrectomy; swift use of IV adrenaline ended up being crucial. It shows how vital it is for the anesthesia team to stay alert, as delays could affect both donor and recipient outcomes (Pal et al., 2020). The event highlights not only the importance of spotting symptoms early but also how these moments can change the course of a transplant procedure. When it comes to managing such allergic episodes, effective strategies are a must to keep surgical risks at bay. Generally speaking, proceeding with surgery after an anaphylactic incident is a tricky call—especially in living donor cases where patient safety is the top concern. After such a reaction, inflammatory mediators might stick around for up to 48 hours, which naturally raises doubts about whether to move forward immediately. In most cases, the literature advises a cautious pace, recommending that surgery only resumes if the patient shows clear hemodynamic stability and solid recovery (Pal et al., 2020). This careful balancing act forces anesthesiologists and surgical teams to navigate a very complex timeline of physiological changes. The fallout from anaphylactic reactions also stretches far beyond the immediate crisis, influencing longer-term patient care and safety protocols. In transplant scenarios, there can even be a transmission of donor allergies to the recipient—an issue that sometimes leads to dangerous intraoperative complications. Thorough preoperative evaluations and consistent monitoring become necessary, as various case reports underline the seriousness of transplant-acquired allergies (Pal et al., 2020). With new advances in anesthesia and drug alternatives, professionals are leaning on a multidisciplinary approach that emphasizes donor safety and a patient-centered care model. Continuous education, regular protocol alters, and a willingness to adapt are key, even if the conversation sometimes gets a bit uneven in its flow (Figure 13.13).

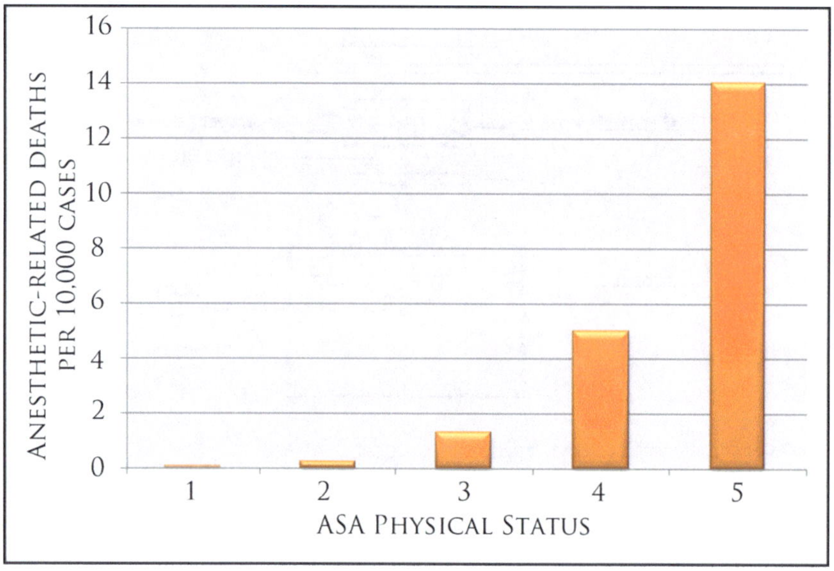

Figure 13.13. Allergic reactions: the secret danger of anesthesia.

Source: By Ian Furst - Own work based on data and graph from Anesthesiology, V 97, No 6, Dec 2002 p1615, CC BY-SA 3.0, https://commons.wikimedia.org/w/index.php?curid=31268864.

13.4.2. Cardiac Arrest

Sometimes, during surgeries there's a real risk of the heart suddenly stopping—an event that demands everyone in the OR stays on high alert. The operating room can feel like a whirlwind of shifting patient conditions and high-pressure moments where every move counts. Spotting early signs that a patient is declining is vital because a quick, clear response can make the difference. Simulation training, for example, goes a long way in building confidence and sharpening decision-making skills. This is especially helpful for Student Registered Nurse Anesthetists (SRNAs), who don't always get enough exposure to real-time crisis events (Lee et al., 2024). Interestingly, the causes behind a cardiac arrest during surgery aren't quite the same as those seen outside the hospital. Generally speaking, factors like gas embolism, an overdose of local anesthetic, or even spinal bradycardia can be the culprits. Because these events are rare and show up in different ways, standard protocols have to change on the fly to address them properly. In most cases, the medical team already knowing a patient's full history gives them a leg up in quickly pinpointing what went wrong, which in turn speeds up remedial action. Relying on solid physiological insights combined with expert opinions—not just sticking to old guidelines—can improve care when it matters most (Moitra et al., 2012). When it comes to handling crises in surgical settings, understanding how unpredictable cardiac arrests can be is key. Often, these incidents are seen coming and leave a very short window for effective intervention. Training that focuses on team dynamics and encourages open, cross-disciplinary communication turns out to be crucial since every second counts when a cardiac arrest occurs. In a setting where decisions need to be made lightning fast, nurturing a teamwork-focused atmosphere pays off. Evidence-based crisis management education, especially when built around simulation, not only boosts readiness but also helps medical teams feel more confident when emergencies hit, ultimately leading to better patient outcomes during an intraoperative crisis (Lee et al., 2024) (Figure 13.14).

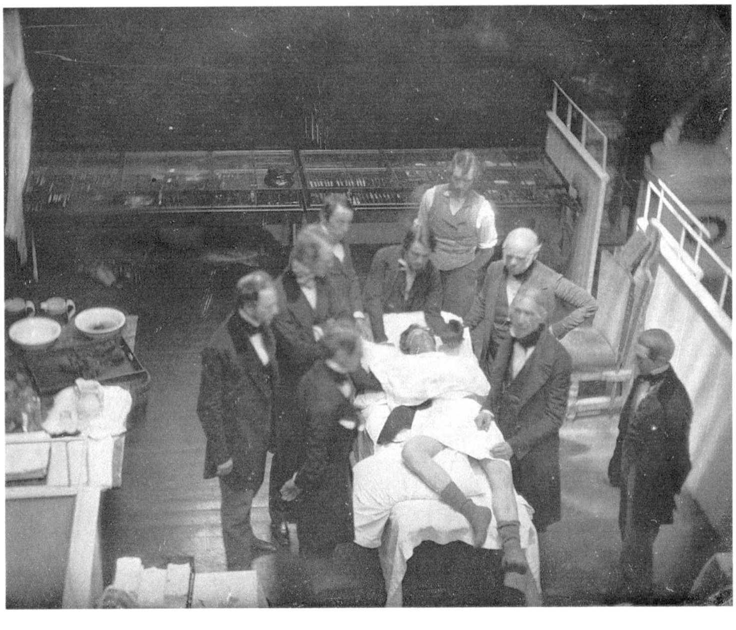

Figure 13.14. Cardiac arrest.

Source: By Southworth & Hawes - https://www.loc.gov/pictures/item/2004667744/Library of Congress Prints and Photographs Division Washington, D.C. 20540 USA.DIGITAL ID: (b&w film copy neg.) cph 3b15373 http://hdl.loc.gov/loc.pnp/cph.3b15373REPRODUCTION NUMBER: LC-USZ62-67905 (b&w film copy neg.)CALL NUMBER: LOT 11662 [item] [P&P], Public Domain, https://commons.wikimedia.org/w/index.php?curid=2220536.

13.4.3. Hemorrhage

Unexpected bleeding during surgery is a serious risk that can quickly lead to major complications and higher rates of morbidity. Controlling blood loss is key to keeping a patient's circulation steady—especially when large vessels are involved or when the dissection extends over wide tissue areas. In the past, checking how much blood was circulating mostly depended on standard formulas and intrusive, fixed methods; while these techniques did provide some info, their accuracy and reliability were often less than ideal. Our growing understanding of bleeding now suggests we need methods that offer real-time updates on how much blood is in play. Generally speaking, this shift nudges both anesthesiologists and surgeons to start using modern monitors that help adjust fluid therapy to match each patient's needs exactly as bleeding happens, thereby reducing the immediate dangers (Gutierrez et al., 2013). When a crisis strikes in the OR, it becomes clear that a broad view of the patient's functions is essential. Both overall and brain-specific blood flow have to be watched closely—particularly in folks who are already at risk for neurological issues. A mix of monitoring techniques can give a more personal glimpse into what each patient is going through, rather than relying on one single strategy, which might miss some signals of trouble. In many cases, using systems that check brain oxygenation together with other bodily variables offers a stronger, more practical support for making decisions in tough moments. In this way, these advanced tools allow surgical teams to better handle the bleeding and its fallout, paving the way for faster, more informed interventions (Kirkman et al., 2016). To summarize, managing bleeding during surgery is one of the trickier parts of handling a crisis—it demands both sharp vigilance and a flexible approach. Combining live monitoring with broad checks of a patient's physical state forms the core of effective care during such critical times. Not only does this approach help clinicians spot and react to problems more quickly, but it also works to keep the body's equilibrium intact when it matters most. As surgical techniques keep evolving and patient safety stays front and center, next-generation monitoring technology is set to play a key role in lowering both how often and how hard bleeding incidents hit. This evolving trend clearly underscores the need for continuous learning and adapting in the surgical field, reflecting the ever-changing connection between monitoring practices and patient care strategies in modern medicine (Gutierrez et al., 2013; Kirkman et al., 2016) (Figure 13.15).

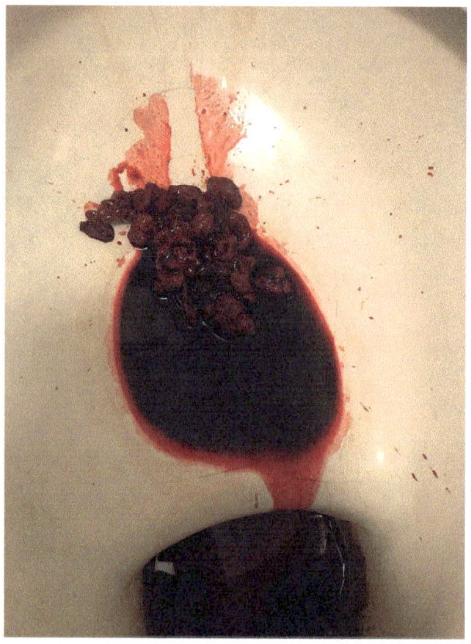

Figure 13.15. Hemorrhage.

Source: By LennBr - Own work, CC BY-SA 4.0, https://commons.wikimedia.org/w/index.php?curid=113338594.

Test Your Knowledge

1. What are the causes of anaphylactic reactions?
2. What can cause cardiac arrest during surgery?

13.5. Crisis Management Protocols

Learning Outcome

1. Understand the immediate response strategies.
2. Learn about the use of emergency medications.
3. Describe the team coordination during crises.

During surgery, situations can shift suddenly into full-bl crises, so having a ready plan is just plain necessary. Medical teams rely on these plans to figure out unexpected events, keeping patient safety at the forefront. Take standard monitoring, for instance—by keeping a close eye during procedures, issues can pop up early enough to stop them from escalating. Tools like continuous intraoperative electroencephalography (EEG) and real-time blood gas checks are crucial for keeping everyone on the same page. Using these approaches means healthcare providers can jump into action when a patient's condition changes, lessening the chance of bad outcomes. Clear communication within the team, too, plays an essential role; when everyone's talking openly and quickly, the overall response is much more effective, as noted in recent literature. Adopting crisis management methods into anesthesia routines isn't optional, especially when the stakes are high. A study out of Bangladesh generally showed that sticking to solid monitoring protocols lowers complications during surgery. By regularly logging vital signs—heart rate, blood pressure, and oxygen saturation—teams manage to keep patients stable. In most cases where protocols were followed closely, the research found complications in only about 10% of patients, which drives home the importance of these strategies. Creating an atmosphere where anesthesia providers routinely follow their checklists not only boosts patient care but also gears them up for sudden emergencies in the OR, aligning with effective crisis management goals. Training and being ready are key parts of any crisis management plan, especially for intraoperative monitoring. Regular simulation exercises and drills can, quite frankly, sharpen a team's response when things go off script. Running through realistic scenarios not only hones clinical skills but also naturally builds better communication and coordination among team members. Studies hint that close collaboration between neurology and neurosurgery groups often leads to even better patient results. Overall, prioritizing ongoing training and proactive measures cultivates a spirit of readiness, equipping healthcare teams with the know-how to tackle emergencies effectively, and ultimately boosting the overall standard of care during operations (Alhayen et al., 2025; Rahman et al., 2024).

13.5.1. Immediate Response Strategies

Modern surgery is tough – sometimes you have to act fast when complications come out of nowhere. In the middle of an operation, unexpected crises can hit without warning, and just a tiny delay might mean the difference between keeping a patient safe or ending up in serious trouble. Teams keep a close eye on vital signs; if things start to fluctuate unpredictably, it could be a sign of a sudden hormone surge or abrupt bleeding, which calls for quick changes in anesthesia and the way the procedure is done. Having a set routine means everyone knows their role, so they can jump in swiftly when things get dicey. Clear, straightforward communication and a spirit of teamwork are key in those split-second moments. Every crew member should feel free to say something if they spot something odd – even if it's just a small observation – because those little things can count when timing is critical. Real-time data from monitors mixed with direct, sometimes a bit uneven, conversation helps clinicians act on the fly. Many teams also run simulation drills to handle high-pressure scenarios safely, allowing them to practice without any risk to patients. Usually, this hands-on approach not only sharpens their crisis response but also builds trust and camaraderie among the group, which, in turn, makes outcomes better for patients. Relying on solid, evidence-informed guidelines is another crucial part of handling surprises during surgery. For instance, updates like the 2023 Guideline for the Management of Patients With Aneurysmal Subarachnoid Hemorrhage underline the need for flexible, adaptive practices in crises (Hoh et al., 2023). Such guidelines serve as a kind of roadmap that helps practitioners quickly spot problems and adjust their plans to fit what each patient uniquely needs. It's important to tell when to stick to a standard routine and when to mix in a more personal touch – after all, patients rarely react exactly the same way. Generally, blending tried-and-true protocols with the unique demands of the moment enables teams to act fast and safely, ultimately boosting patient safety during critical moments (Hoh et al., 2023) (Figure 13.16).

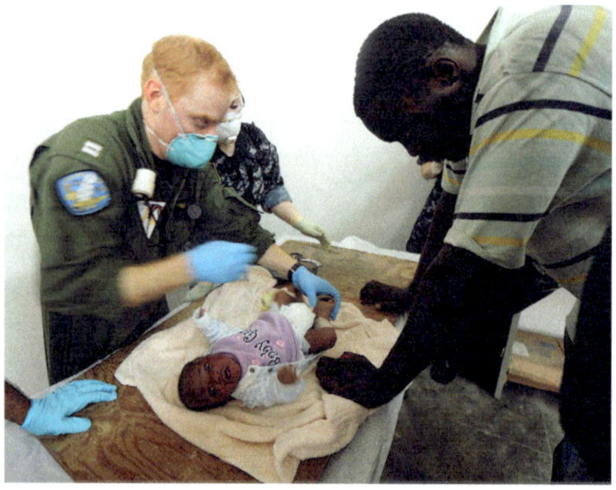

Figure 13.16. U.S. Navy sailors assigned to the aircraft carrier USS Carl Vinson treat a baby injured by 2010 Haiti earthquake.

Source: By Petty Officer 2nd Class Adrian White, U.S. Navy - This image was released by the United States Navy with the ID 100117-N-2953W-832 (next).This tag does not indicate the copyright status of the attached work. A normal copyright tag is still required. See Commons:Licensing. العربية · বাংলা ·Bahaso Jambi ·Deutsch · Deutsch (Sie-Form) · English · español · euskara · فارسی · français · italiano · 日本語 · 한국어 · македонски · മലയാളം · Plattdüütsch · Nederlands · polski · پښتو · português · русский · slovenščina · svenska · Türkçe · українська · 简体中文 · 繁體中文 · +/−, Public Domain, https://commons.wikimedia.org/w/index.php?curid=20714102.

13.5.2. Use of Emergency Medications

When a surgery is underway, acting fast with emergency medications can literally make the difference between recovery and a critical setback. Unexpected issues like unstable heart rhythms or sudden allergic reactions can arise at any moment, so the surgical team must be ready to intervene immediately. It's not uncommon for life-saving drugs—think epinephrine for anaphylaxis or atropine when the heart slows d—to be administered in a flash, often turning a looming crisis into a manageable hiccup. Many current guidelines generally speak to adopting a step-by-step protocol that helps clinicians spot these dangers early and treat them with the right meds (Hoh et al., 2023). Team readiness plays a huge role here too. In the operating room, rehearsed simulations and practical communication tools can bolster the team's ability to respond well under pressure. Training programs like Crew Resource Management (CRM) and TeamStepps, for instance, have been drawing attention because they not only sharpen individual skills but also foster a shared grasp of emergency procedures. When everyone on the team understands their role—even if it means repeating key concepts during drills—the overall response to emergencies becomes more fluid and effective (Samardžić et al., 2020). Overall, the success of emergency medications is tightly linked to continuous monitoring and robust crisis protocols. Keeping a constant check on patients allows any complications to be caught early enough for immediate action. Advanced methods, such as capnography and pulse oximetry, offer real-time insights into a patient's condition, ensuring that medications reach them quickly when needed. This close tie between vigilant monitoring and prompt drug administration underscores why ongoing, hands-on training in the OR is so essential. Aligning everyday clinical practices with established guidelines, while also nurturing natural team dynamics, can significantly boost patient safety and reduce the chance of adverse events during surgery (Hoh et al., 2023) (Figure 13.17).

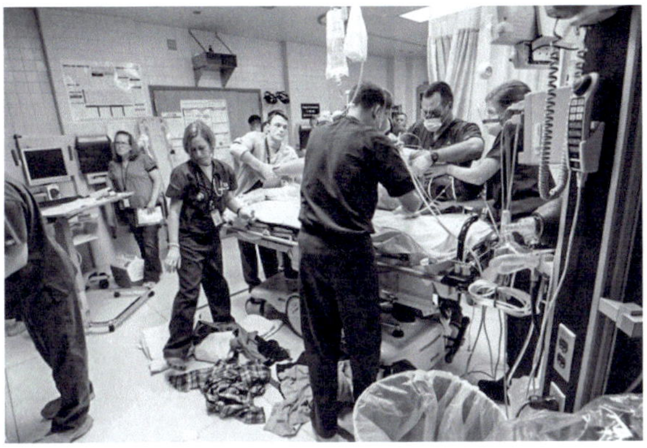

Figure 13.17. Emergency medicine.

Source: https://en.wikipedia.org/wiki/File:10530-banner-Lives625-6-14.jpg.

13.5.3. Team Coordination During Crises

Operating rooms are intense spaces where effective teamwork isn't just a bonus—it's a must, especially when things go sideways unexpectedly. Surgical crews face so many challenges that they can't rely on technical know-how alone; being on the same wavelength is key. When surprises hit and complications arise, roles can be reshuffled in an instant, making quick decisions all the more critical. Sometimes, a bit of cross-professional chatter goes a long way. Trust and spontaneous, open communication let everyone share the vital details quickly, which bumps up patient outcomes and helps reduce crisis risks. Training drills that mimic real emergencies are also crucial—they get teams ready for those split-second moments where coordination truly makes the difference between a win and a loss. The ongoing pandemic made it clear that solid team coordination in surgeries is more important than ever. When elective surgeries were put on hold and everyday routines were thrown out the window, surgical teams suddenly had to deal with challenges they'd never seen before, testing their adaptability and grit. Social distancing and resource shortages forced a reevaluation of old workflows, which in many cases highlighted just how handy robotics and AI could be in handling both pre-op and post-op assessments—and even in surgical training. In that kind of environment, everyone had to quickly get comfortable with new technologies and keep communication channels open to reduce on infection risks, all while still providing top-notch care.

Generally speaking, the pandemic's impact drove home the point that managing crises in surgery means blending technological upgrades with robust teamwork (Feizi et al., 2021). Mixing in recommendations for pain management and more careful opioid use only deepens the picture of why coordinated efforts are key during a crisis in the middle of surgery. Several professional organizations have come out with guidelines designed to improve care after surgery and also scale back opioid use. Still, putting these protocols into everyday practice can stumble because different providers often do their thing in isolation. A more unified, team-based approach usually cuts through that problem. By creating a culture loaded with shared responsibility and a dash of accountability, surgical teams can smooth out pain management processes and truly support patients from surgery right through recovery. Besides keeping everyone more or less on track with the rules, this kind of interprofessional teamwork also boosts the overall resilience of the team during tough times—making it a cornerstone of effective intraoperative monitoring and crisis management (Hyland et al., 2021) (Figure 13.18).

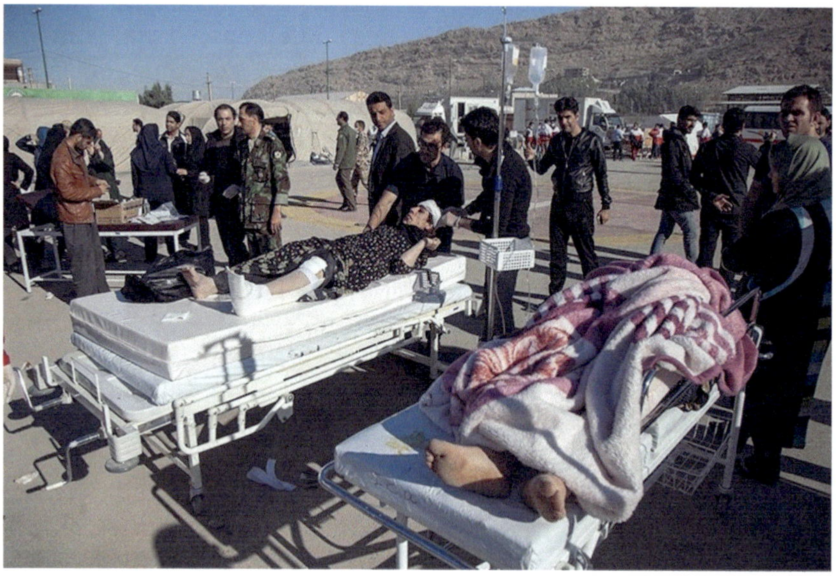

Figure 13.18. Team coordination during crises.

Source: By Tasnim News Agency, CC BY 4.0, https://commons.wikimedia.org/w/index.php?curid=64040671.

Test Your Knowledge

1. What is the immediate response strategy?
2. What is the use of emergency medications?

SUMMARY

Intraoperative monitoring, which is sophisticated, ensures patient safety. Quantitative Train-of-Four (TOF) monitoring, for instance, has emerged as an important piece in the practice of anesthesia—it's being highly effective in the optimization of the reversal of neuromuscular blockade. The move towards evidence-based practice evens out results and lessens the risks of residual paralysis. Evidence seems to illustrate that the application of quantitative TOF leads to more stable control of the blockade, showing its growing applicability in operating rooms nowadays. In short, testing new monitoring techniques can make procedures safer and more effective, since even a momentary lapse can have disastrous consequences. Crisis management, along the same lines, relies heavily on the speed and accuracy with which medical staff handle unexpected challenges. Earlier public health crises, in the majority of cases, have taught us that an active approach—highlighted by current data and robust information systems—is essential for making wise choices. Regularly reviewing earlier data seems to engender a culture of preparedness and resilience among teams. Apparently, the synthesis of robust monitoring habits and data-driven methods sparks the development of more practical crisis management programs. Creating mechanisms for data integration and real-time communication not only improves intraoperative monitoring but also improves responses to adverse events taking place during surgery. Finally, the ongoing development of monitoring technologies and crisis management techniques offers a chance to transform the practice of anesthesia and surgery. Health organizations with a culture of interdisciplinary teamwork appear better able to respond to the challenges of modern surgical practice. Prioritizing standardized data protocols and adequate training for clinicians can help the community utilize resources more effectively during times of need. Current research, for example, supports that adopting quantitative TOF monitoring is an important move towards updating anesthetic safety—reducing on adverse effects during surgical emergencies. Cumulatively, these observations portend a future where technology and intelligent methods inexorably converge to drive patient care and operational excellence in the surgical arena (Adekugbe et al., 2024; Yadav, 2025).

Real-time monitoring during surgery is a crucial part of keeping procedures safe and effective. Gone are the days when doctors relied solely on those old invasive methods—instead, we're now seeing a shift toward simpler, minimally invasive techniques that give updates as things happen. In high-risk cases, for example, these dynamic methods often guide fluid therapy in a way that beats the old static approach. It just so happens that even such dependable volume indicators are no longer as dependable (Gutierrez et al., 2013). With the inclusion of these high-tech tools in their process, surgical teams can make instantaneous decisions in the moment and minimize surprise setbacks. This type of point-by-point surveillance not only helps patients to recover sooner but also enhances the overall quality of the operation. Another very important piece of the puzzle is pain management. The traditional methods have issues—some get too little or too much opioid, and that interrupts recovery and satisfaction. Not long ago, some mention has been made of AI stepping onto the stage to transform the way we treat pain. By analyzing data in real time, AI applications, on the whole, can tailor pain management to each patient's individual needs (Jacob et al., 2024). This trend is pushing us toward more data-centered, patient-focused care, and as the medical field leans more into new tech, AI's role in refining pain protocols becomes all the more important. Bringing together these smarter monitoring techniques and AI-powered pain management reflects a larger push to upgrade intraoperative care overall. Both approaches remind anesthesiology and surgery personnel that it is significant to stay updated with new technology—a point oft reiterated during continuing education courses. When these new technologies are understood and utilized, they plug the gaps left by earlier techniques and even eliminate some of the associated old woes. Continuing education in this manner encourages practitioners to adopt these procedures, which further ensures better teamwork among staff. The latest studies, for example (Jacob et al., 2024), illustrate that an educated, sometimes even improvisational approach can optimize clinical performance. All this contributes to the improvement of care standards and, ultimately, making operating rooms safer for everyone.

KEY TERMS FROM THIS CHAPTER

- Anesthesiology control tower
- Artificial intelligence
- Blood pressure
- Blood volume
- Capnography
- Cardiology
- Communication
- Crisis management
- Electromagnetic interference
- Erratic heartbeat
- Heart rate
- Machine learning
- Modern surgery
- Neuromuscular monitoring

CRITICAL THINKING QUESTIONS

1. **Which of the following is a mandatory monitor according to the American Society of Anesthesiologists (ASA) standards?**
   a. Bispectral index (BIS)
   b. End-tidal CO_2 ($ETCO_2$)
   c. Electroencephalography (EEG)
   d. Pulse oximetry
2. **Intraoperative bradycardia is most effectively treated with:**
   a. Epinephrine
   b. Atropine
   c. Phenylephrine
   d. Lidocaine
3. **The primary purpose of capnography during general anesthesia is to:**
   a. Monitor oxygen saturation
   b. Measure tidal volume
   c. Assess ventilation and detect apnea
   d. Measure arterial blood gases
4. **The first step in managing intraoperative hypotension is:**
   a. Administering vasopressors
   b. Assessing the cause of hypotension
   c. Increasing anesthetic depth
   d. Administering fluids
5. **During an airway crisis involving laryngospasm, the first-line treatment is:**
   a. Administration of a muscle relaxant
   b. Increasing the depth of anesthesia
   c. Positive pressure ventilation with 100% oxygen
   d. Emergency tracheostomy

Short Answer Questions

1. What is intraoperative monitoring?
2. Why is crisis management important in surgical settings?
3. List the types of intraoperative monitoring.
4. What are the techniques used in intraoperative monitoring?
5. What are the roles of anesthesiologist?

Answers to Critical Thinking Questions

1. (d); 2. (b); 3. (c); 4. (b); 5. (c)

REFERENCES

1. Adekugbe, A. P., & Ibeh, C. V. (2024). Harnessing data insights for crisis management in U.S. public health: Lessons learned and future directions. *International Medical Science Research Journal, 4*(4). https://doi.org/10.51594/imsrj.v4i4.998.
2. Alfaifi, J. (2024). The impact of using next-generation pulse oximetry on the outcomes of preterm babies admitted to the NICU: A randomized controlled trial. *Signa Vitae*. https://www.semanticscholar.org/paper/0c9542b6ea1989438d9d90a9390d93b7dccf1308 (accessed on 20 May 2025).
3. Alhayen, B. I., Abdel-Bari, S. H. H., Mohammad, M. E., Ayoub, B. M., & Ali, R. A. K. (2025). Indications and surgical management for movement disorders. *South Eastern European Journal of Public Health*. https://www.semanticscholar.org/paper/267a56b39be1210da284a41c57e711dcb2f6f06a (accessed on 20 May 2025).
4. Alonso Alonso, M., Casteras Román, A., De Miguel Negro, M., Loaiza Aldean, et al. (2021). Intraoperative adenosine for pheochromocytoma with myocardial infarction and SARS-CoV-2: Case report. https://core.ac.uk/download/548544507.pdf (accessed on 20 May 2025).
5. Antonelli, M., Aurilio, C., Baroncini, S., Carron, M., Cataldo, R., Chiumiento, F., Cinnella, G., et al. (2016). Perioperative and periprocedural airway management and respiratory safety for the obese patient: 2016 SIAARTI Consensus. https://core.ac.uk/download/621419161.pdf (accessed on 20 May 2025).
6. Borges, E. S., & Ferreira, S. C. M. (2016). Validation of instrument for control and prevention and infection of surgical site in neurosurgery. *Journal of Nursing UFPE Online, 10*, 4778–4787. https://www.semanticscholar.org/paper/75c215663211a97ae01aea0fdca389971e4c6165 (accessed on 20 May 2025).
7. Boszczyk, B., Breedon, P., Siena, F. L., Sizer, et al. (2020). Monitoring and alleviating the effects of pressure related injuries for spinal surgery–A need for improvement? https://core.ac.uk/download/328708929.pdf (accessed on 20 May 2025).
8. Buljac-Samardžić, M., Doekhie, K. D., & van Wijngaarden, J. D. H. (2020). Interventions to improve team effectiveness within health care: A systematic review of the past decade. *Human Resources for Health, 18*, Article 13. https://doi.org/10.1186/s12960-019-0411-3.
9. Coêlho de Sá, H. D., Farah, V. C. M., Alevato, L. F., Pinheiro, T. Z., Sobrinho, P. V. E., Neto, J. S. M., Lima, P. A. R. R., et al. (2024). Impact of advanced hemodynamic monitoring on myocardial revascularization surgery in high-risk patients. *Health and Society*. https://www.semanticscholar.org/paper/7cae28e03e4cb4e71fc7c350da7f8c84e3245e2c (accessed on 20 May 2025).
10. Domi, R., Coniglione, F., Abdyli, A., Huti, G., Lilaj, K., & Bilotta, F. (2025). Anesthesia considerations on pediatric neurosurgery. *Turkish Journal of Anesthesiology and Reanimation, 53*, 34–41. https://www.semanticscholar.org/paper/8a1e56ce88f4f73fb04e1445455dd55b78e85824 (accessed on 20 May 2025).
11. Douma, A. (2019). ESRA19-0605 Opioid free anesthesia with RA techniques: What is the concept? *Regional Anesthesia & Pain Medicine, 44*, A41–A43. https://www.semanticscholar.org/paper/dff89d7ba9680421686024c0765fd2a363f09737 (accessed on 20 May 2025).

12. Faisal Irwanda, & Anggraeni, N. (2025). Successful anesthetic management of pheochromocytoma in a patient with preoperative hypertension: A case report. *Bio Scientia Medicina: Journal of Biomedicine and Translational Research, 9*(3), 6681–6695. https://doi.org/10.37275/bsm.v9i3.1222.

13. Feizi, N., Tavakoli, M., Patel, R. V., & Atashzar, S. F. (2021). Robotics and AI for teleoperation, tele-assessment, and tele-training for surgery in the era of COVID-19: Existing challenges and future vision. *Frontiers in Robotics and AI, 8*, Article 610677. https://doi.org/10.3389/frobt.2021.610677.

14. Franson, H. (2020). *A Pain Control Optimization Pathway to Reduce Acute Postoperative Pain and Opioid Consumption Postoperatively: An Approach to Battling the Opioid Epidemic.* https://core.ac.uk/download/389488233.pdf (accessed on 20 May 2025).

15. Grant, M. C., Suffredini, G., & Cho, B. C. (2021). Is it time to eliminate the use of opioids in cardiac surgery? *JTCVS Open, 7*, 247–252. https://doi.org/10.1016/j.xjon.2021.03.022.

16. Gregory, S., Murray-Torres, T. M., Fritz, B. A., et al. (2018). Study protocol for the Anesthesiology Control Tower—Feedback Alerts to Supplement Treatments (ACTFAST-3) trial: A pilot randomized controlled trial in intraoperative telemedicine [version 2; peer review: 2 approved]. *F1000Research, 7*, 623. https://doi.org/10.12688/f1000research.14897.2.

17. Gutierrez, M. C., Liu, H., & Moore, P. G. (2013). *Goal-Directed Therapy in Intraoperative Fluid and Hemodynamic Management.* https://core.ac.uk/download/323069925.pdf.

18. Hoh, B. L., Ko, N., Amin-Hanjani, S., Chou, S., Cruz-Flores, S., Dangayach, N., Derdeyn, C. P., et al. (2023). 2023 Guideline for the management of patients with aneurysmal subarachnoid hemorrhage: A guideline from the American Heart Association/American Stroke Association. *Stroke, 54*. https://doi.org/10.1161/str.0000000000000436.

19. Hyland, S. J., Brockhaus, K. K., Vincent, W. R., Spence, N. Z., Lucki, M. M., Howkins, M. J., & Cleary, R. K. (2021). Perioperative pain management and opioid stewardship: A practical guide. *Healthcare, 9*(3), 333. https://doi.org/10.3390/healthcare9030333.

20. Ike, C. C., Ige, A. B., Oladosu, S. A., Adepoju, P. A., & Afolabi, A. I. (2024). Advancing real-time decision-making frameworks using interactive dashboards for crisis and emergency management. *International Journal of Management & Entrepreneurship Research, 6*(2). https://doi.org/10.51594/ijmer.v6i12.1762.

21. Iorio-Morin, C., Hodaie, M., Sarica, C., Dea, N., Westwick, H. J., Christie, S., McDonald, P. J., et al. (2020). Letter: The risk of COVID-19 infection during neurosurgical procedures: A review of SARS-CoV-2 modes of transmission and proposed neurosurgery-specific mitigation measures. *Neurosurgery, 87*, E178–E185. https://doi.org/10.1093/neuros/nyaa157.

22. Izakovicova, P., Borens, O., & Trampuž, A. (2019). Periprosthetic joint infection: Current concepts and outlook. *EFORT Open Reviews, 4*(9), 482–494. https://doi.org/10.1302/2058-5241.4.180092.

23. Jacob, C. B., & Diaz, V. J. (2024). Utilization of artificial intelligence algorithms in the perioperative management and reduction of pain: An evidence-based educational module. *Nicole Wertheim College of Nursing Student Projects, 199*. https://digitalcommons.fiu.edu/cnhs-studentprojects/199 (accessed on 20 May 2025).

24. Kirkman, M. A., & Smith, M. (2016). Multimodality neuromonitoring. *Anesthesiology Clinics, 34*(3), 511–523. https://doi.org/10.1016/j.anclin.2016.04.005.

25. Law, J. A., Duggan, L. V., Asselin, M., Baker, P., Crosby, E. T., Downey, A., Hung, O., et al. (2021). Canadian Airway Focus Group updated consensus-based recommendations for management of the difficult airway: Part 1. Difficult airway management encountered in an unconscious patient. *Canadian Journal of Anesthesia / Journal Canadien D'Anesthésie, 68*, 1373–1404. https://doi.org/10.1007/s12630-021-02007-0.

26. Lee, M. (2024). *Enhancing SRNA Confidence: Integrating Simulation-Based CRM Training with Didactic Education to Improve Intraoperative Recognition, Communication, and Management of Intraoperative Cardiac Arrest.* https://core.ac.uk/download/616421823.pdf (accessed on 20 May 2025).

27. Li, Z., Cai, H., Yan, Y., Liu, X., & Zhao, J. (2025). IoC2 monitoring versus standard practice in reducing opioid consumption in elderly patients undergoing laparoscopic colorectal surgery: A study protocol for a randomized controlled trial. *BMJ Open, 15*(1), e093322. https://doi.org/10.1136/bmjopen-2024-093322.

28. Madian, F. A., Ebrahim, G., Salah, M. M., & Abdelaal, M. A. (2024). An intelligent data analytics approach for crisis management in healthcare systems. *2024 International Conference on Computer and Applications (ICCA)*. https://www.semanticscholar.org/paper/c94a56f5acadbcb6f3bbd459de495690e85b81c7 (accessed on 20 May 2025).

29. Mahendran, V., Turpin, L. E., Boal, M., & Francis, N. (2024). Assessment and application of non-technical skills in robotic-assisted surgery: A systematic review. *Surgical Endoscopy, 38*, 1758–1774. https://doi.org/10.1007/s00464-024-10713-1.

30. Moitra, V. K., Gabrielli, A., Maccioli, G. A., & O'Connor, M. F. (2012). Anesthesia advanced circulatory life support. *Canadian Journal of Anesthesia = Journal Canadien D'Anesthésie, 59*(6), 586–603. https://doi.org/10.1007/s12630-012-9699-3.

31. Pal, A., & Muralidhar, V. (2020). Intraoperative anaphylaxis—Highlighting the dilemmas in living donor nephrectomy. *Indian Journal of Anesthesia, 64*, 236. https://doi.org/10.4103/ija.ija_414_19.

32. Rahman, A., & Azad, A. K. (2024). Management and monitoring of anesthesia during the perioperative period in a tertiary hospital in Bangladesh. *World Journal of Biology Pharmacy and Health Sciences.* https://www.semanticscholar.org/paper/81f66c7aeb6d7f9ec45821ae83c1577e708e4177 (accessed on 20 May 2025).

33. Ramirez, A. Y., Howes, S., Sanchez, K., Mullin, J., & Chilton, R. J. (2025). Anesthesia and EMI: Ensuring safe CIED management during surgical procedures. *Journal of Cardiothoracic and Vascular Anesthesia.* https://www.semanticscholar.org/paper/8ff6371167f6c2cb8b6a4fe963c26af0afce57e9 (accessed on 20 May 2025).

34. Rosendo, L. M., Rosado, T., Zandonai, T., Rincon, K., Peiró, A., Barroso, M., & Gallardo, E. (2024). Opioid monitoring in clinical settings: Strategies and implications of tailored approaches for therapy. *International Journal of Molecular Sciences, 25.* https://www.semanticscholar.org/paper/32546471fd4a3dc0e522f714080cc27ed5dad7b8 (accessed on 20 May 2025).

35. Schwenk, E. S., Pozek, J. J., & Viscusi, E. R. (2018). Managing prolonged pain after surgery: Examining the role of opioids. *The Journal of Arthroplasty, 33*(11), 3389–3393. https://doi.org/10.1016/j.arth.2018.08.005.

36. Shiraboina, M., Garre, S., Chandrasekaran, A. C., Ayya, S. S., Gajagouni, N., Shashikanth, T., & Ramachandran, G. (2025). Evolution of perioperative hemodynamic monitoring from the hand on pulse to hypotension prediction index. *Anesthesia and Critical Care Medicine Journal*. https://www.semanticscholar.org/paper/475f90febbf991b7960f334259802bb6ef1d61f9 (accessed on 20 May 2025).

37. Sneyd, J. R. (2022). Developments in procedural sedation for adults. *BJA Education, 22*(9), 258–264. https://doi.org/10.1016/j.bjae.2022.02.006.

38. Sosnick, M. S. M. (2024). *Improving Anesthesia Technician Workflow: Implementation of A Standardized Checklist and Formal Handoff Communication Tool to Enhance Management of The Pediatric Portable Anesthesia Lockers Recommendation* (Master's thesis, University of San Francisco). https://repository.usfca.edu/capstone/1816 (accessed on 20 May 2025).

39. Staibano, P., McKechnie, T., Thabane, A., Xie, M., Zhang, H., et al. (2024). Trends in using intraoperative parathyroid monitoring during parathyroidectomy: Protocol and rationale for a cross-sectional survey study of North American surgeons. https://www.semanticscholar.org/paper/de86f2a24993d9329ebd657ae0d182f576dda322 (accessed on 20 May 2025).

40. Williams, M., & Miller, A. (2023). An educational module on the clinical effectiveness of magnesium sulfate in the perioperative period (Student Project No. 246). Nicole Wertheim College of Nursing. https://digitalcommons.fiu.edu/cnhs-studentprojects/246 (accessed on 20 May 2025).

41. Yadav, R. (2025). Clinical guidelines and best practices for neuromuscular blockade monitoring: Ensuring patient safety and optimal outcomes. *Middle East Journal of Applied Science & Technology*. https://www.semanticscholar.org/paper/746b79e034a1a7c7132d765d3c2e8433638fb050 (accessed on 20 May 2025).

POST-ANESTHESIA CARE AND PAIN MANAGEMENT

14

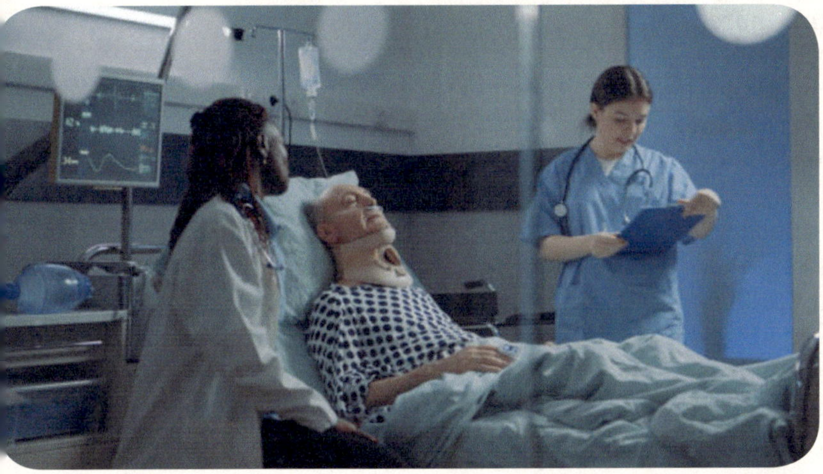

LEARNING OBJECTIVES

After studying this chapter, you will be able to:

1. Understand the role of post-anesthesia care units (PACUs).
2. Learn about pain assessment techniques.
3. Describe the pain management strategies.
4. Describe the challenges in post-anesthesia care.

Introduction

The movement from the operating room to PACU is a turning point in the recovery of a patient—routine monitoring and prompt pain medication become key. As anesthesia fades away, patients experience a mix of pain and distress, and the situation gets a little more complicated based on the length and nature of the surgery. Physicians are no longer just working to relieve pain at this stage; they're also watching for any side effects of the anesthesia. In the majority of cases, pairing intelligent pain relief with good post-op care makes patients more comfortable and allows them to heal faster. It implies treatments should be broad in scope—a blend of medication and non-medication methods—to deal with both stinging pain and apprehensive sensations. A careful, step-by-step analysis of pain afterwards serves as the basis for individualized care plans that address every patient's unique requirements, desires, and situation. Clear, concise communication between health care providers and patients is at the heart of effective post-anesthesia care. Poor management of pain can easily delay recovery, increase lengths of stay, and leave patients feeling abandoned. In most instances, being fully transparent in regards to what sort of pain relief to expect and some self-care fundamentals is a world of difference. Nonetheless, new paradigms like telemedicine open up channels for unimaginable scale for informed patients and permit quick and immediate consults in occasions of need (Kamdar et al., 2020). Adopting these technological advancements has the potential to upend pain management in the PACU and beyond; they facilitate both immediate response and more accountability on the part of caregivers. Simply put, integrating technology with honest, plain-English communication in post-op care is quite necessary to obtaining the best outcomes and having patients feel secure after anesthesia. Today, pain management is moving in a direction that is highly dynamic, and it may transform the quality of post-anesthetic care. Recent studies have all been leaning toward basically requiring individualized strategies based on a patient's background, personal likes and dislikes, and even the feeling that things are painful to them.

There's increasing evidence that a combination of rigorously designed medications—not to mention other support techniques—can be more effective at managing pain while curbing opioid overuse (Kertai et al., 2020). And with anesthesiologists, surgeons, and nurses all teaming up, finding pain problems and intervening with Band-Aid solutions can be much simpler. If the big picture is considered, teams can institute protocols that not only treat the immediate pain but also set the stage for future improvement in the long term. Overall, having a flexible, sometimes unorthodox, approach to pain management in the recovery unit is essential for enhancing both patient safety and patient satisfaction, even if it means occasional small inconsistency along the way (Figure 14.1).

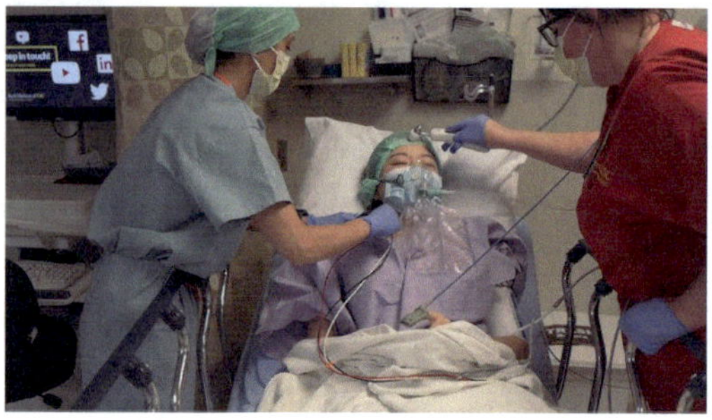

Figure 14.1. Post Anesthesia Care Unit (PACU).

Source: https://i.ytimg.com/vi/ETjo7Ja3qpU/hq720.jpg?sqp=-oaymwE7CK4FEIIDSFryq4qpAy0IARUAAAAAGAElAADIQj0AgKJD8AEB-AH-DoACuAiKAgwIABABGGUgXChPMA8=&rs=AOn4CLAqPki7aCmDTyfSGYLJTnv50ycEFQ.

Definition of Post-Anesthesia Care

Moving from the operating suite to the PACU is a real switch in gear in a patient's process. Here, patients are closely watched as the anesthetic effect wears off, with the treatment staff keeping tabs on vital signs, consciousness, and overall stability – and standing by to act at a moment's notice if any hiccups occur. This is not a recovery room but rather a vital connection within the entire surgery process that enables physicians to modify pain relief maneuvers at will. Anesthesiologists, in particular, come into play to sort out pain control plans that can affect the patient's overall good-feeling factor after surgery. Pain control is significant because, in most cases, uncontrolled pain can be at fault for an entire array of issues. Studies show that an acceptable proportion of patients continue to experience pain well after surgery, especially those that are more vulnerable. Generally speaking, tailoring pain management plans lowers on opioid usage – because relying too much on them may cause chronic pain or even addiction to opioids. Clinicians often use a rotation and combination of various painkillers in follow-ups, which works to reduce the total dose of opioids. This overall approach not only helps in alleviating short-term pain but also reduces long-term exposure to opioids, as research on opioid-related problems today proves (Wenzel et al., 2016). Multidisciplinary collaboration comes into play here. Anesthesiologists and the rest of the operating team take a seat in order to improve post-anesthesia care, working together to treat pain from various angles. There is evidence that, by coordinating everybody's work during the procedure, recovery will go more smoothly. For example, more effective recovery pathways offer a sort of flexible map to deal with post-op issues, even when the steps occasionally vary. For consideration of individual idiosyncrasies—e.g., preop opioid consumption or even nervousness—doctors are in a position to craft care plans that enable pain relief and enable returning to life in a bit of an easier fashion. The individualization lessens prolonged complications and mirrors the emerging focus on surgical recovery today (Schwenk et al., 2018) (Figure 14.2).

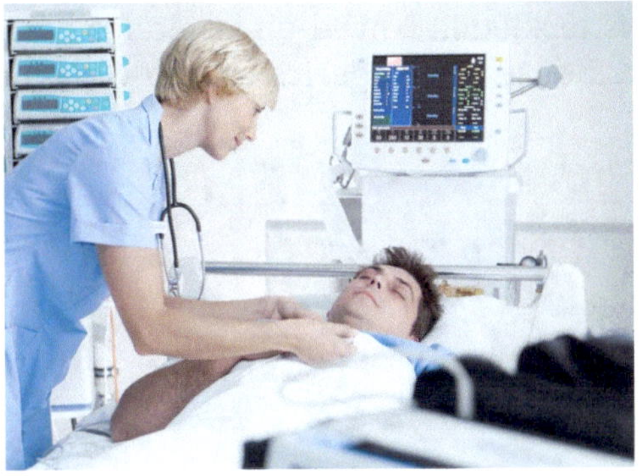

Figure 14.2. Post-anesthesia care.

Source: https://www.ziprecruiter.com/svc/fotomat/public-ziprecruiter/cms/91156502PACURN.jpg=ws720x480.

Importance of Effective Pain Management

After surgery, proper pain relief is something of monumental concern to patients' recovery and ultimately their sense of well-being. When pain is not directed the exactly right way, however, it can hinder recovery—delay healing, extend hospital stays, and even open the door to chronic pain. Studies have a tendency to emphasize that tailoring pain relief according to each person's response can ease the way to recovery. A standout example shows how the use of machine learning models to determine post-cesarean section pain care enabled individuals to learn adding certain anesthetic approaches, like esketamine, helps to improve pain relief and decreases opioid use (Sivakumar et al., 2024). Such a development unequivocally shows that the personalization of pain protocols in the post-anesthesia setting isn't nice to have—it's necessary. Pain management is not just a matter of comfort for one patient; its impacts ripple through many types of patients. Diverse physical and psychological factors determine how people deal with pain. Take transgender men and non-binary individuals receiving gender-affirming surgeries, for instance—case in point is why specialized pain practices are sometimes needed. Several studies have demonstrated that the use of pectoral nerve blocks is able to decrease d opioid use and lower pain scores compared to more traditional methods (Sivakumar et al., 2024). By considering the particular problems these populations bring, practitioners are better able to develop pain plans that treat the short-term pain and manage long-term health. In the majority of cases, fitting in on a customized level is what creates the difference when it comes to fair and efficient care. Pain that is not controlled results not only in misery for the patient—tacking on economic and social expenses in addition. As healthcare expenditures rise, the implications of not getting pain in check go far beyond an individual patient. Hospitals that do pain management correctly tend to report fewer readmissions and less time spent in the hospital, which of course reduces overall costs. Additionally, good pain care has a tendency to increase patient activation and overall satisfaction, even if that is a few more commas or pauses along the way. Overall, pain management needs to be considered an integral aspect of postoperative care and not an add-on; not only is it a shortcut to recovery but it also maximizes hospital resources (Figure 14.3).

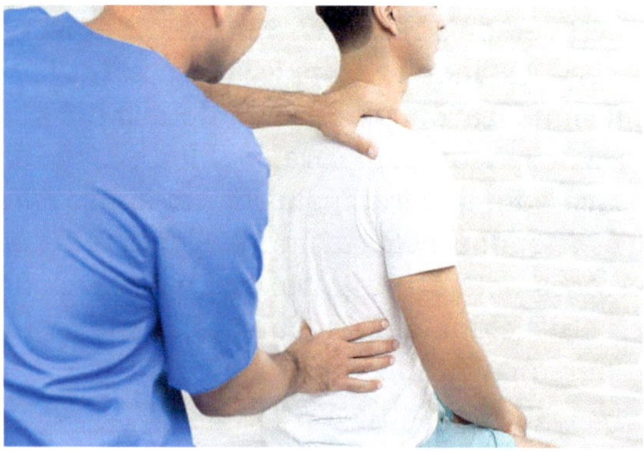

Figure 14.3. The importance of proper pain management after surgery.

Source: https://painandspinespecialists.com/wp-content/uploads/Back-Pain-Specialists-1024x684.jpeg.

14.1. The Role of Post-Anesthesia Care Units (PACUs)

Learning Outcome

1. Understand the purpose and function of PACUs.
2. Describe the staffing and resources in PACUs.
3. Understand the monitoring protocols in the PACU.

After surgery, most people take for granted how essential PACUs (Post-Anesthesia Care Units) really are. At the exact time patients wake up from anesthesia and are especially vulnerable, these units take over, bridging that gap to recovery. Patients, still a bit out of it, need quick and watchful monitoring—a sharp eye that picks up on unexpected complications like respiratory trouble, bleeding, or even uncontrolled pain. Overall, by maintaining a peaceful, focused atmosphere, PACUs reduce risks that may seep in after an individual is recuperating from a procedure, never losing sight of the end goal of a trouble-free recovery. Nurses in these units are the unsung heroes, doing more than just routine checks. They get into everything—from hands-on patient examinations (research on nursing attitudes has stated this, by the way) to keeping a running record of how things develop throughout a patient's stay. In most cases, their conscientious record-keeping and repeated, often revisited observations, work to link care between different teams. They communicate the highs and lows of every patient's condition, nothing being lost in translation as medical personnel work together to guide recovery. This sort of record-keeping, while sometimes a little sloppy, speaks to a diligent attitude toward both safety and restoring patients to good health. Besides the clinical function, PACUs play a big part in patients' attitudes toward their overall recovery. Surgery is not just a physical procedure—many nerves are also agitated. With the timeliness of intervention in these units, whatever fears one has also dissipate the instant pain is tackled in a head-on fashion; a carefully titrated dose of analgesics can do wonders.

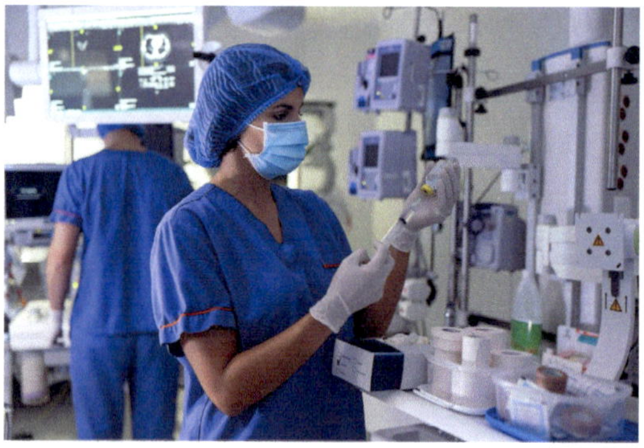

Figure 14.4. Role of post-anesthesia care units (PACUs).

Source: https://cdn.prod.website-files.com/5babc11099f97ea5dbcf24d5/65b829131c46647c8f3729de_pacu-nurse.jpg.

The hands-on, in-the-moment treatment adjustments not only soothe the physical discomfort but address the emotional upset a patient may have, reaffirming that their overall well-being matters. In short, the extra going around that is done by these units—some rough edges notwithstanding—underscores their essential role, and points to the ongoing need for innovations that make recuperation as personalized and as comforting as possible (Figure 14.4).

14.1.1. Purpose and Function of PACUs

Postoperative care depends a lot on how Post-Anesthesia Care Units, or PACUs, are set up and run. Right after surgery, these units become the go-to spots where patients slowly wake from anesthesia, and staff keep a watchful eye on them to make sure everything's safe and comfortable. In many cases, doctors and nurses can quickly jump in if a patient shows signs of trouble—say, a breathing hiccup or a shaky blood flow. There's a kind of relaxed yet focused vibe in these rooms that not only helps reduce on complications but also builds trust in the whole recovery process. Overall, PACUs serve as a place where healing isn't just physical; patients also leave feeling more confident about the care they received. But it isn't only about keeping an eye on recovery; these units also bring together a thoughtful approach to pain management. Tools like the OPIAID Zone Tool are put into play, aiming to improve how pain is handled while, in most cases, reducing the risk of adverse drug events. This tool keeps track of how intense pain is and whether opioid side effects might sneak in, offering on-the-spot guidance to clinicians. Research generally hints that mixing both opioid and non-opioid options can lead to a more balanced strategy, which often means better outcomes and faster recovery times. In a sense, PACUs turn into testing grounds for evolving pain management tactics that boost the overall effectiveness of postoperative care. Beyond managing the immediate after-effects of surgery, PACUs also have a hand in guiding patients through their recovery journey. In these settings, healthcare providers share advice tailored to each patient, explaining pain management in everyday terms that help lessen anxiety and speed up the return to normal activities. Studies have shown that when patients understand what to expect, they usually feel more at ease—even if the instructions might repeat a point here and there. For example, research focusing on oral surgery recovery sometimes points out that clear, continuous patient education can ease worries about both pain and potential setbacks. Ultimately, PACUs do more than just oversee physical recovery; they empower patients with knowledge, fostering a more holistic care experience that leaves a lasting, reassuring impression.

14.1.2. Staffing and Resources in PACUs

Staffing PACUs isn't just a checklist—it's about making sure patients stay safe and that pain is handled well from the get-go. Having the right mix of nurses can be tricky, especially when each patient's needs differ after surgery. One study, for instance, shows that a nursing intensity tool offers a clear picture of varying care demands; it highlights what's needed when patients move from the operating room into recovery. Using this tool helps set the right nurse-to-patient balance, mixing physical care with safety needs in a way that makes a difference for those coming out of anesthesia (Rauta et al., 2019). It's not only about people either. A PACU runs best when it's stocked with essential meds, monitoring gadgets, and safety gear—all of which play a big role in how smoothly a patient bounces back. Research over the years hints that patient satisfaction often comes d to how well the whole setup functions. In most cases, investing in quality and well-kept resources not only spurs better recovery outcomes but also builds trust and comfort among patients (Fortier et al., 2019). When you look at it, a successful PACU keeps its human and material assets on equal footing, setting up an environment that supports healing. Then there's the whole mix of staffing, resources, and training that ties everything together. It's clear that when nurses know exactly how to handle the available tools—and they get regular, hands-on training—it pays off in the form of better pain management and smoother recoveries. Ongoing education ensures that staff stay in the loop with best practices and new technologies, even if sometimes informal chats or quick huddles are all it takes to realign care goals. To summarize, a PACU that nails both team skills and resource readiness tends to create an atmosphere that boosts patient safety and overall satisfaction (Fortier et al., 2019) (Figure 14.5).

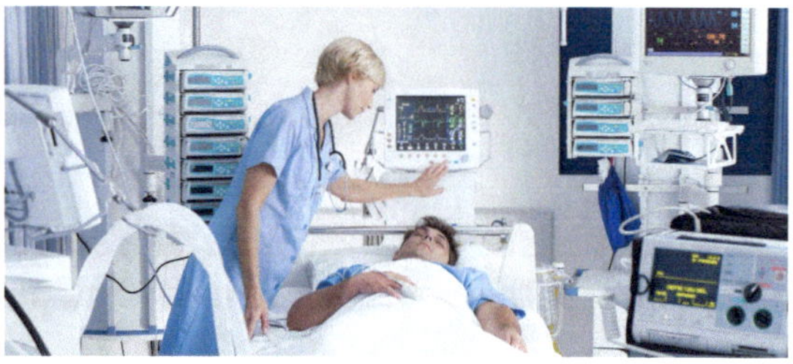

Figure 14.5. PACU nurse.

Source: https://images.aspen.edu/wp/uploads/2022/12/PACU-post-anesthesia-care-unit-Nurses-Job-Description-and-Outlook-a-picture-of-a-nurse-checking-on-her-patient.-1.jpg.

14.1.3. Monitoring Protocols in the PACU

Switching from the operating room to the PACU marks a pivotal moment in surgery. Right off the bat, patient safety and effective pain relief take center stage. Doctors, nurses, and other care staff run through an array of checks that look at vital signs, neurological alertness, and how well the patient's breathing is holding up – sometimes all at once. They follow a kind of unwritten checklist; patients need to have steady vitals and enough pain control before they're cleared to leave. Every case is a bit different, though—factors like age, past medical issues and even the type of anesthesia all influence how quickly someone recovers. Generally speaking, if the team sticks closely to these monitoring protocols, they can catch signs of complications early, which in turn improves overall outcomes and helps ward off later issues. Enhanced Recovery After Surgery (ERAS) has reshaped how things are handled in the PACU. Instead of just following routine checks, ERAS pushes for using multiple pain management methods and keeping a close eye on any side effects, however small they might be. Most studies these days suggest that when hospitals follow these ERAS pathways, outcomes tend to improve, partly because teams can step in sooner if something goes off track. Setting up these standards builds a sort of built-in safety net among surgical teams, making everyone a bit more alert and in tune with what modern care demands.

And as these procedures get woven into everyday practice, you sometimes see shorter hospital stays and, well, happier patients when they finally leave the PACU. When it comes to kids undergoing procedures like tonsillectomy, the story is quite similar but with some extra care. Research shows that premedicating with bronchodilators (say, albuterol) can sometimes reduce on breathing problems during recovery. Clinical trials have hinted that keeping a close watch in the PACU can help reduce complications like laryngospasm or drops in oxygen levels—even if every patient is a little different. The blend of using smart drug interventions alongside traditional monitoring not only boosts the overall quality of care but also fits neatly with modern post-anesthesia standards. To summarize, these advanced monitoring steps help balance immediate recovery needs with long-term health goals, creating a safer environment, especially for most vulnerable patients (Figure 14.6).

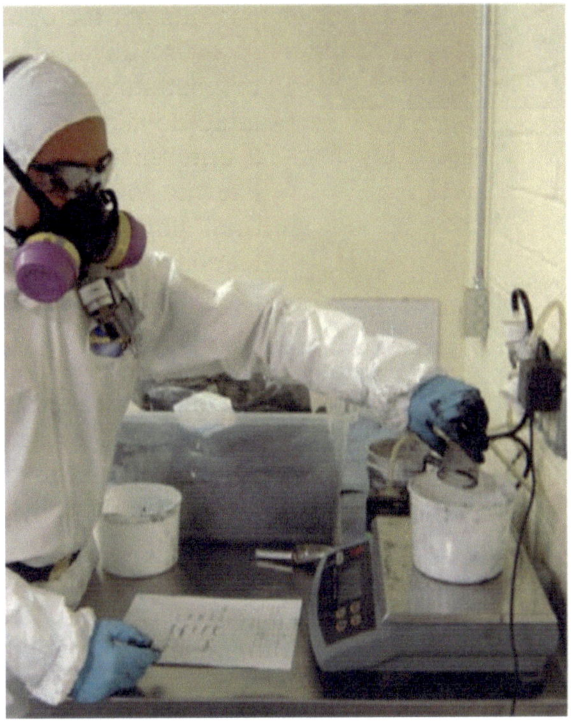

Figure 14.6. The importance of patient monitoring in the PACU.

Source: By U.S. National Institute for Occupational Safety and Health - General Safe Practices for Working with Engineered Nanomaterials in Research Laboratories (in en-us). U.S. National Institute for Occupational Safety and Health pp. 10–28 (May 2012). Retrieved on 2017-03-05., Public Domain, https://commons.wikimedia.org/w/index.php?curid=57175188.

Test Your Knowledge

1. What are the purpose and function of PACUs?
2. What are the monitoring protocols in the PACU?

14.2. Pain Assessment Techniques

Learning Outcome

1. Discuss subjective versus objective pain assessment.
2. Describe the common pain scales used in clinical practice.
3. Understand the importance of timely pain assessment.

Effective pain management right after anesthesia starts with nailing down how much pain a patient feels – it's the groundwork, for a smooth recovery. Many say evidence-based protocols are a must, and generally speaking, they play a huge role in determining how patients do afterwards. Yet, studies show that sometimes these guidelines aren't followed as closely as they should, especially in specialized spots like Anesthesia Intensive Care Units (AICUs). For instance, one teaching hospital in Hefei, China, found that adherence was less than ideal, which led to an intervention aimed at bumping things up. They introduced a structured framework that, unsurprisingly, led to a noticeable jump in compliance – proving that focused strategies can directly elevate postoperative pain management (Liu al., 2025). A go-to method for checking pain is the Visual Analog Scale (VAS). This tool lets patients mark out their pain intensity in a way that's both clear and immediate, giving clinicians a quick snapshot of how someone's feeling. The VAS essentially lays out pain on a continuous scale, and its simplicity helps in evaluating how well different pain control techniques work. For example, a recent study compared bupivacaine and ropivacaine in Transversus Abdominis Plane (TAP) blocks for Cesarean delivery; it turned out that patients receiving bupivacaine recorded significantly lower VAS scores – a result that subtly suggests a preference for that anesthetic. These direct measurements aren't just numbers; they're a key part of making sure patients get the optimal care they need as they recover (Goyal et al., 2025). When it comes to post-surgery care, mixing things up with multiple methods of pain assessment can make a difference. Blending subjective evaluations like the VAS with more objective measures – think physiological indicators or direct patient feedback – provides a broader picture of a patient's status. Educational initiatives for healthcare providers also come into play here, sharpening how pain is assessed on the ground. As seen in the study mentioned earlier, boosting adherence to evidence-based pain assessment methods via such programs can have a clear positive impact. By nurturing an environment of ongoing learning and improvement, hospitals better equip their teams to carry out detailed pain checks and custom-fit interventions, which, in turn, lifts patient satisfaction and overall outcomes in post-anesthesia care (Liu et al., 2025).

14.2.1. Subjective Versus Objective Pain Assessment

Right after anesthesia, figuring out pain isn't as clear-cut as you might think. Patients rate their discomfort using tools like the VAS or NRS, and that self-reporting provides insights not just into the intensity but also into how each person tolerates what they feel. Pain, by its nature, is messy—with moods, emotions, and even slight variations in perception chipping in—so what patients say matters when doctors try to shape treatments that fit each unique recovery. In most cases, leaning on these personal reports is key for crafting pain relief plans that seem to work best for every individual. On the flip side, numbers don't lie entirely either. Doctors often turn to measurable signs: a jump in heart rate, changes in blood pressure, or even a fleeting frown can all point to discomfort. These objective checks come in handy especially when someone is too disoriented or overwhelmed to explain their pain in words. Blending these physical cues with what patients report gives a broader picture of the whole experience—even if sometimes the hard data might miss some of the subtleties that a patient personally feels. Recent studies generally back up the idea of mixing both sides when it comes to pain management. For instance, some research suggests that simple relaxation techniques can shift how pain is perceived, even though the measurable indicators don't always show obvious changes (Weekes et al., 2019). Similarly, a combined analgesic approach has been seen to not only lower the pain levels that can be observed visually but also to reduce on opioid use (Lucas et al., 2019). This kind of combined outlook deepens our understanding of postoperative pain and, in most cases, helps refine treatment protocols to match what each patient truly needs (Figure 14.7).

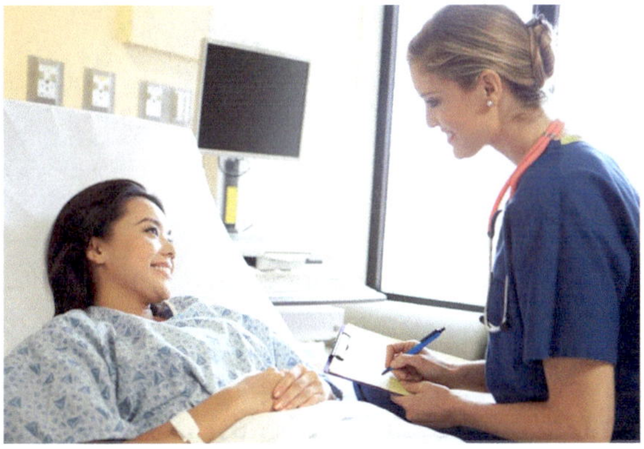

Figure 14.7. Subjective versus objective pain assessment.

Source: https://www.nursingprocess.org/bimg/subjective-vs-objective-nursing-data.webp.

14.2.2. Common Pain Scales Used in Clinical Practice

In post-surgery settings, handling pain starts with getting a real sense of how someone's feeling. One common method is asking patients to mark their pain along a 10-centimeter line – this so-called Visual Analog Scale offers a simple, visual picture of their discomfort. Then there's the straightforward 0-to-10 Numeric Rating Scale that asks patients to pick a number, making it easier for both them and their caregivers to chat about what they're experiencing. And if a patient finds words hard to come by—like young kids or anyone with communication issues—the Wong-Baker FACES series steps in with different expressions. These simple tools, repeated time and again in hospitals, help shape pain management plans and boost recovery during that delicate phase after anesthesia wears off. Even though these scales generally work well, putting them into everyday practice isn't always smooth. Many healthcare providers sometimes feel underprepared when choosing the right tool, and this lack of knowledge can lead to less-than-ideal pain handling.

A study even highlighted real hurdles – for instance, insufficient staff training and spotty documentation in electronic health records (Bixio et al., 2024). On top of that, individual differences like varying pain thresholds or cultural backgrounds can alter what those numbers or faces actually mean. In most cases, targeted educational programs and regular training sessions help bridge that gap, gradually building caregivers' confidence and ensuring that pain management sticks to best practices while honoring each patients unique pain experience. When resources are tight, evaluating pain can get even more complicated. In environments where decisions need to be made fast, as noted by the Italian Society of Anesthesia, Analgesia, Resuscitation and Intensive Care (SIAARTI) (Bixio et al., 2024), simple, easy-to-use scales become even more crucial. Under pressure, these straightforward tools let healthcare professionals quickly figure out pain levels and tailor treatment plans—balancing what's available with what each patient needs. Mixing and matching different pain management approaches in such settings means that even when things are hectic, reliable assessments help improve both immediate relief and overall patient care outcomes.

14.2.3. Importance of Timely Pain Assessment

Getting a handle on pain right after surgery is key. Quick pain checks help set the stage for the right kind of treatment, knowing that delays can crank up the discomfort and complicate recovery. When pain isn't promptly measured, patients can end up suffering more and hospital stays might stretch out, which drives costs up too. Regular pain assessments—something many have started to introduce—do help smooth out these issues. By gauging pain levels early, doctors can swiftly tailor pain relief options that usually speed up recovery and keep patient comfort front and center (Liu et al., 2025). Timely checks do more than just ease immediate suffering; they also support the whole team effort in post-surgery care. In most cases, a dependable pain management routine brings everyone on board, whether it's nurses, doctors, or specialists. One report from an Anesthesia Intensive Care Unit noticed that better adherence to scheduled pain evaluations led to noticeably improved outcomes (Liu et al., 2025). This shows that when hospitals invest in steady pain assessments, patients benefit right away, and the care team finds it easier to work together toward recovery. It's even more noticeable in ERAS settings. Spotting pain early allows for quick fixes that help ward off complications and encourage patients to get moving sooner. For example, some studies in post-caesarean care have seen that fast pain evaluation supports early feeding and bonding with newborns—a boost for both physical and emotional recovery. A focused, routine approach to monitoring pain helps highlight the weak spots in current practices, pushing for improvements that lift maternal and neonatal outcomes along with overall patient satisfaction (Figure 14.8).

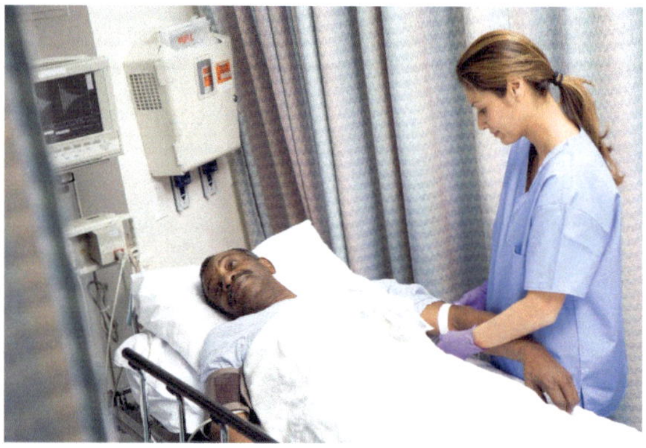

Figure 14.8. Importance of Timely Pain Assessment.

Source: https://cdn.ps.emap.com/wp-content/uploads/sites/3/2003/07/hospital_bed_ward_patient.jpg.

Test Your Knowledge

1. What is the difference between subjective and objective pain assessment?
2. What is the importance of timely pain assessment?

14.3. Pain Management Strategies

Learning Outcome

1. Understand the pharmacological interventions for pain relief.
2. Understand the non-pharmacological approaches to pain management.
3. Describe the multimodal pain management techniques.

Pain control after anesthesia is key to making sure patients recover well. Nowadays, care teams mix different expertise, and you see this a lot in programs treating older adults with fractures. A look back at patient records shows that when hospitals tried these new plans, emergency room pain relief for fragile hip fractures in seniors improved a lot. They ended up using more techniques like fascia iliaca compartment blocks (FICB) and acetaminophen – which, incidentally, helped reduce the usual reliance on opioids. Patients even got their first pain relief sooner after these changes, pointing to how a well-organized strategy can drop risks in vulnerable groups (Casey et al., 2017). The opioid crisis still looms, so mixing various painkillers is becoming a major move in managing pain. Generally speaking, this idea is all about using a variety of drugs to hit different pain points, instead of just leaning on opioids – which, let's be honest, come with a fair share of side effects. These plans don't just tackle pain right after surgery; in most cases, they're also aiming to reduce long-term opioid use. By altering medication choices for each patient and their specific surgery, healthcare providers can often get better results while keeping unwanted effects in check. Studies back this up, showing that spreading the load across several medications often lowers complications linked to opioids (Schwenk et al., 2018). Doctors, anesthesiologists, and pain specialists have to team up on this front. Especially now, with shortages in opioid alternatives and other medications causing extra headaches, it's more important than ever for experts to work together. They juggle these supply issues while still trying to give patients the pain control they need during those critical recovery moments. On top of that, pushing locally and nationally can help keep a steadier supply of analgesics and spark new ideas for alternatives. In short, as pain management keeps shifting, consistently reviewing and adjusting these plans is essential for better patient experiences during post-anesthesia care (Schwenk et al., 2018) (Figure 14.9).

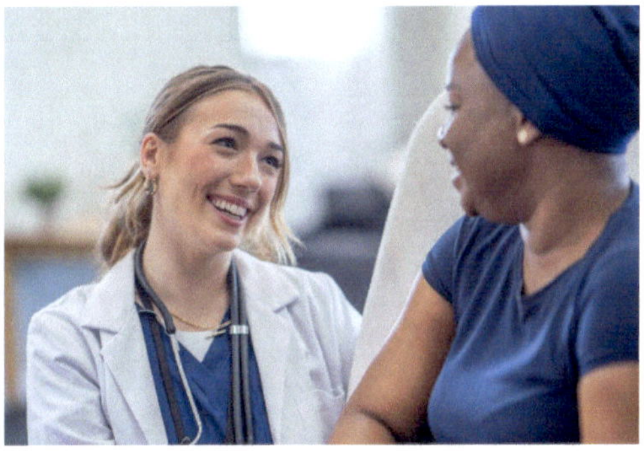

Figure 14.9. Post-Surgical pain management strategies for a smooth recovery.

Source: https://www.woosterhospital.org/wp-content/uploads/sites/229/2023/12/iStock-1438404344-1.jpg.

14.3.1. Pharmacological Interventions for Pain Relief

Pain management after anesthesia isn't just a one-trick pony—it's a mix of different methods to ease discomfort in a few unexpected ways. Non-opioid drugs like NSAIDs and acetaminophen kick off the relief process, often teaming up with opioids to keep the overall opioid dose lower and, in turn, reduce side effects. Sometimes, local anesthetics are used regionally or infiltratively to zero in on painful spots right after surgery. This combination not only makes patients feel more at ease but can also speed up recovery.

In most cases, weaving these pharmacological techniques together shows a deeper, more nuanced grasp of managing post-anesthesia pain. Opioids have their place, sure, but they come with their baggage. They're mighty effective for severe pain; however, they bring risks like respiratory depression, sedation, and even addiction. So, striking a careful balance between effectiveness and safety is necessary. Increasingly, clinicians are leaning on multimodal analgesia—mixing a variety of drugs—to boost pain relief while keeping opioid use in check. There's been a growing conversation about preemptive analgesia, where medications are given before pain even sets in, such as ahead of surgery, to target those pain pathways more directly.

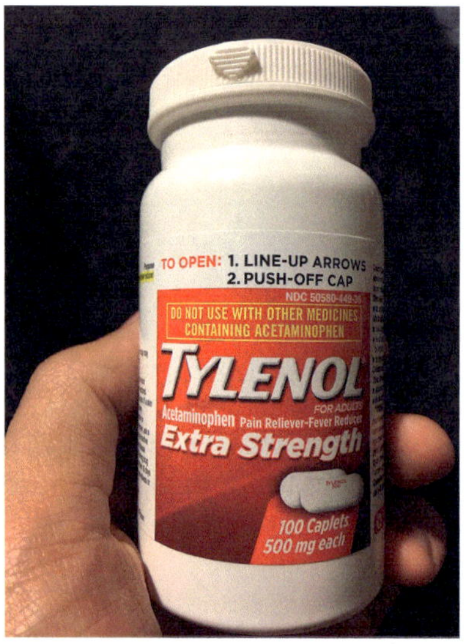

Figure 14.10. Pain control after surgery: pain medicines.

Source: By Mrbeastmodeallday - Own work, CC BY-SA 4.0, https://commons.wikimedia.org/w/index.php?curid=76917486.

The result? A better chance at managing pain successfully without leaning too heavily on opioids, which is pretty much in line with today's best practices. When it comes to children, pain management gets even trickier because it's not just the body that hurts—the mind feels it too. Kids can be extra anxious before invasive procedures, and that anxiety makes it all the more important to get the pain relief right. Doctors might use a mix of local anesthetics and conscious sedation for procedures like lumbar punctures or bone marrow aspirations, and sometimes even throw in psychological approaches like cognitive-behavioral therapy or hypnosis. Research, for instance, shows that hypnosis can reduce on procedure-related pain. In short, blending these drug-based methods with non-drug strategies seems to offer a more complete solution, ultimately enhancing the overall healthcare experience for young patients (Kendrick et al., 2016; Liossi et al., 1999) (Figure 14.10).

14.3.2. Non-Pharmacological Approaches to Pain Management

Bringing in treatments that don't rely solely on drugs is reshaping how we deal with pain after anesthesia. Instead of defaulting to standard medications, patients are now trying out methods like CBT sessions and music therapy; these approaches work gradually to build long-term coping skills rather than offering the quick hit of traditional painkillers. In most cases, merging these lifestyle changes with drug-based treatments seems to boost overall satisfaction and pain relief (Raja et al., 2025). This mix not only tackles the pain in the moment but also creates an environment that values each patient's comfort—even if it feels a bit less formulaic. TENS—short for transcutaneous electrical nerve stimulation—has lately caught the eye of many as a helpful supplement in managing pain after operations. Research generally agrees that HFHI TENS can ease pain in minutes, making it a valuable option right after anesthesia. Patients' feedback often reveals that using TENS leaves them feeling more in control and reassured about managing their pain (Angelini et al., 2025). Combining TENS with conventional treatments gives patients a bit of self-administration power, which sits well with today's goals for pain care. Non-drug methods don't stop at easing pain; they also reach into the psychological and emotional sides of recovery. Techniques like guided imagery, mindfulness, and even simple relaxation exercises pop up as useful tools in reducing anxiety during surgical recovery. In most cases, these approaches help speed up healing while offering a sense of security in the post-op days (Raja et al., 2025). As more healthcare providers notice that recovery isn't just about physical relief, blending these natural techniques with regular pain management is gradually becoming a key part of comprehensive postoperative care.

14.3.3. Multimodal Pain Management Techniques

Effective pain management after anesthesia isn't just about using one method—it's about mixing many approaches. Multimodal analgesia, for instance, doesn't simply rely on one drug but blends common meds like NSAIDs and acetaminophen with extras such as gabapentinoids or even NMDA receptor blockers. Using this mix lets clinicians target various pain routes, which tends to boost relief while reducing on opioid use; in many cases, this combo even speeds up recovery and makes patients feel better overall (Ismail, 2025). It's a kind of "do-it-all" strategy, where merging different treatments creates a fuller picture of care, sometimes repeating the idea of diversity in pain control. Regional anesthesia (RA) adds another layer to this picture, especially for surgery patients. Techniques like nerve blocks and neuraxial methods jump in to offer strong pain relief, and they can also speed up rehab and lower the risk of long-term, post-op pain—plus, they help avoid the downsides of systemic opioids, like respiratory issues and nausea. In most protocols (think Enhanced Recovery After Surgery, for example), this targeted approach not only lets patients get moving sooner but also bumps up overall satisfaction (Kim, 2025). To be clear, these regional tactics work in tandem with broader methods to provide a safety net that almost feels like a backup plan, even if sometimes the details can get a bit repetitive. Still, challenges persist that keep these techniques from being used as widely as they might be. Differences in clinician expertise and limited resources can get in the way, and patients often aren't fully clued in on why these approaches might work better for them; this leads to underuse. A real team effort—where anesthesiologists, surgeons, and pain specialists share ideas and insights—is generally needed to overcome these hurdles. By nurturing an environment of teamwork and continuous learning, the industry can gradually weave these evidence-based pain management strategies into everyday practice, ultimately making post-surgery care and overall patient recovery that much better (Ismail, 2025) (Figure 14.11).

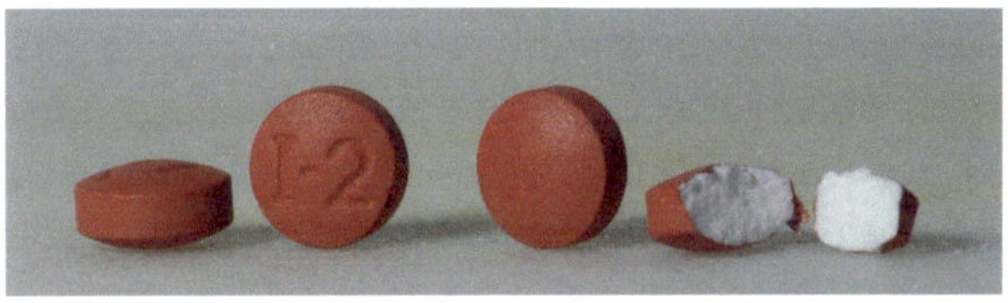

Figure 14.11. Multimodal analgesia pain management.

Test Your Knowledge

1. Describe the pharmacological interventions for pain relief.
2. What is multimodal pain management techniques?

14.4. Challenges in Post-Anesthesia Care

Learning Outcome

1. Understand the variability in patient responses to anesthesia and pain.
2. Manage complications and side effects in post-anesthesia care.
3. Address the opioid crisis in pain management.

Coming off anesthesia can bring a whole load of unexpected challenges that shape how patients do afterward. Responses to pain management can be all over the map, coming from things like a person's physical state, their mental outlook, or even the kind of surgery they had. Standard protocols, though useful, often don't address these differences. In most cases, recent observations imply that mixing in newer tactics—like using machine learning to fine-tune treatment for each patient might be the key to handling the messy business of pain perception and relief. It's clear that as the medical world starts to see these issues more clearly, tailoring care to the individual keeps coming up as a top priority (Sivakumar et al., 2024). Pain after anesthesia, especially in busy intensive care settings, is even more of a tough nut to crack. Managing it isn't just about the tricky medical side of things; it's also about juggling limited resources, like having enough staff and reliable pain assessment tools on hand. When pain management guidelines miss the mark, patients can either end up with too little relief or suffer from the downsides of too many drugs, like problems with opioids. Some researchers even point to non-drug methods—think music therapy or relaxation techniques as helpful companions to traditional medication. On top of that, bringing together different experts, from nurses and anesthesiologists to physical therapists, helps catch the little nuances in what each patient might need. Generally speaking, this kind of team approach is crucial for building better plans that mix both medicinal and alternative strategies. And with ongoing research into fresh ways of looking at pain management, we might just keep raising the bar for patient care long after the surgery is done (Zakeri et al., 2024) (Figure 14.12).

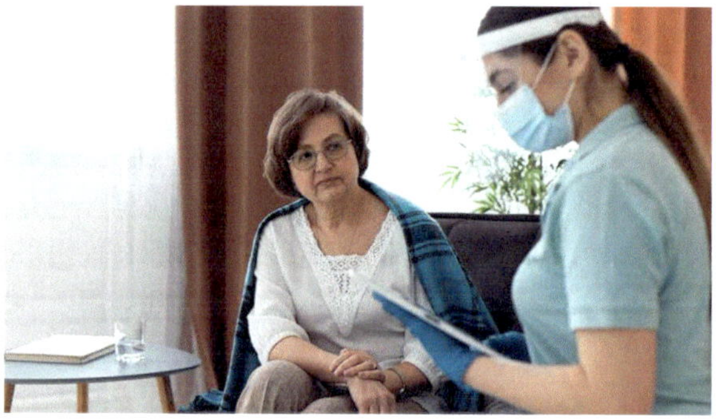

Figure 14.12. Post-surgery psychological challenges for seniors.

Source: https://ghost-cms.s3.ap-south-1.amazonaws.com/2024/05/Post-Surgery-Psychological-Challenges-For-Seniors_the-wellness-corner.jpg.

14.4.1. Variability in Patient Responses to Anesthesia and Pain

Patients can react very differently to anesthesia and pain meds; it's not a one-size-fits-all deal. Many things are at play—genetics, our body's workings, and even what's happening in our heads all mix together to change how drugs get broken down and how pain is felt. Sometimes, a specific genetic twist can mean a drug works too strongly, or maybe barely at all. Health issues like obesity or heart conditions can further throw a wrench in the works by messing with how pain control methods do their job. All these bits and pieces mean that the care after anesthesia has to be tailor-made to each person for the best, safest results. Pain, by its very nature, is a deeply personal experience, and people don't just feel it the same way—they also cope with it uniquely. Think about how things like anxiety, past pain episodes, or even cultural views on suffering shape what someone considers painful. Studies tend to show that when pain management is built around a person's story and preferences, it not only lifts their spirits but also speeds up recovery. A patient-focused setup, where doctors and patients have an easy back-and-forth chat, can end up making pain treatment feel much more effective and in tune with what each individual needs. On top of that, clinical guidelines are key players in managing these differences.

For example, the Enhanced Recovery After Surgery (ERAS) protocol tosses out solid, research-backed tips to standardize care—while still leaving wiggle room for adjustments based on who exactly is in the room (Nelson et al., 2019). And when you look at what groups like the American College of Cardiology and American Heart Association suggest, the importance of teaming up with patients—making decisions together—jumps out, boosting how likely patients are to stick with the plan (Stout et al., 2018). By weaving these guidelines into everyday practice, healthcare folks can better handle the messy mix of individual differences, aiming for smoother recoveries after anesthesia.

14.4.2. Managing Complications and Side Effects

Managing care after anesthesia isn't just about checking off boxes—it's a real balancing act where you have to keep an eye on many potential issues. Pain that isn't kept under control can sneak up on you; patients might feel more dissatisfied and their recovery can stretch on longer than expected. Sometimes, this unmanaged pain doesn't just fade—it can stick around and develop into something chronic. This is especially tricky with opioid-tolerant patients, who generally need some careful dosing changes.

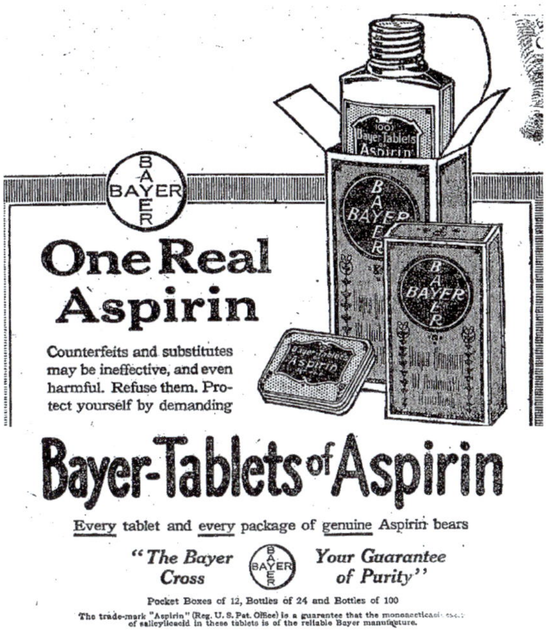

Figure 14.13. Reduce your risk of side effects from anesthesia.

Source: By New York Times, February 19, 1917, p. 6 (via ProQuest Historical Newspapers: "Display Ad 26 -- No Title"), Public Domain, https://commons.wikimedia.org/w/index.php?curid=3661828.

Using patient-specific strategies that start during preoperative assessments and stretch all the way to discharge seems key, putting anesthesiologists in the middle of a web of coordinating comprehensive pain plans (Wenzel et al., 2016). There's also a growing trend in mixing different types of painkillers instead of sticking with a one-drug approach. In most cases, multimodal analgesia—where you use several classes of pain relievers—hits multiple pain pathways at once. This usually boosts overall effectiveness and cuts back on the odd side affects you might see when relying on a single medication. Think of it less like following a strict recipe and more like checking off a customizable list that adapts to the patient's needs and the surgical situation. Often, this strategy isn't just about better pain relief; it can also lower the dependency on opioids, which is a big deal given today's concerns over opioid misuse and long-term addiction (Schwenk et al., 2018). On top of all that, the whole landscape of pain management gets even messier thanks to ongoing shortages of key drugs. Anesthesiologists and acute pain specialists now, in many cases, find themselves having to push for a wider range of analgesics, not just opioids but also non-opioid alternatives and various adjuncts. It often comes down to a collaborative, sometimes patchy effort at both the local and national levels to ensure that no matter what, patients have access to the full spectrum of pain relief options. All of these challenges mean that, to keep patients both safe and satisfied, innovative and flexible thinking in pain management is more necessary than ever (Schwenk et al., 2018) (Figure 14.13).

14.4.3. Addressing the Opioid Crisis in Pain Management

Pain management today asks us to revisit old opioid-heavy methods, especially in post-anesthesia settings. Rising rates of addiction and fatal overdoses have, generally speaking, pushed both clinicians and researchers to look beyond standard opioid use. Alternative drugs like NSAIDs and local anesthetics offer one route to reduce on opioid risks, while treatments such as physical therapy and cognitive-behavioral approaches slip in as useful non-drug options. Addressing opioid dependence not only lifts the well-being of patients but also ties into broader public health goals to slow the epidemic's impact. Clinicians, in many cases, are finding that mixing these strategies can lead to effective relief and better overall care (Borode et al., 2024). When it comes to reducing opioid reliance, getting patients involved turns out to be crucial. Collaborative care models—where, say, interdisciplinary teams join forces to build care plans—encourage patients to be active in managing their pain. Some programs, for example, wedded behavioral health to rehab services, thereby bridging the gap between diverse healthcare experts and the individuals they serve. This kind of teamwork tackles persistent issues like stigma and decision-making challenges. By embracing a more holistic way to assess the many shades of pain, providers can fine-tune treatments to match what each patient needs. In most cases, such engagement not only boosts satisfaction but also builds a sense of ownership over their health outcomes, ultimately helping patients stick with their treatment plans (Overman, 2021). Health systems, grappling with the persistent opioid crisis, are now pressed to maintain interventions that combine different pain management tactics. Crafting a care model that mixes both drugs and non-drug therapies is key—especially in the tricky arena of post-anesthesia care. Small shifts, like altering scheduling or reworking documentation practices, can help teams communicate better, while giving patients straightforward education on self-management helps them deal with pain more confidently. Take, for instance, standardized reviews of chronic pain; such evaluations can let caregivers map out treatment paths that are as individual as the patients themselves. These systematic yet flexible approaches not only promise improved clinical outcomes but also work to replace overdependence on opioids with a more sustainable method of care (Borode et al., 2024; Overman, 2021).

Test Your Knowledge

1. How do you manage side effects of anesthesia?
2. How to address the opioid crisis in pain management?

SUMMARY

One step closer to the forces behind post-surgery recovery, it is obvious that performing well on pain management is more or less the focal point of recovery. Simple steps in pain scoring have routinely led to wonderfully better outcomes. For example, in a study at Hefei Teaching Hospital in China, they discovered that after some special education workshops and focus groups, the rate of adherence to these guidelines increased from 66% to 92%. That is a positive sign that hospitals need to keep on educating their nurses—improving nurses' skills while helping patients navigate a delicate time (Liu et al., 2025).

Having in mind now the many facets of pain after surgery, it is assured that dealing with its multifaceted character is the only method to reduce both acute and lingering discomfort. Researchers have a tendency to point out that pragmatic steps—like the use of IV pain medications and nerve blocks—play a huge role in reducing severe pain and allowing patients to be discharged from post anesthesia care units sooner. Audits performed in large and small hospitals somehow show that possessing a simple framework for pain control is sheer magic, with everybody taking precautions to mold care to what each patient really needs (Jayanth et al., 2025).

Lastly, the incorporation of proven research with routine pain management practice promotes recovery and overall satisfaction. Systematic pain assessment and thoughtfully designed management regimens promise better outcomes and may even lower costs by minimizing prolonged hospital stays. In most cases, creating a sense of ongoing progression by sticking to proven and authentic methods paves the way for genuine progress in pain management. Continuous education of health professionals, along with regular monitoring of pain management practices, thus forms a robust foundation for outstanding post-anesthesia care (Jayanth et al., 2025; Liu et al., 2025).

Optimal recovery for patients from anesthesia depends on the synthesis of a series of techniques rather than a formula. Instead of following a recipe, theater teams observe vital signs, communicate findings openly, and explain matters clearly to patients. Regular observation of things like heart rate or pain levels during the recovery phase means that the team can pick up on early warning signs or determine if a pain trick is working. Nowadays, increasingly more recovery protocols bring together a mix of different techniques - sometimes non-opioid pain medications, nerve blocks, or RA are combined—to manage pain and restrict on opioid use, which also averts negative side effects and other issues that still manifest in clinics today.

There is no single schedule fits all; who you are is an important factor in experiencing pain. Age, prior health issues, or even the nature of the procedure all play some part in affecting every patient's pain experience and reaction to pain relievers. It so happens that observing these details and crafting a plan just for that person works better. For example, noting that someone is already experiencing chronic pain or even anxiety can change the whole dynamic of what will and will not be effective.

This is why doctors, surgeons, nurses—and sometimes other experts—have to come together, adjusting their strategy as the situation evolves day by day. Finally, keeping up with new ideas and training is absolutely essential for any practitioner working with post-anesthesia treatment. Staying current with items such as adjuvant therapies, new twists on RA, and even looking over the latest pain assessment tools gives caregivers greater decision-making confidence. Most guidelines now suggest evaluating how pain care is going on a regular basis, which can lead to changes that keep care in a more dynamic state. Cumulatively, this commitment to ongoing learning not only enhances professional competency but also makes recovery a more relaxed, confident experience for patients, demonstrating how vital informed, evolving care is.

KEY TERMS FROM THIS CHAPTER

- Anesthesia intensive care units
- Enhanced recovery after surgery
- Monitoring gadgets
- Numeric rating scale
- Pain management
- Post-anesthesia care
- Anxiety
- Esketamine
- Non-opioid drugs
- Opioids
- Personal preferences
- Post-anesthesia care units

CRITICAL THINKING QUESTIONS

1. **The primary goal of monitoring in the post-anesthesia care unit (PACU) is to:**
   a. Detect and treat respiratory and cardiovascular complications
   b. Provide complete pain relief
   c. Monitor urine output and fluid balance
   d. Administer antibiotics
2. **The most common cause of airway obstruction in the immediate postoperative period is:**
   a. Laryngospasm
   b. Tongue falling back due to muscle relaxation
   c. Tracheal edema
   d. Aspiration
3. **Which of the following scales is commonly used to assess pain in the postoperative setting?**
   a. APGAR Score
   b. Visual Analog Scale (VAS)
   c. Glasgow Coma Scale (GCS)
   d. Modified Bromage Scale
4. **Which drug is commonly used for patient-controlled analgesia (PCA)?**
   a. Ibuprofen
   b. Morphine
   c. Acetaminophen
   d. Diazepam
5. **In patient-controlled analgesia (PCA), the primary advantage is:**
   a. Reduced need for nursing staff
   b. Improved patient satisfaction by allowing self-administration of analgesia
   c. Elimination of side effects from opioids
   d. Increased duration of pain relief

Short Answer Questions

1. What is post anesthesia care?
2. Why is pain management important?
3. Describe the role of post-anesthesia care units (PACUs).
4. What are the pain management strategies?
5. What are the challenges in post-anesthesia care?

Answers to Critical Thinking Questions

1. (a); 2. (b); 3. (b); 4. (b); 5. (b)

References

1. Angelini, E., Josefsson, C., Ögren, C., Andréll, P., Wolf, A., & Ringdal, M. (2025). Patients' experiences of TENS as a postoperative pain relief method in the post-anesthesia care unit after laparoscopic cholecystectomy: A qualitative study. *BMC Anesthesiology, 25*. https://www.semanticscholar.org/paper/355822190538d8f2a6aefdcc6b0359a9a4eda918 (accessed on 20 May 2025).
2. Bixio, M., Carenzo, L., Accurso, G., Balagna, R., Bazurro, S., Chiarini, G., Cortegiani, A., et al. (2024). Management of critically ill patients in austere environments: Good clinical practice by the Italian Society of Anesthesia, Analgesia, Resuscitation and Intensive Care (SIAARTI). *Journal of Anesthesia, Analgesia and Critical Care, 4*. https://www.semanticscholar.org/paper/9b202bcd64f43d07e5241da96b9324a623dc37f8 (accessed on 20 May 2025).
3. Borode, A. S., & Wadaskar, D. R. (2024). Navigating opioid alternatives in spine surgery: A comprehensive review. *Cureus, 16*. https://www.semanticscholar.org/paper/41e8aa169c56bcae1a541a41293686c64eff6db9 (accessed on 20 May 2025).
4. Br, J., Singh, K., Dumitru, R., Chan, E. Y., & Kim, M. P. (2018). The benefits of Enhanced Recovery After Surgery programs and their application in cardiothoracic surgery. *Methodist DeBakey Cardiovascular Journal, 14*(2), 77–77. https://doi.org/10.14797/mdcj-14-2-77.
5. Calkins, H., Hindricks, G., Cappato, R., Kim, Y. H., Saad, E., Aguinaga, L., Akar, J. G., et al. (2017a). 2017 HRS/EHRA/ECAS/APHRS/SOLAECE expert consensus statement on catheter and surgical ablation of atrial fibrillation: Executive summary. *Journal of Arrhythmia, 33*(4), 369–409. https://doi.org/10.1016/j.joa.2017.08.001.
6. Calkins, H., Hindricks, G., Cappato, R., Kim, Y. H., Saad, E., Aguinaga, L., Akar, J. G., et al. (2017b). 2017 HRS/EHRA/ECAS/APHRS/SOLAECE expert consensus statement on catheter and surgical ablation of atrial fibrillation: Executive summary. *EP Europace, 20*(1), 157–208. https://doi.org/10.1093/europace/eux275.
7. Casey, S. D., Hirsch, C. H., Mumma, B. E., Slee, et al. (2017). Emergency department pain management following implementation of a geriatric hip fracture program. https://core.ac.uk/download/323071629.pdf.
8. Fortier, M. A., Kain, Z. N., & Trinh, L. N. (2019). Primer on adult patient satisfaction in perioperative settings. *Core*. https://core.ac.uk/download/287622490.pdf.
9. Goyal, A., Sharma, P., Zaki, T., & Gohiya, S. (2025). To compare the analgesic efficacy of 0.25% bupivacaine and 0.25% ropivacaine in TAP block as a part of a multimodal analgesia regimen for post caesarean delivery pain management. *Global Journal for Research Analysis, 14*(3). https://doi.org/10.36106/gjra.
10. Grant, M. C., Suffredini, G., & Cho, B. C. (2021). Is it time to eliminate the use of opioids in cardiac surgery? *JTCVS Open, 7*, 247–252. https://doi.org/10.1016/j.xjon.2021.03.022.
11. Ismail, M. F. (2025). Opioid-sparing strategies in perioperative pain management: Current evidence, challenges, and future directions. *Asian Journal of Medicine and Health, 23*(2), 107–119. https://doi.org/10.9734/ajmah/2025/v23i21181.
12. Jayanth, T. B., Aithal, R. R., & Rao, S. T. (2025). A prospective clinical audit into the management of postoperative pain in the post anesthesia care unit of a tertiary care teaching hospital in Coastal Karnataka, India. *Annals of African Medicine*. https://www.semanticscholar.org/paper/82df8ff6482c80bedbb9b22d749d286f4b0fad62 (accessed on 20 May 2025).

13. Kaefer, C. T., Arboit, J., Dill, M. C. P., & Arboit, É. L. (2018). Perceptions about an instrument used for patients' evaluation and discharge from post-anesthesia care units / Percepções acerca de um instrumento para avaliação e alta da sala recuperação pós-anestésica. https://core.ac.uk/download/429988732.pdf (accessed on 20 May 2025).

14. Kamdar, N., & Jalilian, L. (2020). Telemedicine: A digital interface for perioperative anesthetic care. *Anesthesia & Analgesia, 130*, 272–275. https://doi.org/10.1213/ane.0000000000004513.

15. Kamel, B., Cyrine, K., & Hayene, M. (2024). Post-caesarean rehabilitation: Evaluation of practices. *Journal of Health and Rehabilitation Research, 4*(1), 1214–1218. https://doi.org/10.61919/jhrr.v4i1.439.

16. Karlsen, A. P. H., Tran, T. X. M., Mathiesen, O., Jakobsen, J. C., Meyhoff, C. S., Lunn, T. H., & Olsen, M. H. (2024). The OPI•AID Zone Tool as a composite outcome for postoperative pain management quality–A protocol for an observational pilot study. *Acta Anesthesiologic Scandinavica, 68*(7), 960–974. https://doi.org/10.1111/aas.14422.

17. Kendrick, C., Sliwinski, J., Yu, Y., Johnson, A., Fisher, W., Kekecs, Z., & Elkins, G. (2016). Hypnosis for acute procedural pain: A critical review. *The International Journal of Clinical and Experimental Hypnosis, 64*(1), 75–115. https://doi.org/10.1080/00207144.2015.1099405.

18. Kim, Y. D. (2025). Association between postoperative pain management and long-term patient outcomes. *Journal of the Korean Medical Association, 68*(1), 6–8. https://www.semanticscholar.org/paper/bb46f1c64120a483ad1dcee92e42e1a36acdd0fe (accessed on 20 May 2025).

19. Ley, E. J., Br, C. V. R., Moore, E. E., Sava, J., Peck, K. A., Ciesla, D. J., Sperry, J. L., et al. (2020). Updated guidelines to reduce venous thromboembolism in trauma patients: A Western Trauma Association critical decisions algorithm. *Journal of Trauma and Acute Care Surgery, 89*, 971–981. https://doi.org/10.1097/ta.0000000000002830.

20. Liu, C., Li, S., Zhou, J., Zhao, H., Zhou, R., Zhu, C., Chen, S., et al. (2025). Enhancing pain assessment among post-surgery patients at a tertiary hospital in China: A best practice implementation project. *Journal of Nursing Care Quality*. https://www.semanticscholar.org/paper/e6f4d29cd400bb2c8886a9bcb540d81b6a957557 (accessed on 20 May 2025).

21. Lucas, J., Gross, M., Yafi, F., El-Khatib, F., DeLay, K., & Simhan, J. (2019). PD44-02 A multi-institutional assessment of multimodal analgesia in penile implant recipients demonstrates dramatic narcotics reduction. *The Journal of Urology, 201*, e821. https://www.semanticscholar.org/paper/fa4a1dfd493f1a83c3d7d1c2f48324012d4ba131 (accessed on 20 May 2025).

22. Lv, S., Sun, N., Hao, C., Li, J., & Li, Y. (2025). Development and validation of machine learning models for predicting post-cesarean pain and individualized pain management strategies: A multicenter study. *BMC Anesthesiology, 25*. https://www.semanticscholar.org/paper/81a8ea8cbef8cdb8d0b8825832998a2930079bc3 (accessed on 20 May 2025).

23. Nelson, G., Bakkum-Gamez, J. N., Kalogera, E., Glaser, G., Altman, A. D., Meyer, L. A., Taylor, J., et al. (2019). Guidelines for perioperative care in gynecologic/oncology: Enhanced Recovery After Surgery (ERAS) Society recommendations—2019 update. *International Journal of Gynecological Cancer, 29*(5), 651–668. https://doi.org/10.1136/ijgc-2019-000356.

24. Overman, S. (2021). Integrated team assessment and patient perspective pain paradigm in primary pain care pain management: A new language for provider-provider and provider patient communication. *International Journal of Integrated Care, 20*, 31. https://www.

semanticscholar.org/paper/9c2ae19c2ba8feef8cd66179f331e7677abdf2c2 (accessed on 20 May 2025).

25. Patel, S., & Raymond, B. (2025). Interactions between anesthesia and sleep: Optimizing perioperative care to improve sleep quality and surgical recovery outcomes. *Cureus, 17.* https://www.semanticscholar.org/paper/143dc86e0c82a8147255338d89bccadaacf4ba4f (accessed on 20 May 2025).

26. Raja, J., Parmar, D., Subramaniam, S. D., Nagella, S. P., Pappulwar, S. M., Mehlawat, R., & Maini, A. (2025). Anxiety and pain management in dental patients: A systematic review of pharmacological and non-pharmacological approaches. *Journal of Pharmacy and Bioallied Sciences.* https://www.semanticscholar.org/paper/7bd514d588d36e550c4118f5129b16d9e1f9e236 (accessed on 20 May 2025).

27. Rauta, S. (2019). Nursing intensity and nurse staffing in perioperative settings. https://core.ac.uk/download/198017163.pdf (accessed on 20 May 2025).

28. Rifat, M., Nahiduzzaman, N., Haque, M., & Azad, M. (2024). A retrospective study on the post-operative complications of bipolar diathermy tonsillectomy in a rural setting of Bangladesh. *Annals of International Medical and Dental Research, 10*, 142–150. https://doi.org/10.53339/aimdr.2024.10.1.17.

29. Ruiz González, S., López Rico, T., Arribas Arauzo, E., García Prieto, J., & Albornos Muñoz, L. (2025). Improving post-operative pain management after total hip and knee replacement in a special care unit: A best practice implementation project. *JBI Evidence Implementation.* https://www.semanticscholar.org/paper/c64505f651d857931749c611fbfbd5206f4760c9 (accessed on 20 May 2025).

30. Sabu, N., Raipure, A., Balasubramanian, B., & Thappa, P. (2024). Treading on thin ice: Anesthesia management of a neonate with Pierre Robin sequence for feeding gastrostomy and diagnostic bronchoscopy–A case report. *Journal of Neonatal Critical Care and Anesthesia.* https://www.semanticscholar.org/paper/d6b72048eb63399d0e2bf66a89bd30289f5a17af (accessed on 20 May 2025).

31. Schwenk, E. S., & Mariano, E. R. (2018). Designing the ideal perioperative pain management plan starts with multimodal analgesia. *Korean Journal of Anesthesiology, 71*(5), 345–352. https://doi.org/10.4097/kja.d.18.00217.

32. Schwenk, E. S., Pozek, J. J., & Viscusi, E. R. (2018). Managing prolonged pain after surgery: Examining the role of opioids. *The Journal of Arthroplasty, 33*(11), 3389–3393. https://doi.org/10.1016/j.arth.2018.08.005.

33. Silow-Carroll, S., & Lashbrook, A. (2009). *St. Charles Hospital: Improving Surgical Care Through Best-Practice Literature and Order Sets.* The Commonwealth Fund.

34. Sivakumar, S., Kressel, A., Mendonca, R., & Girshin, M. (2024). Battle of the blocks: Which pain management technique triumphs in gender-affirming bilateral mastectomies? *Journal of Clinical Medicine Research, 16*, 284–292. https://www.semanticscholar.org/paper/0decde4257af19543f4fc08b1956ff91192d7119 (accessed on 20 May 2025).

35. Stout, K., Daniels, C. J., Aboulhosn, J., Bozkurt, B., Broberg, C. S., Colman, J. M., Crumb, S. R., et al. (2018). 2018 AHA/ACC guideline for the management of adults with congenital heart disease: A report of the American College of Cardiology/American Heart Association Task Force on Clinical Practice Guidelines. *Circulation, 139.* https://doi.org/10.1161/cir.0000000000000603.

36. von Ungern-Sternberg, B. S., Sommerfield, D., Slevin, L., Drake-Brockman, T. F. E., Zhang, G., & Hall, G. L. (2019). Effect of albuterol premedication vs placebo on the occurrence of respiratory adverse events in children undergoing tonsillectomies. *JAMA Pediatrics, 173*, 527. https://doi.org/10.1001/jamapediatrics.2019.0788.

37. Weekes, D. G., Wicks, E. D., Campbell, R. E., Hadley, C. J., Carter, A., Chaudhry, Z. S., Pepe, M., et al. (2019). Do relaxation exercises decrease postoperative pain after rotator cuff repair? A randomized controlled trial. *Orthopedic Journal of Sports Medicine, 7*. https://www.semanticscholar.org/paper/3a5ea8c0008160ae3dcf911c0e55acb4481f2a6f (accessed on 20 May 2025).

38. Wenzel, J. T., Schwenk, E. S., Baratta, J. L., & Viscusi, E. R. (2016). Managing opioid-tolerant patients in the perioperative surgical home. *Anesthesiology Clinics, 34*(2), 287–301. https://doi.org/10.1016/j.anclin.2016.01.005.

39. Youssef, H. A., Abdel-Ghaffar, H. S., Mostafa, M. F., Abbas, Y. H., Mahmoud, A. O., & Herdan, R. A. (2021). Sphenopalatine ganglion versus greater occipital nerve blocks in treating post-dural puncture headache after spinal anesthesia for cesarean section: A randomized clinical trial. *Pain Physician, 24*(4), E443–E451. https://www.semanticscholar.org/paper/bd82e8bb1a05298ba142cbf747c63f6e3c0a8153 (accessed on 2025).

40. Zakeri, H., Mahtosh, P., Radmehr, M., Rahbani, R., Montazeri, L., Moalemi, S., Mahdiyar, P., et al. (2024). Pain management strategies in intensive care unit: Challenges and best practice. *Galen Medical Journal, 13*. https://www.semanticscholar.org/paper/433d730667138f05d7b82b2fb2afc1ede8c0c115 (accessed on 20 May 2025).

41. Zhang, Q., Tang, H., Yao, Z., & Han, W. (2023). The construction of patient quality management model in oral post anesthesia care unit in China: A grounded theory approach. *BMC Anesthesiology, 23*. https://www.semanticscholar.org/paper/fa39775483f631fc5e79734d5e8bf0a1e477c1d8 (accessed on 20 May 2025).

ANESTHETIC COMPLICATIONS

15

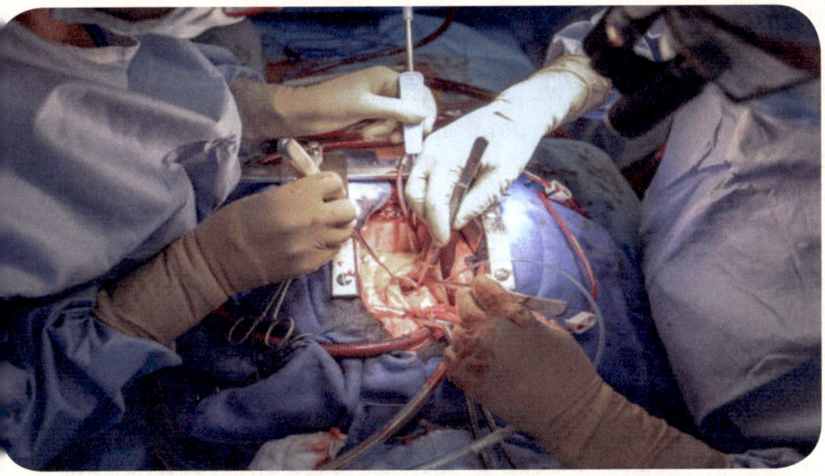

LEARNING OBJECTIVES

After studying this chapter, you will be able to:

1. Learn about common anesthetic complications.
2. Understand the risk factors for anesthetic complications.
3. Understand the prevention strategies of anesthetic complications.
4. Discuss on management of anesthetic complications.

Introduction

Anesthesia is complex; you need to know what each drug does during surgery. New sedatives like dexmedetomidine (DEX) are changing the landscape, especially when dealing with sick patients. Current studies show that these drugs help to calm the nerves, ease the passage into surgery, and even guide outcomes in measurable ways. However, when it comes to elderly patients they need extra care – they're more likely, in most circumstances, to develop complications. We might not have all the data on side effects for this group, but current research still points out that safety profiles differ between sedatives, and it becomes clear that treatments need to fit each patient's particular state of health (Paschoal et al., 2025). Doctors are constantly adapting anesthesia techniques; it's crucial to know how these sedatives move and work in the body. Elderly people, with their physical quirks and other complicating conditions, only add to the puzzle. Some studies stress that it's not just a question of how effectively a sedative works, but also of keeping an eye out for side effects, especially in the more vulnerable. Reports even suggest that choosing a sedative entails trial of its effect on heart and lungs - which in the elderly can be unstable. In brief, research and sensible, practical judgment need to combine in the process of choosing an apt sedative (Paschoal et al., 2025). New approaches to anesthesia are also spoken of, ones that may improve care for older persons. For example, the use of evidence-based protocols can regulate sedative use for patients of different ages, keeping complications at a minimum. There is a big push for additional training in geriatric anesthesia - for sure, the subtleties do make a difference when working with older individuals. Through methods that emphasize patient safety, medical practitioners can reduce risks connected with anesthesia and give elders the utmost care they can during operations. Ultimately, conformity to up-to-date research and a commitment to education should make anesthesia procedures safer, blending positive outcomes with a candid understanding of each patient's needs (Figure 15.1).

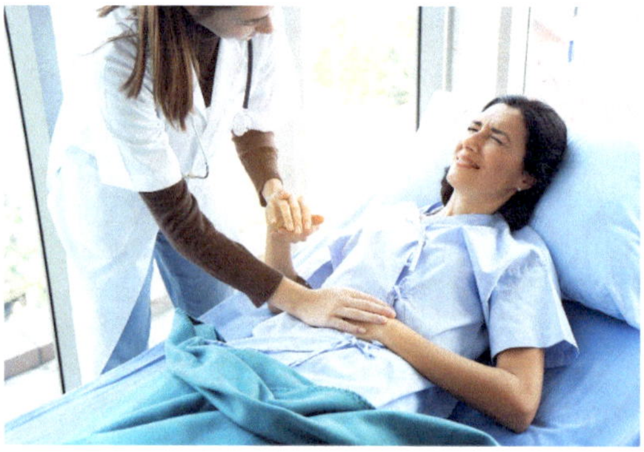

Figure 15.1. Anesthetic Complications.

Source: https://twincitiespainclinic.com/wp-content/uploads/2022/12/Dark-haired-female-wincing-in-pain-while-lying-in-a-hospital-bed-and-being-attended-to-by-a-doctor.jpg.

Definition of Anesthetics

Anesthetics play a crucial role in preventing pain and controlling complications during the process of performing medical procedures. They're drugs that knock you out or numb an area, making it possible for doctors to work on you without injuring you. Practically, you learn about two categories: one that puts your whole body out, general anesthetics, and the other that just numbs an isolated area, local anesthetics.

Which of the two will be used most frequently will be based upon the nature of the procedure, what have been the patient's past medical issues, and how these drugs might interact with any other medication. A pre-op checkup is, in most cases, a necessity. While we can trust that anesthetics are safe, things do sometimes go wrong. Sometimes the reaction is as benign as headache or nausea, but sometimes more severe side effects like cardiac complications or respiratory distress can occur. Children, for example, need special precautions when sedation is to be given to them; strict vital sign monitoring is just required. Professional organizations have offered safety measures—like conducting a pre-sedation evaluation and choosing patients carefully (Coté et al., 2019)—and these guidelines highlight just how crucial monitoring of drug actions and effects is along the way. In addition to the physical issues, anesthetic selection and management can raise ethical and clinical concerns, particularly in complex cases. Evidence-informed policies guide doctors to balance the benefits with the drawbacks in a general sense, and to promote a team-based approach where the patient's care is specialized to the individual case. The American Society of Colon and Rectal Surgeons, for instance, sees that reaching a consensus that stems from sound, research-based recommendations is crucial (Davis et al., 2018). By combining tried and true protocols with practice refinements that keep coming, the medical community is still working to minimize complications and ensure that pain gets dealt with appropriately—sometimes with a little trial and error added in along the way (Figure 15.2).

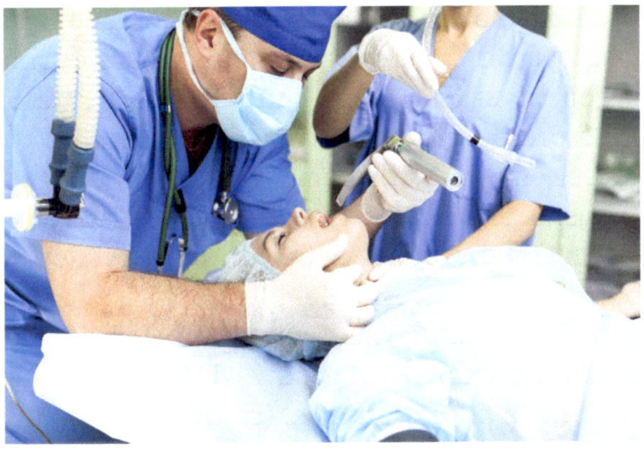

Figure 15.2. Anesthetics.

Source: https://external-content.duckduckgo.com/iu/?u=http%3A%2F%2Fphotos.demandstudios.com%2Fgetty%2Farticle%2F99%2F128%2F489120943.jpg&f=1&nofb=1&ipt=aec71f49c5433500272a744ace3be7dfbca4d513712c36868c4833bbf9fc115f.

Importance of Understanding Complications

Anesthesia is a fine art; it always tries to walk the thin line between working well and safeguarding patients. Complications can result from a whole range of reasons, and for everyone who is giving anesthesia, knowing these traps inside and out is necessary to catch trouble early and moving promptly. Take, for example, local anesthetic systemic toxicity (LAST)—it usually signals itself with neurologic issues, but every now and again it surprises you by having unexplained cardiovascular spasms. Doctors who pay attention to these varied signs are able to come up with strategies that reduce on the risks involved in anesthetic use. Being in the loop about what causes LAST means they can depend on methods like ultrasound-guided injections and close monitoring of doses to avoid what can be a life-threatening condition, which goes some way to show that knowing your way around things can really make a difference to patient care (El Boghdadly et al., 2018). The field of anesthetics isn't simple either. Generally speaking, it means having to acquire both the pros and the cons. For instance, the typical individual will remember ketamine as simply that drug causing dissociation, but it also has adverse effects that render it problematic to administer in the clinic. The practitioners have to watch for cognitive stumblings or even psychomimetic responses—issues that can affect immediate safety and recovery potential in the long term. Taking a closer examination of the way ketamine is metabolized by the body and exactly what it does is going to make the practitioners more in charge of its use. Frequently, even taking this closer examination brings with it the potential for trying other therapies that can bring the same benefit without all the added baggage (Zanos et al., 2018). Finally, having a solid understanding of the pitfalls of anesthesia is not some theoretical idea—its a real game-saver when it comes to patient safety and overall quality of care. If healthcare providers are aware of these dangers, it's easier for them to see if something is going to go wrong and to respond before disaster strikes, based on evidence-based practice. Remaining up to speed with the latest research in this area also fosters a culture of continuous learning, which is comparatively necessary given all the new challenges that continually seem to be emerging. This new knowledge can even lead to modifications to anesthesiologist procedures and education, ultimately impacting patient outcomes for a wide range of surgeries. Short answer: truly understanding these complications is not an option; it's just part of delivering safe, effective anesthesia care—when things aren't always perfectly planned, that is.

15.1. Common Anesthetic Complications

Learning Outcome

1. Understand the allergic reactions in anesthesia.
2. Describe the respiratory complications and cardiovascular complications.

Anesthetic procedures can be a bit finicky—unexpected issues sometimes pop up that clearly affect how well patients bounce back and how they feel about their overall care. Postoperative pain, for example, is a pretty common hiccup; it often stems from minor nerve irritation during surgery (knee arthroscopy being one case in point). Generally speaking, the way we handle pain relief matters a lot. One study compared intra-articular local anesthetic infiltration with an ultrasound-guided adductor canal block; interestingly, the latter often gave better results in terms of pain control and patient satisfaction (Hefni et al., 2023). This kind of evidence nudges clinicians to think hard about using effective pain management strategies, even if it means being a bit more creative with their approach. There's also the issue of neuromuscular complications, which—let's be honest—can be a serious worry. Spinal anesthesia (SA) is favored for its reliability, but it isn't completely risk-free; adding something like Butorphanol to local anesthetics can, in most cases, ramp up pain relief and even stabilize blood pressure a bit better, thus reducing risks like hypotension or a motor blockade lasting too long (Garg et al., 2022). Sometimes mixing and matching the right agents, along with subtle alters in dosing and careful monitoring, makes a difference; it kind of reminds you that a little extra caution goes a long way when it comes to patient comfort. Then you have cardiovascular complications that might crop up during anesthetic administration—especially when agents such as bupivacaine are involved. Cardiac toxicity may be rare, but it is no small matter for patient safety. Keeping a close eye on hemodynamic parameters during surgery is crucial since shifts in heart rate or blood pressure can subtly signal something off. Studies, albeit with some variability, suggest that using levobupivacaine instead of its racemic cousin might offer a better cardiovascular profile with fewer side effects (Garg et al., 2022). To summarize, when you personalize anesthetic choices and stay vigilant, you not only anticipate potential complications but also tailor the approach to suit each patient's needs—something that can tip the scales toward a smoother recovery (Figure 15.3).

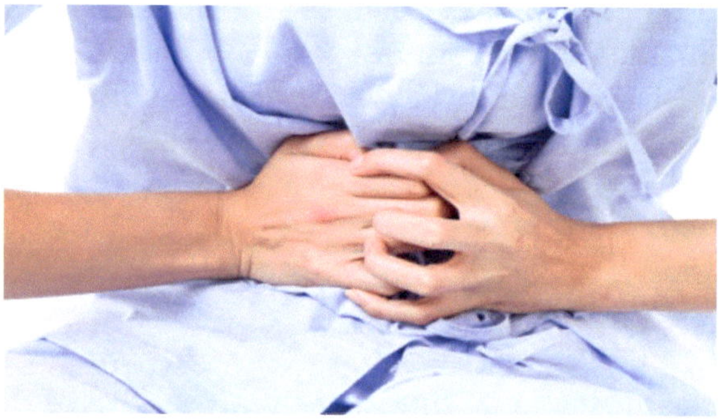

Figure 15.3. Postoperative pain.

Source: https://www.clinicalpainadvisor.com/wp-content/uploads/sites/15/2019/01/thinkstockphotos513110688pos_964277.jpg.

15.1.1. Allergic Reactions

Allergic reactions in anesthesia aren't just an oddity – they can upend a surgery when you least expect it. Sometimes you get nothing more than a bothersome rash or a bit of itching, but other times it ramps up to full-blown anaphylaxis, which puts patient safety on edge. It turns out these responses often boil down to intricate immune triggers fired up by the anesthetic agents, so clinicians have to keep a close watch. For example, even though allergic responses to local anesthetics show up pretty rarely, they still mean that surgical teams need to stay extra alert. Patients with a history of sensitivities or an atopic background tend to be more at risk, so going over their history in detail isn't just a nice idea—it's often essential. Recording any previous allergic events can reduce repeat issues and make sure the right steps are taken during anesthesia administration, especially in higher-risk cases (Islam et al., 2024). Tech improvements in anesthetic techniques have upped the safety game for lots of agents, yet the possibility of an allergic reaction is still there. New options – whether inhaled or given intravenously – have reshaped the landscape of anesthesia in ways we might not have expected. In most cases, serious reactions have become less common over time; still, the unpredictable behavior of these allergies means each patient needs individual care. Doctors, for instance, are encouraged to tread carefully when testing novel agents or when handling patients known to have allergies. A thorough preoperative review coupled with ready-to-go plans for managing allergic episodes can make a big difference in outcomes. Also, continual studies into genetic clues behind these sensitivities may lead to more personalized anesthetic strategies, which could further reduce the risks during surgeries (Dalamagka, 2024). After an operation, keeping an eye out for allergy signs remains crucial – sometimes issues crop up several hours or even days after the anesthetic is given. Late-onset symptoms like urticaria or respiratory troubles can throw a wrench in recovery if they aren't caught quickly. It's important for healthcare folks to be on guard not just for standard side effects like nausea and vomiting but also for these unpredictable allergic reactions. Teaching patients about what to watch for empowers them to speak up when something seems off. Simple, clear communication channels and pre-planned responses to allergic events can help lower the risks. As medical practices continue to shift and grow, the ongoing need for training and research on spotting and managing allergic reactions remains as pressing as ever (Rahib et al., 2024) (Figure 15.4).

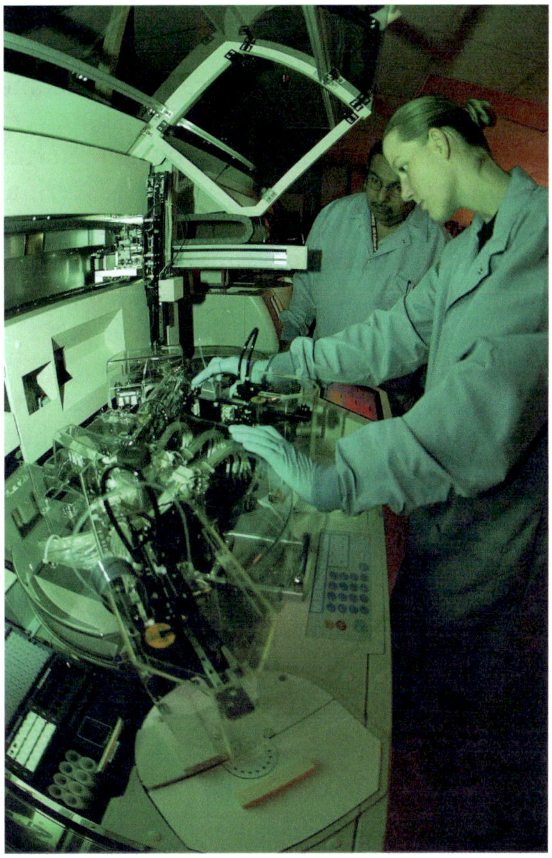

Figure 15.4. Allergic reactions.

Source: By U.S. Air Force photo/Senior Airman Erin M. Peterson - USAF Photographic Archives (image permalink), Public Domain, https://commons.wikimedia.org/w/index.php?curid=3292807.

15.1.2. Respiratory Complications

Anesthesia plays a huge role in surgeries, even though it comes with its set of breathing risks. When patients wake up, they can show signs of airway problems like aspiration or blockage—issues that seem to pop up more often in kids because their lungs and air passages are still developing. The type of anesthetic used can change how fast these reflexes bounce back; for instance, some studies suggest sevoflurane might help airway reflexes return more quickly than isoflurane, reducing the time between taking out the breathing tube and getting those protections back (Rasool et al., 2025). During recovery, keeping an eye on breathing becomes vital to ward off any problems from poor airway management. Delaying the return of normal breathing after anesthesia can have serious, sometimes even dangerous, effects—especially in patients with pre-existing conditions. Kids with congenital issues like D syndrome face extra challenges due to the differences in their anatomy, which can make them more likely to experience breathing distress after surgery. It's important to adjust anesthetic care to these special needs. Strategies such as the Enhance Recovery After Surgery (ERAS) protocol are showing promise by mixing various pain management techniques and careful fluid control to ease the recovery process (Lucía et al., 2024).

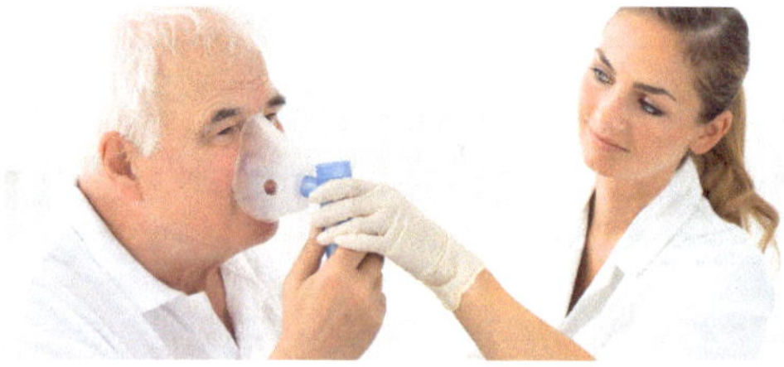

Figure 15.5. Post-surgery respiratory complications.

Source: https://www.hearthugger.com/sites/default/files/image-uploads/nurse-helps-patient-with-oxygen-mask.jpg.

In most cases, reducing surgical stress is key, as too much stress can further impair respiratory function after surgery. The kind of anesthesia and even the intubation method used can seriously shape a patient's breathing outcome. Sometimes, rapid sequence intubation is chosen—especially in emergencies or with patients known to have gastroparesis—to lower the risk of aspiration. A thorough check before surgery, looking at things like lung function and oxygen levels, is essential for crafting a tailored anesthetic plan. Different techniques have been seen to impact how breathing recovers postoperatively, showing that a one-size-fits-all approach just doesn't work (Rasool et al., 2025). Ultimately, working together with a team, planning carefully, monitoring vigilantly, and managing things effectively goes a long way toward keeping anesthesia-related breathing issues to a minimum and improving overall patient care (Figure 15.5).

15.1.3. Cardiovascular Complications

Cardiovascular issues can suddenly pop up during surgery and mess with how things turn out. Anesthesia may throw off the blood flow—especially for people with existing heart troubles—even when you think everything's under control. Take, for example, doing a total endovascular aortic arch repair; this is a procedure that, while aiming to fix things, can bring along sudden kidney stress and brain complications, among other risks. Surgeons and anesthesiologists often end up working side-by-side, checking every patient's unique risks (and yes, sometimes rechecking them) by weighing both the surgical plan and any anesthesia quirks. Each case gets its plan, mixing in pre-surgery heart checks to help steer outcomes right (Martins et al., 2024). Patient positioning is another factor that can sneak up and cause issues. A recent study shows that patients who end up sitting during surgery tend to hit snags like lower blood pressure and other anesthesia troubles, whereas those in the so-called park-bench position seem to fare better (Radu et al., 2024). In cases like neurosurgery or complex heart interventions, it turns out the way you set up the patient can be just as important as the procedure itself. The idea here is simple in most cases: fine-tune your monitoring and anesthesia tricks to the patient's position, and you might just dodge some heart-related hiccups along the way. Bringing it all together, the mix between how anesthesia is managed and how the heart holds up is a bit like a dance that never quite follows a set routine. Anesthesiologists stay on their toes, constantly watching for any sudden changes, and adjusting their approach as needed to keep risks in check. At the same time, keeping an eye on how patients are positioned—and getting input from all sides of the team—seems to boost overall safety. In most cases, staying flexible and working together means that even when challenges pop up, patient care stays a step ahead, ensuring that heart complications don't steal the spotlight from a successful surgery (Radu et al., 2024) (Figure 15.6).

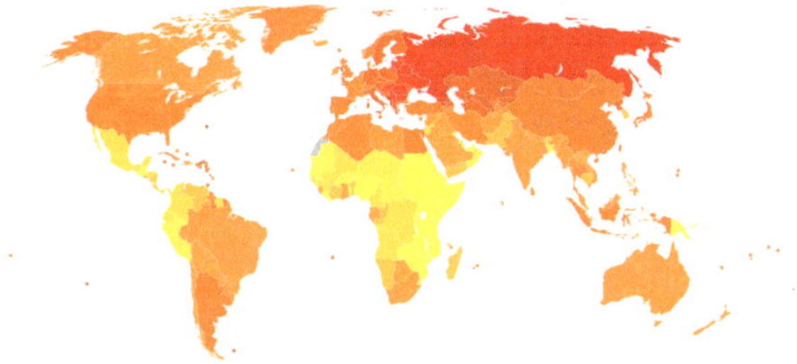

Figure 15.6. Cardiovascular complications.

Source: By Chris55 - Data from World Health Organization Estimated Deaths 2012 Vector map from BlankMap-World6, compact.svg by Canuckguy et al., CC BY-SA 4.0, https://commons.wikimedia.org/w/index.php?curid=50287978.

Test Your Knowledge

1. What are the most common allergic reactions in anesthesia?
2. What are the common respiratory complications?

15.2. Risk Factors for Anesthetic Complications

Learning Outcome

1. Understand the patient health history.
2. Describe the type of surgery.
3. Understand the anesthetic technique used.

Patients come into surgery with many different things that can bump up the risks when using anesthesia, so doctors typically check everything out thoroughly before getting started. Age, for instance, is a big deal—older patients often have extra health problems like heart or lung issues that may complicate how anesthesia works. Obesity, too, can stir up breathing problems and might even lead to more issues after surgery. Sometimes, if someone already has challenges like low blood pressure or wobbly heart rhythms, things can get tricky and close observation becomes necessary. In many cases, the anesthesia plan ends up being custom-fit to deal with each patient's unique risks; tailoring treatment this way is pretty important to help lower the chance of difficulties and boost overall safety during surgery. Another layer of complexity is the patient's overall health, especially when it comes to their heart and lungs. People with conditions like pulmonary hypertension (PH) face a higher risk for events while under anesthesia—generally speaking, this means a more detailed game plan is needed while the surgery is happening. With better treatments these days, more folks with PH are making it to surgery, so anesthesiologists have to be on their toes managing these intricate cases. Understanding how PH can be broken down into different types and recognizing related risk factors lets clinicians come up with a plan that might sidestep some complications. This whole process usually means doctors from various specialties pooling their expertise together to keep circulation steady, reduce risks, and deal with any issues that pop up along the way, as noted in recent studies (Seo et al., 2019). The way the surgery itself is done, along with choices about anesthesia, can also add to the potential for trouble. Take thoracic surgeries like lung resection—here, specialized techniques can require extra care to ward off lung complications. Sometimes, simply adjusting the way a patient is ventilated or keeping the operation shorter can make a noticeable difference in recovery. In most cases, research points out that protective ventilation strategies help reduce lung injury overall, even if dealing with one-lung ventilation isn't always straightforward (Lederman et al., 2019). As surgical methods keep evolving, so too must the approaches to anesthesia, with a focus on speeding up recovery and keeping complications at bay. To summarize, by mixing up the latest research with everyday sense, healthcare teams can work toward better patient outcomes and minimize many of the downsides that sometimes come with anesthesia.

15.2.1. Patient Health History

A patient's past health is often where things start to go awry with anesthesia. Rather than simply ticking boxes, providers dig into details like old medical issues, earlier surgeries, and the meds someone's taken over the years. Certain conditions can shift how the body handles anesthetic drugs. Sometimes, especially with older adults or those juggling several problems, the mix of past ailments calls for extra attention. In most cases, tying a full health history into planning isn't just useful—it's downright necessary for keeping risks low (Argo et al., 2019). Every person's unique makeup means that one standard approach just won't do. Their history, which might include a rough reaction to anesthesia before or even stuff that runs in the family, pushes the team to craft more personalized plans. For example, if someone has had breathing troubles, the team might lean toward extra careful airway management, aiming to dodge ventilation issues. Looking back on past surgeries can also hint at how well a patient might handle anesthesia now, and sometimes it even warns of surprises later. Without these thoughtful checks, providers can end up ramping up the risk during surgery (Henshaw et al., 2017). Beyond just the immediate concerns, the way anesthesia evolves nowadays rests a lot on understanding this connection between health history and outcomes. As perioperative care generally marches forward, the push for quality control means that detailed patient backgrounds are front and center.

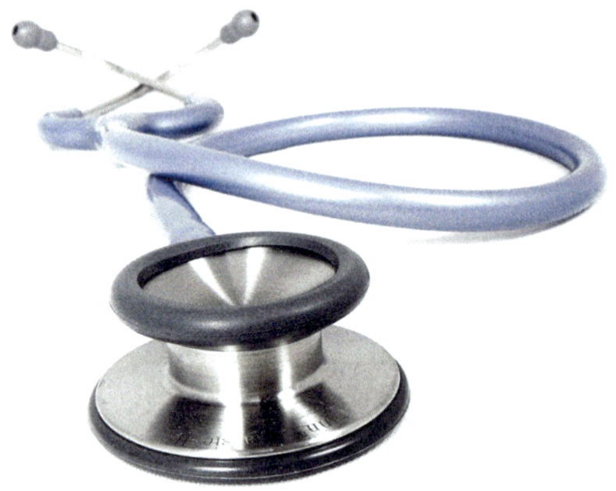

Figure 15.7. Patient health history.

Source: By Stethoscopes - Own work, CC BY-SA 3.0, https://commons.wikimedia.org/w/index.php?curid=4540865.

A thorough pre-op check might even reveal that a regional approach fits a patient better than a full-blown general anesthetic, reducing the chance of complications. Ongoing monitoring of how patients fare after anesthesia plays a key role in trimming preventable errors, and in most cases, knowing a patient's story doesn't just guide anesthetic decisions—it lifts the whole quality of surgical care (Argo et al., 2019) (Figure 15.7).

15.2.2. Type of Surgery

Surgical interventions come in all shapes and sizes, and each one brings its anesthesia puzzles. Take open procedures like posterior component separation (PCS) for example – these operations are big and often call for advanced techniques like thoracic epidural analgesia (TEA). TEA can help ease pain after surgery, though people still argue whether it speeds up recovery. One study even pointed out that when systemic opioids aren't used, TEA might help the bowels get back to normal sooner (Henshaw et al., 2017); however, when mixed with opioids, the extra benefit just doesn't show up. These kinds of results make it clear that how we handle anesthesia depends on the kind of surgery and the patient's specific needs. Surgery for skin tumor removals is usually pretty straightforward, but those procedures aren't without their anesthesia twists either. Sometimes a simple local infiltration does the job, while at other times a nerve block might be a better bet. Studies generally suggest that although both local infiltration and nerve blocks can manage pain just fine, nerve blocks might give a little extra comfort during the operation and reduce on risks from larger cuts (Arrico et al., 2018). This kind of difference shows that the type of surgery itself plays a big role in deciding which anesthesia to use and what complications might pop up. It's a reminder that surgeons and anesthesia experts do need to talk through these details together. At the same time, the choice of anesthesia needs to match how demanding the surgery is expected to be. Longer, more intense operations like PCS, with lots of tissue work, naturally increase the chances of issues such as breathing problems or a longer recovery period. Some studies even show that by fine-tuning pain relief – say, sticking with pure TEA – the time patients spend in the hospital afterward can be shortened (Henshaw et al., 2017). In most cases, adjusting anesthesia to fit the surgery not only helps keep patients more comfortable but might also lower the chance of complications. All of this points to the importance of knowing the ins and outs of each surgical procedure when planning the best anesthesia approach (Figure 15.8).

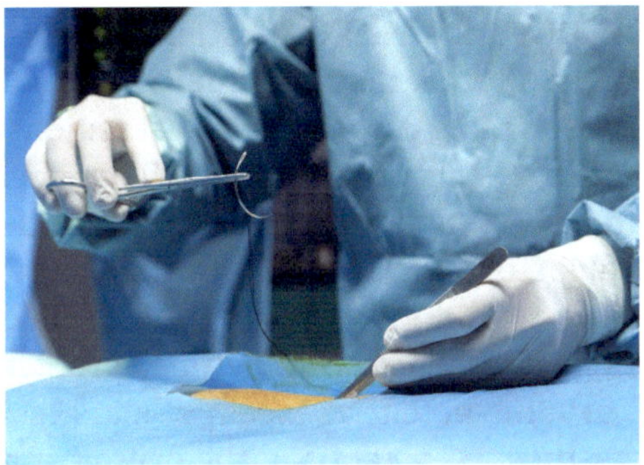

Figure 15.8. Type of surgery.

Source: https://www.addmoretolives.com/wp-content/uploads/2022/12/surgical-procedure-made-by-doctor-scaled.jpg.

15.2.3. Anesthetic Technique Used

Anesthesia has long been at the heart of surgical care – its many subtle details can shape how well a patient recovers. In outpatient settings, choosing the right local anesthetic isn't just routine; it's a careful balancing act intended to boost comfort and reduce on complications. Take, say, the debate over using the H-block versus the V-block for ingrown toenail removal. Research generally shows that the V-block kicks in quickly and does a solid job on routine pain relief, while the H-block sometimes offers a more sustained, even rounded, effect in tougher cases. This goes to show that anesthetic methods need to be tailored to the unique demands of each surgical situation (Farooqi et al., 2024). Nowadays, as techniques evolve, there's a growing focus on various sedative approaches, especially when it comes to ambulatory surgeries. The choice between mixing local anesthesia with a bit of sedation or opting for full-on general anesthesia (GA) often boils down to the complexity of the procedure and some pretty individual patient factors. This nuanced decision-making is particularly crucial in ENT procedures – airway management is tricky when anatomical considerations overlap, for example. Modern agents like propofol and remifentanil have, in most cases, improved recovery times and even helped lower the risk of postoperative issues such as respiratory distress (Shetti, 2024). Then there's the whole preoperative assessment side of things. It isn't only the anesthetic method that matters; understanding each patient's medical history and any extra health challenges is equally vital. By using a tailored evaluation approach, clinicians can sometimes predict and work around potential hiccups, making both the anesthesia's impact and the overall surgery run more smoothly. To summarize, combining the right anesthetic technique with a clear, comprehensive look at each patient's situation tends to cut complications and boost surgical success (Figure 15.9).

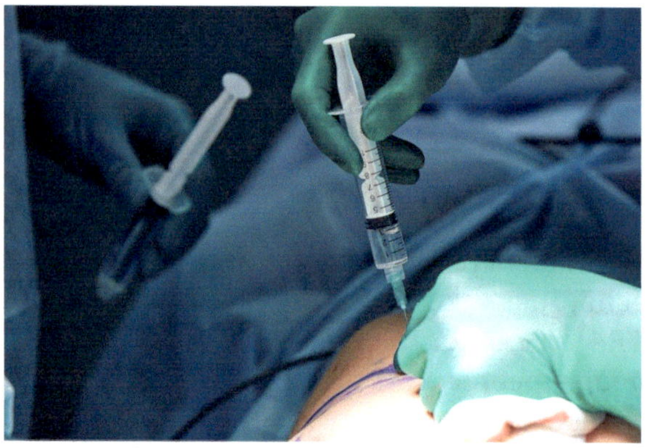

Figure 15.9. Anesthetic Technique.

Source: https://philadelphiaanesthesiaservices.com/wp-content/uploads/2024/11/fieldblock.jpg.

Test Your Knowledge

1. Describe the patient health history.
2. List the type of surgery.

15.3. Prevention Strategies

Learning Outcome

1. Perform preoperative assessment.
2. Monitor during anesthesia.
3. Describe the postoperative care.

Anesthetic mishaps come in many shapes and sizes, and handling them means tackling problems from all sides. A big piece of the puzzle is setting up quality control measures around the time of surgery. Generally speaking, even though deaths from these issues have dropped over the years, preventable losses still happen—often because of bad drug reactions or not managing patient conditions well enough (Argo et al., 2019). Tightening up how patients get checked before and during anesthesia, for example, cuts risks by a fair margin. Thorough pre-surgery tests and getting the patient in the best possible shape go a long way in stopping problems before they start. New tech is another game changer in this area. Tools like telemedicine decision support systems have begun to shift the whole approach, and a standout example is the Anesthesiology Control Tower (ACT), which watches over things in real-time. With ACT in place, clinicians get guidance based on a solid mix of live data (Gregory et al., 2018). This setup deals not only with things like blood sugar and body temperature during a procedure, but it also steps in to help manage issues like drops in blood pressure and breathing troubles after the operation. In most cases, leaning on technology in this way has boosted overall safety and shown just how important innovative support can be. Keeping skills fresh is yet another key factor. Continuous learning for anesthesiologists and the whole team builds a culture that values safety above all. Regular simulations, workshops, and crisis drills—especially in dealing with airway problems and drug mishaps (Argo et al., 2019)—help sharpen vital skills. It's important too to foster an environment where mistakes can be openly discussed and learned from, even if that means a few awkward moments here and there. This honest dialogue not only helps everyone remember the best practices but also cements a strong commitment to top-notch patient care, which ultimately brings down the number of anesthetic complications in real-world settings.

15.3.1. Preoperative Assessment

A strong preoperative check can make all the difference in surgery. Often, it starts with more than a simple review of a patient's history—it's about spotting little risk factors that might otherwise be missed. In many cases doctors look into known conditions like heart or lung troubles to fine-tune the anesthesia plan for each person. Sometimes, the careful eye that catches these details early on ends up reducing post-surgery complications and even boosting overall patient satisfaction. It even sets up room for planning out pain management because, quite frankly, uncontrolled pain just invites more trouble (Wenzel et al., 2016). There's also the whole angle of adding in drug strategies before the procedure. Generally speaking, giving preoperative dexamethasone, for example, tends to ease the body's inflammatory response after surgery. This approach has shown that by lowering signs like the systemic inflammatory response (SIR) — often seen in operations such as those for colorectal cancer — patients can avoid a host of subsequent issues. A deep dive into a patient's specific situation lets doctors figure out just how effective and safe a drug might be for them. In several studies, such targeted use of dexamethasone has led to notable drops in high C-reactive protein levels as well as the overall rate of post-surgery hiccups (Horgan et al., 2017). This underscores that thorough assessments can open the door to extra therapies that boost recovery and trim anesthesia risks. And then there's the chat with the patient. A preoperative check isn't all about clinical numbers; it also involves making sure patients understand what's coming. Explaining the surgical process, the risks involved and why sticking to the pre-op routines matters can help a lot in getting patients mentally ready. Sometimes, the conversation isn't perfectly polished—but those small, human touches encourage patients to speak up, ask questions, and feel more involved in their care. This back-and-forth not only clears up any confusion but may also help lower the chance of surprises later on (Horgan et al., 2017; Wenzel et al., 2016). Overall, by blending clear explanations with a bit of genuine dialogue, preoperative assessments help pave the way for smoother, safer surgeries (Figure 15.10).

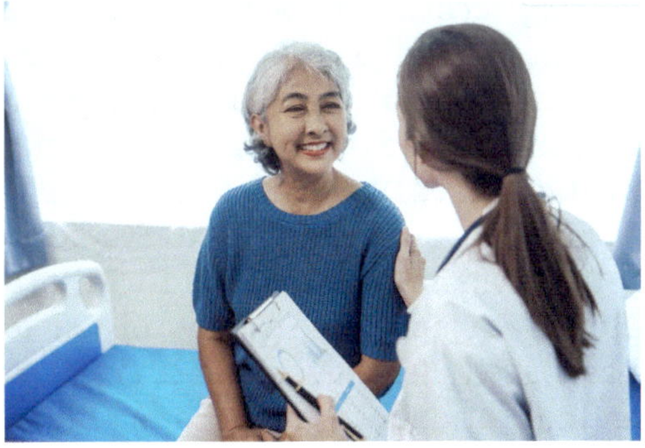

Figure 15.10. Preoperative Assessment.

Source: https://sa1s3optim.patientpop.com/filters:format(webp)/assets/production/practices/377012814fbb4323f1bc0008126ef1d839c9f69f/images/2710485.jpeg.

15.3.2. Monitoring During Anesthesia

Watching patients closely during surgery lowers anesthesia problems. You need to keep an eye on things like heart rate, blood pressure and oxygen saturation throughout the procedure so any unexpected changes can be caught in time. In one study with pygmy goats treated for obstructive urolithiasis, careful monitoring picked up minor issues—like a slower heartbeat and low blood pressure—that later helped avoid worse complications (Cremer et al., 2018). This clearly shows that steady oversight isn't just about immediate safety but also about managing anesthesia as a whole. Strict observation routines seem to lower the risk of anesthesia mishaps quite a bit. When data from different anesthesiology departments is looked at, there's generally a clear link between solid real-time checks and fewer complications. For instance, a review at the General Hospital Karlovac noted that with detailed monitoring during both the anesthesia and recovery phases, complication rates dropped from 5.4% to around 1.25% (Henshaw et al., 2017). Such regular checks, in most cases, not only keep patients safer but also build a sense of accountability and constant improvement among the team. New monitoring tech has upped the safety game even further. Techniques like ultrasound-guided regional anesthesia (RA) have changed how patients are handled by reducing the amount of anesthetic needed, which in turn lowers risks like toxicity and other side effects. Studies even show that, when RA is combined with proper monitoring, complication rates can fall to as little as 0.31% (Henshaw et al., 2017). Overall, these innovations highlight how blending modern monitoring methods into anesthesia practice can lead to better outcomes and open the door for continuous advances in patient care.

15.3.3. Postoperative Care

Postoperative care is incredibly important—especially when you consider the many twists anesthesia can bring to a patient's recovery. Sometimes, anesthesia ends up causing a whole mix of issues that only show up later, like pain that just won't quit. Keeping that pain under control is a big deal, since unmanaged discomfort not only makes getting better harder but can also extend hospital stays. Take TEA for example; using this method in surgeries—say, in cases like open posterior component separation surgery—has been linked to a noticeably faster return of bowel function compared to sticking with systemic opioids alone (Henshaw et al., 2017).

In most cases, tailoring pain relief in this way shapes both the immediate and longer-term recovery journey. Watching over a patient's heart and blood pressure during recovery is another matter that shouldn't be taken lightly. Anesthetic drugs can sometimes nudge blood pressure or heart rate into unexpected territory, which can be tricky for people who are already vulnerable. A neat trick here is the TAP block, or transversus abdominis plane block, which tends to lower the overall need for heavy stuff like propofol and remifentanil. This approach does more than just reduce on anesthetic use—it also seems to foster quicker extubation and steadier vitals. In fact, the numbers suggest that patients receiving TAP blocks experience way fewer wobbles requiring intervention than those on standard GA (Jiang et al., 2018). Generally speaking, combining solid surgical techniques with smart anesthetic tricks goes a long way. Then there's the broader picture of spotting and handling other bumps along the recovery road—not just pain or unstable vitals. It's important to catch things like postoperative nausea and vomiting (PONV) early because these issues can drag down patient comfort and delay getting better. By putting in place layered and often flexible care plans that blend different pain relief options with early nausea control, healthcare teams can make things feel a lot smoother. It's all about keeping a close, sometimes improvised, watch on recovery signals and altering care as needed, which not only helps dodge the risks that come with anesthetic complications but also makes the path back to health a bit less bumpy (Figure 15.11).

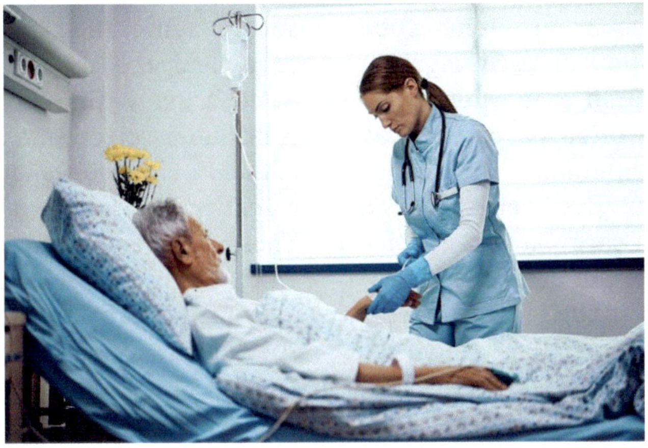

Figure 15.11. Importance of post-operative care.

Source: https://sukinohealthcare.com/wp-content/uploads/2023/06/Post-operative-cares-1024x683.jpg.

Test Your Knowledge

1. What to monitor during anaesthesia?
2. What is the postoperative care?

15.4. Management of Anesthetic Complications

Learning Outcome

1. Understand the immediate response protocols.
2. Understand the long-term management strategies.
3. Describe the role of the anesthesiologist.

Managing anesthetic complications isn't just about following a strict checklist—it comes down to knowing each patient's quirks and the risks baked into different anesthetic methods. Preoperative checks, for example, should zero in on potential issues like tricky airways (kids, in particular, often throw extra curveballs). Recent work generally suggests that congenital issues and systemic diseases tend to make keeping the airway open a real challenge, sometimes even turning dangerous if things go awry. In most cases, using newer airway tools and keeping a nearly constant eye on patients during and after the procedure helps dodge problems like failed intubation, among other mishaps. Clearly, a detailed look-over combined with hands-on, proactive planning is key to keeping patients safe and sorting out these knotty anesthetic issues (Lepik et al., 2024). It's also vital that everyone on the medical crew stays in the loop when it comes to tackling these complications. In a multidisciplinary setting—where anesthesiologists, surgeons, and nursing staff all pitch in—a steady, informal back-and-forth can make a difference. Continuous talk ensures all team members know the patient's condition and any sudden twists during the procedure. For instance, setting up quick-response plans might cover problems such as difficult mask ventilation or early signs of hypoxia. Open communication, even when things aren't perfectly scripted, often paves the way for faster decisions and minimizes the chance of lingering complications (Casey et al., 2017). After surgery, the kind of care patients receive becomes just as crucial; it can even shape how well they bounce back over the long haul. This phase is all about keeping a vigilant watch for problems like breathing struggles or tricky pain control. Combining various pain relief methods not only eases discomfort but can also reduce on too much opioid use—a point that recent studies have underscored by showing improved analgesic results with techniques like fascia iliaca compartment blocks. Such tactics tend to speed up recovery and might prevent issues like unnecessarily long hospital stays or slow rehabilitation. In short, effective postoperative management boosts patient satisfaction and, in most cases, leads to better overall outcomes (Casey et al., 2017; Lepik et al., 2024).

15.4.1. Immediate Response Protocols

Managing anesthetic mishaps calls for quick, decisive actions to keep patients safe and get the best results. When things start going wrong, medical staff need to pinpoint the issue right away and jump in with specific fixes. It all begins with getting everyone talking—surgeons, anesthesiologists, nurses—all sharing what they see so that emergency steps can kick in fast. Mixing these actions into everyday routines can pay off, especially when every second matters and regular drills help keep everyone on their toes. Different emergencies, like a blocked airway or a sudden allergic reaction, need their kind of response. In a breathing crisis, time is everything; spotting an obstruction quickly and using methods like bag-mask ventilation or intubation can make a huge difference. For cases of anaphylaxis, a swift dose of epinephrine is often the game changer needed to reverse severe symptoms. These focused moves not only clear the chaos in the moment but also build trust within the team. In most cases, continuous review and altering—based on fresh clinical evidence—ensure these plans stay on track with what's considered best practice. These on-the-spot strategies work even better when they form part of a broader, team-based approach that brings together different medical specialties. By working in close collaboration, anesthesiologists, surgeons, and pain experts can create a smoother overall perioperative experience. For example, when multimodal pain relief is combined, it not only tackles immediate post-surgery pain but also lowers opioid use, thereby reducing risks tied to those drugs. The spirit of teamwork carries on after the operating room too, with follow-up visits for patients still dealing with lingering pain. All these efforts underline the importance of a well-organized, collaborative response to hitting the best possible surgical outcomes (Kim et al., 2015; Schwenk et al., 2018) (Figure 15.12).

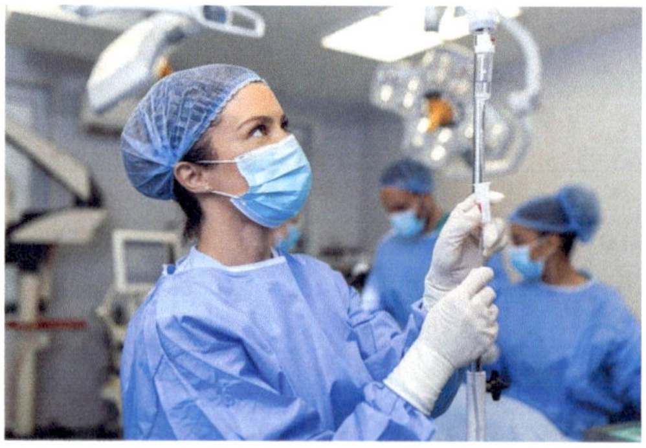

Figure 15.12. Immediate response protocols.

Source: https://external-preview.redd.it/ama-opposes-nurse-anesthesiologist-title-for-crnas-in-v0-TjsfLHnIbQYc2QIGD7v6l3Y7aCrmiTsh6RJnOpxjvbE.jpg?width=640&crop=smart&auto=webp&s=99f53b7eba6c20cb40f34f9ccf25bbdd28e21041.

15.4.2. Long-Term Management Strategies

Managing long-term issues is crucial to easing anesthesia-related problems that sometimes arise during and after surgery. One promising approach involves using Multidisciplinary Geriatric Fracture Programs (GFP); these programs, in many cases, have been linked with better outcomes. Research suggests that early and varied pain management—kicking off treatment sooner rather than later—can help lower both illness and death rates among older patients with fragile hip fractures. For example, after a GFP was introduced, patients generally experienced a quicker start to pain relief, made greater use of acetaminophen, and saw a clear rise in the use of fascia iliaca compartment blocks. Mixing different methods of pain control shows how important it is to tailor interventions to each person's needs while cutting back on opioid use after the operation (Casey et al., 2017). Pharmacological measures also play a major role in long-term care; we can't overstate their importance, especially when it comes to taming the body's inflammatory response during recovery. Studies generally indicate that administering dexamethasone before surgery—particularly in elective colorectal cancer cases—can markedly improve outcomes. By keeping the SIR in check, dexamethasone tends to lower complications like infections and extended recovery times. In one carefully matched cohort study, patients getting this corticosteroid had notably lower C-reactive protein levels on days after surgery, hinting at a milder inflammatory reaction. Fewer patients even topped the established CRP limits, which, in most cases, underscores the drug's promise for fostering a better long-term recovery environment (Horgan et al., 2017). Long-term care doesn't stop at medications and programs; it also means continuously checking in on pain management strategies based on what patients tell us. Regular assessments of pain levels and side effects pave the way for adjustments in postoperative care. Adding educational tools and supportive networks into the mix encourages patients to get more involved in their recovery, even if that means a few hiccups along the way. When healthcare teams listen and adapt, they can fine-tune treatments to fit individual needs, potentially boosting both adherence and satisfaction. All these proactive steps—blending insights from GFPs with smart pharmacological choices—come together to build a pretty solid framework for managing anesthesia issues in the long run, ultimately aiming to raise quality of life and improve surgical outcomes for a wide range of patients.

15.4.3. Role of the Anesthesiologist

Modern anesthesia today has grown complex, and anesthesiologists now have to handle way more than just giving a shot of anesthetic. They not only check on patients before surgery and watch over them afterward, but they also adjust drug plans based on how medicines work in the body—considering everything from how fast a drug moves to how it actually affects the patient. This tailored approach lowers risks when things go awry during anesthesia; take airway issues, for example, which perfectly show why these skills matter. In short, these experts create a safe surgical setup by keeping the right balance between deep sedation and steady patient stability, which is key to successful surgery (Coté et al., 2019). Anesthesiologists also play a huge part in building bridges between different members of the healthcare team. As operating rooms and procedures keep changing, these doctors find themselves naturally stepping into roles that mix surgery, nursing, and other support services. They help smooth out the whole process, coordinating everything from post-op care to recovery routines to fend off issues like infections or longer hospital stays. With the system slowly shifting toward value-based care—generally speaking meaning more focus on outcomes—these specialists are even taking on leadership roles in managing patient pathways.

Their broader contributions extend well beyond the operating room, enabling better resource use and boosting overall patient satisfaction (Prielipp et al., 2015). When complications with anesthesia come up, their role grows even more critical, especially during sedation processes for different patient groups. Kids, for instance, bring their set of challenges that call for extra careful checks and custom sedation plans to keep things safe. These doctors look into underlying conditions, pay close attention to airway issues, and even consider how drugs might interact, all to set up a safe protocol. Being ready to act fast when unexpected things happen—like a sudden airway blockage or an unexpected drug reaction—shows just how central their work is in protecting patients. Their deep expertise in handling these sudden twists not only keeps folks safe but also helps surgeries run smoother. This ever-growing responsibility for quick decision-making is a big part of moving anesthesiology forward, all with a focus on better patient outcomes and fewer complications (Coté et al., 2019) (Figure 15.13).

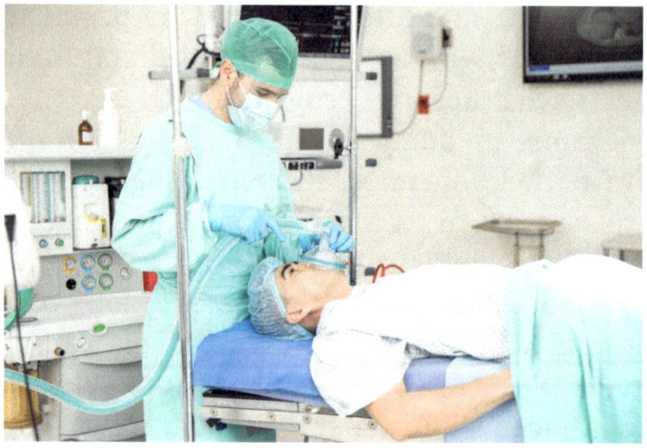

Figure 15.13. Role of the Anesthesiologist.

Source: https://www.onlinedegree.com/wp-content/uploads/2016/11/anesthesiologist.jpg.

Test Your Knowledge

1. What are immediate response protocols?
2. What is the role of the anesthesiologist?

SUMMARY

The choice of how to administer anesthesia can be a factor when surgery is carried out. Recent research shows that the use of monitored anesthesia care (MAC) has clear benefits in risky procedures like transcatheter aortic valve implantation. MAC has a tendency to decrease mortality and hospitalization and also addresses complications like stroke or even paravalvular leakage (Xie et al., 2024). This means that anesthesiologists will need to be highly careful regarding their monitoring habits; knowing which approach is most superior will aid physicians in varying their technique according to patient. Risk evaluation is also a major consideration. The American Society of Anesthesiologists (ASA) classification—means of assessing a patient's preoperative risk—is often synonymous with higher scores equating to higher complications and even a higher risk of death (Al-Husinat et al., 2024).

For instance, studies in geriatric hip fracture patients have noted that patients who were in higher ASA classes spent more time in the hospital and had more thromboembolic events. In most cases, this trend reflects the need for detailed, in some cases even multiple, pre-surgical assessments so that patients' treatment would be tailored accordingly. Research and constant developments in how we provide anesthesia are still key to reducing surgery complications. More and more evidence exists that enhancing surveillance technology and altering anesthetic methods based on ASA data can, in the end, lead to safer procedures. Working amongst different medical teams – although the process at times feels rather imbalanced – allows new data to be integrated into standard practice (Al-Husinat et al., 2024; Xie et al., 2024). Ultimately, a respect for the complex dynamic between anesthetic choices, patient health, and potential complications makes way for safer surgery and smoother recoveries.

Anesthesia issues can readily undermine patient outcomes. It's a matter of understanding what does the trick. As an example, having the puncture right in procedures like hemodialysis is crucial—especially when beginning to develop an autologous arteriovenous fistula (AVF). Studies have found that if staff receive proper training, achieve the first puncture correctly, and do a good pre-procedure check before proceeding, problems decrease considerably. Best practices formulated through systematic reviews and expert consensus seem to make the process more secure and efficient for performing vascular access procedures. The hybrid method of mixed bag for most cases helps the nurses maintain evidence-based action in constant coordination with each patient's specific situation, enhancing safety and therapy effectiveness (Zhang et al., 2025). Familiarizing oneself with subtle details of medical conditions that affect anesthesia is important as well. Carcinoid tumors, although rare, can provoke odd challenges—especially if they involve carcinoid heart disease (CaHD).

Treatment of such patients entails becoming knowledgeable about the behavior and potential complications of the disease. A judicious plan based on good hemodynamic monitoring and skillful anesthetic tricks can minimize the complications during the operative procedure. For the most part, newer research even suggests preoperative somatostatin use reduces heart-related hiccups, indicating that a decision-making algorithm of incremental steps should be used when treating such patients (Ussel et al., 2024). In terms of anesthetic complications, it is helpful if everyone works together. Not only anesthesiologists, but also surgeons, nurses, and other experts contribute their input to patient treatment, particularly when surgeries become complex. Merging multiple perspectives produces a more obvious analysis of each patient's needs and helps guide anesthesia maneuvers that keep issues on track. And that is not all—a regular review of old protocols and merging with new evidence is essential to patient safety. Keeping health professionals current with new research and anesthetic developments is a key factor in enhancing outcomes and ensuring high safety levels (Ussel et al., 2024; Zhang et al., 2025.

KEY TERMS FROM THIS CHAPTER

- Allergic reactions
- Blockage
- Body temperature
- Complex heart interventions
- Local anesthetic systemic toxicity
- Neurosurgery
- Patient positioning
- Postoperative pain
- Aspiration
- Blood sugar
- Cardiovascular issues
- D syndrome
- Medical practices
- Obesity
- Posterior component separation
- Pulmonary hypertension

CRITICAL THINKING QUESTIONS

1. **Which of the following is the most common cause of intraoperative hypotension?**
   a. Anaphylaxis
   b. Blood loss
   c. Decreased anesthetic depth
   d. Vasodilation due to anesthetic agents
2. **The earliest sign of malignant hyperthermia during anesthesia is:**
   a. Hyperthermia
   b. Increased end-tidal CO_2 ($ETCO_2$)
   c. Tachycardia
   d. Muscle rigidity
3. **The most common cause of intraoperative anaphylaxis is:**
   a. Antibiotics
   b. Muscle relaxants
   c. Volatile anesthetics
   d. Latex
4. **Postoperative cognitive dysfunction is most commonly seen in:**
   a. Pediatric patients
   b. Elderly patients
   c. Healthy adults
   d. Patients with a history of epilepsy
5. **The best method to prevent intraoperative awareness is:**
   a. Use of muscle relaxants
   b. Monitoring bispectral index (BIS)
   c. Administering high doses of opioids
   d. Avoiding regional anesthesia

Short Answer Questions

1. What is the most common complication of anesthesia?
2. What are the cardiovascular complications?
3. Describe the risk factors for anesthetic complications.
4. What are the prevention strategies of anesthetic complications?
5. How to manage anesthetic complications?

Answers to Critical Thinking Questions

1. (d); 2. (b); 3. (b); 4. (b); 5. (b)

REFERENCES

1. Al-Husinat, L., Azzam, S., Al Sharie, S., Al Hseinat, L., Araydah, M., Al Modanat, Z., Balawi, A. R., et al. (2024). Impact of the American Society of Anesthesiologists (ASA) classification on hip fracture surgery outcomes: Insights from a retrospective analysis. *BMC Anesthesiology, 24*. https://www.semanticscholar.org/paper/15f81427f421980938bd98f30431d23b53896df1 (accessed on 20 May 2025).
2. Argo, A., Buscemi, R., Karch, S. B., Lanzarone, A., Roccuzzo, R., & Zerbo, S. (2019). Perioperative and anesthetic deaths: Toxicological and medico-legal aspects. Retrieved from: https://core.ac.uk/download/224993621.pdf (accessed on 2025).
3. Arrico, L., Brancadoro, D., Collini, S., Grippaudo, et al. (2018). Local anesthetic infiltration vs. nervous blocks in face's skin lesions: What's new. Retrieved from: https://core.ac.uk/download/188827411.pdf (accessed on 20 May 2025).
4. Beltran Paschoal, J. F., Pinheiro Santos, I., Malaquias, D. M., de Freitas, K. C., Barbosa Leão, M. E., Carvalho Silva, A., Lins da Silva, K., et al. (2025). Comparative analysis of the best drug of choice for sedation in a surgical procedure in elderly patients: Pros and side effects of sedatives. *Journal of Anesthesia*. https://www.semanticscholar.org/paper/04fed51def341c6feb9a4c7efec75f092c6236ea (accessed on 20 May 2025).
5. Bretzman, J. P., Ziegelmann, M., & Reisenauer, C. J. (2025). Selective penile artery angioembolization for high flow priapism–A step-by-step overview for the non-radiologist. *The Journal of Sexual Medicine*. https://www.semanticscholar.org/paper/a8bb66d0137b207d8e139f89d8fd340eaa7729fd (accessed on 20 May 2025).
6. Casey, S. D., Stevenson, D. E., Mumma, B. E., Slee, C., Wolinsky, P. R., Hirsch, C. H., & Tyler, K. (2017). Emergency department pain management following implementation of a geriatric hip fracture program. *The Western Journal of Emergency Medicine, 18*(4), 585–591. https://doi.org/10.5811/westjem.2017.3.32853.
7. Coté, C. J., & Wilson, S. (2019). Guidelines for monitoring and management of pediatric patients before, during, and after sedation for diagnostic and therapeutic procedures. *Pediatrics, 143*(6), e20191000. https://doi.org/10.1542/peds.2019-1000.
8. Dalamagka, M. (2024). Anesthesiology complications in children. *International Journal of Science and Research Archive*. https://www.semanticscholar.org/paper/b7e4efc9530c5de4d82d01b3d2ef5fd601ec5de1 (accessed on 20 May 2025).
9. Davis, B. R., Lee-Kong, S. A., Migaly, J., Feingold, D. L., & Steele, S. R. (2018). The American Society of Colon and Rectal Surgeons clinical practice guidelines for the management of hemorrhoids. *Diseases of the Colon & Rectum, 61*(3), 284–292. https://doi.org/10.1097/DCR.0000000000001030.
10. El-Boghdadly, K., Pawa, A., & Chin, K. J. (2018). Local anesthetic systemic toxicity: Current perspectives. *Local and Regional Anesthesia, 11*, 35–44. https://doi.org/10.2147/LRA.S154512.
11. Farooqi, A., Zaheer, F., Salman, S., Sadia, Shaikh, S., & Rimsha, S. (2024). A comparative study of anesthetic block techniques (V-block vs. H-block) for removal of ingrown toenail. *Biological and Clinical Sciences Research Journal*. https://www.semanticscholar.org/paper/ac1d8c925d6f6e0af24bd984da0f8a2db955897c (accessed on 20 May 2025).

12. Garg, A., Pathak, A., Gupta, A., & Agrawal, M. (2022). Comparison of 0.5% levobupivacaine alone and 0.5% levobupivacaine with butorphanol given intrathecally in infraumbilical surgeries. *International Journal of Medical Reviews and Case Reports, 6*(20), 39–47. https://doi.org/10.5455/IJMRCR.172-1657087612.

13. Gregory, S., Murray-Torres, T. M., Fritz, B. A., et al. (2018). Study protocol for the Anesthesiology Control Tower—Feedback Alerts to Supplement Treatments (ACTFAST-3) trial: A pilot randomized controlled trial in intraoperative telemedicine [version 2; peer review: 2 approved]. *F1000Research, 7*, 623. https://doi.org/10.12688/f1000research.14897.2.

14. Hefni, A., Abd El Rahman, W. A., Moris, K., & Nabieh, M. M. (2023). Post-operative analgesic effect of intra-articular local anesthetic infiltration versus adductor canal block after knee arthroscopic surgeries. *QJM: An International Journal of Medicine*. https://www.semanticscholar.org/paper/926084f5c37a49678d270eaa088df3c960ec9f61 (accessed on 20 May 2025).

15. Henshaw, D. S., Edwards, C. J., Sellers, A. R., Russell, G. B., & Weller, R. S. (2017). Benefits of thoracic epidural analgesia in patients undergoing an open posterior component separation for abdominal herniorrhaphy. *Journal of Pain & Palliative Care Pharmacotherapy, 31*(3, 4), 204–211. https://doi.org/10.1080/15360288.2017.1313354.

16. Horgan, P. G., McMillan, D. C., McSorley, S. T., Roxburgh, C. S., et al. (2017). The impact of preoperative dexamethasone on the magnitude of the postoperative systemic inflammatory response and complications following surgery for colorectal cancer. Retrieved from: https://core.ac.uk/download/80696883.pdf (accessed on 20 May 2025).

17. Islam, R. K., Tong, V. T., Robicheaux, C., Tageant, H., Haas, C. J., Kline, R. J., & Islam, K. N. (2024). The impact of anesthesia on dermatological outcomes: A narrative review. *Cureus, 16*. https://www.semanticscholar.org/paper/8e56fe6bcf52fd98948309e41ac01c50cfc4322b (accessed on 20 May 2025).

18. Jiang, M. R., Li, T., Liu, G. G., Liu, Y., et al. (2018). Transversus abdominis plane block reduces remifentanil and propofol consumption, evaluated by closed-loop titration guided by bispectral index. Retrieved from: https://core.ac.uk/download/323067899.pdf.

19. Kim, M., Cheok, S., Chung, L. K., Ung, N., Thill, K., Voth, B., Kwon, D. H., Kim, J. H., Kim, C. J., Tenn, S., Lee, P., & Yang, I. (2015). Characteristics and treatments of large cystic brain metastasis: Radiosurgery and stereotactic aspiration. *Brain Tumor Research and Treatment, 3*(1), 1–7. https://doi.org/10.14791/btrt.2015.3.1.1.

20. Łepik, M., Uszok, Z., Rosiak, K., Płeska, K., Reguła, K., Waloch, K., Wojtania, J., Piaszczyński, S., Czajka, A., & Szymański, B. (2024). Difficult pediatric airway in anesthesia practice and future sport performance. *Quality in Sport, 18*, 50920. https://doi.org/10.12775/QS.2024.18.50920.

21. Michielsen, A., Proost, K., Pardon, B., De Cremer, L., & Schauvliege, S. (2018). General anesthesia for surgical treatment of urethral obstruction in nine goats. *Vlaams Diergeneeskundig Tijdschrift, 87*, 314–325. https://doi.org/10.21825/vdt.v87i6.16049.

22. Prielipp, R. C., Morell, R. C., Coursin, D. B., Brull, S. J., Barker, S. J., Rice, M. J., Vender, J. S., et al. (2015). The future of anesthesiology. *Anesthesia & Analgesia, 120*(5), 1142–1148. https://doi.org/10.1213/ane.0000000000000711.

23. Radu, O. M., Balaci, G. M., Leucuța, D., Moisescu, V. I., Munteanu, C., & Florian, I. (2024). Outcomes and complications of posterior fossa surgery in sitting versus park-bench positions.

Medicina, 60. https://www.semanticscholar.org/paper/44d7b1558856a3306ebcde53a2012158b90fbfa6 (accessed on 20 May 2025).

24. Rasool, N., Shounthoo, R. S., Rashid, P., & Farooq, B. (2025). Comparing the recovery characteristics between sevoflurane and isoflurane following removal of laryngeal mask airway under deeper planes of anesthesia in pediatric surgical patients: An observational study. *Asian Journal of Medical Sciences*. https://www.semanticscholar.org/paper/aaba7a1bee31b9247fc70cad41861205550c1a8b (accessed on 20 May 2025).
25. Schwenk, E. S., Pozek, J. J., & Viscusi, E. R. (2018). Managing prolonged pain after surgery: Examining the role of opioids. *The Journal of Arthroplasty, 33*(11), 3389–3393. https://doi.org/10.1016/j.arth.2018.08.005.
26. Segovia-Medina, L. G., Noguera-Echeverría, A. E., & Basulto-Castro, C. (2024). Utility of the Enhanced Recovery after Surgery Protocol (ERAS Protocol) in anesthetic management for pediatric surgery in patients with D Syndrome: Case report. *International Journal of Medical Science and Clinical Research Studies*. https://www.semanticscholar.org/paper/525ce97aa59d76f021842661f8ae3a8f85c96fb1 (accessed on 20 May 2025).
27. Seo, J., So, K., & Kim, S. H. (2019). Perioperative anesthetic considerations in patients with pulmonary hypertension undergoing non-cardiac and non-obstetric surgeries. *Medical Biological Science and Engineering*. https://www.semanticscholar.org/paper/6a3394bd88dccebf949ed00c3d50e7139d9bf315 (accessed on 20 May 2025).
28. Shetti, A. N. (2024). Sedation and anesthesia in ambulatory ENT procedures–A review. *Journal of Otorhinolaryngology Allied Sciences, 7*(4), 69–73.
29. Van Ussel, K., Leonard, D., Watremez, C., & Robu, C. B. (2024). Anesthetic key points in a patient with a terminal ileum neuroendocrine tumor and a rare carcinoid left heart disease presented for non-cardiac surgery: Case report. *BMC Anesthesiology, 24*. https://www.semanticscholar.org/paper/00705f81786861f2fc182b2ca823ab9c9bb4fc5f (accessed on 20 May 2025).
30. Wenzel, J. T., Schwenk, E. S., Baratta, J. L., & Viscusi, E. R. (2016). Managing opioid-tolerant patients in the perioperative surgical home. *Anesthesiology Clinics, 34*(2), 287–301. https://doi.org/10.1016/j.anclin.2016.01.005.
31. Xie, L., Lang, Z., Liu, Y., Yue, H., Chen, Q., & Tao, G. (2024). Whether monitored anesthesia care is the optimal anesthetic strategy for transcatheter aortic valve implantation surgery? A meta-analysis and systematic review. *BMC Anesthesiology, 24*(1), 429. https://www.semanticscholar.org/paper/1b49fdc36940254183eb564837a2fd42e6b74035 (accessed on 20 May 2025).
32. Zanos, P., Moaddel, R., Morris, P. J., Riggs, L. M., Highland, J. N., Georgiou, P., Pereira, E. F. R., et al. (2018). Ketamine and ketamine metabolite pharmacology: Insights into therapeutic mechanisms. *Pharmacological Reviews, 70*(3), 621–660. https://doi.org/10.1124/pr.117.015198.
33. Zhang, X., Liu, J., Wang, J., Ma, T., & Zhang, H. (2025). Summary of the best evidence for puncture management during the early stage of autologous arteriovenous fistula in maintenance hemodialysis patients. *Journal of Clinical and Nursing Research, 8*, 234–243. https://doi.org/10.26689/jcnr.v8i12.9077.
34. Žunić, J., Belavić, M., & Lončarić-Katušin, M. (2013). Reducing the incidence of adverse events in anesthesia practice. *Periodicum Biologorum, 115*(2), 145–148. https://core.ac.uk/download/14468892.pdf (accessed on 20 May 2025).

INDEX

A

Absorption 38, 52
Acetaminophen 357, 359
Adjunctive anesthetic agents 52
Airway management 20, 112, 113, 114, 116, 119, 120, 121, 123, 126, 128, 130, 131, 134, 136
Airway swelling 259
Allergic reactions 374, 375, 388
Altered drug metabolism 246
American Society of Anesthesiologists (ASA) 300
American Society of Anesthesiologists-Physical Status (ASA-PS) 294
Anesthesia consultation 95, 104
Anesthesia education 94
Anesthesia induction 142, 162
Anesthesia intensive care units 364
Anesthesia Intensive Care Units (AICUs) 354
Anesthesia patients 1
Anesthesia techniques 20
Anesthesiology 1, 2, 3, 13, 14, 19, 20, 22, 23, 24, 25
Anesthesiology control tower 340
Anesthesiology Control Tower (ACT) 322
Anesthesiology residency programs 1
Anesthetic care 195, 209
Anesthetic drugs 78, 79, 140, 141, 157
Anesthetic medicine 27
Anesthetic practice 137
Anesthetic science 52
Anesthetic selection 28
Anesthetics numb pain 29
Angiotensin-converting enzyme 2 (ACE2) 296
Antibiotics 104
Anxiety 364, 368
Apnea 194, 197, 202
Arteries 63, 79
Artificial intelligence 340
Artificial intelligence (AI) 321
Aspiration 388
Automatic body reactions 28

B

Bioelectrical impedance analysis 287
Bioelectrical impedance analysis (BIA) 266, 291
Bleeding 259
Blockage 388
Blocking pain 28
Blood pressure 69, 79, 80, 340
Blood sugar 388
Blood vessel 79
Blood volume 340
Body composition 268, 287
Body mass index 61, 259
Body temperature 388
Brain cells 157
Brain diseases 79
Brain health 266, 284
Breathing rhythms 234
Bronchi 131

Bronchioles 131
B-type natriuretic peptide (BNP) 301
Bupivacaine 52
Burn dressing changes 189, 194, 199, 203

C

Calming nerves 27
Capnography 325, 326, 340
Cardiac implantable electronic devices (CIEDs) 319
Cardiology 340
Cardiovascular diseases 296, 311
Cardiovascular issues 376, 388
Cardiovascular system 287
Central nervous system 62, 64, 65, 66, 67, 79, 84
Central venous catheters 320
Cerebral blood flow (CBF) 60, 139
Cerebral oximetry 137, 157
Cerebrospinal fluid 183
Certified Registered Nurse Anesthetists (CRNAs) 94
Change management 299, 311
Chemistry 216, 217
Childbirth 248, 251, 253, 259
Chloroprocaine 183
Chronic pain 164, 165, 167, 173, 177
Ciprofol 157
Clinical anesthesiology 2, 3, 4, 13, 19
Clinical competencies 2
Clinical practice 164, 186
Cognitive-behavioral therapy 234, 358
Cognitive hiccups 287
Cognitive impairment 268
Combined spinal-epidural 259, 260
Combined spinal-epidural (CSE) block 244
Communication 328, 340, 344, 345
Complex heart interventions 388
Computer-driven systems 104
Contemporary medical practice 3
Continual monitoring 28
Continuing education 29, 43
Creatinine levels 298
Crisis management 320, 339, 340
CRNAs (certified registered nurse anesthetists) 245

D

Deep sedation 28, 192, 194, 195, 209, 210
Delirium 266, 267, 268, 269, 272, 280, 281, 282, 283, 284, 288, 289, 292
Dexmedetomidine 267, 287
Dexmedetomidine (DEX) 7
Diabetes 104, 298, 311
Diagnostic testing 301, 302, 311
Distribution 38, 52
Drug dosage 217
Drug metabolism 259
Drug processing 79
D syndrome 376, 388
Dual-energy X-ray absorptiometry 287
Dual-energy X-ray absorptiometry (DXA) 266
Dynamical system 79

E

Educational programs 234
E-learning 225
Electroencephalography 287
Electroencephalography (EEG) 270
Electromagnetic interference 340
Emergency cesarean 259
Emergency medicine 4
Emergency situations 250, 255
Emotional health 20
Emotional support 234
Endoscopic Retrograde Cholangiopancreatography (ERCP) 192
Endotracheal intubation 124, 131
Enhanced recovery after surgery 364
Enhanced Recovery After Surgery (ERAS) 195, 352, 361, 367
Epidural anesthesia 172, 177, 183, 184
Erratic heartbeat 340
Esketamine 364
Evidence-based practices 234
Evidence-based protocols 354
Evidence-based screening 2

Excitatory circuits 157
Excretion 52, 259
Extracorporeal membrane oxygenation 234

F

Fascia iliaca compartment blocks (FICB) 357
Fetal distress 259
Flooding 164
Fluid balance 268
Full-blown anaphylaxis 374

G

Gabapentinoids 359
General anesthesia 137, 139, 157, 158, 159
General anesthesia (GA) 3
Geriatric anesthesia 266, 280, 287
Global health crises 317
Glomerular filtration rate 268, 287
Glycine receptors 157

H

Headaches 183, 298
Healthcare 97, 98, 104
Healthcare environment 317
Health crises 113, 131
Heart 59, 60, 61, 62, 66, 68, 69, 70, 71, 74, 75, 76, 77, 78, 83
Heart disease 88
Heart failure 311
Heart injuries 296
Heart irregularities 20
Heart problems 104
Heart rate 79, 80, 340
Hemodynamics 183
Hemodynamic stability 138, 209
High blood pressure 311
High-risk pregnancies 247, 250, 251
Human breathing system 115
Hyomental gap 114
Hypertension 259
Hypnosis 358
Hypotension 183, 194
Hypoxemia 193

I

Infection control 131
Infections 183
Infectious diseases 296
Inhalational anesthetics 287
Inhaled agents 157
Integrated Behavior Model (IBM) 86
Intraoperative monitoring 317, 319, 339
Intravenous anesthetics 273, 287
Intubation 113, 124, 127, 131, 135
Invasive arterial lines 320

K

Kidney problems 296
Kidneys 268

L

Labor analgesia 259, 262
Laryngomalacia 311
Levobupivacaine 6
Lidocaine 52
Lipid solubility 145
Local anesthesia 4, 7
Local anesthetic systemic toxicity 388, 390
Low- and middle-income countries (LMIC) 222
Lower airway 131
Lungs 59, 62, 71, 72, 73, 74, 77, 78
Lung ultrasonography 3, 20

M

Machine learning 340
Machine learning (MI) 321
Maternal care 259
Maternal health 243, 247, 259
Medical fraternity 4
Medical history 92, 104
Medical practices 388
Medical professionals 29, 50
Medication management 87
Memory 266, 267, 272, 281
Metabolism 37, 39, 52, 219, 234
Microglia 142, 157
Midline glossoepiglottic fold 131

Midline glossoepiglottic fold (MVF) 113
Minimal sedation 192, 193, 209, 210
Moderate sedation 192, 209, 210
Modern medicine 1, 4, 21, 28, 293
Modern surgery 318, 335, 340
Monitored Anesthesia Care 189, 190, 195, 196, 198, 209
Monitoring gadgets 364
Multimodal analgesia 359
Multimodal anesthesia 28
Multiscale entropy (MSE) 147
Muscles 1
Musculoskeletal pain 311
Musculoskeletal system 61

N

Near-infrared spectroscopy 234
Near-infrared spectroscopy (NIRS) 217, 239
Nerve blocks 4
Nerves 1, 6
Nervous system 65, 79, 234
Neural activity 64
Neurocommunication 52
Neurological health 157
Neuromuscular blocking drugs 30
Neuromuscular disorders 183
Neuromuscular monitoring 321, 322, 340
Neuropathic pain 27, 54
Neurostimulation 165
Neurosurgery 388
Neutrophil gelatinase-associated lipocalin (NGAL) 298
Nicotinic acetylcholine receptors 157
Nitrous oxide 28
Nociception Level 323
Non-opioid drugs 357, 364
Noonan syndrome 249, 262
Numeric rating scale 364
Nutrition 91, 104

O

Obesity 377, 388
Obstetric anesthesia 241, 242, 246, 251, 252, 254, 255, 256, 258, 259
Obstetric surgeries 249
Obstructive sleep apnea 311
Obstructive sleep apnea (OSA) 3
Opioid dependence 164
Opioid-free anesthesia 209, 213
Opioid-free anesthesia (OFA) 195
Opioids 358, 364
Orthopedic interventions 209
Outpatient Nursing Nutritional Intervention (ONNI) 91
Oxygen flow 131
Oxygen levels 60, 62, 73, 74, 75, 76, 79, 194, 202, 203

P

Pain assessment 347, 354, 355, 356, 360, 363, 364, 367
Pain care 183
Pain control 165, 166, 167, 169, 170, 172, 177
Pain management 5, 6, 7, 8, 15, 16, 17, 18, 22, 25, 218, 230
Pain relief 27, 29, 32, 33, 35, 37, 41, 42, 43, 45, 50
Paralytic drugs 131
Paraventricular thalamus 157
Patient care 2, 3, 4, 20
Patient-centered care 86, 91
Patient comfort 189, 200
Patient consent 209
Patient experience 5
Patient positioning 376, 388
Patient safety 20
Patient satisfaction 183, 294, 299
Paying attention 29
Pedagogy 4
Pediatric anesthesia 216, 217, 225, 228, 230, 232, 233, 234
Pediatric anesthesiologists 215, 216
Pediatric care 220, 222, 234
Pediatric operations 216
Pediatric patients 218, 219, 220, 224, 226, 227, 230, 232, 235, 236, 237, 238
Pediatric physical exams 225

Pediatric surgical care 222
Peripheral nerve blocks 176, 181, 183
Peripheral nervous system 66, 79
Personalized medication 234
Personalized medicine 3, 10
Personal preferences 364
Pharmacodynamics 29, 30, 51, 183
Pharmacokinetics 183
Physical examination 93, 104, 311
Physical response 28
Plan-Do-Study-Act 95, 104
Post-anesthesia care 349, 364
Post-anesthesia care unit 157
Post dural puncture headaches 259
Posterior component separation 388
Posterior component separation (PCS) 379
Postoperative pain 374, 388
Postoperative residual curarization (PORC) 1
Post-surgery recovery 1
Post-surgical cognitive changes 2
Practitioners 189, 193, 199
Precision medicine 294, 311
Preeclampsia 245, 256, 259
Prehabilitation strategy 91
Preoperative anesthesia 94, 104
Preoperative assessments 94, 104
Preoperative evaluation 311
Preoperative screening clinics (PSCs) 94
Pre-surgery evaluations 90
Prolonged anesthesia 142
Propofol 144, 145, 150, 157, 158
Public health 131
Pulmonary edema 2, 22
Pulmonary hypertension 388
Pulse oximetry 325, 341

R

Radiofrequency ablation 311
real-time adjustments 28
Recovery process 20
Regional anesthesia 163, 165, 183, 184, 185, 186
Regional anesthesia (RA) 3, 6
Respiratory disorders 297, 311
Respiratory function 209
Respiratory rate 62
Respiratory rehabilitation 131
Respiratory system 270
Rhinovirus 131
Ropivacaine 6, 168, 183

S

Sacral neuromodulation 209
Sacral neuromodulation (SNM) 195
Safety standards 209
Scholarship 4
Sedation 189, 191, 192, 193, 194, 196, 197, 199, 200, 202, 203, 209, 210, 211, 212, 214
Sensation 28, 32
Sevoflurane 157, 158
Smart monitoring 234
Social media 131, 133
Solid preoperative check 224
Special healthcare needs (SHCN) 221
Special needs children 29
Spinal anesthesia 63, 79, 169, 183, 184
Spinal anesthesia (SA) 4
Spinal canal 79
Spontaneous breathing trials (SBTs) 117
State-of-the-art drug developments 28
Student Registered Nurse Anesthetists (SRNAs) 190
Succinylcholine 30, 255
Supraglottic devices 131
Surgical care 85
Surgical Pleth Index 323
Surgical practices 196, 209
Surgical procedures 91, 100, 104
Surgical setting 27, 47
Surgical-site infections 104
Systemic inflammatory response (SIR) 381
Systemic opioids 165, 169, 170, 172, 175, 176, 177

T

Task-management 209, 213
the Anesthesiology Control Tower (ACT) 3, 14

Thoracic epidural analgesia (TEA) 379
Tidal volume 62
Time to loss of consciousness (TLOC) 138
Trachea 131
Tracheal intubation 131
Transesophageal echocardiography 157
Transesophageal echocardiography (TEE) 137
Transpulmonary thermodilution 3

U

Ultrasound technology 165
Unexpected respiratory drop-offs 193
Upper airway 131

V

Veins 79
Video-assisted thoracic surgery 164
Video laryngoscopy 114, 124, 127, 128, 131, 133, 136
Visual Analog Scale (VAS) 354, 365
Vital signs 59, 79
Von Willebrand disease 263

W

Wellness programs 2, 23